Diabetes: From Research to Diagnosis and Treatment

Diabetes: From Research to Diagnosis and Treatment

Edited by

Itamar Raz MD
Professor of Internal Medicine
Hadassah University Hospital
Jerusalem, Israel

Jay S Skyler MD
Professor of Internal Medicine
University of Miami School of Medicine
Miami, Florida, USA

Eleazar Shafrir PhD MMedSc
Professor of Biochemistry
Hadassah University Hospital
Jerusalem, Israel

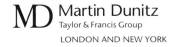
Martin Dunitz
Taylor & Francis Group
LONDON AND NEW YORK

© 2003 Martin Dunitz, an imprint of the Taylor & Francis Group

First published in the United Kingdom in 2003
by Martin Dunitz, an imprint of the Taylor & Francis Group, 11 New Fetter Lane, London EC4P 4EE

Tel: +44 (0) 20 7583 9855
Fax: +44 (0) 20 7842 2298
E-mail: info@dunitz.co.uk
Website: http://www.dunitz.co.uk

Although every effort has been made to ensure that all owners of copyright material have been acknowledged in this publication, we would be glad to acknowledge in subsequent reprints or editions any omissions brought to our attention.

Although every effort has been made to ensure that drug doses and other information are presented accurately in this publication, the ultimate responsibility rests with the prescribing physician. Neither the publishers nor the authors can be held responsible for errors or for any consequences arising from the use of information contained herein. For detailed prescribing information or instructions on the use of any product or procedure discussed herein, please consult the prescribing information or instructional material issued by the manufacturer.

A CIP record for this book is available from the British Library.

ISBN 1 184184 151 X

Distributed in the USA by
Fulfilment Center
Taylor & Francis
10650 Tobben Drive
Independence, KY 41051, USA
Toll Free Tel: +1 800 634 7064
E-mail: taylorandfrancis@thomsonlearning.com

Distributed in Canada by
Taylor & Francis
74 Rolark Drive
Scarborough, Ontario M1R 4G2, Canada
Toll Free Tel: +1 877 226 2237
E-mail: tal_fran@istar.ca

Distributed in the rest of the world by
Thomson Publishing Services
Cheriton House
North Way
Andover, Hampshire SP10 5BE, UK
Tel: +44 (0)1264 332424
E-mail: salesorder.tandf@thomsonpublishingservices.co.uk

Composition by Scribe Design, Gillingham, Kent, UK
Printed in Spain by Grafos SA

Contents

CONTENTS

Foreword

Diabetes is now a world wide pandemic affecting 151 million people in 2001. Numbers are set to rise inexorably over the next two decades unless drastic action is taken. In the meanwhile, there is a tremendous health burden to be dealt with. The days of just a few specialists coping with patients are over. Now it is a question of teams of health care professionals (specialists, primary care physicians, educators, nurses, dieticians, psychologists, podiatrists and patients themselves) trying to deal with the rising workload. Prevention of complications is feasible and vital if health economies are to prevent bankruptcy, and people with diabetes are to be afforded a normal life.

Education is the fulcrum of all these activities. The present volume makes a major contribution and gives an international perspective. It covers recent advances in major clinical areas. It gives the latest in therapeutic developments. There is a focus on the complications of diabetes which sadly still commonly occur and where interesting developments are taking place.

Overall *Diabetes: from research to diagnosis and treatment* is refreshing in that the editors have not attempted to be fully comprehensive, but have focused on what they describe as 'hot' topics. This saves the volume from the torpor and excessive weight of other text books. As such the book is useful to all, be it a health worker wanting to check on the latest on oral insulin or a scientist interested in anti-oxidant actions. It can be recommended to all.

Professor Sir George Alberti
President, International Diabetes Federation
Professor of Medicine, University of Newcastle
Professor of Metabolic Medicine,
Imperial College,
London, UK

Preface

Diabetes is spreading globally and is now accepted by world health authorities as a major morbidity hazard. Even though the last decade has seen tremendous progress in the diagnosis and treatment of diabetes and its complications, we have to brace ourselves to avert and surmount the evolving epidemic of diabetes. As related in Chapter 1, the number of newly diagnosed cases of diabetes worldwide will double within the next 25 years. This raises the need for better screening measures and more effective treatment to prevent the progression of patients with impaired glucose tolerance to overt diabetes with its complications, particularly heart disease and atherosclerosis. The St Vincent Declaration was a milestone in the efforts to prevent long-standing diabetes complications, however a more aggressive approach is needed. New drugs and transplantation techniques need to be developed to enhance our capacity to delay and halt the spread of this disease. These subjects are dealt with in several chapters of this book.

In spite of all the progress made over 100 years of research, the basic pathophysiology of diabetes and insulin resistance has not been completely resolved. Research in animal models exhibiting various patterns of diabetes is paving the way toward elucidation of these enigmas. Proper care of patients with diabetes still needs considerable improvement, and new strategies to prevent the development of complications have promising preliminary outcomes and many of these are described here. This book screens most of the new data available regarding the pathogenesis and development of Type 1 and Type 2 diabetes. Novel treatments to prevent diabetes are presented. The role of glucose, lipoproteins, as well as other metabolic and cardiovascular risk factors in diabetes morbidity are discussed.

The book comprises 31 chapters written by foremost international authorities. Rather than being a systematic textbook that covers all topics, we have selected 'hot' topics in diabetes to enhance the transfer of recent achievements in research into improved diagnosis and clinical practice. The chapters are provided with up-to-date references to facilitate easy access to specific publications.

This book is aimed not only at professional diabetologists but is also for endocrinologists, laboratory personnel, pharmaceutical researchers, epidemiologists, geneticists, and pathologists particularly interested in the investigation of diabetic tissue lesions.

We are grateful to all authors for their excellent contributions. Our thanks are also due to Martin Dunitz and Pete Stevenson who have been efficient and helpful in the preparation of this volume for publication.

Itamar Raz
Jay Skyler
Eleazar Shafrir

Michael Berger: A tribute

Professor Michael Berger was born in Thüringen, Germany in June 1944 and
died in August 2002 in Düsseldorf, following a severe illness.

He studied at the Medical Schools of Wurzburg Germany, Galway, Ireland and Düsseldorf,
Germany and received his MD degree in 1970. He continued his postgraduate education in the
Departments of Medicine at Düsseldorf, Joslin Research Centre, Boston and at the Institute de
Biochimie, Geneva under AE Renold. From 1978, Michael Berger was Professor of Internal
Medicine at the Heinrich-Heine University, Düsseldorf and Director of the Department for
Metabolic Diseases and Nutrition from 1985. Michael Berger received numerous scientific awards
and honorary doctorates from universities in Europe and other parts of the world. He was Chief
Editor of Diabetologia from 1983 to 1988, President of the German Diabetes Society from 1989
to 1990 and President of the EASD from 1995 to1998.

Michael Berger published 600 scientific articles, several textbooks on diabetes and was a member
of editorial boards of many scientific journals. His contribution to European diabetes research
covered a wide range of activities, including laboratory research, evaluation of clinical care and
patient education. Michael Berger will be remembered for his outstanding commitment to EASD,
a physician dedicated to his patients and a strong advocate of evidence-based medicine.

List of contributors

Dorit Adler RD MPH
Dietitian; Head, Dietetic Department
Hadassah University Hospital
Jerusalem
Israel

Joyce Akwe Akwi MD
Research Fellow
Department of Internal Medicine
University of Perugia
Perugia
Italy

Mary Ann Banerji MD
SUNY Health Sciences Center
Department of Medicine
Brooklyn NY
USA

Hanoch Bar-On MD
Professor, Diabetes and Geriatric Units
Division of Medicine
School of Public Health and Community
Medicine
Hadassah University Hospital
Jerusalem
Israel

Luca Benzi MD
Department of Endocrinology and
Metabolism, Section of Diabetes
School of Medicine
University of Pisa
Pisa
Italy

†Michael Berger MD
Professor of Medicine
Director, Department of Metabolic Diseases
and Nutrition
WHO Collaborating Center for Diabetes
Henrich-Heine University
Düsseldorf
Germany

Elliot M Berry MD FRCP
Professor of Internal Medicine; Head
Department of Human Nutrition and
Metabolism
Hebrew University
Hadassah Medical School
Jerusalem
Israel

Geremia B Bolli MD
Professor of Internal Medicine
Department of Internal Medicine
University of Perugia
Perugia
Italy

Andrew JM Boulton MD FRCP
Professor of Medicine
Department of Medicine
Manchester Royal Infirmary
Manchester
UK

† Deceased

Reinhard G Bretzel MD PhD
Chairman, Internal Medicine
Endocrinology and Diabetology;
Head, Third Medical Department and
Policlinic;
Director, International Islet Transplant
Registry
University Hospital Giessen
Giessen
Germany

Sonia Brichard MD PhD
Professor, Division of Endocrinology and
Metabolism
Faculty of Medicine
University of Louvain
Brussels
Belgium

Paul G Cassell PhD
Research Fellow
Department of Diabetes and Metabolic
Medicine
Barts and The London
Queen Mary's School of Medicine and
Dentistry
University of London
London
UK

Alice YY Cheng MD FRCPC
Endocrinology Fellow, Postgraduate Trainee
Department of Medicine
Division of Endocrinology
University of Toronto
Ontario
Canada

Irun R Cohen MD
Mauerberger Professor of Immunology
Director, Robert Koch-Minerva Center for
Research in Autoimmune Disease
Weizmann Institute of Science, Rehovot;
Director, Center for the study of Emerging
Diseases,
Jerusalem
Israel

Mark E Cooper MD PhD FRACP
Professor, Baker Heart Research Institute
St Kilda
Melbourne
Australia

Rosa Corcoy MD PhD
Consultant, Endocrinology Department
Hospital de Sant Pau
Barcelona
Spain

Net Daş-Evcimen PhD
Assistant Professor
Pharmacy Faculty
Biochemistry Department
Ankara University
Tandogan, Ankara
Turkey

Jacqueline M Dekker PhD
Associate Professor
EMGO Institute
VU University Medical Center
Amsterdam
The Netherlands

Alberto de Leiva MD PhD
Director and Professor of Medicine
Endocrinology Department
Hospital de Santa Pau
Barcelona
Spain

Stefano Del Prato MD
Chief, Section of Diabetes; Professor of
Endocrinology
Department of Endocrinology and
Metabolism, Section of Diabetes
School of Medicine
University of Pisa
Pisa
Italy

Gal Dubnov MD MSc
Research Associate
Department of Human Nutrition and
Metabolism
Hebrew University
Hadassah Medical School
Jerusalem
Israel

Sol Efroni MSc
Research Student
Departments of Immunology, and
Computer and Applied Mathematics
The Weizmann Institute of Science
Rehovot
Israel

Joseph L Evans PhD
Vice President, Research and Development
Chief Scientific Officer
Medical Research Institute
San Bruno CA
USA

Carmine G Fanelli MD PhD
Clinical Researcher in Internal Medicine
DIMISEM
University of Perugia
Perugia
Italy

Piero Ferolla MD
Doctorate on Physiopathology of
Metabolism
Department of Internal Medicine
University of Perugia
Perugia
Italy

Robert N Frank MD
Professor of Ophthalmology and of
Anatomy and Cell Biology
Wayne State University School of Medicine
Kresge Eye Institute
Detroit MI
USA

Ira D Goldfine MD
Professor, Diabetes and Endocrine Research
Department of Medicine
Mount Zion Medical Center
University of California
San Francisco CA
USA

Robert J Heine MD PhD
Professor of Diabetology
Department of Endocrinology
Academic Hospital Vrije University
Amsterdam
The Netherlands

Keren Hershkop RD MSc
Staff Dietitian, Dietetic Department
Hadassah University Hospital
Jerusalem
Israel

Graham A Hitman MD FRCP
Professor of Molecular Medicine,
Consultant Diabetologist
Department of Diabetes and Metabolic
Medicine
Barts and the Royal London Hospital
Queen Mary's School of Medicine and
Dentistry
London
UK

Philip D Home DM DPhil
Professor of Diabetes and Medicine;
Vice President, International Diabetes
Federation,
University of Newcastle upon Tyne
Newcastle upon Tyne
UK

Judith RC Jacobs MS
Research Fellow
Research Division
Joslin Diabetes Center
Harvard Medical School
Boston MA
USA

Edward B Jude MD MRCP
Honorary Lecturer
Manchester University;
Consultant Diabetologist
Tameside General Hospital
Ashton-Under-Lyme
Lancashire
UK

Norma Sue Kenyon PhD
Director of PreClinical Research
Diabetes Research Institute
Miami FL
USA

Mogher Khamaisi MD PhD
Diabetes Center and Department of Internal
Medicine
Hadassah University Hospital
Jerusalem
Israel

Miriam Kidron PhD
Research Associate
Diabetes Research Unit
Division of Medicine
Hadassah University Hospital
Jerusalem
Israel

George L King MD
Research Director, Professor of Medicine
Research Division
Joslin Diabetes Center
Harvard Medical School
Boston MA
USA

Andrew P Levy MD PhD FACC
Senior Lecturer
Department of Anatomy and Cell Biology
Bruce Rappaport Faculty of Medicine
Technion-Israel Institute of Technology
Haifa
Israel

Edmund J Lewis MD
Director
Rush Presbyterian St Luke's Medical Center
Division of Nephrology
Chicago IL
USA

Julia Lewis MD
Professor of Medicine
Division of Nephrology
Vanderbilt University Medical Center
Nashville TN
USA

Betty A Maddux PhD
Research Fellow,
Diabetes and Endocrine Research
Department of Medicine
University of California at San Francisco
Mount Zion Medical Center
San Francisco CA
USA

Massimo Massi Benedetti MD
Chairman IDF European Region; Associate
Professor
Department of Internal Medicine
University of Perugia
Perugia
Italy

Roberto Miccoli MD
Department of Endocrinology and
Metabolism, Section of Diabetes
School of Medicine
University of Pisa
Pisa
Italy

Ingrid Mühlhauser MD
Professor of Health Sciences
Unit for Health Sciences and Education
University of Hamburg
Hamburg
Germany

Matthew D Oldfield MD
Department of Medicine
University of Melbourne
Austin and Repatriation Hospital
Heidleberg
Melbourne
Australia

Marco Orsini Federici MD
Doctorate on Physiopathology of
Metabolism
Department of Internal Medicine
University of Perugia
Perugia
Italy

Daphne Owens MA PhD
Research Lecturer
Department of Diabetes and Endocrinology
Trinity College Dublin
The Adelaide and Meath Hospital
Dublin
Ireland

Samson O Oyibo MRCP
Clinical Research Fellow
Department of Medicine
Manchester Royal Infirmary
Manchester
UK

Marian A Parrott MD MPH
Director and Associate Professor of
Medicine
Division of Geriatrics
Department of Medicine
George Washington University Medical
Faculty Associates
Washington DC
USA

Giuseppe Penno MD
Department of Endocrinology and
Metabolism, Section of Diabetes
School of Medicine
University of Pisa
Pisa
Italy

Simone Pampanelli MD
Clinical Researcher in Internal Medicine
DIMISEM
University of Perugia
Perugia
Italy

Francesca Porcellati MD PhD
Clinical Researcher in Internal Medicine
DIMISEM
University of Perugia
Perugia
Italy

Alberto Pugliese MD
Associate Professor of Medicine
Microbiology and Immunology
Head, Immunogenetics Program
Diabetes Research Institute
University of Miami School of Medicine
Miami FL
USA

Itamar Raz MD
Professor of Internal Medicine
Department of Internal Medicine
Hadassah University Hospital - Ein Kerem
Kiryat Hadassah
Jerusalem
Israel

Bernd Richter MD
Clinical Pharmacologist
Review Coordinator, Cochrane Review
Group Metabolic and Endocrine Disorders;
Registrar, Department of Metabolic
Diseases and Nutrition, WHO
Collaborating Center for Diabetes,
Henrich-Heine University of Düsseldorf,
Düsseldorf
Germany

Matthew C Riddle MD
Professor of Medicine
Division of Endocrinology, Metabolism and
Clinical Nutrition
Oregon Health and Science University
Portland OR
USA

Eleazar Shafrir PhD MMedSc
Professor
Department of Biochemistry and Diabetes
Center
Hadassah University Hospital
Jerusalem
Israel

Jonathan Shaw MD MRCP
Director of Research
International Diabetes Institute
Melbourne, Victoria
Australia

Jay S Skyler MD
Professor of Medicine,
Pediatrics and Psychology
University of Miami
Miami FL
USA

Gerald H Tomkin MD FRCP FRACP
Consultant Physician, Director, Associate
Professor of Medicine
Department of Diabetes and Endcrinology
Adelaide and Meath Hospital
Trinity College
Dublin
Ireland

Isaiah Wexler MD PhD
Diabetes Center
Department of Paediatrics, Mount Scopus
Hadassah Hospital
Jerusalem
Israel

Dan Ziegler MD
Professor of Internal Medicine, Consultant
Physician, German Diabetes Research
Institute at the Henrich-Heine University
Düsseldorf
Germany

Paul Zimmet MD PhD FRACP FRCP
Professor and Director
International Diabetes Institute
Melbourne
Victoria
Australia

Bernard Zinman MDCM FRCPC FACP
Director, Leadership Sinai Centre for
Diabetes; Sam and Judy Pencer Family
Chair in Diabetes; Professor of Medicine
University of Toronto
Mount Sinai Hospital
Ontario
Canada

Ehud Ziv PhD
Associate Professor
Diabetes Research Unit
Division of Medicine
Hadassah University Hospital
Jerusalem
Israel

Abbreviations used

ACE	angiotensin converting enzyme	IPTR	International Pancreas Transplant Registry
ACE-I	angiotensin converting enzyme inhibitor	ITR	International Islet Transplant Registry
ADA	American Diabetes Association	LDL	low density lipoproteins
AGE	advanced glycation end products	MCT	mean circulation time
BD	bladder drainage	MIT	multiple insulin injection treatment
c/n/aPKC	conventional/novel/atypical PKC	NCD	non-communicable disease
CFA	complete Freund's adjuvant	NEFA	non-esterified free fatty acids (see also FFA)
CIT	conventional insulin injection treatment	NO	nitric oxide
CM	congenital malformations	NOD	non-obese diabetic (mice)
CSA	cyclosporin A	NPH	neutral protamine hagedorn
CTGF	connective tissue growth factor	PA	phosphatidic acid
CVD	cardiovascular disease	PAI-1	plasminogen activator inhibitor-1
DAG-PKC	diacylglycerol activated PKC	PAK	pancreas after kidney
DCCT	Diabetes Control and Complications Trial	PC	phosphatidylcholine
DECODE	Diabetes Epidemiology Collaborative Analysis of Diagnostic Criteria in Europe	PDK-1	phosphoinositide-dependent protein kinase-1
DI	duct injection	PET	positron emission tomography
DM	diabetes mellitus	PKC	protein kinase C
ECM	extracellular matrix	PLC	phospholipase C
ED	enteric drainage	PLD	phospholipase D
ET-1	endothelin-1	PS	phosphatidylserine
FFA	free fatty acids	PTA	pancreas transplants alone
GLUT	glucose transporter	PVN	paraventricular nucleus
GS	glycogen synthase	RACKs	receptors for activated C kinase
HLA	human leukocyte antigen	ROS	reactive oxygen species
HOPE	Heart Outcomes Prevention Evaluation Study	SIK	simultaneous islet kidney
IAK	islet after kidney	SPK	simultaneous pancreas-kidney
ID	intestinal drainage	TAC	tetracain, epinephrine, cocain
IDNT	Irbesartan and Diabetic Nephropathy Trial	TGF	transforming growth factor
		TNF	tumor necrosis factor
IFG	impaired fasting glucose	UKPDS	United Kingdom Prospective Diabetes Study
IGT	impaired glucose tolerance	VEGF	vascular endothelial growth factor
IMT	intima-media thickness	VLDL	very low density lipoproteins
		VNTR	variable number of tandem repeats
		VPF	vascular permeability factor

1

Diabetes on six continents – ethnic and geographic differences: views on the future

Paul Zimmet, Jonathan Shaw

Diabetes: an epidemic in full flight

Over the past few decades, we have seen a global reappearance of communicable diseases, both old ones such as tuberculosis and newer ones such as HIV-AIDS, Legionnaire's disease and the Ebola virus. This resurgence has come at a time when there has also been a dramatic rise in prevalence of cardiovascular diseases (CVD), Type 2 diabetes, obesity and other non-communicable diseases (NCD) in developing and newly developed nations on all six inhabited continents of the globe.[1]

In the early 1970s, Bennett and co-workers reported on the extraordinarily high prevalence of Type 2 diabetes in the Pima Indians.[2] This finding and then our own reports of high prevalence in the Micronesian Nauruans in the Pacific in 1975[3] followed by similar findings in other Pacific and Asian Island populations,[4] highlighted the potential for a future global epidemic. The predictions we made at that time have now proven to be correct.[5] Type 2 diabetes has now reached epidemic proportions in many developing and most developed nations. Not only have we already witnessed a dramatic increase, but also the epidemic of Type 2 diabetes will continue to escalate around the world in the coming decades.[6]

Over the past 30 years, Type 2 diabetes has changed from being considered as a relatively mild ailment associated with ageing and the elderly ('just a touch of sugar') to one of the major contemporary causes of premature morbidity and mortality.[7] In virtually every developed nation, diabetes ranks as one of the two top causes of blindness, renal failure, and lower limb amputation.[7] Through its effects on CVD (nearly 80% of people with diabetes die of CVD), it is also now one of the leading causes of death.[8] This chapter discusses the development of the epidemic and highlights some disturbing trends, such as the appearance of Type 2 diabetes in children and adolescents. It also addresses the increasing burden of impaired glucose tolerance (IGT) and the associated Metabolic Syndrome (or Insulin Resistance Syndrome), and the related CVD burden.

Diabetes: a view over six continents

The changing perceptions of diabetes as a public health threat relate partly to a better appreciation of its devastating complications, but mainly to the rapid rise in its prevalence that occurred in the latter part of the twentieth century.[9] The evidence for this global rise is more and more apparent. In Native American and Pacific Island populations, Type 2 diabetes affects up to 40% of adults but was virtually unknown 50 years ago.[2,3] Between 1976 and 1988, the prevalence of diabetes

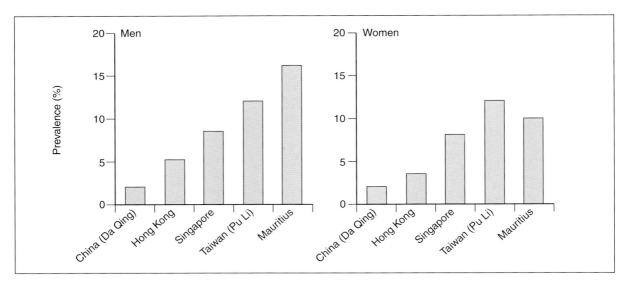

Figure 1.1
Prevalence of Type 2 diabetes in Chinese populations around the world.

(among people age 40–74) rose from 11.4% to 14.3% in the USA.[10] In China, a prevalence figure of 3.1% in 1994 (in the over 25 years of age group), was almost two and a half times higher than a figure from the Chinese province of Da Qing eight years earlier.[11] Two cross-sectional studies in an urban South Indian population showed that the prevalence in the over 20s had risen from 8.3% in 1989 to 11.6% in 1995.[12] In Denmark, a 38% rise in diabetes prevalence has been reported over a 22-year period.[13] In a recent national study in Australia, 7.4% of adults were found to have diabetes compared with an estimated 3.4% in 1981.[14] Data from Mauritius provide the guide to the magnitude of the global diabetes epidemic.[9] Its population of about 1.3 million has three ethnic groups: Asian Indian, Creole (Black) and Chinese. These ethnic groups account for over two-thirds of the world's population. Mauritius has a high diabetes prevalence[15] and a 40% secular increase

occurred between 1987 and 1992 in Asian Indians and Creoles[9] and the highest yet reported prevalence in Chinese.[15] With the evidence that the prevalence of Type 2 diabetes doubled between 1984 and 1992 in Singaporean Chinese, and the high prevalence in Taiwan,[16] this is an alarming indicator of the potential size of the future epidemic in the People's Republic of China (PRC).[9] In the PRC, the prevalence of Type 2 diabetes was, until recently, less than 1%. Recent studies show a three-fold increase in prevalence in certain areas of China within the last two decades.[11] The potential scenario can be understood from the data in Figure 1.1 comparing the prevalence of diabetes in Chinese populations in China, Singapore, Taiwan and Mauritius. If China were to experience just one-half the current rate of diabetes in Taiwan, the number of individuals with diabetes will increase dramatically from 8 million in 1996 to over 32 million by 2010.

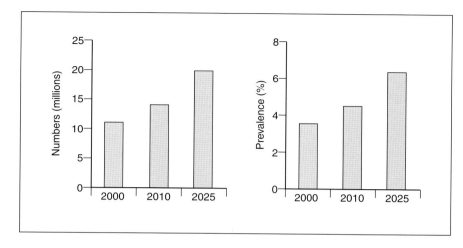

Figure 1.2
Estimated increases in numbers of people with and prevalence of diagnosed diabetes in the USA for the years 2000, 2010 and 2025.
Note: The data apply to the whole population, including both adults and children, and assume both growth in the population and a rise in the age-specific prevalence of diabetes. Data are based on ref. 51.

The highest rates of Type 2 diabetes are seen in Native Americans and Pacific Islanders, followed by Hispanics or Mexican Americans, people originating from the Indian subcontinent, South East Asians and African Americans. In addition, relatively high prevalence has been reported from some of the Middle East Arab states,[1] as well as in disadvantaged minorities in the developed countries, e.g. Australia's indigenous population.[1,9] In fact, the only people for whom Type 2 diabetes remains rare are indigenous peoples living a traditional lifestyle.

It is estimated that globally, the number of people with diabetes will rise from 151 million in the year 2000, to 221 million by the year 2010,[5] and to 300 million by 2025.[6] This rise is predicted to occur in virtually every country in the world, with the greatest increases expected in developing countries. The projections of increasing numbers of people with diabetes are driven mainly by the anticipated world population growth, especially amongst the middle-aged and elderly. Indeed, the estimates are conservative, as they have not fully accounted for increases in the prevalence

A. Genetic factors
Genetic markers, Family history, 'Thrifty gene(s)' etc.

B. Demographic characteristics
Sex, age, ethnicity

C. Behavioural and lifestyle-related risk factors
Obesity (including distribution of obesity and duration)
Physical inactivity
Diet
Stress
'Westernization, urbanization, modernization'

D. Metabolic determinants and intermediate risk categories of Type 2 diabetes
Impaired glucose tolerance
Insulin resistance
Pregnancy-related determinants (parity, gestational diabetes, diabetes in offspring of women with diabetes during pregnancy, intra-uterine mal- or over-nutrition)

Table 1.1
Aetiological determinants and risk factors of Type 2 diabetes

of diabetes within each age group. Such age-specific rises have been documented over the last 20 years,[10] and have recently been incorporated into projections for the USA (Figure 1.2). This spectacular increase in the frequency of Type 2 diabetes is being paralleled by a similarly alarming increase in obesity.[17] Obesity is one of the major risk factors for Type 2 diabetes (Table 1.1) and because these two conditions are so closely linked, the term 'diabesity' has been suggested by Shafrir.[17]

The epidemiological transition

The rising burden of Type 2 diabetes and other NCDs which has occurred with modernization can be understood in the context of 'epidemiological transition'.[18] Over the past 100 years, improved nutrition, better hygiene and the control of many communicable diseases have resulted in dramatically improved longevity. Yet, these benefits have unmasked many age-related NCDs including Type 2 diabetes and CVD.[9] These formerly uncommon NCDs have replaced many communicable diseases and are now major contributors to ill-health and death.

This phenomenon of shifting disease patterns, termed epidemiological transition, initially occurred in developed countries and subsequently spread to developing nations.[9] Arthur Koestler coined the term 'Coca-colonization' to describe the impact of the lifestyle of Western societies on developing countries.[19] The devastating results of intrusion by Western society into the lives of traditional-living indigenous communities can now be seen across the globe.

Many once idyllic atolls in the Pacific region now show the disastrous results of epidemiological transition. During the nineteenth century early European voyagers brought many infectious diseases such as measles, whooping cough, tuberculosis, influenza and venereal diseases to the Pacific Island communities.[20] In the nineteenth century, nearly all of the islands suffered a drastic reduction in population as a result of these imported diseases. The transition has seen Type 2 diabetes catapulting from a rare disease at the beginning of the twentieth century to its current position as one of the major epidemics of the twenty-first century and a major global contributor to disability and death.[17]

While the threat of communicable diseases has reduced, rapid socio-economic development and 'Coca-colonization' have resulted in a lifestyle transition from traditional to modern. In virtually all populations, higher fat diets and decreased physical activity have accompanied the benefits of modernization. Exercise has been engineered out of our daily lives, both in the workplace and at leisure.[1] These lifestyle changes have been well documented in Canadian[21] and Native American communities, Pacific and Indian Ocean Island populations,[4] as well as in Australian Aboriginal communities,[1,9] and when combined with increasing longevity, form the basis of the dynamic Type 2 diabetes epidemic that we are witnessing today.

Genes or environment?

The explosion of Type 2 diabetes in Native American and Pacific Island populations points the finger squarely at environmental causes albeit in populations with a high genetic susceptibility to Type 2 diabetes.[1] The rise has taken place too quickly to be due to altered gene frequencies. On the other hand, the large differences in prevalence between ethnic groups when exposed to similar environments also implicates a significant genetic contribution. Jared Diamond, a leading American biologist

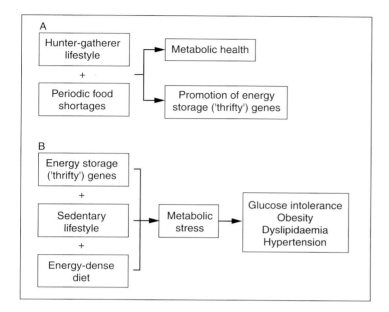

Figure 1.3
The development of the thrifty genotype and its role in epidemiological transition. Panel A shows how a traditional lifestyle may have both maintained metabolic health and selected for thrifty genes. Panel B shows the impact of a modern lifestyle in the presence of thrifty genes.

and author, has suggested that the lifestyle-related diabetes epidemic in Native Americans and Pacific Islanders probably results from the collision of our old hunter-gatherer genes with the new twentieth century way of life.[22] The Western lifestyle must have unmasked the effects of pre-existing genes because the consistent result has been diabetes within a few decades.

The former dependency on hunting and gathering in these societies, and later subsistence agriculture, was replaced with a modern pattern characterized by a sedentary lifestyle and a diet of energy-dense processed foods, high in saturated fat. These were usually imported from neighbouring and perhaps well-meaning developed nations.[9] In the Pacific region, nations such as Australia and New Zealand still export large quantities of consumable products rich in animal fats, e.g. canned meats and fatty joints, to the Pacific Islands. These are foodstuffs that their own populations would be loathe to eat.

Another way to explain the epidemic is through Neel's 'thrifty genotype' hypothesis, which proposes that the genes selected over previous millennia to allow survival in times of famine by efficiently storing all available energy during times of feast, are the very genes that lead to obesity and Type 2 diabetes when exposed to a constant high energy diet[23,24] (Figure 1.3).

In recent years, an observation of the association between low birth weight and abnormal glucose tolerance (as well as with hypertension and CVD) has led to a competing hypothesis of the 'thrifty phenotype'. Studies have shown that middle-aged people with abnormal glucose tolerance were, on average, lighter at birth than the healthy controls. It has been suggested that intra-uterine malnutrition slows fetal growth, causing low birth weight, insulin resistance and defects in insulin secretory function.[25] When these metabolic abnormalities combine with advancing age and obesity, abnormal glucose tolerance develops. Therefore, environmental influences affecting the intra-uterine environment are suggested to be more important than genetic factors in causing Type 2 diabetes. It seems more likely that a *combination* of genetic factors and environment affect the intra-uterine environment and the fetal response to it.[1] Furthermore, low birth weight does not account for more than 35% of cases of diabetes in any population studied.[26] Thrifty phenotype and thrifty genotype may not be 'competing' hypotheses at all, but may both contribute to what is clearly a multifactorial problem.

The changing age profile: Type 2 diabetes in childhood and adolescents

Several decades ago, Type 2 diabetes was typically regarded as a disease of the middle aged and elderly. While it is still true that this age group maintains a higher relative risk (in relation to younger adults), there is accumulating and disturbing evidence that onset in the 20 to 30 years of age group is increasingly seen.[27,28] Even children are now being caught up in the diabetes epidemic. Although Type 1 diabetes remains the main form of the disease in children worldwide, it is likely that Type 2 diabetes will be the predominant form within 10 years in many ethnic groups and potentially in Europid groups,[28] having already been reported in children from Japan, the USA, Pacific Islands, Hong Kong, Australia and the United Kingdom.[27,28]

This new phenomenon brings a serious new aspect to the diabetes epidemic and heralds an emerging public health problem of major proportions. Among children in Japan, Type 2 diabetes is already more common than Type 1 diabetes, accounting for 80% of childhood

diabetes; the incidence almost doubled between 1976–80 and 1991–5.[29] The rising prevalence of obesity and Type 2 diabetes in children is yet another symptom of the effects of globalization and industrialization affecting all societies, with sedentary lifestyle and obesity the predominant factors involved.[28]

This fall in the age of onset of Type 2 diabetes is an important factor influencing the future burden of the disease. Onset in childhood heralds many years of disease and an accumulation of the full range of both micro- and macrovascular complications. The American Diabetes Association and the American Academy of Pediatrics have recently issued a consensus statement on the problem.[30] The report addresses the issue of compliance in diet and tablet and insulin therapies. Recently, a number of pharmaceutical companies have embarked on clinical trials of oral hypoglycaemic agents to check their safety and efficacy in this age group as they may face up to 40–50 years of therapy.

Views on the future: the concealed burden of impaired glucose tolerance

There is increasing interest concerning subjects with IGT. IGT is defined as hyperglycaemia (with glucose values intermediate between normal and diabetes) following a glucose load.[31] There are at least 200 million people worldwide with IGT. The prevalence of IGT varies widely, being 3–10% in Europid populations.[32] It is much higher in some newly industrialized nations and high Type 2 prevalence groups such as Asian Indians, Native Americans, Pacific Islanders and indigenous Australians. Recent data now suggest increasing rates in Europids, for example in the recent national Australian diabetes study the preva-lence of IGT was 10.6%.[14] It represents a key stage in the natural history of Type 2 diabetes, as these people are at much higher future risk than the general population for developing diabetes. Approximately 40% of subjects progress to diabetes over 5–10 years, but some revert to normal or remain IGT.

Subjects with IGT also have a heightened risk of macrovascular disease[8] because of the association with other known CVD risk factors, including hypertension, dyslipidaemia and central obesity. A diagnosis of IGT, partic-ularly in apparently healthy and ambulatory individuals, has important prognostic implica-tions. Impaired fasting glucose (IFG) was intro-duced recently as another category of abnormal glucose metabolism.[31] It is defined on the basis of a fasting glucose concentration of 6.1–6.9 mmol/l and, like IGT, it is associated with risk of CVD and future diabetes.[33]

Importantly, recent studies have shown the potential for intervention in IGT subjects to reduce progression to Type 2 diabetes. One such study is the recently completed Diabetes Prevention Program in the USA.[34] This showed that over three years, lifestyle intervention (targeting diet and exercise) reduced the risk of progressing from IGT to diabetes by 58%, while the oral hypoglycaemic drug, metformin, reduced the risk by 31%. Two other large-scale studies have also demonstrated the efficacy of lifestyle interventions – from Da Qing, China[35] and from Finland.[36] In the Finnish study, the cumulative incidence of diabetes after four years was 11% in the intervention group and 23% in the control group. During the trial, the risk of diabetes was reduced by 58% in the intervention group. The reduction in the incidence of diabetes was directly associated with changes in lifestyle.

The recently defined category of IFG recog-nizes the fact that elevated but non-diabetic levels of fasting glucose also carry a higher risk of future diabetes, and probably also of CVD.[33] It is now clear that, while in a broad sense IFG and IGT represent disorders with similar impli-cations, significant differences exist. Although the risk of progressing to diabetes for an individual is similar for both IGT and IFG, many more progressors can be identified by IGT.[37] The majority of people with either IGT or IFG do not have the other condition, and indeed approximately 20% of people with a fasting glucose in the IFG range already have diabetes on the 2-h glucose.[37] Finally, and perhaps most importantly, the 2-h post-challenge glucose appears to be a better predic-tor of CVD and mortality than is the fasting glucose.[38,39]

In a study in Mauritius, we showed that there was a definite gender difference in preva-lence of IFG and IGT. IGT was more common in women, and IFG more common in men and only a small but equal proportion of men and women were found to have both IFG and IGT co-existing.[40] Other recent epidemiological studies have also reported similar sex differ-ences in the prevalence of IFG and IGT.[10,14,16] The observation that IFG is more prevalent in males and IGT is usually more prevalent in females raises important questions as to the underlying aetiology of IFG and IGT and to the ability of the current glucose thresholds to identify high-risk categories equally amongst men and women.

Thus, future interest for intervention focuses not only on Type 2 diabetes but also on other areas of glucose intolerance such as IGT, IFG and gestational diabetes. In a sense, the defini-tion of diabetes is artificial and based on cut-off points associated with risk of compli-cations.[31,33] For example, as a CVD risk factor, glucose is a continuous variable with no sudden increase in risk.[41] The possibility of preventing Type 2 diabetes by interventions that target the lifestyles of subjects at high risk for the disease is now complemented by ongoing studies that are investigating pharmacological interventions.

Type 2 diabetes and the cardiovascular disease epidemic

Type 2 diabetes is a multifactorial disease and shows heterogeneity in numerous respects.[31,42,43] Our understanding of Type 2 diabetes and related disorders such as IGT and IFG is undergoing a radical change, particularly as there are data that suggest that the risk of complications, at least from macrovascular disease, commences many years before the onset of clinical diabetes.[44] Previously it was regarded as a relatively distinct disease entity, but in reality, Type 2 diabetes is a descriptive term and a manifestation of a much broader underlying disorder.[45,46] This includes the Metabolic Syndrome, also referred to as the Insulin Resistance Syndrome, a cluster of CVD risk factors which apart from glucose intolerance includes hyperinsulinaemia, dyslipidaemia, hypertension, visceral obesity, hypercoagulability and microalbuminuria.[1] This combination of risk factors is partly responsible for the increased risk of CVD in people with diabetes.[47] Attention has recently been drawn to the CVD epidemic now seen in many developing nations.[8,9]

While IGT is predictive of future diabetes, it also carries a substantial risk of CVD.[8] Evidence suggests that those with IGT who have one or more components of the Metabolic Syndrome are more likely to progress to diabetes.[48] While we do not yet know whether treatment of IGT can delay or prevent the appearance of CVD, it is sensible to establish whether any individual IGT subject has other CVD risk factors. If they do, consideration for treating those abnormalities with either lifestyle measures or pharmacological interventions such as statin or antihypertensive therapy should be given, as macrovascular disease is the major cause of morbidity and mortality in Type 2 diabetes.

Conclusions

As diabetologists, we face some new and pressing challenges at the start of this millennium. The appearance of Type 2 diabetes in earlier age groups, the escalating numbers of patients to be treated and the problem of what to do with persons with IGT are all top priorities. The cost of diabetes and its treatment and prevention have the potential to cripple the budgets of both developed and developing nations.[28,49] There needs to be a much more aggressive and global approach to tackling the diabetes epidemic by international agencies and national governments. While there may be differences in genetic susceptibility to Type 2 diabetes, its complications and the Metabolic Syndrome, environmental factors are a very important driving force. Socio-economic factors have a major influence on nutrition, physical activity and health, and as a result, on individual and community disease patterns.[50] Globalization with its social, cultural, economic and political aspects has had a major impact on community health. The prevention of Type 2 diabetes cannot come through traditional medical approaches alone.[9] Major and dramatic changes in the socio-economic and cultural status and structure of nations and their people in developing countries, and the disadvantaged, minority groups in developed nations must take place.

References

1. Zimmet P. Diabetes epidemiology as a trigger to diabetes research. Diabetologia 1999; 42: 499–518.

2. Bennett P, Burch T, Miller M. Diabetes mellitus in American (Pima) Indians. Lancet 1971; 2: 125–8.

3. Zimmet P, Taft P, Guinea A et al. The high prevalence of diabetes mellitus on a Central Pacific island. Diabetologia 1977; 13: 111–15.

4. Zimmet P. Type 2 (non-insulin-dependent) diabetes – an epidemiological overview. Diabetologia 1982; 22: 399–411.

5. Amos A, McCarty D, Zimmet P. The rising global burden of diabetes and its complications: estimates and projections to the year 2010. Diabet Med 1997; 14: S1–S85.

6. King H, Aubert R, Herman W. Global burden of diabetes, 1995–2025. Prevalence, numerical estimates and projections. Diabetes Care 1998; 21: 1414–31.

7. World Health Organization. Prevention of Diabetes Mellitus. Geneva: World Health Organization, 1994.

8. Zimmet P, Alberti K. The changing face of macrovascular disease in non-insulin dependent diabetes mellitus in different cultures: an epidemic in progress. Lancet 1997; 350: S1–S4.

9. Zimmet P. Globalization, coca-colonization and the chronic disease epidemic: can the doomsday scenario be averted? J Intern Med 2000; 247: 301–10.

10. Harris MI, Flegal KM, Cowie CC et al. Prevalence of diabetes, impaired fasting glucose, and impaired glucose tolerance in U.S. adults. The Third National Health and Nutrition Examination Survey, 1988–1994. Diabetes Care 1998; 21: 518–24.

11. Pan XR, Yang WY, Li G, Liu J. Prevalence of diabetes and its risk factors in China, 1994. Diabetes Care 1997; 20: 1664–9.

12. Ramachandran A, Snehalatha C, Latha E et al. Rising prevalence of NIDDM in an urban population in India. Diabetologia 1997; 40: 232–7.

13. Drivsholm T, Ibsen H, Schroll M et al. Increasing prevalence of diabetes mellitus and impaired glucose tolerance among 60–year-old Danes. Diabet Med 2001; 18: 126–32.

14. Dunstan DW, Zimmet PZ, Welborn TA et al. The rising prevalence of diabetes mellitus and impaired glucose tolerance: the Australian diabetes, obesity and lifestyle study. Diabetes Care 2002; 25: 829–34.

15. Dowse G, Gareeboo H, Zimmet P et al. High prevalence of NIDDM and impaired glucose tolerance in Indian, Creole and Chinese Mauritians. Diabetes 1990; 39: 390–6.

16. Chen KT, Gregg EW, Williamson DF, Narayan KMV. High prevalence of impaired fasting glucose and type 2 diabetes in Pehghu Islets, Taiwan: evidence of a rapidly emerging epidemic? Diabetes Res Clin Pract 1999; 44: 59–69.

17. Zimmet P, Alberti K, Shaw J. Global and societal implications of the diabetes epidemic. Nature 2001; 414: 782–7.

18. Omran A. The epidemiologic transition: a theory of the epidemiology of population change. Milbank Q 1971; 49: 509–38.

19. Koestler A. The Call Girls. London and Sydney: Pan Books, 1976.

20. Zimmet P, Dowse G, Finch C et al. The epidemiology and natural history of NIDDM – lessons from the South Pacific. Diabetes Metab Rev 1990; 6: 91–124.

21. Harris S, Gittelsohn J, Hanley A et al. The prevalence of NIDDM and associated risk factors in native Canadians. Diabetes Care 1997; 20: 185–7.

22. Diamond JM. Human evolution. Diabetes running wild. Nature 1992; 357: 362–3.

23. Neel J. Diabetes mellitus: a thrifty genotype rendered detrimental by 'progress'? Am J Hum Genet 1962; 14: 353–62.

24. Neel J. The thrifty genotype revisited. In: Kobberling J, Tattersall R, eds. The Genetics of Diabetes Mellitus. Proceedings of the Serono Symposium. London: Academic Press, 1982: 283–93.

25. Hales C, Desai M, Ozanne S. The thrifty phenotype hypothesis: how does it look after 5 years? Diabet Med 1997; 14: 189–95.

26. Boyko EJ. Proportion of type 2 diabetes cases resulting from impaired fetal growth. Diabetes Care 2000; 23: 1260–4.

27. Fagot-Campagna A, Narayan K. Type 2 diabetes in children. BMJ 2001; 322: 377–87.

28. Zimmet P. The rise and rise of diabetes. A

public health challenge for the 21st century. Novartis Journal Pathways 2002; 3: 4–9.

29. Kitagawa T, Owada M, Urakami T, Yamanchi K. Increased incidence of non-insulin dependent diabetes mellitus among Japanese school children correlates with an increased intake of animal protein and fat. Clin Pediatr 1998; 37: 111–16.

30. American Diabetes Association. Type 2 diabetes in children and adolescents. Diabetes Care 2000; 23: 381–9.

31. World Health Organization. Definition, Diagnosis and Classification of Diabetes Mellitus and its Complications; Part 1: Diagnosis and Classification of Diabetes Mellitus. Geneva: Department of Noncommunicable Disease Surveillance, WHO, 1999.

32. King H, Rewers M. Global estimates for prevalence of diabetes mellitus and impaired glucose tolerance in adults. Diabetes Care 1993; 16: 157–77.

33. American Diabetes Association. Report of the expert committee on the diagnosis and classification of diabetes mellitus. Diabetes Care 1997; 20: 1183–97.

34. Knowler WC, Barrett-Connor E, Fowler SE et al. Reduction in the incidence of type 2 diabetes with lifestyle intervention or metformin. N Engl J Med 2002; 7: 393–403.

35. Pan X, Li G, Hu Y et al. Effects of diet and exercise in preventing NIDDM in people with impaired glucose tolerance: the Da Qing IGT and Diabetes Study. Diabetes Care 1997; 20: 537–44.

36. Tuomilehto J, Lindstrom J, Eriksson J et al. Prevention of type 2 diabetes mellitus by changes in lifestyle among subjects with impaired glucose tolerance. New Engl J Med 2001; 1343–50.

37. Shaw J, Zimmet P, de Courten M et al. Impaired fasting glucose or impaired glucose tolerance. What best predicts future diabetes in Mauritius? Diabetes Care 1999; 22: 399–402.

38. Shaw J, Hodge A, de Courten M et al. Isolated post-challenge hyperglycaemia confirmed as a risk factor for mortality. Diabetologia 1999; 42: 1050–4.

39. DECODE Study Group. Glucose tolerance and mortality: comparison of WHO and American Diabetes Association diagnostic criteria. Lancet 1999; 354: 617–21.

40. Williams J, De Courten M, Cox H et al. Coexisting IFG and IGT confer greatest risk of progressing to diabetes. Diabetes 2000; 49(suppl 1): A25.

41. Shaw JE, Zimmet PZ, Hodge AM et al. Impaired fasting glucose: how low should it go? Diabetes Care 2000; 23: 34–9.

42. Zimmet P. The pathogenesis and prevention of diabetes in adults. Genes, autoimmunity, and demography. Diabetes Care 1995; 18: 1050–64.

43. Groop L. The molecular genetics of non-insulin dependent diabetes mellitus. J Intern Med 1997; 241: 95–110.

44. Haffner SM, Stern MP, Hazuda HP et al. Cardiovascular risk factors in confirmed prediabetic individuals. Does the clock for coronary heart disease start ticking before the onset of clinical diabetes? JAMA 1990; 263: 2893–8.

45. Zimmet P. Non-insulin-dependent (Type 2) diabetes mellitus – does it really exist? Diabet Med 1989; 6: 728–35.

46. Zimmet P. Challenges in diabetes epidemiology – from West to the rest. Diabetes Care 1992; 15: 232–52.

47. Isomaa B, Almgren P, Tuomi T et al. Cardiovascular morbidity and mortality associated with the metabolic syndrome. Diabetes Care 2001; 24: 683–9.

48. Boyko E, de Courten M, Zimmet P et al. Features of the Metabolic Syndrome predict higher risk of diabetes and impaired glucose tolerance. Diabetes Care 2000; 23: 1242–8.

49. American Diabetes Association. Economic consequences of diabetes mellitus in the U.S. in 1997. Diabetes Care 1998; 21: 296–309.

50. Drewnowski A, Popkin B. The nutrition transition: new trends in the global diet. Nutr Rev 1997; 55: 31–43.

51. Boyle JP, Honeycutt AA, Narayan KM et al. Projection of diabetes burden through 2050: impact of changing demography and disease prevalence in the U.S. Diabetes Care 2001; 24: 1936–40.

2

Genetics of Type 1 diabetes
Alberto Pugliese

Introduction

Type 1 diabetes mellitus (T1DM), or insulin-dependent diabetes mellitus (IDDM), is a chronic condition of insulin deficiency resulting from the autoimmune destruction of pancreatic β-cells.[1] The disease is most common in childhood and adolescence but it can occur at any age showing significant heterogeneity in its clinical presentation and evolution. A large proportion of patients with T1DM lack a positive family history for the disease, but first degree relatives, most commonly siblings or twins, have a higher risk of developing T1DM than the general population. Within families, individual susceptibility depends on the degree of genetic identity with the proband, and the risk of diabetes in families has a non-linear correlation with the number of alleles shared with the proband. The highest risk is therefore observed in monozygotic twins (100% sharing) followed by first, second, and third degree relatives (50%, 25%, 12.5% sharing, respectively). Identical twins have a concordance rate for T1DM development ranging between 30 and 50% with rates of 70% reported in studies with longest follow-up.[2,3] The average prevalence of T1DM is 6% in siblings compared to 0.4% in the US Caucasian population. The familial clustering (λs) can be calculated as the ratio of the risk to siblings over the disease prevalence in the general population. It has

been estimated that for T1DM, the familiar clustering has a λs of 15 (λs = 6/0.4 = 15).[4,5]

These simple epidemiological observations imply that genetic factors play a role in the multifactorial origin of this complex disease. Over the years numerous studies have accumulated a large body of evidence indicating that genetic factors influence both susceptibility and resistance to T1DM. There appear to be several categories of genetic factors and mechanisms that modulate diabetes susceptibility: inherited gene polymorphisms, epigenetic mechanisms regulating the transmission and expression of inherited genes, and post-transcriptional regulatory mechanisms. This chapter will review the current knowledge about these various factors and mechanisms and discuss the likely mechanisms of genetic susceptibility to T1DM.

Inherited susceptibility loci

Both association studies and linkage analysis using various analytical methods have been used to identify susceptibility loci, and these are noted using the abbreviation *IDDM* and a number, e.g. *IDDM1*, *IDDM2*, etc. Using the candidate gene approach, association studies provided evidence for two susceptibility loci, the HLA region (*IDDM1*) and the insulin gene (*INS*) locus (*IDDM2*), approximately 20 years ago. However, these two loci only contribute a

Locus	Chromosome	Candidate genes	Markers
IDDM1	6p21.3	HLA DR/DQ	-
IDDM2	11p15.5	INSULIN VNTR	-
IDDM3	15q26	Unknown	D15S107
IDDM4	11q13.3	MDU1, ZFM1, RT6, ICE, LRP5, FADD, CD3	FGF3, D11S1917
IDDM5	6q25	MnSOD	ESR, a046Xa9
IDDM6	18q12-q21	JK (Kidd), ZNF236	D18S487, D18S64
IDDM7	2q31-33	NEUROD	D2S152, D251391
IDDM8	6q25-27	Unknown	D6S281, D6S264, D6S446
IDDM9	3q21-25	Unknown	D3S1303, D10S193
IDDM10	10p11-q11	Unknown	D10S565
IDDM11	14q24.3-q31	ENSA, SEL-1L	D14S67
IDDM12	2q33	CTLA-4	(AT)n 3' UTR, A/G Exon 1
IDDM13	2q34	IGFBP2, IGFBP5, NEUROD, HOXD8	D2S137, D2S164, D2S1471
IDDM15	6q21	Unknown	D6S283, D6S434, D6S1580
IDDM17	10q25	Unknown	D10S1750, D10S1773
IDDM18	5q31.1-33.1	IL12B	IL12B

Notes: Candidate gene abbreviations are explained in the text. The IDDM14 and IDDM16 denominations have not been assigned to any locus.

Table 2.1
Susceptibility loci for Type 1 diabetes

portion of the disease familial clustering, suggesting the existence of additional loci. The increasing availability of polymorphic markers (microsatellites, single nucleotide polymorphisms (SNPs)) and the development of fluorescence-based automated typing technology has greatly facilitated studies in large collections of families with affected sib-pairs, including those in the Human Biological Data Interchange (HBDI) and British Diabetic Association (BDA) Warren repositories. A number of genome-wide scans have been performed in an effort to map IDDM loci, and approximately 20 chromosomal regions have been linked with the disease suggesting that T1DM is a polygenic disorder. A comprehensive list of the known susceptibility loci is shown in Table 2.1. Of the linked loci, nine lie on just three chromosomes (6, 2 and 11). Chromosome 6 contains IDDM1 on 6p21.3, IDDM5 on 6q25, IDDM8 on 6q25-27, and IDDM15 on 6q21. Chromosome 2 contains IDDM7 on 2q31-q33, IDDM12 on 2q33, and IDDM13 on 2q34. Chromosome 11 contains IDDM2 on 11p15.5 and IDDM4 on 11q13.3. Moreover, susceptibility loci on chromosomes 2 and 6 seem to cluster within fairly small distances. This may facilitate co-inheritance of susceptibility and epistatic interactions.

Most of the loci identified through linkage analysis provide only a modest contribution to the familial clustering of diabetes, and no other major susceptibility locus has been reported besides IDDM1. This is consistent with a model that predicted that diabetes susceptibility may be linked to a major locus and that several other minor loci contribute to diabetes risk in an epistatic way.[6] However, genetic heterogeneity has been consistently reported among and within different data sets, and this could decrease the probability that other major susceptibility genes, if heterogeneous and occurring in a minority of families, could be identified with the current analytical power and study design. The identification of *IDDM17* in a large pedigree may reflect this phenomenon, and also suggests the alternative hypothesis that T1DM may be oligogenic rather than polygenic.[7] Moreover, not all studies have consistently reproduced evidence for linkage, and a second-generation genome-wide scan performed in a large data set of US and UK families combined using multipoint linkage methods has failed to confirm linkage for most of the previously identified loci.[8] In contrast, another study of 263 UK pedigrees found confirmation for many of the same loci.[9] Thus, a definitive confirmation of linkage will require the analysis of additional and larger data sets and, as recently suggested, more powerful analytical methods involving linkage disequilibrium-based and haplotype mapping approaches.[9] Consistent with the interpretation that discrepant results may often result from inadequate sample size, a third genome scan was recently performed using a new collection of 225 multiplex families and merging the data from all three major genome scans.[10] The combined sample of 831 affected sibling pairs provided 90% power to detect linkage for loci with $\lambda s = 1.3$ at $p = 7.4 \times 10^{-4}$. Three chromosomal regions showed significant evidence of linkage (LOD scores >4): 6p21 (*IDDM1*), 11p15 (*IDDM2*), and 16q22-q24. Four additional regions showed suggestive evidence (LOD scores ≥2.2): 10p11 (*IDDM10*), 2q31 (*IDDM7*, *IDDM12*, and *IDDM13*), 6q21 (*IDDM15*), and 1q42. Additional analyses that included the presence of specific high-risk HLA genotypes and age at disease onset provided

evidence of linkage for additional loci, including the putative *IDDM8* locus on chromosome 6q27. It is now expected that international collaborations such as the 13th International HLA Working Group (http://www.ihwg.org), the European Consortium for IDDM Studies[11] and the Type 1 Diabetes Genetic Consortium (http://www.t1dgc.org) will allow studying larger and diversified data sets, thus improving our ability to identify susceptibility genes. A review of the current knowledge about the susceptibility loci identified thus far follows.

The major susceptibility locus, IDDM1

The major susceptibility locus lies within the HLA (human leukocyte antigen) region on the short arm of chromosome 6[12] and it provides up to 40–50% of the inheritable diabetes risk.[13] The HLA complex is classically divided in three regions known as class I, class II, and class III. Alleles, modes of inheritance and putative mechanisms of susceptibility encoded for at the *IDDM1* locus are discussed below. A schematic representation of the HLA region and its association with [...] is shown in Figure 2.1.

The HLA class [...]

There is evidence [...] DR, DQ and DP loci contribute to [...] diabetes susceptibility.[14–19] The g[...] ority of patients carry the HLA-DR3 or [...] class II antigens and approximately [...]% of patients are DR3/DR4 heterozygotes. The DR3/DR4 genotype confers the highest diabetes risk with a synergistic mode of action, followed by DR4 and DR3 homozygosity, respectively.[20] The HLA-DQ locus was later found to be the most strongly associated with diabetes susceptibility. This locus encodes for several variants of the HLA-DQ molecule, a heterodimer consisting of two glycoproteic chains (α and β) involved in immune recogni-

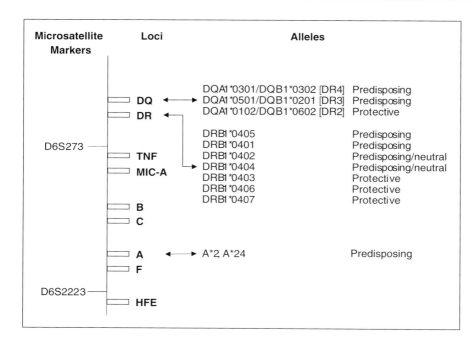

Figure 2.1
Schematic representation of the HLA region showing microsatellite markers, loci, and alleles associated with T1DM susceptibility. Inter-locus distances are approximated.

tion and antigen presentation to CD4 T-cells. In Caucasians, the HLA-DQ heterodimers (the α-chains are labeled DQA1 and the β-chains DQB1) encoded by the DQA1*0301, DQB1*0302 and DQA1*0501, DQB1*0201 alleles have the strongest association with diabetes. These alleles are in linkage disequilibrium with the HLA-DR4 and -DR3 alleles (Table 2.2), respectively.[21-23] Allelic variation at the DQB1 locus differentiates IDDM susceptibility among the two most common HLA-DR4 haplotypes found in Caucasians based on the presence of the DQB1*0302 or DQB1*0301 alleles. In fact, most patients with DR4 carry the DQB1*0302 allele. The fact that both the DQ α- and β-chains are polymorphic and that trans-complementation from opposite haplotypes has been recently demonstrated, significantly increases the diversity of class II antigens participating in the immune response and the potential for HLA-DQ contribution to T1DM

susceptibility. A trans-complementing DQ αβ heterodimer would be unique to a heterozygous individual and usually it would not be expressed in their parents. This may explain the increased risk observed in DR4, DQA1*0301, DQB1*0302/DR3, DQA1*0501, DQB1*0201 heterozygotes.[24,25]

The DQ locus also harbors diabetes-protective alleles. The DQA1*0102, DQB1*0602 heterodimer found on HLA-DR2 haplotypes confers dominant protection from the development of T1DM (reviewed in ref. 26). Among four common DR2 haplotypes observed in Caucasians (Table 2.2), the DQA1*0102, DQB1*0602, DRB1*1501 haplotype is negatively associated with T1DM and is reported in less than 1% of patients in most populations studied, including those of Caucasian (both European and North-American),[21,27,28] Asian,[29-32] African–American,[32,33] and Mexican–American origin.[34,35] The DQB1*0602 allele in particular is

DQA1	DQB1	DRB1	Susceptibility
0102	0602	1501 (DR2)	Protective
0102	0502 (AZH)	1601 (DR2)	Predisposing
0103	0601	1502 (DR2)	Neutral
0501	0201	0301 (DR3)	Predisposing
0301	0302	0401 (DR4)	Predisposing
0301	0302	0402 (DR4)	Predisposing
0301	0302	0403 (DR4)	Neutral
0301	0302	0404 (DR4)	Neutral
0301	0302	0405 (DR4)	Neutral
0301	0301	0401 (DR4)	Neutral
0301	0301	0403 (DR4)	Neutral
0201	0303	0701 (DR7)	Protective
0101	0503	1401 (DR1)	Protective

Table 2.2
Allele linkage patterns at the HLA class II DR-DQ loci patterns in Caucasians and relation to disease susceptibility

the only class II allele exclusively found on protective DR2 haplotypes while all the other alleles (DQA1*0102, DQA1*0103, DQB1*0601, DQB1*0502, DRB1*1501, DRB1*1502, DRB1*1601) can be found on neutral or moderately predisposing DR2 haplotypes. Moreover, a few rare patients with T1DM have been described carrying mutated DQB1*0602 alleles or unusual DQA1/DQB1 alleles in *cis* with the usual DRB1*1501 allele.[36–39]

Thus, the available evidence suggests that the diabetes-protective effect associated with DR2 haplotypes may be mostly mapped within the DQ locus and in particular to the DQB1*0602 allele. Although a number of patients with DQB1*0602 have been identified,[39] the overall number is small. Protection appears to be dominant since DQB1*0602 protects from diabetes even in the presence of high-risk HLA alleles,[40–42] but in the Swedish population the protective effect seems to attenuate with age.[43] Two additional haplotypes that are strongly protective are DRB1*1401, DQA1*0101, DQB1*0503 and DRB1*0701, DQA1*0201, DQB1*0303. The DRB1*1401 haplotype is particularly interesting in that the DRB1 allele shows a dramatic reduction in transmission to affected children that can be compared to that of DQB1*0602.[44]

HLA-DQ heterodimers are antigen-presenting molecules, and there is evidence that polymorphisms at the HLA-DQ locus may affect the structure and binding characterisitics of the molecules. For example, DQB1*0302 differs from DQB1*0301 at position 57, where it lacks an aspartic acid residue, similar to the I-A molecule of the NOD (non-obese diabetic) mouse (reviewed in ref. 45). The DQB1*0201 allele also lacks aspartic acid at position 57, and it has been proposed that this residue may be involved in the molecular mechanism underlying *IDDM1*-encoded susceptibility.[21,23] In fact, the amino acid residue at position 57 of the DQ-β chain appears to be critical for peptide binding and recognition.[46] Other residues of the DQ-β chain may influence peptide binding and diabetes susceptibility, in particular the combined variation of residues at positions 57 and 70[38,47,48] and an arginine residue at position 52 of the DQ-α chain.[24] By using X ray crystallography, investigators have recently determined the three-dimensional structure of the DQ8 molecule (encoded by DQA1*0301/ DQB1*0302) complexed with an immuno-dominant peptide of the insulin molecule.[49] The DQ8 structure suggests that the residue at position 57 contributes to the shaping of the P9 pocket, which together with the P1 and P4 pockets appear relevant to diabetes susceptibility. Moreover, the binding pockets of DQ8 were similar to those of DQ2 (encoded by DQA1*0501/DQB1*0201) and to those of the I-Ag7 molecule (corresponding to human DQ) from NOD mice. This finding suggests that diabetes may depend on an antigen presentation event(s) that may be similar in humans and NOD mice.

It remains unclear, however, whether genetically determined differences in peptide binding and presentation affect the shaping of the T-cell repertoire in the thymus or modulates immune responses in the extra-thymic periphery. A poor presentation in the thymus could impair mechanisms of negative selection, allowing autoreactive T-cells to escape deletion. In contrast, a protective HLA-DQ molecule could promote tolerance to β-cell molecules by eliciting more efficient antigen presentation and negative selection in the thymus. There is evidence for thymic deletion as a mechanism of protection associated with HLA genes in transgenic mice[50] and the recent demonstration that insulin and other islet cell antigens are expressed in human thymus[51,52] indirectly supports the hypothesis that thymic self-antigen presentation and thymic deletion mechanisms may be affected by the affinity and binding properties of HLA-DQ and HLA-DR molecules. An alternative hypothesis is that DQ molecules may control presentation in the periphery during the effector phase of the immune response and also influence regulatory immune responses associated with peripheral tolerance. Such responses may

control the balance between Th1 and Th2 lymphocytes, and a predominance of Th2 responses is usually associated with lack of progression to overt diabetes (reviewed in ref. 53). There is evidence that a non-diabetogenic immune response, mostly limited to the production of autoantibodies against the GAD autoantigen, may occur in first degree relatives with DQB1*0602[42] in whom the presence of DQB1*0602 and DQA1*0102 has been confirmed by direct sequencing.[39] The presence of GAD autoantibodies, often at high titers, may reflect the predominance of Th2 responses in relatives with DQB1*0602. A similar response has been reported in patients with Type 1 autoimmune polyendocrine syndrome who do not invariably progress to overt diabetes.[54,55] A protective effect has also been reported in first degree relatives participating in the ongoing Diabetes Prevention Trial (DPT-1), although different degrees of protection may occur in different ethnic groups.[56,57] Finally, the two hypotheses are not mutually exclusive, and DQB1*0602-associated protection could be mediated both in the thymus and the periphery.

The HLA class I region

A number of observations indicate that class II genes cannot explain all of the HLA association with T1DM. In fact, the class I region was the first HLA region to be linked to diabetes when associations with several HLA class I antigens (HLA-B8, -B18, and -B15) were discovered by serological typing.[58,59] Subsequently, Robinson et al.[60] examined affected sib-pairs with parents homozygous for the DR3 haplotype and used the HLA class I B locus to distinguish between the 2 DR3 haplotypes of the homozygous parent. The observation of significant deviation from 50% sharing implicated other HLA loci in T1DM susceptibility besides HLA-DR. Several other reports suggest that HLA class I genes may also influence susceptibility and particular clinical aspects of the disease such as age of onset[61,62] and the rate of β-cell destruction.[63–68] More recently, a T1DM-associated locus has been found in the class I region, telomeric to HLA-F.[69] By considering the transmission ratios of microsatellite variation from parents homozygous for the HLA class II DR-DQ genes (using the Homozygous Parent Transmission Disequilibrium Test), the possible confounding effect of linkage disequilibrium was removed. Evidence for a second T1DM locus in this region was demonstrated, near the HFE (hemochromatosis) gene and 8.5 Mb distal to the HLA class II loci. Analyses from three independent family data sets from Norway, Denmark, and the UK suggested the presence of additional T1DM gene(s). Allele 3 of marker D6S2223, 5.5 Mb telomeric of the class II region, was associated with T1DM when the haplotype was fixed for HLA-DRB1*03-DQA1*0501-DQB1*0201. In a case–control study, allele 3 at D6S2223 was found to be reduced among DRB1*03-DQA1*0501-DQB1*0201 homozygous patients with T1DM compared to DR-DQ matched controls, thus corroborating the results of the family analysis.[70] The protective effects seem to be inherited as a recessive trait. Further studies are necessary to confirm these observations in multiple ethnic groups and to better characterize these putative additional HLA region susceptibility loci. Such an effort has recently been launched by the 13th International HLA Working Group, which is currently studying a large data set collected with the collaboration of many laboratories throughout the world to dissect finely the contribution of other loci besides HLA-DQ/DR to T1DM susceptibility.

The HLA class III region

Moghaddam et al.[71] provided strong evidence that another critical region for IDDM susceptibility, approximately 200 kb in size, lies around the microsatellite locus D6S273 which is located between the *TNF* and *HSP70* genes. Another study has independently confirmed linkage with marker D6S273, showing evidence for non-random transmission from DRB1*03-DQA1*0501-DQB1*0201 homozygous parents.[69] The *TNF* gene is a strong candidate since polymorphisms of this gene may affect the production of TNF-α (tumor necrosis factor), a potent cytokine, and in turn the magnitude of immune responses. It has also been reported that TNF-α polymorphisms are associated with age of onset and may influence the inflammatory process leading to the destruction of pancreatic β-cells and the development of T1DM.[72] In addition, the class I chain-related MIC-A and MIC-B genes, located between the HLA-B and the TNF-α genes, may also affect T1DM susceptibility. In a recent case–control study of Italian patients, the frequency of the MIC-A5 allele was increased in patients while none of the TNF-α alleles were statistically significantly associated with the disease. In this study, the MIC-A5 allele was associated with T1DM independently of class II alleles, suggesting an independent contribution of this locus to diabetes risk.[73] A contribution of MIC-A was also reported in Basque families.[74]

The insulin gene-VNTR locus, IDDM2

The *IDDM2* locus has been mapped to a variable number of tandem repeats (VNTR) located ~0.5 kb upstream of the insulin gene (*INS*) (reviewed in ref. 75) (Figure 2.2). This polymorphic repeat, also known as the insulin gene minisatellite or ILPR (insulin-linked polymorphic region),[76] consists of a 14–15 bp unit consensus sequence (ACAGGGGTCT GGGG) with slight variations of the repeat sequence. Allele frequencies tend to cluster in the 30–60 repeat range (class I alleles) or at 120–170 repeats (class III alleles). The intermediate class II alleles are rare in Caucasians and less rare in individuals of African descent. Shortly after its discovery, the insulin VNTR was found to be associated with T1DM.[77] Extensive studies involving cross-match haplotype analysis and multiple DNA variant association analysis involving polymorphisms in the neighboring *HUMTHO1* (tyrosine hydroxylase) and *IGF2* genes provided strong evidence that the VNTR is the main susceptibility determinant in this region[78–82] (Figure 2.2), although the influence of nearby loci was not formally excluded by all genetic analyses.[83,84] Homozygosity for the short class I VNTR alleles is found in ~75–85% of the patients compared to a frequency of 50–60% in the general population, suggesting that it predisposes to T1DM. In contrast, the longer class III VNTR alleles are rarely seen in patients and are believed to confer a dominant protective effect.[77,85,86] The relative risk ratio of the I/I genotype versus I/III or III/III has been reported to be moderate (in the 3–5 range) and it accounts for about 10% of the familial clustering of T1DM.[75] Metcalfe et al.[87] showed that homozygosity for the predisposing *INS* genotype increases the likelihood that identical twins will be concordant for T1DM.

There is evidence that VNTR alleles are quite heterogeneous and may differ in their ability to modulate disease susceptibility. Further classification of VNTR alleles is indeed possible according to size differences, and at least 21 class I and 15 class III VNTR alleles were described by fluorescence-based DNA fragment-sizing technology[81] (Figure 2.2). Bennett et al. grouped the 15 class III VNTR alleles identified according to two main modes of transmission based on the linkage disequilibrium pattern with alleles at the *HUMTHO1*

locus on chromosome 11p15. Thus, by taking both size and flanking haplotypes into account, class III VNTR alleles linked to the *HUMTHO1* Z-8 allele were found more protective (very protective haplotype or VPH) than those linked to the *HUMTHO1* Z allele (protective haplotype or PH) (Figure 2.2).[81,86] However, certain VNTR alleles can be found in linkage disequilibrium with either the Z or Z-8 alleles. The variable degree of protection observed for these alleles may also be influenced by sequence heterogeneity and its effects on the VNTR physical state and transcriptional activity. The VNTR sequence is particularly G-rich, and forms unusual DNA structures *in vitro* and *in vivo*, presumably through the formation of G-quartets.[88–91] Sequencing studies have indeed identified several variants of the commonest VNTR repeat sequence that characterize yet another level of heterogeneity.[76,92–95]

Recent studies analyzed the variant repeat distribution within the VNTR using minisatellite variant repeat mapping by PCR (MVR-PCR).[96] Some of the variation within the repetitive sequence most probably arises by mitotic replication slippage at an estimated frequency of 10^3 per gamete. However, sperm DNA analysis revealed a second class of mutation occurring at a frequency of approximately 2×10^5 that involved highly complex intra- and inter-allelic rearrangements, which are probably meiotic in origin.[97] These events may help explain the heterogeneity of the VNTR locus. The combined analysis of the variant repeat distribution and of the haplotypes flanking the VNTR has allowed defining five new ancestral allele lineages.[97] Class III VNTR alleles can be divided into two diverging lineages, IIIA and IIIB (Figure 2.2). These two lineages correspond to the PH and VPH haplotypes previously defined by Bennett et al.[81] Class I alleles can also be divided into

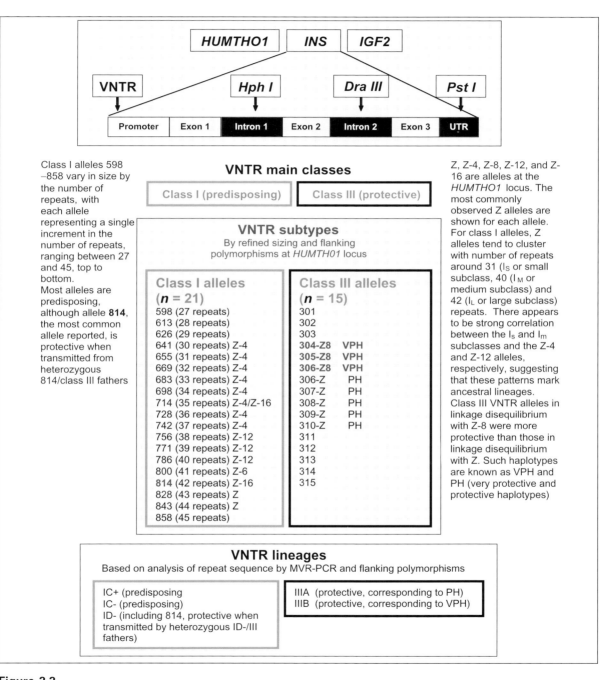

Class I alleles 598 –858 vary in size by the number of repeats, with each allele representing a single increment in the number of repeats, ranging between 27 and 45, top to bottom. Most alleles are predisposing, although allele **814**, the most common allele reported, is protective when transmitted from heterozygous 814/class III fathers

VNTR main classes

Class I (predisposing)	Class III (protective)

VNTR subtypes
By refined sizing and flanking
polymorphisms at *HUMTH01* locus

Class I alleles (*n* = 21)
598 (27 repeats)
613 (28 repeats)
626 (29 repeats)
641 (30 repeats) Z-4
655 (31 repeats) Z-4
669 (32 repeats) Z-4
683 (33 repeats) Z-4
698 (34 repeats) Z-4
714 (35 repeats) Z-4/Z-16
728 (36 repeats) Z-4
742 (37 repeats) Z-4
756 (38 repeats) Z-12
771 (39 repeats) Z-12
786 (40 repeats) Z-12
800 (41 repeats) Z-6
814 (42 repeats) Z-16
828 (43 repeats) Z
843 (44 repeats) Z
858 (45 repeats)

Class III alleles (*n* = 15)
301
302
303
304-Z8   VPH
305-Z8   VPH
306-Z8   VPH
306-Z   PH
307-Z   PH
308-Z   PH
309-Z   PH
310-Z   PH
311
312
313
314
315

Z, Z-4, Z-8, Z-12, and Z-16 are alleles at the *HUMTHO1* locus. The most commonly observed Z alleles are shown for each allele. For class I alleles, Z alleles tend to cluster with number of repeats around 31 (I$_S$ or small subclass, 40 (I$_M$ or medium subclass) and 42 (I$_L$ or large subclass) repeats. There appears to be strong correlation between the I$_s$ and I$_m$ subclasses and the Z-4 and Z-12 alleles, respectively, suggesting that these patterns mark ancestral lineages. Class III VNTR alleles in linkage disequilibrium with Z-8 were more protective than those in linkage disequilibrium with Z. Such haplotypes are known as VPH and PH (very protective and protective haplotypes)

VNTR lineages
Based on analysis of repeat sequence by MVR-PCR and flanking polymorphisms

IC+ (predisposing IC- (predisposing) ID- (including 814, protective when transmitted by heterozygous ID-/III fathers)	IIIA (protective, corresponding to PH) IIIB (protective, corresponding to VPH)

Figure 2.2
The IDDM2 *susceptibility locus. Top to bottom, the figure shows the* HUMTHO1, INS *and* IGF2 *loci, as well as a schematic structure of the insulin gene with the approximate location of some of the most characterized polymorphic loci (VNTR,* Hph I, Dra III, Pst I*) in relation to the promoter region, introns, exons, and UTR (untranslated region). Also shown are VNTR classes, alleles and lineages.*

three lineages, IC+, ID+ and ID−. The lineage denomination reflect the class of alleles, noted by the letter 'I', while the letters 'C' or 'D' identify two different lineages defined by the very different distribution of variant repeats noted by multidimensional scaling.[97] The notation '+' or '−' refers to the presence (+) or absence (−) of a *MspI* restriction site at position +3,850, so that depending on this haplotypic analysis lineages could either be IC+, ID+ or ID−. IC+ and ID+ alleles are all predisposing to T1DM. In contrast, ID− alleles are protective when transmitted from ID−/III heterozygous fathers. Similar findings were reported for the class I allele termed 814 (42 repeats), which is included in the ID− lineage. The analysis of class ID− alleles into those of 42 repeats and those of other sizes suggested that the protective effect was a feature of all ID− alleles, irrespective of size. However, ID− alleles are clearly distinguished from all other alleles by a *MspI* variant within the *IGF2* gene. This suggests that susceptibility conferred by class I ID− VNTR alleles may be modified by nearby sequences, and that in this case *IDDM2* susceptibility may have a multilocus origin.[97]

Collectively, the above studies suggest that the VNTR locus is extremely polymorphic, and that not only the size of the VNTR but also sequence variation may play a significant role in modulating *INS* transcription and diabetes susceptibility. It has also been shown that single nucleotide differences in the VNTR sequence can affect *INS* transcription and correlate with the ability to form unusual DNA structures, both at the inter- and intramolecular levels.[91] These findings have led to the hypothesis that VNTR variants may differ in their ability to stimulate transcription as a function of the binding of inter- and intramolecular quartets with the transcription factor Pur1.

Studies on the transcriptional effects of the VNTR *in vivo* showed that the *INS* transcript in *cis* with the class III VNTR was expressed at lower levels (15–20%) than the class I transcript in fetal[98] and adult pancreas.[81] However, these studies report only marginal differences in pancreatic *INS* transcription, and the lower transcription associated with diabetes-protective class III VNTR alleles does not fit well with their dominant protective effect. It seems unlikely that such minor differences may influence susceptibility to a form of diabetes resulting from the autoimmune destruction of pancreatic β-cells. A mechanistic hypothesis consistent with this assumption was formulated following the discovery that *INS* is actively transcribed in the thymus. Thymic *INS* transcription has now been reported in mouse,[99] rat,[100] and humans during fetal development and childhood[51,52,101] as well as in adult life.[102] Overall, genes encoding for several self-molecules have been found to be expressed in the thymus, including pancreatic and thyroid hormones, neuroendocrine molecules and other peripheral proteins.[103,104] Increasing evidence suggests that thymic expression of self-antigens may be crucial for the development of self-tolerance during the maturation of the immune system. The fact that negative selection of autoreactive thymocytes is dose-dependent suggested the hypothesis that different VNTR alleles may modulate tolerance to insulin by affecting insulin expression levels in the thymus. Consistent with this hypothesis, *INS* mRNA levels in the thymus were found to correlate with VNTR alleles in opposite fashion to that observed in the pancreas.[81] *INS* transcripts in *cis* with class III VNTR alleles are transcribed at much higher levels (on average 2–3-fold) than those in *cis* with class I VNTR alleles.[51,52] The increased transcription levels detected in the thymus fit well with the dominant protective effect associated with class III VNTR alleles, as higher insulin levels in the thymus may more efficiently induce negative selection of insulin-specific T-lymphocytes (or improved selection of regulatory T-cells). In contrast, homozygosity for diabetes-associated class I VNTR alleles determines lower insulin levels that may be associated with a less efficient deletion of insulin-specific autoreactive T-cells (or impaired selection of regulatory T-cells).

Functional studies in transgenic mice and fetal organ thymic cultures have provided both *in vivo* and *in vitro* data showing that thymic expression of self-antigens and their levels of expression can dramatically affect the development of self-tolerance.[105–114] Direct support for the hypothesis that thymic levels of *INS* expression can influence T1DM susceptibility and immune responsiveness to insulin is provided by recent work in a mouse model with graded thymic insulin expression.[115] In this elegant model, mice expressing low thymic insulin levels presented detectable peripheral reactivity to insulin, whereas mice with normal levels showed no significant response. Additional support for this hypothesis derives from the finding that transgenic expression of increased levels of proinsulin in the thymus (in MHC class II-positive cells) of NOD mice prevents insulitis and diabetes.[116] Proinsulin expression would likely affect tolerance to insulin as well, since most of the known immunodominant epitopes identified as targets of the insulin autoimmune responses in T1DM are shared by both insulin and proinsulin,[117–120] and some proinsulin epitopes are directly targeted.[121] *INS* transcription in human thymus also correlates with protein production in the thymus.[51,52] Proinsulin appears to be the main product of the insulin gene in the thymus.[102] This is not surprising since thymus cells expressing proinsulin are not likely to possess the refined machinery necessary to process proinsulin to mature insulin. Further support for the concept that the expression of proinsulin is relevant to

tolerance comes from the finding that insulin and other self-antigens are expressed in the thymus by a subset of antigen presenting cells that appear to mediate a tolerogenic signal, both in mouse[104,111,112,122] and humans.[102,123] Moreover, similar cells and *INS* transcription have also been demonstrated in peripheral lymphoid organs, suggesting that insulin expression in lymphoid organs may also play a role in maintaining peripheral self-tolerance throughout life.[102,123]

Overall, the studies reviewed here suggest that the *IDDM2* is a quantitative trait resulting from allelic variation and, as discussed in more detail in a later paragraph, from complex parental and epigenetic effects at the VNTR locus. *IDDM2*-associated susceptibility and resistance may derive from quantitative differences in *INS* transcription in the specialized antigen presenting cells found in thymus and peripheral lymphoid tissues, where production of self-antigens such as proinsulin may be crucial for the shaping and maintaining of a self-tolerant T-cell repertoire. Such mechanisms may influence the probability of developing autoimmune responses to insulin, a key autoantigen in T1DM.

Other IDDM loci

Linkage with additional loci has been obtained, but in general with less reproducibility than *IDDM1* and *IDDM2*, as previously discussed. These include loci *IDDM3* through *IDDM17* (Table 2.1) and other loci that have received an official denomination. In most instances the actual gene linked to diabetes remains unknown, and only a few will be discussed here. A more complete review is available on line (http://www.uchsc.edu./misc/diabetes/ bdc.html).

IDDM12 is one of the best studied loci and maps on chromosome 2q33,[124] a chromosomal region containing the CTLA-4 (cytotoxic T-lymphocyte associated-4) and CD28 genes. Both genes encode molecules involved in T-cell activation and proliferation and differential regulation of these molecules could easily affect T-cell function. However, the *IDDM12* locus is likely to correspond to either CTLA-4 or to an unknown gene in very close proximity based on linkage with three markers within CTLA-4 and two immediate flanking markers (D2S72 and D2S105) on each side of CTLA-4, but not with more distant markers including CD28.[125] The linked markers encompass a region containing an (AT)n microsatellite located in the 3' UTR of the CTLA-4 gene. Moreover, the analysis of an A–G transition in the first exon of the CTLA-4 gene, coding for a Thr/Ala substitution in the leader peptide, also showed preferential transmission to the affected siblings.[124] Although linkage was not observed in every population studied, there are numerous studies demonstrating linkage between diabetes and *IDDM12* in numerous populations (especially mediterranean ones) and in combined data sets.[126–129]

Chromosome 6q25[130–135] contains the *IDDM5* locus. The best candidate gene to explain susceptibility at this locus is the Mn-superoxide dismutase (MnSOD), as polymorphisms affecting the function of MnSOD could render β-cells more susceptible to free oxygen radicals damage.

Chromosome 2q may also harbor a susceptibility locus, *IDDM7*.[131,136,137] The available evidence places *IDDM7* within two centiMorgans of D2S152, a chromosomal region that is synthenic with the non-obese diabetic (NOD) mouse chromosome 1 region containing the Idd5 susceptibility gene.[132,136] The *HOXD8* gene has been proposed as a possible susceptibility gene at the *IDDM7* locus.[138] Another potential candidate gene in this chromosomal region is *NEUROD*, a

transcription factor regulating the expression of the insulin gene and playing an important role in the development of pancreatic β-cells. A polymorphism consisting of a nucleotide G–A transition results in the substitution of alanine to threonine at codon 45 (Ala45Thr). The analysis of this polymorphism in Japanese and Danish patients suggested an association with Type 1 but not Type 2 diabetes,[139,140] but a case–control study in France did not find a similar association.[141,142]

IDDM11 appears to lie on chromosome 14q24.3-q31 and may be an important susceptibility locus in families lacking strong HLA predisposition.[143] Two candidate genes have been recently mapped to this chromosomal region. The *ENSA* gene encodes alpha-endosulfine, an endogenous regulator of β-cell K(ATP) channels.[144] The recombinant alpha-endosulfine has been shown to inhibit sulfonylurea binding to β-cell membranes, to reduce cloned K(ATP) channel currents, and to stimulate insulin secretion from β-cells. The *SEL-1L* gene codes for a negative regulator of the *NOTCH*, *LIN-12*, and *GLP-1* receptors, which are required for differentiation and maturation of β-cells as well as cell–cell interactions during development.[145] *SEL-1L* is abundantly expressed only in the pancreas, and appears to be involved in the down-regulation of mammalian Notch signaling, recently shown to be critical for the development of the pancreas and β-cells.[146] However, a study of families from Denmark and Sardinia found no evidence that *SEL-1L* is directly linked to diabetes.[147]

IDDM18 maps to a single base pair change in the 3' UTR (untranslated region) of the *IL-12B* gene and T1DM in two Australian cohorts.[148] The *IL-12* gene is an important candidate in terms of immune function. Unfortunately multiple studies from other populations, including the UK, USA, Sardinia, Finland and Romania have failed to find evidence of association with the reported polymorphism.[10,149] The functional influence of the 3' UTR also remains unconfirmed.

Unlike all the preceding susceptibility loci, which have mostly been pinpointed by studying a large collection of families with affected sibling pairs, evidence for the *IDDM17* locus has been found by studying a large Bedouin Arab family with 19 affected individuals.[7] *IDDM17* maps to the long arm of chromosome 10 (10q25). Remarkably, one chromosome 10 haplotype was transmitted from a heterozygous parent to 13 of 13 affected offspring compared to 10 of 23 unaffected siblings. Moreover, all of the affected members in this family carry one or two high-risk HLA-DR3 haplotypes that are rarely found in other family members. Thus, the study of this family suggests the alternative hypothesis that T1DM may be an oligogenic disease rather than a polygenic one, and that perhaps just two or three genes may suffice to explain all of the inherited susceptibility in a given family.

Parent-of-origin effects on inherited genes expression

The genetics of T1DM is further complicated by the possible existence of parental effects acting on the transmission and expression of inherited genes. Several studies have shown that diabetes risk differs in the offspring of diabetic mothers and fathers, although the results of different studies have been discrepant.[150] It is also controversial whether parent-of-origin effects influence the transmission of *IDDM1* alleles to the diabetic offspring.[151–153] Recent evidence also suggests that parental influences may be operative at the *IDDM8*, *IDDM10*, and *IDDM15* loci.[134,154] Parent-of-origin effects influence the transmission of the VNTR alleles at the *IDDM2* locus.

The first report of linkage at the *IDDM2* locus found evidence, in a small subset of families that were informative for parental origin, that the excess allele sharing was exclusively paternal.[78] Most of the subsequent studies of intra-familial association demonstrated a statistically significant difference only for paternally transmitted alleles.[85,155–157] These observations may be explained by imprinting, a mechanism that regulates gene expression by silencing either the maternal or the paternal allele. The silencing effect results from the epigenetic modification (probably mediated by methylation) of the DNA during the passage from the male or the female germline. This modification of the DNA marks the genetic material as maternal or paternal (parental imprint). Of note, the insulin gene is located in a region of the human genome that is known to be subject to parental imprinting.[157] *INS* is expressed from both copies in the pancreas of mice,[158] human fetuses of 7–20 weeks' gestation[159] and adult humans.[86,160,161] However, we recently observed monoallelic *INS* expression in the pancreas of a 40-week old female fetus.[160,161] *INS* is also expressed monoallelically, and specifically from the paternal chromosome in the mouse yolk sack.[158] In addition, evidence has been recently presented for the imprinted paternal expression of *INS* in the human yolk sac.[162] Thus, imprinted expression can depend on the tissue and possibly the developmental stage.[163] The effects of imprinting on insulin expression may influence insulin expression during development and susceptibility to insulin/growth-related diseases in later life, including insulin resistance and Type 2 diabetes.[161]

Imprinting may also affect the levels of insulin being produced in the thymus. In fact, 5 out of 22 heterozygous thymus samples analyzed to date expressed only one *INS* transcript.[51,52] In all instances, the silenced allele was the one in *cis* with a class III VNTR.

Such monoallelic expression resulting from the silencing of class III VNTR transcripts in the thymus may prevent the protective effect associated with the class III VNTR and explain the parent-of-origin effects discussed above. Vafiadis et al.[164] recently studied in more detail the class III alleles that were silenced in the thymus. They developed a DNA fingerprinting method for identifying the type of alleles corresponding to the class III VNTR alleles that were found silenced in two thymus samples (S1, S2), and then analyzed the parental transmission of these type of class III alleles in a set of 287 diabetic children. Twelve of 18 possible transmissions of alleles matching the fingerprint of the S1 or S2 alleles were transmitted to the diabetic offspring, at a frequency of 0.67, which is significantly higher than the frequency of 0.38 seen in the remaining 142 class III alleles. These findings suggest that certain class III alleles may be predisposing instead of protective, and presumably these alleles are silenced in the thymus with obvious effects on the development of tolerance to insulin. Moreover, we have recently demonstrated monoallelic *INS* expression in the spleen of an 18-year-old Caucasian male, again preventing the expression of the *INS* transcript in *cis* with the class III VNTR allele.[161] Assuming that monoallelic expression in this subject was mediated by imprinting (parents were unavailable to determine the parental origin of the silenced allele), this finding suggests that the imprint status may be maintained beyond development and perhaps throughout life. Thus, imprinting in the thymus could silence the transcription of protective alleles and prevent the protective effect associated with increased levels of insulin in the thymus.

There is also evidence for even more complex mechanisms regulating *INS* transcription. Bennett et al.[165] studied more than 1,300 triads (two parents and affected child) and showed that the most common class I VNTR allele among Caucasians, termed 814 in arbitrary electrophoretic mobility units, has a protective effect similar to that of class III VNTR alleles. A protective effect of the 814 allele was independently confirmed in Basque families.[166] Bennett et al.[165] observed this protective effect only when the 814 allele was inherited from fathers with an 814/III VNTR genotype. In contrast, fathers with an 814/I VNTR genotype transmitted both the 814 and other class I VNTR alleles to their diabetic children at similar frequency. This unusual transmission pattern suggests that the 814 allele may behave differently in the offspring depending on the father's non-transmitted allele. This phenomenon could be explained by paramutation, a mechanism initially described in plants that requires some kind of physical interaction between homologous chromosomal domains in the pre-meiotic nucleus of the male germline.[167] According to this mechanism, the function of the 814 class I VNTR allele can be modified by some interactions with the paternal class III allele that is not transmitted to the offspring. This hypothesis finds additional support in the recent finding that both *cis*- and *trans*-allelic interactions influence imprinting at the *Ins2* locus in the mouse.[168] Morphological evidence for a similar interaction has been presented for another imprinted locus (the Prader-Willi/Angelman syndrome locus on chromosome 15) in somatic cells.[169] The data presented here suggest that besides allelic variation, parent-of-origin effects and complex epigenetic phenomena can dramatically influence *INS* transcription. It is important to notice that these phenomena can only be studied by evaluating *INS* transcription in selected tissues and correlating the subsequent data to the VNTR genotype. Thus, expression studies and genotyping must be combined to dissect fully the contribution of the insulin gene to diabetes susceptibility.

Other regulatory mechanisms of gene expression

Besides parent-of-origin effects and other epigenetic phenomena, there is also evidence that alternative splicing can affect gene expression in a tissue-specific manner and predispose to certain conditions.[170] These include T1DM, multiple sclerosis, and other neurological diseases.[171,172] In the case of T1DM, alternative splicing may affect the probability that one would mount autoimmune responses to the autoantigen IA-2. IA-2 is a tyrosine-phosphatase-like protein enriched in the secretory granules of islet and neuroendocrine cells,[173] and consists of a single transmembrane (TM) region (residues 577–600) and extra- and intracellular domains. A recent study investigated IA-2 expression in islets, thymus and spleen from non-diabetic human tissue donors (no tissues were available from patients) of different ages (from 21 weeks of gestation to 52 years of age) and from diverse racial groups. IA-2 mRNA expression and splicing were evaluated by RT-PCR using primers that amplify both full-length and Δexon 13 transcripts, and the identity of the products was verified by sequencing. All pancreatic samples expressed full-length IA-2 transcript and approximately 50% also expressed the Δexon 13 transcript. Of the lymphoid tissues found to express IA-2 transcripts, all thymus and spleen specimens exclusively expressed the Δexon 13 transcript. Further, this study discovered another alternatively spliced IA-2 transcript in which 129 bp of exon 14 are spliced out, resulting in the deletion of 43 amino acids (aa 653–695) in the intracellular domain. This transcript was detected in about 50% of the pancreatic samples studied but essentially in none of the thymus and spleen specimens. Thus, alternative splicing causes differential IA-2 expression in pancreas compared to lymphoid organs. Such differences may affect immune responsiveness to specific epitopes and help explain why IA-2 and not many other islet proteins become targets of autoimmunity in T1DM. Tolerance to linear or conformational epitopes typical of the full-length protein or of the Δexon 14 variant may not be achieved if these epitopes are expressed in islets but not in lymphoid organs. The specific lack of expression of the TM/Juxta-membrane domains (exon 13) in lymphoid organs helps to explain why epitopes from these domains are often targeted by autoimmune responses in T1DM. Autoantibodies against IA-2 epitopes encoded by exons 13 and 14 have been reported in patients and can precede the appearance of autoantibodies against other intracellular epitopes (epitope spreading). Although T-cell reactivity against IA-2 epitopes encoded by exons 13 and 14 or against epitopes generated by alternative splicing of these exons has not been directly analyzed, there is evidence that the HLA-DR4-restricted, naturally processed 654-674 epitope (exon 14) is recognized by autoreactive T-cells.[174] Similar to the parent-of-origin effects affecting insulin gene expression in thymus[51,52] and peripheral lymphoid organs[160,161] differential IA-2 splicing appears to function as a mechanism regulating gene expression independent of inherited alleles at the insulin and IA-2 loci. Although recent investigations had excluded linkage with *IA-2* polymorphisms,[129] these findings suggest that expression studies for selected candidate genes in tissues relevant to the disease process can help dissect the complex genetics of a multifactorial disease such as T1DM.

Concluding remarks

It is apparent that significant progress has been made in unraveling the complex genetic mechanisms that modulate susceptibility to T1DM, and in dissecting the related molecular pathways controlled by these mechanisms. It is a fair speculation that at least the main component of *IDDM1*, the HLA/DQ/DR loci, is involved in antigen presentation and controls immune responsiveness to one or more islet cell antigens, either in the thymus or in the periphery, or in both. As regards *IDDM2*, VNTR alleles appear to influence *INS* expression in the thymus, and thus may affect the development of tolerance to insulin. Thus, *IDDM1* and *IDDM2* may influence basic immunological functions such as antigen presentation and thymic selection, and appear to control the specificity of the immune response rather than mediate a generic predisposition to autoimmunity. However, there is growing evidence that some loci may be shared by different autoimmune diseases. One would expect that those loci would play a role by affecting less specific mechanisms, for instance the degree of inflammation or the production of certain cytokines. It is also important to note that the susceptibility alleles identified at the best characterized loci (*IDDM1*, *IDDM2*, and *IDDM12*) are commonly observed in the population and all appear to have normal sequence. This suggests that susceptibility may simply derive from polymorphisms affecting the function and expression of certain proteins. It is plausible that a number of loci may map to regulatory sequences (such as VNTRs) and act as quantitative traits. Complex parental effects and other genetic mechanisms, such as alternative splicing, may modify the transmission and expression of inherited genes, further complicating the genetics of diabetes. Future studies are expected to lead to the full identification and characterization of susceptibility and perhaps disease genes, and this will improve our ability to predict disease risk by genetic testing and deepen our understanding of the key mechanisms leading to T1DM. Such improved knowledge should be instrumental for developing successful strategies for prevention and cure.

References

1. Schranz DB, Lernmark A. Immunology in diabetes: an update. Diabetes Metab Rev 1998; 14: 3–29.
2. Leslie RDG, Pyke DA. Escaping insulin dependent diabetes. Characteristic immunological changes don't invariably lead to disease. BMJ 1991; 302: 1103–4.
3. Verge CF, Gianani R, Yu L et al. Late progression to diabetes, evidence for chronic beta cell autoimmunity in identical twins of patients with type 1 diabetes. Diabetes 1995; 44: 1176–9.
4. Risch N, Ghosh S, Todd JA. Statistical evolution of multiple locus linkage data in experimental species and relevance to human studies: application to murine and human IDDM. Am J Hum Genet 1993; 53: 702–14.
5. Todd JA, Farrall M. Panning for gold: genome-wide scanning for linkage in type 1 diabetes. Hum Mol Genet 1996; 5: 1443–8.
6. Rich SS. Mapping genes in diabetes. Diabetes 1990; 39: 1315–19.
7. Verge CF, Vardi P, Babu S et al. Evidence for oligogenic inheritance of type 1 diabetes in a large Bedouin Arab family. J Clin Invest 1998; 102: 1569–75.
8. Concannon P, Gogolin-Ewens KJ, Hinds DA et al. A second-generation screen of the human genome for susceptibility to insulin-dependent diabetes mellitus. Nat Genet 1998; 19: 292–6.
9. Mein CA, Esposito L, Dunn MG et al. A search for type 1 diabetes susceptibility genes in families from the United Kingdom. Nat Genet 1998; 19: 297–300.
10. Cox NJ, Wapelhorst B, Morrison VA et al.

Seven regions of the genome show evidence of linkage to type 1 diabetes in a consensus analysis of 767 multiplex families. Am J Hum Genet 2001; 69: 820–30.

11. Nerup J, Pociot F. A genomewide scan for type 1-diabetes susceptibility in Scandinavian families: identification of new loci with evidence of interactions. Am J Hum Genet 2001; 69: 1301–13.

12. Johnson AH, Hurley CK, Hartzman RJ et al. HLA: The major histocompatibility complex of man. In: Henry JB, ed. Clinical Diagnosis and Management by Laboratory Methods, 18th ed. Philadelphia: WB Saunders, 1991: 761–94.

13. Noble JA, Valdes AM, Cook M et al. The role of HLA class II genes in insulin-dependent diabetes mellitus: molecular analysis of 180 Caucasian, multiplex families. Am J Hum Genet 1996; 59: 1134–48.

14. Sheehy MJ, Scharf SJ, Rowe JR et al. A diabetes susceptible HLA haplotype is best defined by a combination of HLA-DR and DQ alleles. J Clin Invest 1989; 83: 830–5.

15. Nepom GT, Erlich H. MHC class-II molecules and autoimmunity. Annu Rev Immunol 1991; 9: 493–525.

16. Sanjeevi CB, Hook P, Landin-Olsson P et al. DR4 subtypes and their molecular properties in a population-based study of Swedish childhood diabetes. Tissue Antigens 1996; 47: 275–83.

17. Undlien DE, Friede T, Rammensee HG et al. HLA-encoded genetic predisposition in IDDM: DR4 subtypes may be associated with different degrees of protection. Diabetes 1997; 46: 143–9.

18. Noble JA, Valdes AM, Thomson G, Erlich HA. The HLA class II locus DPB1 can influence susceptibility to type 1 diabetes. Diabetes 2000; 49: 121–5.

19. Valdes AM, Noble JA, Genin E et al. Modeling of HLA class II susceptibility to Type I diabetes reveals an effect associated with DPB1. Genet Epidemiol 2001; 21: 212–23.

20. Thomson G, Robinson WP, Kuhner MK et al. Genetic heterogeneity, modes of inheritance, and risk estimates; a joint study of Caucasians with insulin-dependent diabetes mellitus. Am J Hum Genet 1988; 43: 799–816.

21. Todd JA, Bell JI, McDevitt HO. HLA-DQ beta gene contribution to susceptibility and resistance to insulin dependent diabetes mellitus. Nature 1987; 329: 599–604.

22. Horn GT, Bugawan TL, Long CM, Erlich HA. Allelic sequence variation of the HLA-DQ loci: relationship to serology and to insulin-dependent diabetes mellitus susceptibility. Proc Natl Acad Sci USA 1988; 85: 6012–16.

23. Morel PA, Dorman JS, Todd JA et al. Aspartic acid at position 57 of the HLA-DQ beta chain protects against Type I diabetes: a family study. Proc Natl Acad Sci USA 1988; 85: 8111–15.

24. Khalil I, d'Auriol L, Gobet M et al. A combination of HLA-DQB Asp57-negative and HLA-DQA Arg52 confers susceptibility to insulin-dependent diabetes mellitus. J Clin Invest 1990; 85: 1315–19.

25. Khalil I, Deschamps I, Lepage V et al. Dose effect of cis- and trans-encoded HLA-DQalpha/beta heterodimers in IDDM susceptibility. Diabetes 1992; 41: 378–84.

26. Pugliese A. Genetic protection from insulin-dependent diabetes mellitus. Diabetes Nutr Metab 1997; 10: 169–79.

27. Baisch JM, Week T, Giles R et al. Analysis of HLA-DQ genotypes and susceptibility in insulin-dependent diabetes mellitus. N Engl J Med 1990; 322: 1836–41.

28. Sorrentino R, DeGrazia U, Buzzetti R et al. An explanation for the neutral effect of DR2 on IDDM susceptibility in central Italy. Diabetes 1992; 41: 904–8.

29. Awata T, Iwamoto Y, Matsuda A et al. High frequency of aspartic acid at position 57 of HLA-DQ s chain in Japanese IDDM and non-Diabetic subjects. Diabetes 1989; 38: 90A (abstract)

30. Ikegami H, Kawaguchi Y, Yamato E et al. Analysis by the polymerase chain reaction of histocompatibility leucocyte antigen-DR9-linked susceptibility to insulin-dependent diabetes mellitus. J Clin Endocrin Metab 1992; 75: 1381–5.

31. Penny MA, Jenkins D, Mijovic CH et al. Susceptibility to IDDM in a Chinese population. Diabetes 1992; 41: 914–19.

32. Ronningen KS, Spurkland A, Tait BD et al. HLA class II associations in insulin-dependent

diabetes mellitus among Blacks, Caucasoids, and Japanese. In: Tsuji K, Aizawa M, Sasazuki T, eds. HLA 1991. Oxford: Oxford University Press, 1991: 713–22.

33. Mijovic CH, Jenkins D, Jacobs KH et al. HLA-DQA1 and -DQB1 alleles associated with genetic susceptibility to IDDM in a black population. Diabetes 1991; 40: 748–53.

34. Sanjeevi CB, Zeidler A, Shaw S et al. Analysis of HLA-DQA1 and -DQB1 genes in Mexican Americans with insulin-dependent diabetes mellitus. Tissue Antigens 42: 72–7.

35. Erlich HA, Zeidler A, Chang J et al. HLA class II alleles and susceptibility and resistance to insulin dependent diabetes mellitus in Mexican-American families. Nat Genet 1993; 3: 358–64.

36. Erlich HA, Griffith RL, Bugawan TL et al. Implication of specific DQB1 alleles in genetic susceptibility and resistance by identification of IDDM siblings with novel HLA-DQB1 allele and unusual DR2 and DR1 haplotypes. Diabetes 1991; 40: 478–81.

37. Zeliszewski D, Tiercy J, Boitard C et al. Extensive study of DRbeta, DQalpha, and DQbeta gene polymorphism in 23 DR2-positive, insulin-dependent diabetes mellitus patients. Hum Immunol 1992; 33: 140–7.

38. Hoover ML Marta RT. Molecular modelling of HLA-DQ suggests a mechanism of resistance in type 1 diabetes. Scand J Immunol 1997; 45: 193–202.

39. Pugliese A, Kawasaki E, Zeller M et al. Sequence analysis of the diabetes-protective human leukocyte antigen- DQB1*0602 allele in unaffected, islet cell antibody-positive first degree relatives and in rare patients with type 1 diabetes. J Clin Endocrinol Metab 1999; 84: 1722–8.

40. Hagopian WA, Sanjeevi CB, Kockum I et al. Glutamate decarboxylase-, insulin-, islet cell antibodies and HLA typing to detect diabetes in a general population-based study of Swedish children. J Clin Invest 1995; 95: 1505–11.

41. Kockum I, Wassmuth R, Holmberg E et al. HLA-DQ primarily confers protection and HLA-DR susceptibility in type I (insulin-dependent) diabetes studied in population-base affected families and controls. Am J Hum Genet 1993; 53: 150–67.

42. Pugliese A, Gianani R, Moromisato R et al. HLA-DQB1*0602 is associated with dominant protection from diabetes even among islet cell antibody positive first degree relatives of patients with insulin-dependent diabetes. Diabetes 1995; 44: 608–13.

43. Graham J, Kockum I, Sanjeevi CB et al. Negative association between type 1 diabetes and HLA DQB1*0602-DQA1*0102 is attenuated with age at onset. Swedish Childhood Diabetes Study Group. Eur J Immunogenet 1999; 26: 117–27.

44. Redondo MJ, Kawasaki E, Mulgrew CL et al. DR- and DQ-associated protection from type 1A diabetes: comparison of DRB1*1401 and DQA1*0102-DQB1*0602*. J Clin Endocrinol Metab 2000; 85: 3793–7.

45. Bellgrau D, Pugliese A. NOD mouse and BB rat: genetics and immunological function. In: Eisenbarth GS, Lafferty KJ, eds. Type I diabetes. Molecular, Cellular, and Clinical Immunology. New York: Oxford University Press, 1996: 53–75.

46. Kwok WW, Domeier ME, Johnson ML et al. HLA-DQB1 codon 57 is critical for peptide binding and recognition. J Exp Med 1996; 183: 1253–8.

47. Sanjeevi CB, DeWeese C, Landin-Olsson M et al. Analysis of critical residues of HLA-DQ6 molecules in insulin-dependent diabetes mellitus. Tissue Antigens 1997; 50: 61–5.

48. Sanjeevi CB, Landin-Olsson M, Kockum I et al. The combination of several polymorphic amino acid residues in the DQalpha and DQbeta chains forms a domain structure pattern and is associated with insulin-dependent diabetes mellitus. Ann NY Acad Sci 2002; 958: 362–75.

49. Lee KH, Wucherpfennig KW, Wiley DC. Structure of a human insulin peptide-HLA-DQ8 complex and susceptibility to type 1 diabetes. Nat Immunol 2001; 2: 501–7.

50. Schimdt D, Verdaguer J, Averill N, Santamaria P. A mechanism for the major histocompatibility complex-linked resistance to autoimmunity. J Exp Med 1997; 186: 1059–75.

51. Pugliese A, Zeller M, Fernandez AJ et al. The insulin gene is transcribed in the human thymus and transcription levels correlated

with allelic variation at the INS VNTR-IDDM2 susceptibility locus for type 1 diabetes. Nat Genet 1997; 15: 293–7.

52. Vafiadis P, Bennett ST, Todd JA et al. Insulin expression in human thymus is modulated by INS VNTR alleles at the IDDM2 locus. Nat Genet 1997; 15: 289–92.

53. Rabinovitch A. An update on cytokines in the pathogenesis of insulin-dependent diabetes mellitus. Diabetes Metab Rev 1998; 14: 129–51.

54. Gianani R, Verge CF, Moromisato-Gianani RI et al. Limited loss of tolerance to islet autoantigens in ICA+ first degree relatives of patients with type I diabetes expressing the HLA-DQB1*0602 allele. J Autoimmun 1996; 9: 423–5.

55. Tuomi T, Bjorses P, Falorni A et al. Antibodies to glutamic acid decarboxylase and insulin-dependent diabetes in patients with autoimmune polyendocrine syndrome type I. J Clin Endocrinol Metab 1996; 81: 1488–94.

56. Greenbaum CJ, Schatz DA, Cuthbertson D et al. Islet cell antibody-positive relatives with human leukocyte antigen DQA1*0102, DQB1*0602: identification by the Diabetes Prevention Trial-type 1. J Clin Endocrinol Metab 200; 85: 1255–60.

57. Greenbaum CJ, Gaur LK, Noble JA. ICA+ relatives with DQA1*0102/DQB1*0602 have expected 0602 sequence and DR types. J Autoimmun 2002; 18: 67–70.

58. Nerup J, Platz P, Andersen OO et al. HL-A antigens and diabetes mellitus. Lancet 1974; 2: 864–6.

59. Cudworth AG, Woodrow JC. Evidence for HL-A-linked genes in 'juvenile' diabetes mellitus. BMJ 1975; 3: 133–5.

60. Robinson WP, Barbosa J, Rich SS, Thomson G. Homozygous parent affected sib pair method for detecting disease predisposing variants: application to insulin dependent diabetes mellitus. Genet Epidemiol 1993; 10: 273–88.

61. Valdes AM, Thomson G, Erlich HA, Noble JA. Association between type 1 diabetes age of onset and HLA among sibling pairs. Diabetes 1999; 48: 1658–61.

62. Demaine AG, Hibberd ML, Mangles D, Millward BA. A new marker in the HLA class I region is associated with the age at onset of IDDM. Diabetologia 1995; 38: 623–8.

63. Fennessy M, Metcalfe K, Hitman GA et al. A gene in the HLA class I region contributes to susceptibility to IDDM in the Finnish population. Childhood Diabetes in Finland (DiMe) Study Group [see comments]. Diabetologia 1994; 37: 937–44.

64. Langholz B, Tuomilehto-Wolf E, Thomas D et al. Variation in HLA-associated risks of childhood insulin-dependent diabetes in the Finnish population: I. Allele effects at A, B, and DR loci. DiMe Study Group. Childhood Diabetes in Finland. Genet Epidemiol 1995; 12: 441–53.

65. Nakanishi K, Kobayashi T, Murase T et al. Association of HLA-A24 with complete beta-cell destruction in IDDM. Diabetes 1993; 42: 1086–93.

66. Nakanishi K, Kobayashi T, Inoko H et al. Residual beta-cell function and HLA-A24 in IDDM. Markers of glycemic control and subsequent development of diabetic retinopathy. Diabetes 1995; 44: 1334–9.

67. Honeyman MC, Harrison LC, Drummond B et al. Analysis of families at risk for insulin-dependent diabetes mellitus reveals that HLA antigens influence progression to clinical disease. Mol Med 1995; 1: 576–82.

68. Nejentsev S, Reijonen H, Adojaan B et al. The effect of HLA-B allele on the IDDM risk defined by DRB1*04 subtypes and DQB1*0302. Diabetes 1997; 46: 1888–92.

69. Lie BA, Todd JA, Pociot F et al. The predisposition to type 1 diabetes linked to the human leukocyte antigen complex includes at least one non-class II gene. Am J Hum Genet 1999; 64: 793–800.

70. Lie BA, Sollid LM, Ascher H et al. A gene telomeric of the HLA class I region is involved in predisposition to both type 1 diabetes and coeliac disease [In Process Citation]. Tissue Antigens 1999; 54: 162–8.

71. Moghaddam PH, de Knijf P, Roep BO et al. and the Belgian Diabetes Registry. Genetic structure of IDDM1. Two separate regions in the major histocompatibility complex contribute to susceptibility or protection. Diabetes 1998; 47: 263–9.

72. Fukui Y, Nishimura Y, Iwanga T et al. Glycosuria and insulitis in NOD mice expressing the HLA-DQw6 molecule. J Immunogenetics 1989; 16: 445–53.

73. Gambelunghe G, Ghaderi M, Cosentino A et al. Association of MHC Class I chain-related A (MIC-A) gene polymorphism with type I diabetes. Diabetologia 2000; 43: 507–14.

74. Bilbao JR, Martin-Pagola A, Calvo B et al. Contribution of MIC-A polymorphism to type 1 diabetes mellitus in Basques. Ann NY Acad Sci 2002; 958: 321–4.

75. Bennett ST, Todd JA. Human type 1 diabetes and the insulin gene: principles of mapping polygenes. Annul Rev Genet 1996; 30: 343–70.

76. Bell GI, Selby MJ, Rutter WJ. The highly polymorphic region near the insulin gene is composed of simple tandemly repeating sequences. Nature 1982; 295: 31–5.

77. Bell GI, Horita S, Karam JH. A polymorphic locus near the human insulin gene is associated with insulin dependent diabetes mellitus. Diabetes 1984; 33: 176–83.

78. Julier C, Hyer RN, Davies J et al. Insulin-IGF2 region on chromosome 11p encodes a gene implicated in HLA-DR4-dependent diabetes susceptibility. Nature 1991; 354: 155–9.

79. Bain SC, Prins JB, Hearne CM et al. Insulin gene region-encoded susceptibility to type I diabetes is not restricted to HLA-DR4-positive individuals. Nat Genet 1992; 2: 212–5.

80. Owerbach D, Gabbay KH. Localization of a Type I diabetes susceptibility locus to the variable tandem repeat region flanking the insulin gene. Diabetes 1993; 42: 1708–14.

81. Bennett ST, Lucassen AM, Gough SC et al. Susceptibility to human type 1 diabetes at IDDM2 is determined by tandem repeat variation at the insulin gene minisatellite locus. Nat Genet 1995; 9: 284–92.

82. Undlien DE, Bennett ST, Todd JA et al. Insulin gene region-encoded susceptibility to IDDM maps upstream of the insulin gene. Diabetes 1995; 44: 620–5.

83. Doria A, Lee J, Warram JH, Krolewski AS. Diabetes susceptibility at IDDM2 cannot be positively mapped to the VNTR locus of the insulin gene. Diabetologia 1996; 39: 594–9.

84. Mijovic CH, Penny MA, Jenkins D et al. The insulin gene region and susceptibility to insulin-dependent diabetes mellitus in four races; new insights from Afro-Caribbean race-specific haplotypes. Autoimmunity 1997; 26: 11–22.

85. Pugliese A, Awdeh ZL, Alper CA et al. The paternally inherited insulin gene B allele (1,428 FokI site) confers protection from insulin-dependent diabetes in families. J Autoimmun 1994; 7: 687–94.

86. Bennett ST, Wilson AJ, Cucca F et al. IDDM2-VNTR-encoded susceptibility to type 1 diabetes: dominant protection and parental transmission of alleles of the insulin gene-linked minisatellite locus. J Autoimmun 1996; 9: 415–21.

87. Metcalfe KA, Hitman GA, Rowe RE et al. Concordance for type 1 diabetes in identical twins is affected by insulin genotype. Diabetes Care 2001; 24: 838–42.

88. Hammond-Kosack MC, Kilpatrick MW, Docherty K. Analysis of DNA structure in the human insulin gene-linked polymorphic region in vivo. J Mol Endocrinol 1992; 9: 221–5.

89. Hammond-Kosack MC, Dobrinski B, Lurz R et al. The human insulin gene linked polymorphic region exhibits an altered DNA structure. Nucleic Acids Res 1992; 20: 231–6.

90. Hammond-Kosack MC, Docherty K. A consensus repeat sequence from the human insulin gene linked polymorphic region adopts multiple quadriplex DNA structures in vitro. FEBS Lett 1992; 301: 79–82.

91. Lew A, Rutter WJ, Kennedy GC. Unusual DNA structure of the diabetes susceptibility locus IDDM2 and its effect on transcription by the insulin promoter factor Pur-1/MAZ. Proc Natl Acad Sci USA 2000; 97: 12508–12.

92. Ullrich A, Dull TJ, Gray A et al. Variation in the sequence and modification state of the human insulin gene flanking regions. Nucleic Acid Res 1982; 10: 2225–40.

93. Owerbach D, Aagaard L. Analysis of a 1963-bp polymorphic region flanking the human insulin gene. Gene 1984; 32: 475–9.

94. Rotwein P, Yokoyama S, Didier DK, Chirgwin JM. Genetic analysis of the hypervariable region flanking the human insulin gene. Hum Genet 1986; 39: 291–9.

95. Owerbach D, Gabbay KH. The search for IDDM susceptibility genes. Diabetes 1996; 45: 544–51.

96. Stead JD, Jeffreys AJ. Allele diversity and germline mutation at the insulin minisatellite. Hum Mol Genet 2000; 9: 713–23.

97. Stead JD, Buard J, Todd JA, Jeffreys AJ. Influence of allele lineage on the role of the insulin minisatellite in susceptibility to type 1 diabetes. Hum Mol Genet 2000; 9: 2929–35.

98. Vafiadis P, Bennett ST, Colle E et al. Imprinted and genotype-specific expression of genes at the IDDM2 locus in pancreas and leucocytes. J Autoimmun 1996; 9: 397–403.

99. Jolicouer C, Hanahan D, Smith KM. T-cell tolerance toward a transgenic beta-cell antigen and transcription of endogenous pancreatic genes in thymus. Proc Natl Acad Sci USA 1994; 91: 6707–11.

100. Heath VL, Moore NC, Parnell SM, Mason DW. Intrathymic expression of genes involved in organ specific autoimmune disease. J Autoimmun 1998; 11: 309–18.

101. Sospedra M, Ferrer-Francesch X, Dominguez O et al. Transcription of a broad range of self-antigens in human thymus suggests a role for central mechanisms in tolerance toward peripheral antigens. J Immunol 1998; 161: 5918–29.

102. Pugliese A, Brown D, Garza D et al. Self-antigen presenting cells expressing IDDM-associated autoantigens exist in both thymus and peripheral lymphoid organs in humans. J Clin Invest 2001; 107: 585–93.

103. Werdelin O, Cordes U, Jensen T. Aberrant expression of tissue-specific proteins in the thymus: a hypothesis for the development of central tolerance. Scand J Immunol 1998; 47: 95–100.

104. Derbinski J, Schulte A, Kyewski B, Klein L. Promiscuous gene expression in medullary thymic epithelial cells mirrors the peripheral self. Nat Immunol 2001; 2: 1032–9.

105. Heath WR, Allison J, Hoffmann MW et al. Autoimmune diabetes as a consequence of locally produced interleukin-2. Nature 1992; 359: 547–9.

106. Ashton-Rickardt PG, Bandeira A, Delaney JR et al. Evidence for a differential avidity model of T cell selection in the thymus. Cell 1994; 76: 651–63.

107. Sebzda E, Wallace VA, Mayer J et al. Positive and negative thymocyte selection induced by different concentrations of a single peptide. Science 1994; 263: 1615–18.

108. Oehen SU, Ohashi PS, Burki K et al. Escape of thymocytes and mature T cells from clonal deletion due to limiting tolerogen expression levels. Cell Immunol 1994; 158: 342–52.

109. Sprent J, Webb SR. Intrathymic and extrathymic clonal deletion of T cells. Curr Opin Immunol 1995; 7: 196–205.

110. Liblau RS, Tisch R, Shokat K et al. Intravenous injection of soluble antigen induces thymic and peripheral T-cells apoptosis. Proc Natl Acad Sci USA 1996; 93: 3031–6.

111. Smith KM, Olson DC, Hirose R, Hanahan D. Pancreatic gene expression in rare cells of thymic medulla: evidence for functional contribution to T cell tolerance. Int Immunol 1997; 9: 1355–65.

112. Hanahan D. Peripheral-antigen-expressing cells in thymic medulla: factors in self-tolerance and autoimmunity. Curr Opin Immunol 1998; 10: 656–62.

113. Klein L, Kyewski B. 'Promiscuous' expression of tissue antigens in the thymus: a key to T-cell tolerance and autoimmunity? J Mol Med 2000; 78: 483–94.

114. Kishimoto H, Sprent J. A defect in central tolerance in NOD mice. Nat Immunol 2001; 2: 1025–31.

115. Chentoufi AA, Polychronakos C. Insulin expression levels in the thymus modulate insulin-specific autoreactive T-cell tolerance: the mechanism by which the IDDM2 locus may predispose to diabetes. Diabetes 2002; 51: 1383–90.

116. French MB, Allison J, Cram DS et al. Transgenic expression of mouse proinsulin II prevents diabetes in nonobese diabetic mice. Diabetes 1997; 46: 34–9.

117. Alleva DG, Crowe PD, Jin L et al. A disease-associated cellular immune response in type 1 diabetics to an immunodominant epitope of insulin. J Clin Invest 2001; 107: 173–80.

118. Kuglin B, Gries FA, Kolb H. Evidence of IgG autoantibodies against human proinsulin in patients with IDDM before insulin treatment. Diabetes 1988; 37: 130–2.

119. Castano L, Ziegler AG, Ziegler R et al. Characterization of insulin autoantibodies in relatives of patients with type I diabetes. Diabetes 1993; 42: 1202–9.

120. Keilacker H, Rjasanowski I, Besch W, Kohnert

KD. Autoantibodies to insulin and to proinsulin in type 1 diabetic patients and in at-risk probands differentiate only little between both antigens. Horm Metab Res 1995; 27: 90–4.

121. Chen W, Bergerot I, Elliott JF et al. Evidence that a peptide spanning the B-C junction of proinsulin is an early autoantigen epitope in the pathogenesis of type 1 diabetes. J Immunol 2001; 167: 4926–35.

122. Throsby M, Homo-Delarche F, Chevenne D et al. Pancreatic hormone expression in the murine thymus: localization in dendritic cells and macrophages. Endocrinology 1998; 139: 2399–406.

123. Pugliese A. Peripheral antigen-expressing cells and autoimmunity. Endocrinol Metab Clin North Am 2002; 31: 411–30, viii.

124. Nistico L, Buzzetti R, Pritchard LE et al. The CTLA-4 gene region of chromosome 2q33 is linked to, and associated with, type 1 diabetes. Belgian Diabetes Registry. Hum Mol Genet 1996; 5: 1075–80.

125. Marron MP, Zeidler A, Raffel LJ et al. Genetic and physical mapping of a type 1 diabetes susceptibility gene (IDDM12) to a 100-kb phagemid artificial chromosome clone containing D2S72-CTLA4-D2S105 on chromosome 2q33. Diabetes 2000; 49: 492–9.

126. Marron MP, Raffel LJ, Garchon HJ et al. Insulin-dependent diabetes mellitus (IDDM) is associated with CTLA4 polymorphisms in multiple ethnic groups. Hum Mol Genet 1997; 6: 1275–82.

127. Awata T, Kurihara S, Iitaka M et al. Association of CTLA-4 gene A-G polymorphism (IDDM12 locus) with acute- onset and insulin-depleted IDDM as well as autoimmune thyroid disease (Graves' disease and Hashimoto's thyroiditis) in the Japanese population. Diabetes 1998; 47: 128–9.

128. Hayashi H, Kusaka I, Nagasaka S et al. Association of CTLA-4 polymorphism with positive anti-GAD antibody in Japanese subjects with type 1 diabetes mellitus. Clin Endocrinol (Oxf.) 1999; 51: 793–9.

129. Esposito L, Hill NJ, Pritchard LE et al. Genetic analysis of chromosome 2 in type 1 diabetes: analysis of putative loci IDDM7, IDDM12, and IDDM13 and candidate genes NRAMP1 and IA-2 and the interleukin-1 gene

cluster. IMDIAB Group. Diabetes 1998; 47: 1797–9.

130. Luo DF, Buzzetti R, Rotter JI et al. Confirmation of three susceptibility genes to insulin-dependent diabetes mellitus: IDDM4, IDDM5 and IDDM8. Hum Mol Genet 1996; 5: 693–8.

131. Davies JL, Kawaguchu Y, Bennett ST et al. A genome-wide search for human type 1 diabetes susceptibility genes. Nature 1994; 371: 130–6.

132. Buhler J, Owerbach D, Schaffer AA et al. Linkage analyses in type I diabetes mellitus using CASPAR, a software and statistical program for conditional analysis of polygenic diseases. Hum Hered 1997; 47: 211–22.

133. Davies JL, Cucca F, Goy JV et al. Saturation multipoint linkage mapping of chromosome 6q in type 1 diabetes. Hum Mol Genet 1996; 5: 1071–4.

134. Delepine M, Pociot F, Habita C et al. Evidence of a non-MHC susceptibility locus in type I diabetes linked to HLA on chromosome 6. Am J Hum Genet 1997; 60: 174–87.

135. Perez dN, Bilbao JR, Calvo B, Castano L. Analysis of chromosome 6q in Basque families with type 1 diabetes. GEPV-N. Basque-Navarre Endocrinology and Paediatric Group. Autoimmunity 2000; 33: 33–6.

136. Copeman JB, Cucca F, Hearne CM et al. Linkage disequilibrium mapping of a type 1 diabetes susceptibility gene (IDDM7) to chromosome 2q31-q33. Nat Genet 1995; 9: 80–5.

137. Kristiansen OP, Pociot F, Bennett EP et al. IDDM7 links to insulin-dependent diabetes mellitus in Danish multiplex families but linkage is not explained by novel polymorphisms in the candidate gene GALNT3. The Danish Study Group of Diabetes in Childhood and The Danish IDDM Epidemiology and Genetics Group. Hum Mutat 2000; 15: 295–6.

138. Owerbach D, Gabbay KH. The HOXD8 locus (2q31) is linked to type I diabetes. Interaction with chromosome 6 and 11 disease susceptibility genes. Diabetes 1995; 44: 132–6.

139. Iwata I, Nagafuchi S, Nakashima H et al. Association of polymorphism in the NeuroD/BETA2 gene with type 1 diabetes in the Japanese. Diabetes 1999; 48: 416–19.

140. Hansen L, Jensen JN, Urioste S et al. NeuroD/BETA2 gene variability and diabetes: no associations to late-onset type 2 diabetes but an A45 allele may represent a susceptibility marker for type 1 diabetes among Danes. Danish Study Group of Diabetes in Childhood, and the Danish IDDM Epidemiology and Genetics Group. Diabetes 2000; 49: 876–8.

141. Dupont S, Dina C, Hani EH, Froguel P. Absence of replication in the French population of the association between beta 2/NEUROD-A45T polymorphism and type 1 diabetes. Diabetes Metab 1999; 25: 516–7.

142. Dupont S, Vionnet N, Chevre JC et al. No evidence of linkage or diabetes-associated mutations in the transcription factors BETA2/NEUROD1 and PAX4 in Type II diabetes in France. Diabetologia 1999; 42: 480–4.

143. Field LL, Tobias R, Thomson G, Plon S. Susceptibility to insulin-dependent diabetes mellitus maps to a locus (IDDM11) on human chromosome 14q24.3-q31. Genomics 1996; 33: 1–8.

144. Heron L, Virsolvy A, Apiou F et al. Isolation, characterization, and chromosomal localization of the human ENSA gene that encodes alpha-endosulfine, a regulator of beta-cell K(ATP) channels. Diabetes 1999; 48: 1873–6.

145. Harada Y, Ozaki K, Suzuki M et al. Complete cDNA sequence and genomic organization of a human pancreas-specific gene homologous to *Caenorhabditis elegans* sel-1. J Hum Genet 1999; 44: 330–6.

146. Apelqvist A, Li H, Sommer L et al. Notch signalling controls pancreatic cell differentiation. Nature 1999; 400: 877–81.

147. Pociot F, Larsen ZM, Zavattari P et al. No evidence for SEL1L as a candidate gene for IDDM11-conferred susceptibility. Diabetes Metab Res Rev 17: 292–5.

148. Morahan G, Huang D, Ymer SI et al. Linkage disequilibrium of a type 1 diabetes susceptibility locus with a regulatory IL12B allele. Nat Genet 2001; 27: 218–21.

149. Dahlman I, Eaves IA, Kosoy R et al. Parameters for reliable results in genetic association studies in common disease. Nat Genet 2002; 30: 149–50.

150. Warram JH, Krolewski AS, Gottlieb MS, Kahn CR. Differences in risk of insulin-dependent diabetes in offspring of diabetic mothers and diabetic fathers. N Engl J Med 1984; 311: 149–52.

151. Vadheim CM, Rotter JI, Maclaren NK et al. Preferential transmission of diabetic alleles within the HLA gene complex. N Engl J Med 1986; 315: 1314–18.

152. Deschamps I, Hors J, Clerget-Darpoux F et al. Excess of maternal HLA-DR3 antigens in HLA DR3,4 positive type 1 (insulin-dependent) diabetic patients. Diabetologia 1990; 33: 425–39.

153. Bain SC, Rowe BR, Barnett AHTJA. Parental origin of diabetes-associated HLA types in sibling pairs with type I diabetes. Diabetes 1994; 43: 1462–8.

154. Paterson AD, Naimark DM, Petronis A. The analysis of parental origin of alleles may detect susceptibility loci for complex disorders. Hum Hered 1999; 49: 197–204.

155. Polychronakos C, Kukuvitis A, Giannoukakis N, Colle E. Parental imprinting effect at the INS-IGF2 diabetes susceptibility locus. Diabetologia 1995; 38: 715–19.

156. Bui MM, Luo DF, She JY et al. Paternally transmitted IDDM2 influences diabetes susceptibility despite biallelic expression of the insulin gene in human pancreas. J Autoimmun 1996; 9: 97–103.

157. Hoffman AR, Vu TH. Genomic imprinting. Scientific American 1996; 1: 52–61.

158. Giddings SJ, King CD, Harman KW et al. Allele specific inactivation of insulin 1 and 2, in the mouse yolk, indicates imprinting. Nat Genet 1994; 6: 310–13.

159. Polychronakos C, Vafiadis P, Giannoukakis N, Colle E. Imprinting and genotype-dependent gene expression at the IDDM2 locus in pancreas and lymphocytes. Autoimmunity 1995; 21: 16–17.

160. Miceli D, Zeller M, Brown D et al. Insulin gene expression and imprinting in pancreas and lymphoid organs. Diabetes 1999; 48 Suppl. 1: A190 (Abstract)

161. Pugliese A, Miceli D. The insulin gene in diabetes. Diabetes Metab Res Rev 2002; 18: 13–25.

162. Moore GE, Abu-Amero SN, Bell G et al.

Evidence that insulin is imprinted in the human yolk sac. Diabetes 2001; 50: 199–203.

163. Deltour L, Montagutelli X, Guenet JL et al. Tissue- and developmental stage-specific imprinting of the mouse proinsulin gene, Ins2. Develop Biol 1995; 168: 686–8.

164. Vafiadis P, Ounissi-Benkalha H, Palumbo M et al. Class III alleles of the variable number of tandem repeat insulin polymorphism associated with silencing of thymic insulin predispose to type 1 diabetes. J Clin Endocrinol Metab 2001; 86: 3705–10.

165. Bennett S T, Wilson AJ, Esposito L et al. Insulin VNTR allele-specific effect in type 1 diabetes depends on identity of untrasmitted paternal allele. Nat Genet 1997; 17: 350–2.

166. Urrutia I, Calvo B, Bilbao JR, Castano L. Anomalous behaviour of the 5' insulin gene polymorphism allele 814: lack of association with Type I diabetes in Basques. GEPV-N Group. Basque-Navarre Endocrinology and Paediatrics. Diabetologia 1998; 41: 1121–3.

167. Hollick JB, Dorweiler JE, Chandler VL. Paramutation and related allelic interactions. Trends Genet 1997; 13: 302–8.

168. Duvillie' B, Bucchini D, Tang T et al. Imprinting at the mouse Ins2 locus: evidence for cis- and trans-allelic interactions. Genomics 1998; 47: 52–7.

169. LaSalle JM, Lalande M. Homologous association of oppositely imprinted chromosomal domains. Science 1996; 272: 725–8.

170. Black DL. Protein diversity from alternative splicing: a challenge for bioinformatics and post-genome biology. Cell 2000; 103: 367–70.

171. Diez J, Park Y, Zeller M et al. Differential splicing of the IA-2 mRNA in pancreas and lymphoid organs as a permissive genetic mechanism for autoimmunity against the IA-2 type 1 diabetes autoantigen. Diabetes 2001; 50: 895–900.

172. Klein L, Klugmann M, Nave KA, Kyewski B. Shaping of the autoreactive T-cell repertoire by a splice variant of self protein expressed in thymic epithelial cells. Nat Med 2000; 6: 56–61.

173. Solimena M, Dirkx RJ, Hermel JM et al. ICA 512, an autoantigen of type I diabetes, is an intrinsic membrane protein of neurosecretory granules. EMBO J 1996; 15: 2102–14.

174. Peakman M, Stevens EJ, Lohmann T et al. Naturally processed and presented epitopes of the islet cell autoantigen IA-2 eluted from HLA-DR4. J Clin Invest 1999; 104: 1449–57.

3

Genetics of Type 2 diabetes mellitus: current progress and future directions

Paul G Cassell, Graham A Hitman

Epidemiological evidence for a genetic component in T2DM

The first evidence alluding to the possibility of a genetic component in the inter-generational transmission of Type 2 diabetes mellitus (T2DM) was derived from the demonstration of familial correlation in a number of diverse ethnic groups. In particular, families with a T2DM proband have an increased prevalence of disease in their siblings, parents and offspring compared to the population; similarly there is an increased prevalence of diabetes in offspring depending on the parental family history of diabetes.[1–4] Observations in the Pima Indians suggested that an even greater risk to disease was conferred to offspring if the parental diabetic history was maternal in origin, or if either parent had an early onset of disease.[4] Based on findings from the San Antonio Family Diabetes Study it was deduced that there is a varying degree of risk within families and this was dependent on relative kinship with the diabetic proband. First-degree relatives were found to have almost double the population risk.[5]

Epidemiological studies in twin studies have also been exploited to support the paradigm that T2DM has a genetic component. Twin studies theoretically allow for the separation of the genetic component of variance, since monozygotic (MZ) twins share 100% of their genes, whilst non-identical dizygotic twins (DZ) only share half on average. Hence, discordance in the rates of diabetes between MZ twins and DZ twins, with MZ twins having consistently greater concordance rates, can be interpreted as evidence that the disease has a genetic basis, under the assumption that they have been subjected to the same shared environment. Concordance rates in European populations have been recorded between 28.6–34% and 14.3–16% for MZ and DZ twins respectively.[6,7] Studies incorporating follow-ups of 10 and 15 years found the concordance rates elevating to 58% and 76%.[6,8] Two recent studies in Danish and British subjects found that in addition to discordance between MZ and DZ, concordance rates within twins was higher when measurements of glucose tolerance were considered rather than overt diabetes.[8,9] Based on these findings, Poulsen et al.[9] postulated that a genetic predisposition was more important for the development of abnormal glucose tolerance, whereas non-genetic factors predominate in controlling whether a genetically predisposed individual progresses to overt T2DM. However, evidence for a genetic component from these epidemiological studies is mainly conjecture. A true unbiased estimate of heritability (both additive and non-additive combined) could only be achieved if the MZ twins are reared separately, and studies of this kind are rare. Moreover, the inferred genetic component in some of these studies could be inflated due to non-additive genetic effects with also the possibility that a non-genetic mode of disease transmission underlies some if not 'all' the differences in concordance rates.[10]

Further support for a genetic mode of transmission is drawn from the substantial differences in disease prevalence often present in distinct ethnic groups under similar environmental burdens. This is particularly evident in the different racial groups within the USA, with progressive admixture into communities through migration affecting relative risk to disease.[11] Admixed populations comprising of two ethnic groups, one at high risk to T2DM, such as Native American Indians and another at relatively low disease risk such as Caucasians, can generate an intermediate disease rate status.[4,12] Under these circumstances it is hypothesized that the high risk ethnic group have a higher frequency of disease susceptibility genes and the rate of disease in the admixed population is proportional to the percentage of the gene pool derived from this ethnic population. For instance, in full-blooded Nauruans of Micronesia the prevalence of diabetes after the age of 60 years is 83%, whereas it is only 17% in those inhabitants who have a Caucasian ancestral gene admixture.[13]

Mode of inheritance-transmission

The heterogeneity of the T2DM both at phenotypic and pathophysiological levels almost certainly indicates that the genetic component is likely to be heterogeneous with no single locus accounting for the disease. However, the manifestation of the 'common' idiopathic T2DM phenotype is likely to be the result of an interaction of diverse environmental factors on this background of heterogeneous genetic predisposition. The complexity and mechanisms involved in the gene-environment interaction and the mode of inheritance of T2DM is still largely unknown.

A variety of genetic models have been proposed using segregation analyses. In the high T2DM prevalence groups of the Nauruans,[14] Pima Indians[15] and Mexican-Americans[16] modelling has provided evidence for a major T2DM susceptibility gene inherited either as an autosomal dominant or a co-dominant. In other studies in lower prevalence groups either an oligogenic or a combination of an oligogenic model superimposed on a polygenic background has been proposed.[17–19] However, Risch[20] has suggested that these conclusions reflect a geneticist's preference for a oligogenic/multigenic model, as it has a tractable degree of complexity. Complex disease models that have infinite genetic complexity, resulting from numerous effector genes, but each only contributing a modest effect, could represent a monumental task in the identification of susceptibility loci.

Complex diseases are difficult to model with problems in estimating penetrance values, phenocopy rates and allele frequency of the disease mutation. The genetic architecture of diabetes could be further complicated by the contribution of multi-allelic and non-additive dominance effects within loci, and additive, multiplicative and epistasis interactions between loci. It is also likely that different modes of transmission are present in discrete families, with different loci interacting within the same family, so no one overall model of transmission may be an appropriate mode of inheritance. Hence complex diseases are defined as being 'non-Mendelian'. However, this does not obviate the fact that underlying individual susceptibility loci with either major or minor biological effects may be transmitted in a Mendelian manner.

Thrifty genotype versus thrifty phenotype

Despite the strong genetic component of T2DM, of equal importance is the environmental component. Whereas differences in disease prevalence between populations could be the culmination of differences in their complement of susceptibility genes, the rapid and recent global increase in prevalence of T2DM cannot be attributed to a rapidly changing human genome. Previously, in ethnic groups such as the Nauruans, the Pima Indians of Arizona and Western Samoans, T2DM was virtually unknown, and yet in the last 50 years the prevalence of T2DM has dramatically increased to over 30%.[21,22] The 'thrifty genotype' hypothesis proposed by Neel[23] endeavours to explain the increase in prevalence in these populations as a result of Westernization affecting the interaction of both genes and environment. In the last 6–7 million years, humans, committed to their evolutionary survival, would have selected genes as a result of adaptation to a hunter-gatherer existence. Genes responsible for the development of advantageous physiological mechanisms would allow the accumulation of energy stores when food is abundant so as to prevent depletion of body energy stores during periods of starvation or limited/seasonal food resources. A change from this lifestyle to one with a continual and abundant supply of high energy density food unaffected by seasonal availability, combined with improvements in health, hygiene and dietary intake, in human evolutionary terms has been extremely recent. The 'thrifty genotype' favours mechanisms that promote high efficiency in the storage of energy as fat and glycogen, yet under the recent major

shift in human habits these genes could now have deleterious effects. These effects are particularly evident when populations in developing countries migrate and become urbanized.[21,22,24–28] Epidemiological evidence strongly supports a relationship between T2DM and obesity. The WHO in 1980 (WHO expert committee, 1980) cited obesity as the most important risk factor in the development of T2DM, with this association transcending ethnicity, differences in measurements of adiposity and criteria for diagnosis of T2DM.[29] The limited capacity of an individual or an ethnic group to adjust to these recent changes is also likely to be determined by genetic factors.[13,22] This is reflected in the fact that weight gain leading to obesity is also determined by an interaction of genetic and environmental components, some possibly the same as for diabetes.

However, the 'thrifty genotype' concept is considered contentious in some quarters, with another hypothesis being that the transmission of diabetes to subsequent generations is the result of a 'thrifty phenotype'.[10] Studies in rodents and humans show that the development of a fetus in an abnormal intrauterine environment can have major consequences on the metabolism of the offspring in later life, including the possible development of diabetes.[30–32] Furthermore, the offspring themselves later in adulthood can also develop abnormal intrauterine environments during gestation, providing a means of transmission of a diabetogenic effect to subsequent generations without genetic interference[33,34]. In a Danish twin study, the diabetic co-sibling within both discordant MZ and DZ twins had a lower birthweight compared to their unaffected co-sibling providing further evidence that the development of diabetes could occur independently of a genetic cause.[35] The increased concordance rates observed in MZ twins could be attributable to differences in the intrauterine environment, as MZ twins more frequently share a chorion and amnion than DZ twins.[36]

However it is also debatable whether the individual phenotypic outcome of these epigenetic effects is not also the result of an interaction with genotype. Half of fetal birthweight variation is due to the genotype of the fetus, with 20% related to the parental genome. One alternative explanation for the 'fetal programming' observations is that genetically predetermined dysfunctional insulin secretion and insulin resistance results in impaired insulin-mediated growth in the fetus as well as insulin resistance and diabetes in adult life.[37] Insulin secreted by the fetal pancreas in response to maternal glucose concentrations is a key growth factor. Monogenic diabetic syndromes due to defects in either decreased beta cell function or defects in insulin action are also associated with impaired fetal growth.[37] Single gene defects that have been shown to affect fetal growth detrimentally include insulin growth factors (*IGF*) I and II genes, glucokinase (*GCK*), *IGFI* receptor gene, and insulin gene 5' VNTR.[38–41]

Genetic evidence for an inherited susceptibility

The plausibility of a genetic contribution to T2DM is further strengthened through the study of animal models and human monogenic syndromes of T2DM.

Animal models

Animal models can be found that support all possible proposed aetiologies of diabetes from entirely environmental to wholly genetic and multifactorial in origin. Amongst the genetic models monogenic and polygenic models are represented. However, the manifestation of different phenotypes between strains of the same species and between species with the same gene defects emphasizes the complexity of the physiological processes involved.

The study of monogenic models of diabetes potentially enables the uncovering of novel metabolic pathways in the disease pathogenesis. One example of this is displayed by the *ob/ob* mouse, which develops both massive obesity and T2DM. The gene defect is a mutation in the *ob* gene leading to leptin deficiency, a hormone that hitherto had not been known until the work on the *ob/ob* mouse.[42] This quickly led to the discovery of the leptin receptor and host of post-receptor signalling pathways involved in feeding behaviour, energy expenditure and fertility. Furthermore, if the *ob/ob* mouse is treated with leptin from a young age then not only does the animal not develop obesity but also it does not develop diabetes. Thus the knowledge that has followed the discovery of the genetic basis of one animal model has suggested a number of different possible therapeutic approaches to the prevention of obesity and subsequent diabetes.

Many groups are concentrating on polygenic models of diabetes since they are more likely to be applicable to man. The foremost studied model is that of the Goto-Kakizaki (GK) rat.[43,44] At least seven loci controlling diabetes-related sub-phenotypes have been identified in the GK rat. Moreover, one locus, the *GK2*, is found in the syntenic region on human chromosome 1 in which linkage with T2DM has been found in several genome scans (Table 3.2).

Monogenic syndromes of T2DM in man

In humans, a substantial part of the knowledge of the genetic component of diabetes has been based on relatively uncommon early age onset of diabetic conditions that result from single

MODY sub-group	Gene	Chromosome	MODY frequency
MODY1	HNF4α (TCF1)	20q	Rare
MODY2	GCK	7p	10–65%
MODY3	HNF1α	12q	20–75%
MODY4	IPF1	13q	Rare
MODY5	HNF1β (TCF2)	17q	Very rare
MODY6	NeuroD/Beta2	2q32	Rare–unknown

Table 3.1

Sub-genotypes of maturity onset diabetes of young (MODY)

gene defects. Presently, there are two main sub-groups of monogenic diabetes: firstly, maturity onset diabetes of the young (MODY) in which diabetes primarily occurs as result of β-cell dysfunction[45–48] and secondly a sub-group which is defined by mutations occurring in the mitochondrial genome.[49,50]

Maturity onset diabetes of young (MODY)

MODY is clinically defined as having an age of onset before the age of 25 years in at least two family members with an autosomal dominant mode of inheritance.[48] MODY accounts for approximately 2–5% of T2DM in Caucasians and mutations have been identified in five or six different genes so far (Table 3.1). These genes are mainly transcription factors, particularly from the hepatocyte nuclear factor (HNF) family of genes. The search for MODY genes has encompassed many of the different approaches used to find genes in T2DM, including a candidate gene approach (glucokinase), genome search (hepatic nuclear factor 1α) and subsequent knowledge of the biochemical pathway (hepatic nuclear factors 1β and 4α). The two most common genes with mutations that lead to MODY are glucokinase (GCK) and hepatic nuclear factor (HNF)1α and both lead to clinically distinct syndromes.[51] Thus patients harbouring HNF1α mutations resemble lean subjects with Type 2 diabetes, but with advancing adiposity increasing the severity of the hyperglycaemia. There is also a progressive pancreatic β-cell failure over time with the eventual requirement for oral hypoglycaemic agents or insulin, and in addition there are frequently microangiopathic complications of the diabetes. In contrast, patients with GCK mutations have 'mild diabetes' in its truest sense. Although there is a gradual deterioration of β-cell function over time, it mirrors that of a non-diabetic. The diabetes is commonly treated with diet and indeed is frequently an incidental diagnosis found at health or family screening, or it presents with gestational diabetes. Furthermore, patients with GCK mutations are unlikely to develop the complications of diabetes. The differentiation of these two types of diabetes is therefore important as patients with GCK mutations do not require as intensive monitoring as those with HNF1α mutations or T2DM and these patients can be reassured that they are unlikely to require insulin treatment in the future nor will they develop the vascular complications of diabetes. A third distinct MODY clinical syndrome (although rare) can also be differentiated by molecular diagnosis of patients with MODY. Patients with HNF1β mutations in addition to diabetes also have renal cysts and are at risk of renal failure.[52]

It has also been proposed that mutations in the MODY genes might also predispose to late onset diabetes. Homozygous mutations of the insulin promoter factor 1 gene (*IPF1*) give rise to the MODY4 phenotype, however, in contrast subjects that are heterozygous for certain variants appear to be more predisposed to the late onset form of T2DM.[48,53,54] A similar effect also occurs with the basic helix-loop-helix transcription factor, neurogenic differen-tiation 1 (NeuroD1/Beta2-MODY6), involved in pancreatic endocrine cell differentiation and the tissue-specific regulation of the insulin gene.[55,56] One variant (residue 206+C) that generates a truncated polypeptide lacking the C-terminal transactivation domain, a region that associates with the two co-activators, CBP and p300, produces a more severe clinical profile in patients that is reminiscent of MODY. In contrast, compound heterozygosity for both this variant and a second missense variant (Arg111Leu) that disrupts the DNA-binding domain and abolishes the E-box-binding activity of NeuroD1 associates with the development of T2DM.[57] However, similar observations have not been found with the other MODY genes, with mutations in the genes for *HNF4α*, glucokinase (*GCK*), *HNF1α*, and *HNF1β* not implicated in polygenic T2DM in any ethnic population so far studied.[58] However, studies so far only rule out coding mutations of these genes and it might be that regulatory variants of some of the MODY genes may be important in the pathogenesis of T2DM.

Maternally inherited diabetes and deafness (MIDD)

MIDD is also another early onset form of T2DM, frequently characterized by progressive β-cell degeneration and deafness. Variants within the mitochondrial genome are associ-ated with the disruption of oxidative phospho-rylation processes consequently affecting intracellular calcium levels and exocytosis of insulin granules by depolarization of the cell membrane. Mitochondrial DNA (mtDNA) is only maternally inherited because the sperm contributes almost no cytoplasm to the zygote.[59] Consequently mtDNA-associated diseases have a maternal dominant inheritance pattern with variable penetrance and clinical phenotypes due to heteroplasmy. The most prevalent characterized mutation is at position 3243 tRNA (Leu, UUR).[60] This mutation is impli-cated in several disease phenotypes including the neurological disorder MELAS mitochon-drial syndrome (myopathy, encephalopathy, lactic acidosis and stroke-like episodes), and both chronic progressive external ophthalmo-gepia (CPEO) and Kearns-Sayre syndrome (KSS).[61] However, the 3243 mutation although it has a frequency of 1–3% in French and Japanese subjects with family histories of diabetes, it is relatively rare in other popula-tions with a frequency of 0.1–0.2% in British Caucasian T2DM patients and is virtually absent in South Indians.[62–64]

The hunt for genes contributing to T2DM of multifactorial origin

The identification of genes responsible for human monogenic diabetes and genetic studies in animal model studies has advanced our knowledge of the underlying physiology involved in the pathogenesis of diabetes. However, neither approach has currently culminated in the identification of any common genes that predispose to polygenic T2DM in man. A number of strategies have been employed to identify disease susceptibility loci, although they are essentially based on two statistical approaches. The first approach is based on pedigree methods and involves either the application of classical linkage analysis

Ethnic population	Chromosomal region	Reference	Linkage
Mormon Caucasian USA	1q21–23	Elbein 1999[79]	N
French Caucasian	1q21–24	Vionnet 2000[132]	N
UK Caucasian	1q24.2	Wiltshire 2001[78]	N
Pima Indian	1q25.3	Hanson 1998[133]	S
Indigenous Australian	2q24.3	Busfield 2002[80]	S
Mexican-American	2q37 (*NIDDM1*)	Hanis 1996[84]	S
French Caucasian	2q37	Hani 1997[134]	N
Mexican-American	3q27	Ehm 2000[81]	S
French Caucasian	3q27	Vionnet 2000[132]	S
Ashkenazi Jews	4q	Permutt 2001[135]	N
Botnian Finnish	4q32–q33	Lindgren 2002[136]	N
USA European	5q13	Ehm 2000[81]	N
UK Caucasian	5q13	Wiltshire 2001[78]	N
UK Caucasian	5q32	Wiltshire 2001[78]	N
French Caucasian	5q31–33	Vionnet 2000[132]	N
UK Caucasian	8p21.3–22	Wiltshire 2001[78]	S
Mormon Caucasian USA	8p21.3	Elbein 1999[79]	N
Indigenous Australian	8p22	Busfield 2002[80]	N
Botnian Finnish	9p13–q21	Lindgren 2002[136]	S
UK Caucasian	10q23.3	Wiltshire 2001[78]	N
Finnish (FUSION)	10q23.33–24.32	Ghosh 2000[137]	S
French Caucasian	10q26.3	Vionnet 2000[132]	N
Mexican-American	10q26.12	Duggirala 1999[130]	N
Mexican American	11p15.4	Stern 1996[139]	S
Pima Indian	11q22–23	Hanson 1998[133]	N
Caucasian	12q15	Bektas 1999[140]	S
USA European	12q15	Ehm 2000[81]	N
Botnian Finnish	12q24 (*NIDDM2*)	Mahtani 1996[141]	S
Botnian Finnish	12q24	Bowden 1997[142]	N
Australian	12q24	Shaw 1998[72]	S
USA White	12q24	Ehm 2000[81]	N
USA European	12q24	Lindgren 2002[136]	N
Finnish (FUSION)	20p12	Ghosh 2000[137]	N
USA European	20q12–13 (*NIDDM3*)	Bowden 1997[142]	N
USA European	20q12–13	Ji 1997[143]	S
Finnish	20q12–13	Ghosh 2000[137]	S
USA European	20q12–13	Zouali 1997[144]	N
Mormon Caucasian	20q12–13	Elbein 1995[145]	N
French Caucasian	20q12–13	Hani 1997[134]	N
Ashkenazi Jews	20q12–13	Permutt 2001[135]	N
USA European	20q13.1–13.2	Klupa 2000[146]	S

Notes: Regions included either have suggestive linkage, replicated nominal evidence of linkage, or had maximum evidence for linkage within the given study. S = LOD (or equivalent) > 3.0; N = LOD (or equivalent) > 1.0

Table 3.2
Autosomal chromosome regions with evidence of linkage for T2DM susceptibility genes

using recombination information or a non-parametric linkage method in affected sibling pairs (ASP). Alternatively strategies have also been used in both families and population samples that utilize the phenomenon of genetic linkage disequilibrium.

Genome searches and T2DM

Whilst there have been remarkable successes in identifying mutations in genes that lead to monogenic diseases, cystic fibrosis, familial polyposis, BBS6 and MODY, to name but a few, there has been limited success in multifactorial disease.[48,65–67] Linkage analysis in monogenic disease requires the specification of various aspects of the disease model. In complex disorders individual families may have several different modes of transmission operative. Moreover, the late age of onset of T2DM and the increased disease-related mortality hampers the collection of typical large multigeneration pedigrees.[68] Furthermore, patients with younger onset of T2DM have a large proportion (83%) of both parents affected and are therefore less informative.[69] To overcome some of these limitations a model-free non-parametric linkage analysis approach using affected sibling pairs has now been widely used in the search for diabetogenic genes. However, this method is also disadvantaged in that large numbers of ASPs are required to achieve sufficient power to detect disease loci. Currently, in excess of 20 genome scans for T2DM have been performed on both ASP sets and extended families. They are showing an emerging pattern of evidence of linkage in the human genome, although studies are predominantly in Caucasian–European ethnic populations (Table 3.2).

The limitation of most linkage-based methods stems from a reduced power to detect genes under many polygenic models of disease.

Disappointingly no scans for T2DM have found an equivalent genetic effect similar to that of the HLA in T1DM. Nonetheless, at least one genome scan has been taken to completion with the identification of the calpain-10 gene (*CAPN10*) as a major susceptibility gene in Mexican-Americans.[70] Genome scans in a variety of populations have identified several regions demonstrating excess allele sharing (Table 3.2), many of which, despite individual low levels of linkage (LOD ~1.5), are replicated between ethnic groups. Some of the peaks contain previously studied candidate genes; for instance *HNF4α* (MODY1) to 20q12–13, *HNF1α* to 12q24 and sulphonylurea receptor-1 (*SUR-1*) to 11p15.

The NIDDM3 region at 20q12–13 is the most frequently replicated region, with current evidence for suggestive or nominal linkage in at least eight studies. The MODY1-*HNF4α* gene locates to this region and could be considered a most likely candidate gene. However, association studies in humans do not support a role for *HNF4α* as a common determinant of susceptibility to T2DM.[58] The *NIDDM3* interval also contains numerous other genes including the melanocortin receptor-3 gene (*MCR3*).[71] A study in French Caucasian families has identified two missense mutations in the *MCR3* gene, which were marginally associated with insulin and glucose levels during oral glucose tolerance testing in normoglycaemic subjects. However, family association studies have not supported a role for *MCR3* coding variants in T2DM or obesity.[71] Similarly for the *HNF1α*-MODY3 locus, there is significant evidence of linkage to this locus on 12q24; nonetheless sequencing of the ten exons and promoter region has not identified any causative mutations.[72]

The sulphonylurea receptor-1 (*SUR-1*) locates to 11p15.1 and has been consistently purported as a strong contender for a T2DM susceptibility locus with linkage further providing supporting evidence in several genome scans.[73,74] SUR-1 is a high affinity receptor for sulphonylureas; it is expressed on pancreatic β-cells and plays a crucial role in regulating glucose-induced insulin secretion by controlling K+-ATP channel activity of the β-cell membrane with an ATP-sensitive potassium channel Kir6.2.[75] In humans, sequence variants within the cytoplasmic domain have been shown to disrupt the regulation of insulin secretion. Furthermore, a splice variant that results in protein truncation, through the removal of the second nucleotide-binding fold, causes a rare autosomal recessive disorder familial persistent hyperinsulinaemic hypoglycaemia of infancy (PHHI).[76] Although gene variants are rare, often specific to one family, over 20 mutations have been identified in the SUR-1 gene. Homozygotes for these variants are invariably hyperinsulinaemic. In addition, another common coding variant in exon 16 appears to associate with T2DM in Dutch Caucasians but at present supporting replicate studies are lacking.[74,77]

One possibly interesting area is that on 8p22, which in one of the largest genome scans to be performed in European Caucasians, had the strongest evidence of linkage, and was the only region in this particular study that could not be excluded at a λs of 1.87.[78] Linkage has been replicated to this region in other Caucasian and indigenous Australian populations (Table 3.2). Within this interval lies the lipoprotein lipase gene (LPL).[78–80] LPL is a strong candidate gene for disorders associated with diabetes, such as cardiovascular disease and hypertriglyceridaemia and could contribute to both the complications and progression of the disease.

Other candidate genes that can be identified in chromosomal intervals that have evidence of linkage to T2DM include the protein kinase C substrate gene (PEA15) and potassium inwardly rectifying channel sub-family J member 9 gene (KCNJ9) to 1q21–24 and the insulin degrading enzyme (IDE) to 10q23–25.[78,81–83]

The calpain 10 gene story

One of the most promising candidate genes to be identified through the genome search approach is calpain 10 (CAPN10)[70] located to 2q37[84] in Mexican-Americans (MA). In the first genome scan for polygenic T2DM, one region on chromosome 2q showed the overall strongest evidence of suggestive linkage with an MLS of 4.0. Subsequent studies involving stratification according to a linkage peak on chromosome 15[85] and the analysis of several single nucleotide polymorphisms (SNPs) internal to CAPN10 identified the gene as a disease susceptibility locus.[70] A common G allele of one intronic variant (UCSNP43) was increased in both Mexican-American and Botnian Finnish diabetics. Additionally, in Finnish subjects, the uncommon allele of a second variant (UCSNP63) was also associated with disease.[70] The modest association of UCSNP43 in MAs could not alone account for the original linkage data, so haplotypes were tested with combinations of other CAPN10 gene polymorphisms. Two common haplotypes were identified both with the disease-associated G allele (allele1) of UCSNP43, and in combination with two other SNPs. These included UCSNP19 (32bp insertion/deletion), an SNP in near perfect LD with a group of four CAPN10 intronic SNPs, UCSNP56, -59, -30, and -65 and one coding mutation in exon 11, UCSNP48 (silent mutation at codon A620) and the Botnian Finnish-associated UCSNP63 variant. The greatest risk to T2DM was defined by the heterozygous haplotype 112 and 121 combination (order UCSNP43, -19, -63) and this was designated an 'at risk' to T2DM haplotype combination. This 'at risk' haplotype combination conferred an overall 2.8-fold increased risk to T2DM diabetes in MAs, and was also associated with a 2.55- and 4.97-fold increase in risk in Botnian Finns and Germans respectively.[70] These findings have also been confirmed in several other ethnic populations.[86–88] Although it is unknown whether these variants are causative or merely in LD with a causative mutation, there is some evidence to suggest that the intronic UCSNP43 may play a role in the regulation of expression of *CAPN10* or another gene located nearby.[70] The *CAPN10* gene is ubiquitously expressed in humans, including skeletal muscle, liver and pancreas, and has a complex pattern of post-trancription splicing producing at least eight transcripts (calpain 10a to 10h).[70] Studies in normoglycaemic Pima Indians revealed that homozygotes for the G allele of UCSNP43 had reduced (58%) skeletal muscle *CAPN10* mRNA levels compared to heterozygotes, although there was no association with T2DM.[89] The calpain superfamily of proteins are intracellular non-lysosomal neutral cysteine processing proteases that function by cleaving specific substrates at a limited number of sites causing the activation and inactivation of specific proteins. They are widely thought to be dependent on activation by calcium.[90–92] Calpains have been implicated in the regulation of a variety of cellular roles, including influencing intracellular signalling pathways and controlling proliferation and differentiation of preadipocytes,[93] myoblasts,[94] osteoblasts[95] and chondrocytes.[96] Studies using cysteine protease inhibitors have implicated members of the calpain family, although not specifically CAPN10, with either the promotion[97] or inhibition[98] of protein secretion depending on the cell type. Subsequent *in vitro* studies have implicated CAPN10 in influencing both insulin secretion and insulin resistance. Inhibition of all calpain protease activity results in reduced insulin-mediated glucose transport and diminished incorporation of glucose into glycogen in isolated rat muscle.[99] Calpains also appear to influence insulin-induced downregulation of insulin receptor substrate –1, a key mediator in insulin action.[100] Tissue-specific expression of at least one transcript has been observed in pancreatic islets.[70] Studies using cell permeable cysteine protease/calpain inhibitors in mouse pancreatic islets have been used to elucidate the role of calpains in glucose metabolism and secretion. However these studies have produced conflicting results with a short-term exposure (four hours) of the islets to inhibitors leading to doubling of the insulin secretory response, whereas longer exposure (48 hours) results in a major (60%) decrease.[99,101] The elevated secretion of insulin appears to be due to the accelerated exocytosis of insulin granules, and this might suggest that calpains could have a crucial role in cellular vesicle trafficking.

Linkage disequilibrium based methods

Linkage analysis has proven to be a very powerful tool in localizing disease susceptibility loci to chromosomal regions in simple mendelian disorders. However, in complex diseases linkage lacks sufficient genetic resolution as it will only succeed in identifying an aetiological variant if it contributes a moderate to large effect to disease predisposition.[102,103] This was succinctly illustrated in the positional cloning of what may be the first common T2DM susceptibility gene, *CAPN10* in Mexican-Americans.[70] The original genome scan of Hanis et al.[84] identified the NIDDM1 disease susceptibility region but was inadequate in locating the actual gene. The localization of a gene required not only information of epistatic interactions between loci[85] but also the application of linkage disequilibrium methods in those ASPs that were positive for evidence of linkage.[70] Indeed, the subsequent degree of association demonstrated with the *CAPN10* UCSNP43 variant,[70] would render all linkage studies including that of Hanis et al.[84] inadequate, in terms of power to detect the increased risk afforded to the increased frequency of G allele of UCSNP43. In this respect, Altshuler et al.[104] suggested that a population group of 100,000 affected sib pairs would have been necessary to attribute this association with the LOD score of 4.0 originally obtained.[84] Compared to linkage, linkage disequilibrium (LD) is only observable between loci that are tightly linked over short genetic distances. As a consequence, LD theoretically can provide adequate power to identify genes with relatively low sibling relative risks (<1.5) even with stringent levels of significance.[102]

Apart from the use of LD in fine mapping it has also been exploited for sometime in case–control type association studies. To establish an association with the candidate gene of interest and disease or a disease-related sub-phenotypic trait it has been common to perform case–control type studies. The underlying premise for these studies is that a marker/variant allele for a given gene may either be causative of disease or may be in linkage disequilibrium with the causative pathogenic mutation in the same gene or another gene in close proximity. Association studies of this kind investigate whether there are statistically significant differences in allele/genotype frequencies between unrelated ethnically matched unaffected (controls) and affected subjects (cases) for each variant, under the assumption that an increase in frequency in the affected group is indicative of an association with disease.

Case–control studies, however, do have certain drawbacks by commonly producing false-positive results. These anomalies are widely perceived as a result of unseen population stratification. Consequently, an additional approach using family-based association studies has become commonplace. These studies utilize family trios consisting of an affected offspring and both parents. The statistic used in these analyses is the transmission disequilibrium test (TDT), with derivation of significance values based on both linkage and association.[105,106] Power studies have also shown that the detection of linkage in complex traits by tests such as TDT has much greater power than allele sharing methods used by non-parametric linkage analysis.[102] Furthermore, the TDT test theoretically avoids the confounding effects of population stratification by using related individuals from within the families as 'pseudocontrols' that match with cases. The test, however, relies heavily on the parental genotypes being informative (heterozygous for the locus); consequently the test can be inefficient depending on the frequency of the disease allele and disease population prevalence.

We will not comprehensively discuss the many candidate genes studied in T2DM, many of which are likely to turn out to be false positives.[107,108] Indeed over 60 potential candidate genes have been examined and published and no doubt many more unpublished. Only a few have been consistent and/or involve variants that would lead to a change in function. In addition to those previously discussed earlier in this chapter, three others deserve a mention.

The peroxisome proliferator-activated receptor-γ gene (PPARγ)

One of the more interesting genes from a therapeutic point of view is that of PPARγ. Drugs that are agonists of PPARγ are currently being used to treat diabetes. A recent published study that also included a meta-analysis of other studies concluded that a Pro12Ala polymorphism of *PPARγ* is associated with a modest decreased risk of T2DM.[108] Furthermore, because the risk allele is found at such high frequency, its effect translates to a large population attributable risk (as much as 25%).

Insulin receptor substrate-1 gene

A common coding variant of *IRS-1*, Gly972Arg has been implicated in insulin resistance in both human obesity and T2DM, possibly in combination with a variant of *IRS-2* (Gly1057Asp).[109,110] Association studies of these variants have been inconsistent, suggesting that they are either not involved in development of the common form of T2DM or they are only very minor susceptibility loci.[110,111]

Insulin gene VNTR

The class 3 allele of the hypervariable region 5' (VNTR) to the gene has recently been demonstrated to be associated with T2DM, despite earlier inconsistent studies.[112] Furthermore, using family-based association methods there is a suggestion that this susceptibility is paternally transmitted. Allelic variation at the insulin gene VNTR has also been shown to be a determinant of insulin gene transcription and fetal growth, suggesting the association with T2DM is not spurious.[41] Lastly, the class I allele of the insulin gene is a major determinant of Type 1 diabetes, indicating that some candidate genes may contribute to both major types of diabetes.[113]

Future directions

There is an accumulating catalogue of single nucleotide polymorphisms (SNPs) in addition to the numerous microsatellite markers previously identified within the human genome, mainly as a consequence of the Human Genome Mapping project. This has led to the theoretical possibility that genome scan strategies utilizing large-scale SNP genotyping and LD could map genes of complex diseases.[102,103,114] The number of SNPs required for such an entire genome search is highly contentious as this would be dependent on the extent of LD in the human genome. It is predicted that LD may extend between 5kb and 100kb, although others contend that it may be no more than 3kb. However, for any given chromosomal region LD will be influenced by population demographic history. Undoubtedly LD is not uniform across the whole genome but if the lower levels of LD were adopted as an average then as many as 500,000 SNPs and a study population numbered in the thousands would be necessary to achieve adequate power for mapping in complex diseases.[115-118] The selection of isolated founder populations could reduce the number of markers required to detect rare disease alleles, although they may not necessarily offer great advantage when common alleles are related to disease.[119] One possible strategy to improve feasibility of these studies would be to select SNPs with *a priori* knowledge that they are more likely to be causative.[20] It is estimated that there are at least 60,000 non-conservative coding mutations in the human genome in the entire world population, with a substantial fraction of these already known. However, this approach could potentially miss mutations that have other effects, such as those that cause alteration in the gene environment in relation to the more tightly wound heterochromatic structure and less condensed euchromatic states, i.e. Position Effect Variegation (PEV).[120] There could also be problems in regions of chromosomes where there is little or no LD unless a causative mutation is selected in the analysis purely by chance. In contrast to linkage analysis, evidence of no association would not allow to exclude the region for the absence of a disease gene.

The recent publication of the first comprehensive analysis of the human genome with 93% coverage and with 50% in uninterrupted sequence contigs[121] revised the projected total number of human genes from 100,000 to only 32,000.[122] The ramifications of this projection and the added fact that at least 40% of human genes have alternate splice functional isoforms, suggests that there are other orders of genetic complexity to accommodate all necessary proteome function. In other species this appears to be the case, for instance the genome of *Drosophila melanogaster* has less genes than simpler organisms such as *Caenorhabditis elegans*. However, this appears to be compensated by an expanded proteome diversity as a result of alternate splicing generating many transcripts from a single gene.[123] In humans, alternate splice sites are primarily in protein coding regions and are particularly common in genes for membrane receptors, and genes specific for immune and nervous systems.[124] The vascular endothelial growth factor (VEGF) that induces microvascular permeability,[125] the integrin family of transmembrane proteins[126] and a number of cytokines[127] all have a number of distinct splice isoforms that differ not only in their expression patterns but also in their biochemical and biological properties. The putative T2DM susceptibility locus *CAPN10* has at least ten splice variant isoforms that are differentially expressed depending on the tissue.[71] In skeletal muscle, two splice isoforms predominate, and variation in their levels could be related to the polymorphic variants associated with increased risk to T2DM, with some protein isoforms possibly being biologically inactive.[128,129]

Any suspected susceptibility gene derived by whatever method, still requires additional evidence to support a cause and effect relationship with disease. Ultimately the tract of DNA must be sequenced to identify the actual pathogenic variant, and subsequent functional characterization would be necessary to demonstrate that the variant leads to an effect on physiological processes. These types of experiments would be dependent on the localization of the variant within the gene, which would determine possible causality. Until recently these studies have focused mainly on variants within coding, exon splice sites and 5' and 3' untranslated regions responsible for gene transcription regulation. However, the identification of intronic variants in the *CAPN10* gene that are not only associated with T2DM and also the discovery that they can modulate gene transcription, suggests that these DNA segments cannot be disregarded as non-functional as they have been in most previous studies.

Recent new techniques using microarray chip technology and mass spectrometry allied with proteomics now provide the opportunity to gain a cellular snapshot of differences in overall gene expression and total protein content between disease and non-disease tissues. These methods offer new avenues to detect disease-causing genetic aberrations that may implicate genes or proteins that would then require investigation on a broader basis in populations.

Genetics of T2DM and disease prevention

The ultimate rationale for studying a disease is to manage, treat and eventually prevent disorders. The identification of susceptibility genes responsible for the genetic component of T2DM could greatly assist in the elucidation of the underlying pathophysiological mechanisms leading to the disease and is central to the development of more effective preventative and therapeutic strategies for this condition.

An understanding of an individual genetic risk profile in combination with established clinically defined predisposing factors could be used as part of a primary prevention in reducing risk of onset of disease. The identification of the genes responsible for MODY that accounts for 1% of T2DM in the UK (approximately 20,000 people) has allowed the development of diagnostic and predictive genetic tests for 80% of MODY families.[130] Families with a history of T2DM would presumably be enriched in specific T2DM susceptibility alleles/genes and information on the sharing and transmission of a majority of the susceptibility polygenes could possibly allow an overall determination of risk and early preventive measures. In the future, the risk of first-degree relatives may be determined in families with a history of T2DM similar to that of MODY. In terms of both primary and secondary prevention the identification of susceptibility genes could not only identify new biological pathways that may permit specific intervention, but also facilitate the individual tuning of treatments. In the latter case the field of pharmacogenomics is emerging as a relatively new sub-discipline of molecular genetics. Future developments in this field are largely dependent on the information made available through analysis of the human genome. Drug response is under the control of multiple genetic factors, and a better understanding of complex traits would permit stratification of patient populations presenting a single disease phenotype into sub-classes whose disorders might have differing genetic components or different responses to particular therapeutics. Clinical trials to associate genotypes in relation to individual variations in therapeutic drug response and in the occurrence of adverse drug reactions are becoming more common with the eventual view to produce customized drugs and treatments.[131]

References

1. Kobberling J, Tillih H. Empirical risk figures for first-degree relatives of non-insulin dependent diabetics. In: Kobberling J, Tattersall R, eds. The Genetics of Diabetes Mellitus. London: Academic Press, 1982: 201–9.
2. Ramachandran A, Mohan V, Snehalatha C, Viswanathan M. Prevalence of non-insulin-dependent diabetes mellitus in Asian Indian families with a single diabetic parent. Diabetes Res Clin Pract 1988; 4: 241–5.
3. Viswanathan M, Mohan V, Snehalatha C, Ramachandran A. High prevalence of Type 2 (non-insulin-dependent) diabetes among the offspring of conjugal Type 2 diabetic parents in India. Diabetologia 1985; 28: 907–10.
4. Knowler WC, Pettitt DJ, Saad MF, Bennett PH. Diabetes mellitus in the Pima Indians: incidence, risk factors, and pathogenesis. Diabetes Metab Rev 1990; 6: 1–27.
5. Mitchell BD, Kammerer CM, Reinhart LJ, Stern MP. NIDDM in Mexican-American families. Heterogeneity by age of onset. Diabetes Care 1994; 17: 567–73.
6. Newman B, Selby JV, King MC et al. Concordance for Type 2 (non-insulin-dependent) diabetes mellitus in male twins. Diabetologia 1987; 30: 763–8.
7. Kaprio J, Tuomilehto J, Koskenvuo M et al. Concordance for Type 1 (insulin-dependent) and Type 2 (non-insulin-dependent) diabetes mellitus in a population-based cohort of twins in Finland. Diabetologia 1992; 35: 1060–7.
8. Medici F, Hawa M, Ianari A et al. Concordance rate for type II diabetes mellitus in monozygotic twins: actuarial analysis. Diabetologia 1999; 42: 146–50.
9. Poulsen P, Kyvik KO, Vaag A, Beck-Nielsen H. Heritability of type II (non-insulin-dependent) diabetes mellitus and abnormal glucose tolerance: a population-based twin study. Diabetologia 1999; 42: 139–45.
10. Hales CN, Barker DJ. Type 2 (non-insulin-dependent) diabetes mellitus: the thrifty phenotype hypothesis. Diabetologia 1992; 35: 595–601.
11. Harris MI, Flegal KM, Cowie CC et al. Prevalence of diabetes, impaired fasting glucose, and impaired glucose tolerance in US adults.

The Third National Health and Nutrition Examination Survey, 1988–1994. Diabetes Care 1998; 21: 518–24.

12. Brosseau JD, Eelkema RC, Crawford AC, Abe TA. Diabetes among the three affiliated tribes: correlation with degree of Indian inheritance. Am J Public Health 1979; 69: 1277–8.

13. Zimmet P, Canteloube D, Genelle B et al. The prevalence of diabetes mellitus and impaired glucose tolerance in Melanesians and part-Polynesians in rural New Caledonia and Ouvea (Loyalty Islands). Diabetologia 1982; 23: 393–8.

14. Serjeantson SW, Zimmet P. Genetics of non-insulin dependent diabetes mellitus in 1990. Baillieres Clin Endocrinol Metab 1991; 5: 477–93 (Review).

15. Hanson RL, Elston RC, Pettitt DJ et al. Segregation analysis of non-insulin-dependent diabetes mellitus in Pima Indians: evidence for a major-gene effect. Am J Hum Genet 1995; 57: 160–70.

16. Stern MP, Mitchell BD, Blangero J et al. Evidence for a major gene for type II diabetes and linkage analyses with selected candidate genes in Mexican-Americans. Diabetes 1996; 45: 563–8.

17. McCarthy MI, Hitman GA, Shields DC et al. Family studies of non-insulin-dependent diabetes mellitus in South Indians. Diabetologia 1994; 37: 1221–30.

18. Cook JT, Shields DC, Page RC et al. Segregation analysis of NIDDM in Caucasian families. Diabetologia 1994; 37: 1231–40.

19. Rich SS. Mapping genes in diabetes. Genetic epidemiological perspective. Diabetes 1990; 39: 1315–9 (Review).

20. Risch NJ. Searching for genetic determinants in the new millennium. Nature 2000; 405: 847–56 (Review).

21. Zimmet PZ. Kelly West Lecture 1991. Challenges in diabetes epidemiology – from West to the rest. Diabetes Care 1992; 15: 232–52.

22. Hodge AM, Dowse GK, Toelupe P et al. Dramatic increase in the prevalence of obesity in western Samoa over the 13 year period 1978–1991. Int J Obes Relat Metab Disord 1994; 18: 419–28.

23. Neel JV. Diabetes mellitus: a 'thrifty' genotype rendered detrimental by 'progress'? 1962. Bull World Health Organ 1999; 77: 694–703.

24. Taylor R, Bennett P, Uili R et al. Diabetes in Wallis Polynesians: comparison of residents of Wallis Island and first generation migrants to New Caledonia. Diabetes Res Clin Pract 1985; 1: 169–78.

25. Helmrich SP, Ragland DR, Leung RW, Paffenbarger RS Jr. Physical activity and reduced occurrence of non-insulin-dependent diabetes mellitus. N Engl J Med 1991; 325: 147–52

26. Aspray TJ, Mugusi F, Rashid S et al. Rural and urban differences in diabetes prevalence in Tanzania: the role of obesity, physical inactivity and urban living. Trans R Soc Trop Med Hyg 2000; 94: 637–44.

27. Ramachandran A, Snehalatha C, Latha E et al. Rising prevalence of NIDDM in an urban population in India. Diabetologia 1997; 40: 232–7.

28. McKeigue PM,. Shah B, Marmot MG. Relation of central obesity and insulin resistance with high diabetes prevalence and cardiovascular risk in South Asians. Lancet 1991; 337: 382–6.

29. Prentice AM, Jebb SA. Obesity in Britain: gluttony or sloth? BMJ 1995; 311: 437–9.

30. Pettitt DJ, Nelson RG, Saad MF et al. Diabetes and obesity in the offspring of Pima Indian women with diabetes during pregnancy. Diabetes Care 1993; 16: 310–4.

31. Phillips DI, Young JB. Birth weight, climate at birth and the risk of obesity in adult life. Int J Obes Relat Metab Disord 2000; 24: 281–7.

32. Barker DJ, Hales CN, Fall CH et al. Type 2 (non-insulin-dependent) diabetes mellitus, hypertension and hyperlipidaemia (syndrome X): relation to reduced fetal growth. Diabetologia 1993; 36: 62–7.

33. Aerts L, Holemans K, Van Assche FA. Maternal diabetes during pregnancy: consequences for the offspring. Diabetes Metab Rev 1990; 6: 147–67 (Review).

34. Holemans K, Verhaeghe J, Dequeker J, Van Assche FA. Insulin sensitivity in adult female rats subjected to malnutrition during the perinatal period. J Soc Gynecol Investig 1996; 3: 71–7.

35. Poulsen P, Vaag AA, Kyvik KO et al. Low birth weight is associated with NIDDM in discordant

monozygotic and dizygotic twin pairs. Diabetologia 1997; 40: 439–46.

36. Phillips DI. Birth weight and the future development of diabetes. A review of the evidence. Diabetes Care 1998; 21 Suppl 2: B150–5 (Review).

37. Hattersley AT, Tooke JE. The fetal insulin hypothesis: an alternative explanation of the association of low birthweight with diabetes and vascular disease. Lancet 1999; 353: 1789–92 (Review).

38. Hattersley AT, Beards F, Ballantyne E et al. Mutations in the glucokinase gene of the fetus result in reduced birth weight. Nat Genet 1998; 19: 268–70.

39. Woods KA, Camacho-Hubner C, Barter D et al. Insulin-like growth factor I gene deletion causing intrauterine growth retardation and severe short stature. Acta Paediatr Suppl 1997; 423: 39–45.

40. Johnston LB, Leger J, Savage MO et al. The insulin-like growth factor-I (IGF-I) gene in individuals born small for gestational age (SGA). Clin Endocrinol (Oxf) 1999; 51: 423–7.

41. Dunger DB, Ong KK, Huxtable SJ et al. Association of the INS VNTR with size at birth. ALSPAC Study Team. Avon Longitudinal Study of Pregnancy and Childhood. Nat Genet 1998; 19: 98–100.

42. Zhang Y, Proenca R, Maffei M et al. Positional cloning of the mouse obese gene and its human homologue. Nature 1994; 372: 425–32.

43. Gauguier D, Froguel P, Parent V et al. Chromosomal mapping of genetic loci associated with non-insulin dependent diabetes in the GK rat. Nat Genet 1996; 12: 38–43.

44. Galli J, Li LS, Glaser A, Ostenson CG et al. Genetic analysis of non-insulin dependent diabetes mellitus in the GK rat. Nat Genet 1996; 12: 31–7.

45. Froguel P, Vaxillaire M, Sun F et al. Close linkage of glucokinase locus on chromosome 7p to early-onset non-insulin-dependent diabetes mellitus. Nature 1992; 356: 162–4.

46. Yamagata K, Furuta H, Oda N et al. Mutations in the hepatocyte nuclear factor-4 alpha gene in maturity-onset diabetes of the young (MODY1). Nature 1996; 384: 458–60.

47. Yamagata K, Oda N, Kaisaki PJ et al. Mutations in the hepatocyte nuclear factor-1

alpha gene in maturity-onset diabetes of the young (MODY3). Nature 1996; 5384: 455–8.

48. Hattersley AT. Diagnosis of maturity-onset diabetes of the young in the pediatric diabetes clinic. J Pediatr Endocrinol Metab 2000; 13 Suppl 6: 1411–7 (Review).

49. Alcolado JC, Thomas AW. Maternally inherited diabetes mellitus: the role of mitochondrial DNA defects. Diabet Med 1995; 12: 102–8 (Review).

50. Maassen JA. Kadowaki T. Maternally inherited diabetes and deafness: a new diabetes subtype. Diabetologia 1996; 39: 375–82 (Review).

51. Frayling T, Beards F, Hattersley AT. Maturity-onset diabetes of the young: a monogenic model of diabetes. In: Hitman GA, ed. Type 2 Diabetes; Prediction and Prevention. Chichester, UK: John Wiley & Sons Ltd, 1999: 107–26.

52. Stoffers DA, Ferrer J, Clarke WL, Habener JF. Early-onset type II diabetes mellitus (MODY4) linked to IPF1. Nat Genet 1997; 17: 138–9.

53. Hani EH, Stoffers DA, Chevre JC et al. Defective mutations in the insulin promoter factor-1 (IPF-1) gene in late-onset Type 2 diabetes mellitus. J Clin Invest 1999; 104: R41–8.

54. Macfarlane WM, Frayling TM, Ellard S et al. Missense mutations in the insulin promoter factor-1 gene predispose to Type 2 diabetes J Clin Invest 2000; 106: 717.

55. Naya FJ, Stellrecht CM, Tsai M.J. Tissue-specific regulation of the insulin gene by a novel basic helix-loop-helix transcription factor. Genes Dev 1995; 9: 1009–19.

56. Fajans SS, Bell GI, Polonsky KS. Molecular mechanisms and clinical pathophysiology of maturity-onset diabetes of the young. N Engl J Med 2001; 345: 971–80.

57. Malecki MT, Jhala US, Antonellis A et al. Mutations in NEUROD1 are associated with the development of Type 2 diabetes mellitus. Nat Genet. 1999 ; 23: 323–8.

58. Malecki MT, Antonellis A, Casey P et al. Exclusion of the hepatocyte nuclear factor 4alpha as a candidate gene for late-onset NIDDM linked with chromosome 20q. Diabetes 1998; 47: 970–2.

59. Giles RE, Blanc H, Cann HM, Wallace DC. Maternal inheritance of human mitochondrial DNA. Proc Natl Acad Sci USA 1980; 77: 6715–9.

60. van den Ouweland JM, Lemkes HH, Ruitenbeek W et al. Mutation in mitochondrial tRNA(Leu)(UUR) gene in a large pedigree with maternally transmitted type II diabetes mellitus and deafness. Nat Genet 1992; 1: 368–7.

61. Goto Y, Nonaka I, Horai S. A mutation in the tRNA(Leu)(UUR) gene associated with the MELAS subgroup of mitochondrial encephalo-myopathies. Nature 1990; 348: 651–3.

62. Saker PJ, Hattersley AT, Barrow B et al. UKPDS 21: low prevalence of the mitochondrial transfer RNA gene tRNA(Leu)(UUR) mutation at position 3243bp in UK Caucasian Type 2 diabetic patients. Diabet Med 1997; 14: 42–5.

63. McCarthy M, Cassell P, Tran T et al. Evaluation of the importance of maternal history of diabetes and of mitochondrial variation in the development of NIDDM. Diabet Med 1996; 13: 420–8.

64. Smith PR, Dronsfield MJ, Mijovic CH et al. The mitochondrial tRNA[Leu(UUR)] A to G 3243 mutation is associated with insulin-dependent and non-insulin-dependent diabetes in a Chinese population. Diabet Med 1997; 14: 1026–31.

65. Kerem B, Rommens JM, Buchanan JA et al. Identification of the cystic fibrosis gene: genetic analysis. Science 1989; 245: 1073–80.

66. Katsanis N, Beales PL, Woods MO et al. Mutations in MKKS cause obesity, retinal dystrophy and renal malformations associated with Bardet-Biedl syndrome. Nat Genet 2000; 26: 67–70.

67. Groden J, Thliveris A, Samowitz W et al. Identification and characterization of the familial adenomatous polyposis coli gene. Cell 1991; 66: 589–600.

68. Panzram G. Mortality and survival in Type 2 (non-insulin-dependent) diabetes mellitus. Diabetologia 1987; 30: 123–31.

69. O'Rahilly S. Turner RC. Early-onset Type 2 diabetes vs maturity-onset diabetes of youth: evidence for the existence of two discrete diabetic syndromes. Diabet Med 1988; 5: 224–9.

70. Horikawa Y, Oda N, Cox NJ et al. Genetic variation in the gene encoding calpain-10 is associated with Type 2 diabetes mellitus. Nat Genet 2000; 26: 163–75.

71. Hani EH, Dupont S, Durand E et al. Naturally occurring mutations in the melanocortin receptor 3 gene are not associated with Type 2 diabetes mellitus in French Caucasians. J Clin Endocrinol Metab 2001; 86: 2895–8.

72. Shaw JT, Lovelock PK, Kesting JB et al. Novel susceptibility gene for late-onset NIDDM is localized to human chromosome 12q. Diabetes 1998; 47: 1793–6.

73. Inoue H, Ferrer J, Welling CM et al. Sequence variants in the sulfonylurea receptor (SUR) gene are associated with NIDDM in Caucasians. Diabetes 1996; 45: 825–31.

74. Hart LM, de Knijff P, Dekker JM et al. Variants in the sulphonylurea receptor gene: association of the exon 16–3t variant with Type II diabetes mellitus in Dutch Caucasians. Diabetologia 1999; 42: 617–20.

75. Stirling B, Cox NJ, Bell GI et al. Linkage studies in NIDDM with markers near the sulphonylurea receptor gene. Diabetologia 1995; 38: 1479–81.

76. Thomas PM, Cote GJ, Wohllk N et al. Mutations in the sulfonylurea receptor gene in familial persistent hyperinsulinemic hypoglycemia of infancy. Science 1995; 268: 426–9.

77. Nestorowicz A, Glaser B, Wilson BA et al. Genetic heterogeneity in familial hyperinsulinism. Hum Mol Genet 1998; 7: 1119–28.

78. Wiltshire S, Hattersley AT, Hitman GA et al. A genomewide scan for loci predisposing to Type 2 diabetes in a UK population (the Diabetes UK Warren 2 Repository): analysis of 573 pedigrees provides independent replication of a susceptibility locus on chromosome 1q. Am J Hum Genet 2001; 69: 553–69.

79. Elbein SC, Hoffman MD, Teng K et al. A genome-wide search for Type 2 diabetes susceptibility genes in Utah Caucasians. Diabetes 1999; 48: 1175–82.

80. Busfield F, Duffy DL, Kesting JB et al. A genomewide search for Type 2 diabetes-susceptibility genes in indigenous Australians. Am J Hum Genet 2002; 70: 349–57.

81. Ehm MG, Karnoub MC, Sakul H et al. Genomewide search for Type 2 diabetes susceptibility genes in four American populations. Am J Hum Genet 2000; 66: 1871–81.

82. Wolford JK, Bogardus C, Ossowski V, Prochazka M. Molecular characterization of the human PEA15 gene on 1q21–q22 and associa-

tion with Type 2 diabetes mellitus in Pima Indians. Gene 2000; 241: 143–8.

83. Permutt MA, Hattersley AT. Searching for Type 2 diabetes genes in the post-genome era. Trends Endocrinol Metab 2000; 11: 383–93.

84. Hanis CL, Boerwinkle E, Chakraborty R et al. A genome-wide search for human non-insulin-dependent (Type 2) diabetes genes reveals a major susceptibility locus on chromosome 2. Nat Genet 1996; 13: 161–6.

85. Cox NJ, Frigge M, Nicolae DL et al. Loci on chromosomes 2 (NIDDM1) and 15 interact to increase susceptibility to diabetes in Mexican Americans. Nat Genet 1999; 21: 213–5.

86. Evans JC, Frayling TM, Cassell PG et al. Studies of association between the gene for calpain-10 and Type 2 diabetes mellitus in the United Kingdom. Am J Hum Genet 2001; 69: 544–52.

87. Cassell PG, Jackson AE, North BV et al. Haplotype combinations of Calpain 10 gene polymorphisms associate with increased risk to impaired glucose tolerance and Type 2 Diabetes mellitus in South Indians. Diabetes 2002; 51: 1622–8.

88. Schwarz PE, Horikawa Y, Vcelak J et al. Genetic variation of CAPN10 affects susceptibility to Type 2 diabetes in German and Czech population. Diabetes 2001; 50 Suppl 2: 950.

89. Baier LJ, Permana PA, Yang X et al. A calpain-10 gene polymorphism is associated with reduced muscle mRNA levels and insulin resistance. J Clin Invest 2000; 106: R69–73.

90. Sorimachi H, Ishiura S, Suzuki K. Structure and physiological function of calpains. Biochem J 1997; 328 (Pt 3): 721–32 (Review).

91. Saido T, Sorimachi H, Suzuki K. Calpain: new perspectives in molecular diversity and physiological-pathological involvement. FASEB J 1994; 8: 814–822.

92. Carafoli E, Molinari M. Calpain: a protease in search of a function. Biochem Biophys Res Commun 1998; 247: 193–203.

93. Patel YM, Lane DM. Role of calpain in adipocyte differentiation. Proc Natl Acad Sci USA 1999; 96: 1279–85.

94. Ueda Y, Wang MC, Ou BR et al. Evidence for the participation of the proteasome and calpain in early phases of muscle cell differentiation. J Biochem Cell Biol 1998; 30: 679–94.

95. Murray SS, Grisanti MS, Bentley GV et al. The calpain-calpastatin system and cellular proliferation and differentiation in rodent osteoblastic cells. Exp Cell Res 1997; 233: 297–309.

96. Yasuda T, Shimizu K, Nakagawa Y et al. m-Calpain in rat growth plate chondrocyte cultures: its involvement in the matrix mineralization process. Develop Biol 1995; 170: 159–68.

97. Croce K, Flaumenhaft R, Rivers M et al. Inhibition of calpain blocks platelet secretion, aggregation, and spreading. J Biol Chem 1999; 274: 36321–7.

98. Yamazaki T, Haass C, Saido TC et al. Specific increase in amyloid beta-protein 42 secretion ratio by calpain inhibition. Biochemistry 1997; 36: 8377–83.

99. Sreenan SK, Zhou YP, Otani K et al. Calpains play a role in insulin secretion and action. Diabetes 2001; 50: 2013–20.

100. Smith LK, Rice KM, Garner CW. The insulin-induced down-regulation of IRS-1 in 3T3–L1 adipocytes is mediated by a calcium-dependent thiol protease. Mol Cell Endocrinol 1996; 122: 81–92.

101. Zhou Y-P, Sreenan S, Bindokas VP et al. Calpain inhibitors impair insulin secretion after 48-hours: a model for beta-cell dysfunction in Type 2 diabetes? Diabetes 2000; 49 Suppl 1: 324.

102. Risch N, Merikangas K. The future of genetic studies of complex human diseases. Science 1996; 273: 1516–7.

103. Collins FS, Guyer MS, Charkravarti A. Variations on a theme: cataloging human DNA sequence variation. Science 1997; 278: 1580–1.

104. Altshuler D, Daly M, Kruglyak L. Guilt by association. Nat Genet. 2000 Oct; 26: 135–7.

105. Spielman RS, Ewens WJ. The TDT and other family-based tests for linkage disequilibrium and association. Am J Hum Genet 1996; 59: 983–9.

106. Sham PC, Curtis D. An extended transmission/disequilibrium test (TDT) for multi-allele marker loci. Ann Hum Genet 1995; 59: 323–336.

107. Almind K, Doria A, Kahn CR. Putting the genes for type II diabetes on the map. Nat Med 2001; 00: 277–9.

108. Altshuler D, Hirschhorn JN, Klannemark M et

al. The common PPAR Pro12Ala polymorphism is associated with decreased risk of Type 2 diabetes. Nat Genet 2000; 26: 76–80.

109. Almind K, Bjorbaek C, Vestergaard H et al. Aminoacid polymorphisms of insulin receptor substrate-1 in non-insulin-dependent diabetes mellitus. Lancet 1993; 342: 828–32.

110. Hitman GA, Hawrami K, McCarthy MI et al. Insulin receptor substrate-1 gene mutations in NIDDM; implications for the study of polygenic disease. Diabetologia 1995; 38: 481–6.

111. Sesti G, Federici M, Hribal ML et al. Defects of the insulin receptor substrate (IRS) system in human metabolic disorders. FASEB J 2001; 15: 2099–111 (Review).

112. Huxtable SJ, Saker PJ, Haddad L et al. Analysis of parent-offspring trios provides evidence for linkage and association between the insulin gene and Type 2 diabetes mediated exclusively through paternally transmitted class III variable number tandem repeat alleles. Diabetes 2000; 49: 126–30.

113. Bell GI, Horita S, Karam JH. A highly polymorphic locus near the human insulin gene is associated with insulin-dependent diabetes mellitus. Diabetes 1984; 33: 176–83.

114. Roses AD. Pharmacogenetics and the practice of medicine. Nature 2000; 405: 857–65 (Review).

115. Ott J. Predicting the range of linkage disequilibrium. Proc Natl Acad Sci USA 2000; 97: 2–3.

116. Kruglyak L. Prospects for whole-genome linkage disequilibrium mapping of common disease genes. Nat Genet 1999; 22: 139–44.

117. Abecasis GR, Noguchi E, Heinzmann A et al. Extent and distribution of linkage disequilibrium in three genomic regions. Am J Hum Genet 2001; 68: 191–7.

118. Laan M, Paabo S. Demographic history and linkage disequilibrium in human populations. Nat Genet 1997; 17: 435–8.

119. Wright AF, Carothers AD, Pirastu M. Population choice in mapping genes for complex diseases. Nat Genet 1999; 23: 397–404 (Review).

120. Kleinjan DJ, van Heyningen V. Position effect in human genetic disease. Hum Mol Genet 1998; 7: 1611–8 (Review).

121. Nature. Issue 6822, 2001 Feb; 409: 745–964.

122. Lee C. The incredible shrinking human genome. Trends Genet 2001; 17: 187–8.

123. Graveley BR. Alternative splicing: increasing diversity in the proteomic world. Trends Genet 2001; 17: 100–7 (Review).

124. Dredge BK, Polydorides AD, Darnell RB. The splice of life: alternative splicing and neurological disease. Nat Rev Neurosci 2001; 2: 43–50 (Review).

125. Robinson CJ, Stringer SE. The splice variants of vascular endothelial growth factor (VEGF) and their receptors. J Cell Sci 2001; 114 (Pt 5): 853–65 (Review).

126. de Melker AA, Sonnenberg A. Integrins: alternative splicing as a mechanism to regulate ligand binding and integrin signaling events. Bioessays 1999; 21: 499–509 (Review).

127. Atamas SP. Alternative splice variants of cytokines: making a list. Life Sci 1997; 61: 1105–12 (Review).

128. Ma H, Fukiage C, Kim YH et al. Characterization and expression of calpain 10. A novel ubiquitous calpain with nuclear localization. J Biol Chem 2001; 276(30): 28525–31.

129. Yang X, Pratley RE, Baier LJ et al. Reduced skeletal muscle calpain-10 transcript level is due to a cumulative decrease in major isoforms. Mol Genet Metab 2001; 73: 111–3.

130. Shepherd M, Ellis I, Ahmad AM et al. Predictive genetic testing in maturity-onset diabetes of the young (MODY). Diabet Med 2001; 18: 417–21.

131. Marshall A. Laying the foundations for personalized medicines. Nat Biotechnol 1997; 15: 954–7 (Review).

132. Vionnet N, Hani El-H, Dupont S et al. Genomewide search for type 2 diabetes-susceptibility genes in French whites: evidence for a novel susceptibility locus for early-onset diabetes on chromosome 3q27-qter and independent replication of a type 2-diabetes locus on chromosome 1q21-q24. Am J Hum Genet 2000; 67: 1470–80.

133. Hanson RL, Ehm G, Pettitt DJ et al. An autosomal genomic scan for loci linked to type II diabetes mellitus and body-mass index in Pirna Indians. Am J Hum Genet 1998; 63: 1130–8.

134. Hani EH, Hager J, Philippi A et al. Mapping NIDDM susceptibility loci in French families: studies with markers in the region of NIDDM1 on chromosome 2q. Diabetes 1997; 46: 1225–6.

135. Permutt MA, Wasson JC, Suarez BK et al. A genome scan for type 2 diabetes susceptibility loci in a genetically isolated population. Diabetes 2001; 50: 681–5.

136. Lindgren CM, Mahtani MM, Widen E et al. Genomewide search for type 2 diabetes mellitus susceptibility loci in Finnish families: the Botnia study. Am J Hum Genet 2002; 70: 509–16.

137. Ghosh S, Watanabe RM, Timo T et al. The Finland–United States Investigation of Non-Insulin-Dependent Diabetes Mellitus Genetics (FUSION) Study. I. An Autosomal Genome Scan for genes That Predispose to Type 2 Diabetes. Am J Hum Genet 2000; 67: 1174–85.

138. Duggirala R, Blangero J, Almasy L et al. Linkage of type 2 diabetes mellitus and of age at onset to a genetic location on chromosome 10q in Mexican Americans. Am J Hum Genet 1999; 64: 1127–40.

139. Stern MP, Duggirala R, Mitchell BD et al. Evidence for linkage of regions on chromosomes 6 and 11 to plasma glucose concentrations in Mexican Americans. Genome Res 1996; 6: 724–34.

140. Bektas A, Suprenant ME, Wogan LT et al. Evidence of a novel type 2 diabetes locus 50 cM centromeric to NIDDM2 on chromosome 12q. Diabetes 1999; 48: 2246–51.

141. Mahtani MM, Widen E, Lehto M et al. Mapping of a gene for type 2 diabetes associated with an insulin secretion defect by a genome scan in Finnish families. Nature Genet 1996; 14: 90–4.

142. Bowden DW, Sale M, Howard TD et al. Linkage of genetic markers on human chromosomes 20 and 12 to NIDDM in Caucasian sib pairs with a history of diabetic nephropathy. Diabetes 1997; 46: 882–6.

143. Ji L, Malecki M, Warram JH, Yang Y et al. New susceptibility locus for NIDDM is localized to human chromosome 20q. Diabetes 1997; 46: 876–81.

144. Zouali H, Hani EH, Philippi A et al. A susceptibility locus for early-onset non-insulin dependent (type 2) diabetes mellitus maps to chromosome 20q, proximal to the phosphoenolpyruvate carboxykinase gene. Hum Mol Genet 1997; 6: 1401–8.

145. Elbein SC, Chiu KC, Hoffman MD et al. Linkage analysis of 19 candidate regions for insulin resistance in familial NIDDM. Diabetes 1995; 44: 1259–65.

146. Klupa T, Malecki MT, Pezzolesi M et al. Further evidence for a susceptibility locus for type 2 diabetes on chromosome 20q13.1-q13.2. Diabetes 2000; 49: 2212–6.

4

Complication-resistant patients
Andrew P Levy

Introduction

Late or long-term microvascular and macrovascular complications are the leading cause of morbidity and mortality in patients with diabetes mellitus (DM). Considerable evidence has been accumulated over the last 20–30 years linking the degree of glycemic control with the development of diabetic vascular disease. Nevertheless, it is clear that some patients never develop these complications and that hyperglycemia is a necessary but not sufficient condition for the development of these complications. Genetic differences between diabetic patients may thus play an important role in the observed differences in susceptibility to these complications. After briefly reviewing the epidemiology and natural history of specific microvascular and macrovascular complications we will review the current status of our understanding of the role of genetic factors in the development of diabetic vascular disease. Identification of these genetic markers will allow further insights into the pathogenesis of diabetic complications, and possibly the development of novel therapeutic agents for their treatment. It will also allow preventive therapy (more aggressive glycemic control and concomitant risk factor reduction and more frequent health screening) to be directed at those patients with the greatest risk for development of diabetic complications. Finally, identification of the molecular basis for increased susceptibility in a given patient will ultimately allow for individually tailored therapies for each patient to reduce the risk of vascular disease.

Epidemiology and natural history of diabetic vascular disease

1. Diabetic retinopathy

Diabetic retinopathy is the leading cause of new cases of blindness in the USA and the western world between the ages of 20 and 74. The natural history of diabetic retinopathy has been well described in several multicenter clinical trials. Specific stages of the retinopathy, normally progressing in an orderly fashion, are characterized by defined clinical parameters on ophthalmological examination. The prevalence of diabetic retinopathy is related to the age of diabetes onset, the duration of diabetes, the type of diabetes and the level of glycemic control. The peak incidence of retinopathy is between 10–18 years after the onset of the diabetes. After 20 years of diabetes at least 85% of patients with Type 1 and more than 60% of patients with Type 2 diabetes develop some form of retinopathy. A definitive relationship between hyperglycemia and diabetic retinopathy has been demonstrated in the

Diabetes Control and Complications Trial (DCCT)[1,2] and in the United Kingdom Prospective Diabetes Study (UKPDS).[3]

2. Diabetic nephropathy

Approximately one-third of patients with DM will develop end-stage renal disease necessitating renal replacement therapy within 25 years of the onset of the diabetes.[4] Similar to diabetic retinopathy, epidemiological studies have demonstrated the importance of age of onset, duration, type of DM and adequacy of metabolic control to the development and severity of diabetic nephropathy (DN).[5,6] The clinical course of DN proceeds through several clinical stages:

(1) hyperfiltration;
(2) microproteinuria (microalbuminuria) in which the excretion of albumin is 30–300 mg per day;
(3) macroproteinuria; and
(4) steady progressive decline in renal function.

Longitudinal studies have shown that if microalbuminuria is not seen within 10 years of the onset of diabetes the risk of developing end-stage renal disease is small.[7]

3. Atherosclerotic coronary artery disease

DM is associated with a markedly increased prevalence of atherosclerotic disease in virtually all vascular beds. The overall prevalence of atherosclerotic coronary artery disease (CAD) as assessed by various diagnostic methods is as high as 55% among adult patients with DM as compared to 2–4% of the general population.[8] Moreover, the cardiovascular mortality rate is more than doubled in men and more than quadrupled in women who have DM,

compared with their non-diabetic counterparts and post-myocardial infarction outcome is worse in these patients. Considerable data supports a direct role for hyperglycemia and abnormal lipid profile in the pathogenesis of diabetic coronary artery disease. The DCCT and UKPDS studies both suggested potential benefit of controlling hyperglycemia and the development of macrovascular cardiovascular disease, although the reductions seen in cardiovascular morbidity and mortality with aggressive glycemic treatment in these studies failed to reach statistical significance. Furthermore, diabetic microvascular disease can lead to kidney damage and secondary hypertension which is synergistic with these other risk factors for the development of CAD.[8]

4. Restenosis after percutaneous coronary intervention (PCI)

PCI is of tremendous importance in the treatment algorithm for coronary artery stenosis. The long-term success of the procedure is limited by the process of restenosis, in which the coronary artery blockage returns 2–8 months after the procedure. In the general population, the incidence of restenosis after balloon angioplasty (PTCA) is approximately 20–50%. However, the incidence of restenosis in the diabetic population is 50–70% higher.[9] Endovascular stents, implanted today in over 80% of PCI procedures, reduces the incidence of restenosis compared to balloon PTCA, but the diabetic patient still has a markedly higher rate of in-stent restenosis. This is particularly problematic given the increased amount of coronary artery disease in diabetic patients often necessitating treatment of multiple coronary lesions. The increased risk of restenosis is an important reason why PCI has not been shown to be as effective as coronary artery by-pass surgery in the treatment of diabetic patients but is as effective as by-pass surgery in the non-diabetic population.[10]

Causes of diabetic vascular complications

As discussed above, hyperglycemia is essential for the development of diabetic vascular disease. The mechanism whereby hyperglycemia leads to these complications involves an increase in oxidative stress and activation of several convergent signal transduction pathways. Oxidative stress is generated in the hyperglycemic state as a result of glucose auto-oxidation and the formation of advanced glycation end (AGE) products shown to be directly capable of stimulating production of multiple cytokines (such as VEGF) and the pathological morphological changes found in retinopathy and nephropathy. AGE products are potent oxidants and many of their effects can be inhibited with antioxidants. Hyperglycemia also results in the activation of the polyol pathway, whose end product sorbitol has been shown to be toxic, and in the stimulation of protein kinase C, a key regulator of intracellular signaling pathways. Recently, it has been demonstrated that the increase in AGE production, protein kinase C activation and aldol reductase activation seen in the diabetic state is linked via a common pathway involving an increased production of reactive oxygen species in the setting of increased oxidative stress.[11]

Oxidative stress in the diabetic patient is reflected by an increase in the oxidation of a number of cellular lipid and protein moieties resulting in their loss or change in function. An increase in specific protein adducts demonstrating increased oxidative stress has been shown in the retina and kidney of patients with retinopathy and nephropathy.[12-14] Oxidative stress has also been proposed to play an important role in the development of coronary artery disease and restenosis after coronary angioplasty.[15] Animal and prospective human studies have demonstrated an inhibition in some studies of CAD progression and restenosis.[16,17]

Genetic basis for diabetic complications

There exists a growing body of evidence that supports the notion that diabetic vascular complications develop only in those patients who are genetically susceptible. Family studies have underscored the point that hyperglycemia is a necessary but not sufficient condition for the development of diabetic complications. In particular, nephropathy and cardiovascular disease have been shown to cluster within families to a significant degree, suggesting that there is a genetic basis for predisposition to these complications.[18-22] Analysis of specific population groups such as the Pima Indians have further supported a role for genetic susceptibility genes for the development of nephropathy and retinopathy.[23]

Two approaches, sib-pair linkage analysis and association studies using polymorphisms in candidate genes, have been taken in the search for possible complication susceptibility genes. Sib-pair linkage analysis using genome-wide scans with genetic markers spanning the genome have been used to identify several chromosomal regions that are linked to these complications. Four chromosomal regions with some evidence of linkage with complications have been described on chromosomes 3, 7, 9 and 20.[23] Within the regions on these chromosomes delineated by markers there exist many potential candidate genes, some of which have also been implicated in the association studies discussed below.

A large number of candidate genes with known polymorphisms have been studied in the diabetic population and the relative distribution of the different polymorphs correlated with diabetic complication rate (so-called association studies). Likely candidate genes include those for which a functional polymorphism exists in a gene that is important in mediating the molecular pathogenesis of diabetic complications as discussed above. We have grouped these polymorphic loci according to their putative pathophysiological mechanisms as follows:

I. *Genes involved in etiology of hypertension*
Polymorphism in angiotensin converting enzyme I/D
Polymorphism in angiotensin II receptor
Polymorphism in angiotensinogen
Polymorphism in chymase
Polymorphism in beta subunit of G protein (GNB3) (neg)
Polymorphism in beta adrenergic receptor (neg)
Polymorphism in nitric oxide synthetase

II. *Genes involved in basement membrane production/metabolism*
Polymorphism in transforming growth factor-B
Polymorphism in heparan sulfate proteoglycan (neg)
Polymorphism in collagen type IV (neg)

III. *Genes involved in oxidative stress pathway*
Polymorphism in AGE-receptors
Polymorphism in PKC (neg)
Polymorphism in aldose reductase
Polymorphism in glycogen synthase
Polymorphism in Glut-1 transporter
Polymorphism in haptoglobin
Polymorphism in methylenetetrahydrofolate reductase (MTHFR)
Polymorphism in catalase (neg)
Polymorphism in glutathione peroxidase (neg)

Polymorphism in superoxide dismutase (neg)

IV *Genes involved in lipoprotein metabolism*
Polymorphism in paraoxonase
Polymorphism in Apo E
Polymorphism in Apo a
Polymorphism of the peroxisome proliferator-activated receptor (PPAR) (neg)
Polymorphism of plasminogen activator inhibitor
Polymorphism in beta-fibrinogen

V *Growth factors*
Polymorphism in insulin promoter

VI *Genes involved in the inflammatory response*
Polymorphism in complement C4 (neg)
Polymorphism in tumor necrosis factor
Polymorphism in T-cell receptor beta chain
Polymorphism in von Willebrand factor (neg).

Genes for which a single negative association was demonstrated are so indicated and are not discussed in further detail. All polymorphisms for which at least a single study demonstrated an association with diabetic complications are described. Undoubtedly there are many other susceptibility genes that are not listed here that have not yet been studied or identified.

Specific allelic polymorphisms associated with diabetic vascular complications

Genes involved in etiology of hypertension

Polymorphism in angiotensin converting enzyme I/D[24–32]

The ACE gene on chromosome 17q23 has drawn considerable attention due to the central role that this enzyme plays in the regulation of blood pressure, sodium metabolism, and renal hemodynamics. ACE plays a critical role in cardiovascular hemostasis and by activating angiotensin 1 into angiotensin 2 and inactivating bradykinin. These two peptides play antagonistic roles in the cardiovascular system by regulating vascular tone and vascular smooth muscle cell proliferation. The insertion/deletion (ID) polymorphism of the ACE gene is defined by the presence of a 287 base pair Alu sequence in intron 16. The majority of association studies and a recent meta-analysis have failed to find a connection between this polymorphism and diabetic nephropathy and cardiovascular disease. However, this may reflect that the D allele is only linked to nephropathy in the presence of other specific polymorphism in other genes of the renin–angiotensin axis. The ID polymorphism does, however, appear to have a role in response to ACE inhibition, with II homozygotes being the most responsive and DD the least.

Polymorphism in angiotensin II receptor[25,26,33,34]

The angiotensin II receptor gene is located on chromosome 3q25 in a region shown to be linked to diabetic nephropathy (DN) by sib-pair analysis. However, extensive sequencing of the entire locus in affected and unaffected sibs has failed to reveal a specific mutation in this gene contributing to risk of DN. A polymorphism A1166C of this gene (replacement of C (cytosine) for A (adenine) at position 1166) has been shown by a single group to be associated with diabetic retinal complications.

Polymorphism in angiotensinogen[25,28,30,35]

The angiotensinogen gene is located on chromosome 1q42 and the most common polymorphism is the M235T. Several studies have failed to show a connection between a common polymorphism in this gene and DN. However, there does appear to be an association of the M235T polymorphisms with arterial hypertension independent of the degree of renal involvement. It has recently been demonstrated that the T allele is associated with increased risk of nephropathy but only when interaction with the D allele of the ACE-ID polymorphism was considered as shown in a single study. In this study, the T allele was also shown to be associated with retinopathy.

Polymorphism in chymase[36]

The enzyme chymase is an alternative pathway to ACE for conversion of angiotensin 1 to angiotensin 2 and a CMA/B hCC polymorphism has recently been described. A decrease in the incidence of retinopathy has been associated in women only with the GG polymorphism at this locus in a single study.

Polymorphism in nitric oxide synthetase[37–39]

Nitric oxide has an important role in regulating vascular tone in muscular arteries and inhibiting platelet aggregation and monocyte adhesion to endothelium. Several *in vitro* studies have demonstrated a role for nitric oxide in the development of nephropathy in the presence of hyperglycemia. Polymorphisms in the constitutive form of endothelial nitric oxide synthetase (NOS3) are of considerable interest because the NOS3 gene is located at the same cytogenetic location (7q35) that has been shown to be linked to nephropathy by sib-pair analysis. Moreover, several association studies have linked specific polymorphisms in the NOS3 locus and diabetic vascular disease. A polymorphic pentanucleotide repeat (CCTTT)n within the 5' upstream promoter has been linked to diabetic vascular disease presumably by affecting the transcriptional activity of the NOS3 gene. Specifically, in individuals having 14 repeats of this motif decreased retinal, renal and cardiovascular disease has been described. An association with a different NOS3 polymorphism (tandem repeat) has also been recently described with respect to diabetic nephropathy.

Genes involved in basement membrane production/metabolism

Polymorphism in transforming growth factor-B[40–42]

The balance between extracellular matrix formation and degradation is important in the pathogenesis of diabetic vascular disease. TGF-B appears to play a pivotal role in the increased accumulation of extracellular matrix in the kidney as noted by an increase in mesangium. An association of the Thr263Ile TGF-B1 polymorphism with diabetic nephropathy has been described in a single study. Recently, an additional association of a T29C polymorphism in TGF-B1 with increased incidence of myocardial infarction has been reported. The functional basis for these polymorphisms has not been determined.

Genes involved in oxidative stress pathway

Polymorphism in AGE-receptors[43,44]

Excessive production of advanced glycation end products (AGEs) has been demonstrated to be of importance in diabetic vascular disease. These AGE products act via specific membrane receptors, called receptors for AGE or RAGE. A number of functional polymorphisms have been identified that regulate RAGE expression and the 429T/C polymorphism has been shown to be significantly associated with retinopathy in a single study.

Polymorphism in aldose reductase[45–52]

Increased flux through the polyol pathway appears to be important for the pathogenesis

of diabetic complications. In this pathway, elevated glucose concentration results in increased production of sorbitol by the enzyme aldose reductase. Diabetic patients with microvascular disease appear to have an increased gene expression of aldose reductase and increased enzyme activity which may be due to variants in the aldose reductase gene. The gene for aldose reductase is on 7q35, which as noted above has been linked to diabetic vascular disease by sib-pair analysis. Two variants in the promoter ((CA)n repeat located at –2100 and a CT transversion at –106), which appear to increase the transcriptional activity of the gene, have been directly linked to diabetic retinopathy and nephropathy by four independent investigators. Two groups have failed to see an association of these polymorphisms and diabetic kidney disease.

Polymorphism in Glut-1 transporter[53–56]

The Glut-1 transporter has been implicated in renal hypertrophy and extracellular matrix formation in mesangial cells. An Xba 1 polymorphic site in the second intron of the glut1–1 gene has been shown in two out of three independent studies with an increased incidence of diabetic nephropathy. No association was found, however, with diabetic retinopathy or with cardiovascular complications.

Polymorphism in haptoglobin[57–62]

Haptoglobin is a serum hemoglobin-binding protein which functions as an antioxidant by virtue of its ability to bind to hemoglobin and prevent hemoglobin-induced oxidative stress. There exists in man two functionally distinct classes of alleles for the haptoglobin gene, designated 1 and 2. These two classes of alleles are in turn responsible for the existence of three distinct phenotypes in man, 1–1, 2–1, and 2–2. The protein products encoded by these two alleles differ dramatically in their biochemical and biophysical properties. The haptoglobin monomer produced by the haptoglobin gene forms polymeric structures that are found in serum whose structure is determined by the haptoglobin phenotype because the haptoglobin 1 allele protein product is monomeric, while the haptoglobin 2 allele is dimeric. This results in the production of dimers in individuals with haptoglobin 1–1, linear polymers in heterozygotes and cyclic polymers in individuals homozygous for the 2 allele. The effective size of these polymers is dramatically different and may influence the ability of the different haptoglobins to penetrate into the extravascular space to prevent hemoglobin-mediated tissue oxidation. Biochemically, there are functional differences between the different haptoglobin phenotypes. We have shown that haptoglobin 1–1 is a superior antioxidant to haptoglobin 2–2 in preventing hemoglobin-induced oxidation. Furthermore, haptoglobin 1–1 and haptoglobin 2–2 appear to differ dramatically in their immunomodulatory role mediated by the scavenger receptor CD163. This difference results in a greater monocyte/macrophage iron loading and cytokine activation in individuals with CD163.

We have recently demonstrated that the haptoglobin phenotype is a major determinant of susceptibility to diabetic micro- and macrovascular complications. Specifically we have shown that in Type 1 DM, patients with the 1–1 haptoglobin phenotype are remarkably protected from the development of diabetic retinopathy and nephropathy. In a longitudinal population-based study we have shown that Type 2 diabetics, with the haptoglobin 2–2 phenotype, have an odds ratio five times greater than individuals with the haptoglobin 1–1 phenotype of developing cardiovascular disease. In this study we demonstrated that haptoglobin phenotype is an independent risk factor for the development of cardiovascular disease in diabetic patients. Finally, in three independent studies of restenosis after angioplasty we have demonstrated that diabetic patients with the haptoglobin 1–1 phenotype have a significantly lower risk of restenosis after angioplasty than patients with the haptoglobin 2–1 or 2–2 phenotypes.

Polymorphism in MTHFR[63,64]

Elevated homocysteine is an independent risk factor for cardiovascular disease. A common polymorphism C→T677 in the gene coding for MTHFR has been reported to reduce the enzymatic activity of MTHFR and is associated with elevated plasma levels of homocysteine, particularly in patients with low folate intake. This polymorphism has also been associated with diabetic nephropathy in some populations but not in others. A recent report suggested that susceptibility to these complications may only be manifested by allele status in the presence of low folate concentrations.

Polymorphism in NADH dehydrogenase[65]

A polymorphism in the NADH dehydrogenase subunit 2 encoded in the mitochondrial genome involving an A→C transversion at nucleotide 5178 resulting in a Leu to Met substitution has been associated with atherosclerosis in diabetic patients in a single study.

Genes involved in lipoprotein metabolism

Polymorphism in paraoxonase[66–72]

Under oxidative stress which is associated with atherosclerosis, oxidative modifications of LDL take place. There appears to be a direct cause and effect relationship between LDL oxidation and atherosclerosis. The paraoxonase protein is found in HDL particles and has been shown to be an antioxidant by virtue of its ability to hydrolyze lipid peroxides. HDL, via paroxonase is thereby able to protect against the oxidation of LDL. There is a growing body of evidence that genetic polymorphisms of paraoxonase-1, least able to protect LDL against lipid peroxidation (due to changes in the serum level of the protein or its activity), are overrepresented in coronary artery disease, particularly in association with diabetes. Two polymorphisms (promoter TC −109 polymorphism and Met-Leu polymorphism in the coding region) in the paroxonase gene have been identified that modulate the serum concentration of paraoxonase and have been shown to increase susceptibility to CVD in patients with diabetes. A third polymorphism has been shown to affect the activity of the paraoxonase enzyme (Q191R) and to be an additional independent risk factor for the development of heart disease in the diabetic patient. No association has been demonstrated between the paraoxonase polymorphisms and microvascular diabetic complications such as diabetic nephropathy.

Polymorphism in Apo E[73–76]

Four distinct polymorphic alleles have been identified in the Apo E gene, a protein moiety recognized by the LDL receptor, with different potentials for lipoprotein oxidation. While the E4 allele appears to be associated with an increased incidence of cardiovascular disease in non-diabetic patients, no such association has been demonstrated with diabetic patients in two independent studies. With regard to microvascular disease, one study has demonstrated an increased risk of nephropathy associated with the E2 allele while no such association was demonstrated in an independent study of DN.

Polymorphism in Apo a[77]

Apolipoprotein a is the specific apolipoprotein of lipoprotein (a) (Lp(a)) a recognized cardiovascular risk factor with at least 34 isoforms present in plasma. A single study has demonstrated an association between specific isoforms and an increased risk of cardiovascular disease in diabetes, hypertension and hypercholesterolemia.

Polymorphism of plasminogen activator inhibitor (PAI-1)[78,79]

PAI-1 is a key regulator of fibrinolysis and extracellular matrix turnover. Because diabetic nephropathy is characterized by the presence of basement membrane thickening and mesangial expansion, PAI-1 is an excellent candidate susceptibility gene. The PAI G polymorphism was shown to be an independent risk factor for the presence of DN in a single study but was not demonstrated in a second independent study. One group has reported an apparent synergy for the development of DN with the ACE D allele.

Polymorphism of fibrinogen[80]

The beta fibrinogen gene G/A-455 polymorphism has been shown to affect fibrinogen concentrations and to be an independent risk factor for ischemic heart disease in diabetic patients in a single study.

Growth factors

Polymorphism in insulin promoter [81]

Hyperinsulinemia has been suggested to play an important role in micro- and macrovascular diabetic complications. A 5' polymorphism has been described, which was demonstrated to be associated with diabetic nephropathy in a single study.

Genes involved in the inflammatory response

Polymorphism in tumor necrosis factor (TNF)[82]

The TNF Nco allelic polymorphism has been shown to be correlated with an increased incidence of proliferative diabetic retinopathy in Type 2 patients in a single study.

Polymorphism in T-cell receptor beta chain
The TCR gene is of considerable interest for the development of diabetic nephropathy due to its cytogenetic localization to 7q35 and linkage to diabetic nephropathy. A BglII RFLP in the gene has been associated with DN in a single study.

Conclusions

The importance of the allelic polymorphisms described here in the development of diabetic vascular disease is an area of intense study. Analysis of the interaction between these polymorphic variants has been scant due in no small part to the difficulties in mathematically modeling such interactions. Table 4.1 summarizes the polymorphic loci that have been demonstrated by at least three independent groups to be associated with diabetic vascular disease. Discrepancies between studies in the apparent importance of a given polymorphism may be due to several factors: population

stratification; small population size in the study; interacting polymorphic loci, which make the importance of that particular polymorphism only apply in a specific population or ethnic group.

Significance for the individual patient-applications of polymorphic allele determination and theranostics

While population-based prospective studies have established the importance of controlling hyperglycemia, it is readily apparent that individual patients develop these complications in a manner that cannot be entirely explained by glycemic control. Theranostics provides physicians a comprehensive set of tools that can indicate changes in the health status of an individual, both toward the onset of disease or increasingly, with the application of pharmacogenetics and treatments based on genomics, toward a likely response to a particular therapy. The result of this approach will be a transition from health care centered on 'sickness services' to one focused on maintaining wellness.

Patients identified as having any one of the above allelic variants may benefit from more aggressive control of not only their hyperglycemia but also their co-morbid risk factors such as hypertension, hypercholesterolemia and obesity in attempting to reduce their risk of developing vascular disease. For example, it is presently recommended by the American Heart Association that the target level of LDL cholesterol and the level at which the physician begins medical therapy with lipid lowering agents is dependent upon the number of cardiac risk factors. An additional role for influencing the treatment algorithm of an individual patient is in the use of different medical procedures for

Gene	Complication
NOS3	Diabetic nephropathy
Aldose reductase	Diabetic nephropathy
Paraoxonase	Cardiovascular disease
Haptoglobin	Cardiovascular disease (and restenosis)

Table 4.1
Complication candidate genes demonstrated in at least three independent studies

diabetic patients with different genetic backgrounds. For example, the BARI study has shown that diabetic patients do better with CABG (by-pass surgery) as compared to angioplasty, in large part due to the increased risk of restenois in the diabetic patient. However, if it is possible to identify a diabetic cohort that is not at increased risk of restenosis (i.e. haptoglobin Type 1–1) angioplasty may be superior to CABG. This would result in a dramatic reduction in CABG-induced morbidity and health care costs.

We anticipate that health care in the future will become individually tailored to the patient's genetic makeup. His or her genetic makeup will be readily determined by use of currently available gene chip technology, which should permit identification of hundreds of allelic polymorphisms in a given patient from several cc of blood. The functional basis for many of these polymorphisms is still not entirely understood but will be necessary in order to translate this diagnostic information into new treatment stratagems.

References

1. Diabetes Control and Complications Trial Research Group. The effect of intensive treatment of diabetes on the development and progression of long term complications in insulin dependent diabetes mellitus. New Engl J Med 1993; 329: 977–86.
2. Diabetes Control and Complications Trial Research Group. The relationship of glycemic exposure (HbA1c) to the risk of development and progression of retinopathy in the Diabetes Control and Complication Trial. Diabetes 1995; 44: 968–83.
3. UK Prospective Diabetes Study Group. Intensive blood glucose control with sulphonylureas or insulin compared with conventional treatment and risk of complications in patients with Type 2 diabetes (UKPDS). Lancet 1998; 352: 837–53.
4. Ritz E, Orth SR. Nephropathy in patients with type II diabetes mellitus. New Engl J Med 1999; 341: 1127–33.
5. Reichard P, Nilsson BY, Rosenquist U. The effect of long-term intensified insulin treatment on the development of microvascular complications of diabetes mellitus. New Engl J Med 1993; 329: 304–9.
6. Warram JH, Gearin G, Laffel L, Krolewski AS. Effect of duration of type I diabetes on the prevalence of stages of diabetic nephropathy defined by urinary albumin/creatinine ratio. J Am Soc Nephrol 1996; 7: 930–7.
7. Hammoud T, Tanguay JF, Bourassa MG. Management of coronary artery disease: therapeutic options in patients with diabetes. J Am Coll Cardiol 2000; 36: 355–65.
8. Carrozza JP, Kuntz RE, Fishman RF, Baim DS. Restenosis after arterial injury caused by coronary stenting in patients with diabetes mellitus. Ann Intern Med 1993; 118: 344–9.
9. BARI investigators. Comparison of coronary artery bypass surgery with angioplasty in patients with multivessel disease. New Engl J Med 1996; 335: 217–25.
10. BARI investigators. Influence of diabetes on 5-year mortality and morbidity in a randomized trial comparing PTCA and CABG in patients with multivessel disease: the Bypass Angioplasty Revascularization Investigation (BARI). Circulation 1997; 96: 1761–9.
11. Nishikawa T, Edelstein D, Du X et al. Normalizing mitochondrial superoxide production blocks three pathways of hyperglycemic damage. Nature 2000; 404: 787–90.
12. Suzuki D, Miyata T, Saotome N et al. Immunochemical evidence for an increased oxidative stress and carbonyl modification of proteins in diabetic glomerular lesions. J Am Soc Nephrol 1999; 10: 822–32.
13. Suzuki D, Miyata T. Carbonyl stress in the pathogenesis of diabetic nephropathy. Intern Med 1999; 38: 309–14.
14. Horrie K, Miyata T, Maeda K et al. Immunohistochemical colocalization of glycoxidative products and lipid peroxidation products in diabetic renal glomerular lesions. Implications for glycoxidative stress in the pathogenesis of diabetic nephropathy. J Clin Invest 1997; 100: 2995–3004.

15. Pollman MJ, Hall JL, Gibbons GH. Determinants of vascular smooth muscle apoptosis after balloon angioplasty injury. Influence of redox state and cell phenotype. Circ Res 1999; 84: 113–21.

16. Schneider JE, Berk BC, Gravanis MB et al. Probucol decreases neointimal formation in a swine model of coronary artery balloon injury. A possible role for antioxidants in restenosis. Circ 1993; 88: 628–37.

17. Tardif JC, Cote G, Lesperance J et al. Probucol and multivitamins in the prevention of restenosis after coronary angioplasty. Multivitamins and probucol study group. New Engl J Med 1997; 337: 365–72.

18. Chowdhury TA, Kumar S, Barnett AH, Bain SC. Nephropathy in type I diabetes: the role of genetic factors. Diabet Med 1995; 12: 1059–67.

19. Parving HH, Tarnow L, Rossing P. Genetics of diabetic nephropathy. J Am Soc Nephrol 1996; 7: 2509–17.

20. Ruiz J. Diabetes mellitus and late complications: influence of the genetic factors. Diabet Med 1997; 23S2: 57–63.

21. Chowdhury TA, Dyer PH, Kumar S et al. Genetic determinants of diabetic nephropathy. 1999; Clin Sci 96: 221–30.

22. Marre M. Genetics and prediction of complications in type I diabetes. Diabetes Care 1999; 22S: B53–8.

23. Imperatore G, Hanson RL, Pettitt DJ et al. Sib-pair linkage analysis for susceptibility genes for microvascular complications among Pima Indians with Type 2 Diabetes. Diabetes 1998; 47: 821–30.

24. Mallamaci F, Zuccala A, Zoccali C et al. The deletion polymorphism of the angiotensin-converting enzyme is associated with nephro-angiosclerosis. Am J Hypertens 2000; 13: 433–7.

25. van Ittersum FJ, de Man AM, Thijssen S et al. Genetic polymorphisms of the renin-angiotensin system and complications of insulin-dependent diabetes mellitus. Nephrol Dial Transplant 2000; 15: 1000–7.

26. Chistiakov DA, Chugunova LA, Shamkhalova MS et al. Polymorphism of gene encoding vascular angiotensin II receptor and micro-angiopathies in patients with insulin dependent diabetes mellitus. Genetika 1999; 35: 1289–93.

27. Chuang LM, Chiu KC, Chiang FT et al. Insertion/deletion polymorphism of the angiotensin I-converting enzyme gene in patients with hypertension, non-insulin dependent diabetes mellitus, and coronary heart disease in Taiwan. Metabolism 1997; 46: 1211–14.

28. Miura J, Uchigata Y, Yokoyama H et al. Genetic polymorphisms of renin-angiotensin system is not associated with diabetic vascular complications in Japanese subjects with long-term insulin dependent diabetes mellitus. Diabetes Res Clin Pract 1999; 45: 41–9.

29. Kitamura H, Moriyama T, Izumi M et al. Angiotensin 1-converting enzyme insertion/deletion polymorphism: potential significance in nephrology. Kidney Int Suppl 1996; 55: S101–3.

30. Solini A, Giacchetti G, Sfriso A et al. Polymorphisms of angiotensin-converting enzyme and angiotensinogen genes in Type 2 diabetic sibships in relation to albumin excretion rate. Am J Kidney Dis 1999; 34: 1002–9.

31. Nagi DK, Mansfield, MW, Stickland MH, Grant PJ. Angiotensin converting enzyme insertion/deletion polymorphism and diabetic retinopathy in subjects with IDDM and NIDDM. Diabet Med 1995; 12: 997–1001.

32. Hadjadj S, Belloum R, Bouhanick B et al. Prognostic value of angiotensin-I converting enzyme I/D polymorphism for nephropathy in type I diabetes mellitus: a prospective study. J Am Soc Nephrol 2001; 12: 541–9.

33. Doria A, Onuma T, Warram JH, Krolewsi AS. Synergistic effect of angiotensin-II type I receptor genotype and poor glycemic control on risk of nephropathy in IDDM. Diabetologia 1997; 40: 1293–9.

34. Krolewski AS. Genetics of diabetic nephropathy: evidence for major and minor gene effects. Kidney Int 1999; 55: 1582–96.

35. Doria A, Onuma T, Gearin G et al. Angiotensinogen polymorphism M235T, hypertension, and nephropathy in insulin dependent diabetes. Hypertension 1996; 27: 1134–9.

36. Sliwa-Strojek K, Grzeszczak W, Romaniuk W et al. Polymorphism of the chymase gene and development of retinopathy in Type 2 diabetic patients. Pol Arch Med Wewn 2000; 104: 363–9.

37. Warpeha KM, Xu W, Liu L et al. Genotyping and functional analysis of a polymorphic

(CCTTT)(n) repeat of NOS2A in diabetic retinopathy. FASEB J 1999; 13: 1825–32.

38. Neugebauer S, Baba T, Watanbe T. Association of the nitric oxide synthase gene polymorphism with an increased risk for progression to diabetic nephropathy in Type 2 diabetes. Diabetes 2000; 49: 500–3.

39. Fujita H, Narita T, Meguro H et al. Lack of association between an ecNOS gene polymorphism and diabetic nephropathy in Type 2 diabetic patients with proliferative diabetic retinopathy. Horm Met Res 2000; 32: 80–3.

40. Yokota M, Ichihara S, Lin TL et al. Association of a T29→C polymorphism of the transforming growth factor-beta gene with genetic susceptibility to myocardial infarction in Japanese. Circulation 2000; 101: 2783–7.

41. Pociot F, Hansen PM, Karlsen AE et al. TGF-beta gene mutations in insulin-dependent diabetes mellitus and diabetic nephropathy. J Am Soc Nephrol 1998; 9: 2302–7.

42. Freedman BI, Yu H, Spray BJ et al. Genetic linkage analysis of growth factor loci and end-stage renal disease in African Americans. Kidney Int 1997; 51: 819–25.

43. Poirer O, Nicaud V, Vionnet N et al. Polymorphism screening of four genes encoding advanced glycation end-product putative receptors. Association study with nephropathy in Type 1 diabetic patients. Diabetes 2001; 50: 1214–18.

44. Hudson BI, Strickland MH, Futers TS, Grant PJ. Effects of novel polymorphisms in the RAGE gene on transcriptional regulation and their association with diabetic retinopathy. Diabetes 2001; 50: 1505–11.

45. Ng DP, Conn J, Chung SS, Larkins RG. Aldose reductase (AC)n microsatellite polymorphism and diabetic microvascular complications in Caucasian Type 1 diabetes mellitus. Diabetes Res Clin Pract 2001; 52: 21–7.

46. Lee SC, Wang Y, Ko GT et al. Association of retinopathy with a microsatellite at 5' end of the aldose reductase gene in Chinese patients with late-onset Type 2 diabetes. Ophthalmic Genet 2001; 22: 63–7.

47. Ichikawa F, Yamada K, Ishiyama-Shigemoto S et al. Association of an A-C dinucleotide repeat polymorphic marker at the 5' region of the aldose reductase gene with retinopathy but not with nephropathy or neuropathy in Japanese patients with Type 2 diabetes mellitus. Diabet Met 1999; 16: 744–8.

48. Demaine A, Cross D, Millward A. Polymorphisms of the aldose reductase gene and susceptibility to retinopathy in Type 1 diabetes mellitus. Invest Ophthalmol 2000; 41: 4064–8.

49. Iserman B, Schmidt S, Bierhaus A et al. CA dinucleotide repeat polymorphism at the 5' end of the aldose reductase gene is not associated with microangiopathy in Caucasians with long term diabetes mellitus Type 1. Nephrol Dial Transplant 2000; 15: 918–20.

50. Moczulski DK, Scott L, Antonellis A et al. Aldose reductase gene polymorphisms and susceptibility to diabetic nephropathy in Type 1 diabetes mellitus. Diabet Med 2000; 17: 111–18.

51. Kao YL, Donaghue K, Chan A et al. An aldose reductase intragenic polymorphism associated with diabetic retinopathy. Diabetes Res Clin Pract 1999; 46: 155–60.

52. Olmos P, Futers S, Acosta AM et al. AC polymorphism of the aldose reductase gene and fast progression of retinopathy in Chilean Type 2 diabetics. Diabetes Res Clin Pract 2000; 47: 169–76.

53. Hodgkinson AD, Millward BA, Demaine AG. Polymorphisms of the glucose transporter (GLUT1) gene are associated with diabetic nephropathy. Kidney Int 2001; 59: 985–9.

54. Grzeszczak W, Moczulski DK, Zychma M et al. Role of Glut-1 gene in susceptibility to diabetic nephropathy in Type 2 diabetes. Kidney Int 2001; 59: 631–6.

55. Liu ZH, Guan TJ, Chen ZH, Liu LS. Glucose transporter (Glut1) allele Xba-1 associated with nephropathy in non-insulin dependent diabetes mellitus. Kidney Int 1999; 55: 1843–8.

56. Gutierrez C, Vendrell J, Pastor R et al. Glut1 gene polymorphism in non-insulin dependent diabetes mellitus: genetic susceptibility relationship with cardiovascular risk factors and microangiopathic complications in a Mediterranean population. Diabetes Res Clin Pract. 1998; 41: 113–20.

57. Levy AP, Roguin A, Marsh S et al. Haptoglobin phenotype and vascular complications in diabetes. N Engl J Med 2000; 343: 369–70.

58. Nakhoul F, Marsh S, Hochberg I et al. Haptoglobin phenotype and diabetic retinopathy. JAMA 2000; 284: 1244–5.

59. Nakhoul F, Zoabi R, Kantor Y et al. Haptoglobin phenotype and diabetic nephropathy. Diabetologia 2001; 44: 602–4.

60. Roguin A, Hochberg I, Nikolsky E et al. Haptoglobin phenotype as a predictor of restenosis after percutaneous transluminal coronary angioplasty. Am J Cardiol 2001; 87: 330–2.

61. Frank M, Lache O, Enav B et al. Structure function relationship of the antioxidant properties of hapatglobin. Blood 2001; in press.

62. Kristiansen M, Graverson JH, Jacobsen C et al. Identification of the hemoglobin scavenger receptor. Nature 2001; 409: 1998–201.

63. Shpichinetsky V, Raz I, Friedlander Y et al. The association beween two common mutations C677T and A1298C in human methylenetetrahydrofolate reductase gene and the risk for diabetic nephropathy in type II diabetic patients. J Nutr 2000; 30: 2493–7.

64. Gulec S, Aras O, Akar E et al. Methylenetetrahydrofolate reductase gene polymorphism and risk of premature myocardial infarction. Clin Cardiol 2001; 24: 281–4.

65. Matsunaga H, Tanaka Y, Tanaka M et al. Antiatherogenic mitochondrial genotype in patients with Type 2 diabetes. Diabetes Care 2001; 24: 500–3.

66. Garin MC, James RW, Dussoix P et al. Paraoxanase polymorphism Met-Leu54 is associated with modified serum concentrations of the enzyme. A possible link between the paraoxonase gene and increased risk of cardiovascular disease in diabetes. J Clin Invest 1997; 99: 62–6.

67. James RW, Leviev I, Ruiz J et al. Promoter polymorphism T(-107)C of the paraoxonase PON1 gene is a risk factor for coronary heart disease in Type 2 diabetic patients. Diabetes 2000; 49: 1390–3.

68. Araki S, Makita Y, Canani L et al. Polymorphisms of human paraoxonase I gene and susceptibility to diabetic nephropathy in Type 1 diabetes mellitus. Diabetologia 2000; 43: 1540–3.

69. Pininzzotto M, Castillo E, Fiaux M et al. Paroxonase 2 polymorphisms are associated with nephropathy in Type 2 diabetes. Diabetologia 2001; 44: 104–7.

70. Durrington PN, Mackness B, Mackness MI. Paraoxonase and atherosclerosis. Arterioscler Thromb Vasc Biol 2001; 21: 473–80.

71. Osei-Hyiaman D, Hou L, Mengbai F et al. Coronary artery disease risk in Chinese Type 2 diabetics: is there a role for paraoxonase 1 gene (Q192R) polymorphism? Eur J Endo 2001; 144: 639–44.

72. Aviram M. Review of human studies on oxidative damage and antioxidant protection related to cardiovascular disease. Free Radic Res 2000; 33S: S85–97.

73. Araki S, Moczulski DK, Hanna L et al. APOE polymorphisms and the development of diabetic nephropathy in Type 1 diabetes: results of case–control and family-based studies. Diabetes 2000; 49: 2190–5.

74. Vauhkonen I, Nishanen L, Ryynanen M et al. Divergent association of apoliprotein E polymorphism with vascular disease in patients with NIDDM and control subjects. Diabet Met 1997; 14: 748–56.

75. Boemi M, Sirolla C, Amadio L et al. Apolipoprotein E polymorphism as a risk factor for vascular disease in diabetic patients. Diabetes Care 1995; 18: 504–8.

76. Kataoka S, Robbins DC, Cowan LD et al. Apolipoprotein E polymorphism in American Indians and its relation to plasma lipoproteins and diabetes. The Strong Heart Study. Arterioscler Thromb Vasc Biol 1996; 16: 918–25.

77. Gazzaruso C, Garzaniti A, Geroldi D, Finardi G. Genetics and cardiovascular risk: a role for apolipoprotein (a) polymorphism. Cardiologia 1999; 44: 347–54.

78. Wong TY, Poon P, Szeto CC et al. Association of plasminogen activator inhibitor-1 4G/4G genotype and Type 2 diabetic nephropathy in Chinese patients. Kidney Int 2000; 57: 632–8.

79. Tarnow L, Stehouwer CD, Emeis JJ et al. Plasminogen activator inhibitor- and apolipoprotein E gene polymorphisms and diabetic angiopathy. Nephrol Dial Transplant 2000; 15: 625–30.

80. Lam KS, Ma OC, Wat NM et al. Beta fibrinogen gene G/A 455 polymorphism in relation to fibrinogen concentrations and ischemic heart disease in Chinese patients with type II diabetes. Diabetologia 1999; 42: 1250–3.

81. Raffel LJ, VadheimCM, Roth MP et al. The 5' insulin gene polymorphism and the genetics of vascular complications in Type 1 diabetes mellitus. Diabetologia 1991; 34: 680–3.

82. Kankova K, Muzik J, Karaskova J et al. Duration of non-insulin dependent diabetes mellitus and the TNF beta Nco genotype as predictive factors in proliferative diabetic retinopathy. Ophthalmology 2001; 215: 294–8.

5

Substance abuse and diabetes

Marian A Parrott

Introduction

Throughout history, human beings have used a variety of substances to produce or enhance pleasure, or to dull negative emotions and experiences such as pain, fear or ennui. Certainly the most prevalent of these substances is alcohol, followed by tobacco. Other substances, including narcotics, stimulants, sedative hypnotics, tobacco, and hallucinogens, have been used to different degrees by some individuals and subcultures. Even caffeine is a mood-altering and habit-forming drug, and subject to abuse, although generally innocuous for most people in small amounts. Cultural attitudes toward this recreational or non-medicinal drug use vary from strict proscription and severe punishment to tolerance and even inclusion of these substances in religious rituals, from sacramental wine to peyote.

Substance abuse is problematic because it may impair health as well as the ability to perform important motor tasks, such as driving a car, and important social roles such as parenting or being employed. Once again alcohol, perhaps because it is legal and readily available in many cultures, is overwhelmingly the largest offender, causing thousands of deaths from overdose, medical complications such as cirrhosis of the liver, motor vehicle accidents and other trauma as well as losses in productivity and disruption of family life. Nicotine obtained by smoking tobacco is overwhelmingly the most lethal of all abused substances in terms of number of deaths caused by direct effects, although smokers are not as likely to have accidents or to fail to perform adequately in social roles as are alcoholics. Use of alcohol, tobacco and illicit drugs generally begins in adolescence, and research shows that adolescents with diabetes are as likely to engage in use of these substances as are young people in general.[1,2]

Despite the many problems caused by alcohol, there may be benefits to its moderate use that make it acceptable for some people. Caffeine in modest amounts (150 mg/day or the equivalent of three cups of coffee a day or less) is probably safe for most people with diabetes.[3] Other substances commonly abused have no known health benefits. Legal and appropriate prescription use of narcotics, sedative hypnotic and other agents may, like any drugs, impact glycemic control or result in drug–drug interactions, but the purpose of this chapter is to describe the impact of recreational or non-medical uses of these drugs on diabetes patients.

There is an extensive body of literature concerning the role of alcohol in the etiology of diabetes, on glycemic control, and on the incidence of complications. The effects of alcohol on diabetes are complex and dose dependent; alcohol consumption affects the risk of developing diabetes, the day-to-day diabetes management and the development of both short-term and long-term complications. Similarly, there is a considerable body of knowledge concerning the effects of smoking on persons with diabetes. For other forms of substance abuse, the literature is not as extensive and consists mainly of case reports and other anecdotal accounts, as human experimentation of this area is obviously very limited and animal research may not be generalizable to human subjects.

Alcohol and diabetes

Epidemiology

According to the World Health Organization,[4] the prevalence of alcohol use disorders (harmful use and dependence) averages about 2.8% in men and 0.5% in women worldwide. Rates vary across cultures; from very low in some Middle Eastern countries to over 5% in North America and Eastern Europe. Alcohol abuse is an emerging problem in developing countries and among indigenous populations. Epidemiological evidence indicates that people with diabetes may be somewhat less likely to use alcohol than people without diabetes. Approximately 10% of the US population abuses alcohol, with about 50% reporting some alcohol consumption.[5]

The role of alcohol in the etiology of diabetes

There is some evidence of a 'U'- or 'J'-shaped curve relating alcohol consumption and the risk of developing diabetes.[6-8] This may reflect increased insulin sensitivity.[9] That is, persons consuming moderate amounts of alcohol may be slightly less likely than non-drinkers to develop Type 2 diabetes, whereas heavy alcohol users are more likely than non-users or moderate drinkers to develop diabetes. The pathophysiologic mechanisms to account for

these findings are not clear. Alcohol may improve insulin sensitivity when consumed in small amounts. At higher levels of intake, alcohol may interfere with insulin-mediated glucose disposal, causing insulin resistance.[10] A secondary cause of diabetes in heavy drinkers may be chronic pancreatitis or cirrhosis of the liver; here the mechanism is more clear-cut as there is either direct damage to the pancreatic beta cells, as in pancreatitis, or increased insulin resistance associated with cirrhosis[11] from alcohol.

Impact of consumption on the management of diabetes

Alcohol consumption may affect the management of diabetes in a number of ways. Excessive alcohol consumption may cause hyperglycemia initially and may result in hypoglycemia several hours later because of decreased hepatic glucose production. In particular, when alcohol is consumed in moderate amounts or greater (>50 g) in the evening, the fasting or morning postprandial glucose may be low the following morning.[12] This effect is more pronounced if the alcohol is consumed after, not with, the evening meal. This hypoglycemia is not ameliorated by glucagons, as it is not a result of excessive insulin action, but rather reflects depletion of liver glycogen stores.[13] Small amounts of alcohol ingested with food have no acute effect on blood glucose or insulin levels and need not be included in calculations of carbohydrate intake for purposes of insulin adjustment.[3]

Alcohol may also raise blood pressure; hypertension is a common co-morbidity of diabetes, which increases the risk of both micro- and macrovascular complications of diabetes.[14] This effect is dose-related and may occur even at moderate levels of alcohol consumption, generally defined as one drink/day for women and 2 drinks/day for men (1 oz of alcohol, which is the amount in 5 oz wine, 1½ oz liquor or spirits, or 12 oz beer, each of which contains approximately 15 g of alcohol). When patients with diabetes and hypertension experience difficulties in achieving goals for blood pressure control, clinicians should review the patient's alcohol consumption pattern and decrease or eliminate alcohol.

The American Diabetes Association (ADA) has recently published revised nutrition recommendations, including recommendation for alcohol intake.[3] These recommendations are based on an extensive review and analyses of the medical literature. The association's recommendations are presented in Table 5.1.

Indirect effects of alcohol consumption on diabetes management

Alcohol may effect diabetes management indirectly by influencing diet and compliance with insulin or oral antidiabetes agents. Heavy consumers of alcohol may neglect to consume other important nutrients; the neurological complications of diabetes such as peripheral neuropathy and Wernicke-Korsakoff syndrome are thought to be caused at least in part by severe nutritional deficiencies accompanying chronic alcohol abuse, particularly thiamine deficiency. Heavy drinkers are more likely to have poor glycemic control and to be hospitalized for diabetic ketoacidosis, which may occasionally be confused with alcoholic ketoacidosis in patients with hyperglycemia.

Drug–alcohol interactions in diabetes

Alcohol may interact with drugs used to treat diabetes. Patients with alcoholic liver disease, or patients with a drinking pattern which

There is strong evidence for the following statements:
- If individuals choose to drink alcohol, daily intake should be limited to one drink for adult women and two drinks for adult men. One drink is defined as a 12-oz beer, 5-oz glass of wine, or 1.5-oz glass of distilled spirits.
- The type of alcoholic beverage consumed does not make a difference.
- When moderate amounts of alcohol are consumed with food, blood glucose levels are not affected.
- To reduce the risk of hypoglycemia, alcohol should be consumed with food.
- Ingestion of light-to-moderate amounts of alcohol does not raise blood pressure; excessive, chronic ingestion of alcohol raises blood pressure and may be a risk factor for stroke.
- Pregnant women and people with medical problems such as pancreatitis, advanced neuropathy, severe hypertriglyceridemia, or alcohol abuse should be advised not to ingest alcohol.

There is some evidence for the following statement:
- There are potential benefits from the ingestion of moderate amounts of alcohol, such as decreased risk of Type 2 diabetes, coronary heart disease, and stroke.

The following statement is based on expert consensus:
- Alcoholic beverages should be considered an addition to the regular food/meal plan for all patients with diabetes. No food should be omitted.

Table 5.1
Recommendations regarding diabetes and alcohol intake. Reproduced from Franz et al.[3]

places them at risk for acute liver toxicity, should not use metformin as this may increase the risk of lactic acidosis.

Though seldom used today, older sulfonylurea agents may have significant interactions with alcohol. Ethanol may cause induction of the metabolism of tolbutamide, with a resultant reduction in the effectiveness of the medication. Approximately 30% of patients who take chlorpropamide and consume alcohol experience a disulfiram (Antabuse®)-like reaction. Heavy consumption of alcohol is a risk factor for metabolic acidosis. The use of metformin in a patient who binge drinks may place the patient at a high risk for acidosis; hence, metformin should be used with caution in patients who consume excessive amounts of ethanol.[15]

Alcohol and diabetes complications

Alcohol can contribute to the development of both acute and chronic diabetes complications. Acute complications of diabetes include diabetic ketoacidosis (DKA), hyperosmolar nonketotic states, and hypoglycemia. In addition to direct effects of alcohol on glucose metabolism, the impairments in judgment and motor skills accompanying alcohol intoxication may result in missed doses of insulin or oral agents with resulting DKA or hyperosmolar coma, or may be associated with decreased food intake and hypoglycemia. In some populations, such as the urban poor, non-compliance with drug therapy and dietary recommendations related to heavy alcohol consumption may play a major role in the development of DKA.[16]

Patients with diabetes, especially Type 1, who are using insulin regimens to achieve tight glycemic control, may experience hypoglycemia, either immediately after drinking or as a later consequence. Evening alcohol consumption has been shown to result in delayed hypoglycemia. In one study, both fasting and morning postprandial glucose levels were lowered, and several subjects required treatment for symptomatic hyperglycemia after 10 a.m. the following morning. This effect may be caused by a decrease in growth hormone secretion.[17] Patients who choose to use alcohol should be warned of this possibility and counseled to take appropriate precautions, such as decreasing evening doses of long acting insulin or eating a bedtime snack as well as limiting intake to no more than the recommended amounts of 1 drink/day for women and 2 drinks/day for men. Alcohol should never be consumed in a fasting state by patients using insulin or insulin secretogogues because of the risk of hypoglycemia caused by decreased hepatic gluconeogenesis. Patients experiencing severe hypoglycemia are more likely to drink ethanol than patients who do not have severe hypoglycemia.[18]

Alcohol influences the development of chronic diabetes complications in a number of ways. Moderate alcohol intake has been associated with a decreased incidence of CAD in a substantial number of observational studies.[19] The mechanism of this reduction is postulated to be an increase in high-density lipoprotein as well as possibly a decrease in insulin resistance.

Caution must be used when interpreting these results however, as they are subject to the same bias common to all observational studies. Results may be biased by the presence of unmeasured differences between moderate drinkers and non-drinkers, or the adjustment for observed differences may be incomplete. For example, non-drinkers may be persons who avoid alcohol because of known health problems; nevertheless, these findings have been replicated in many studies in different parts of the world, and have biological plausibility. In contrast, excessive use of alcohol is clearly associated with increased cardiovascular events and stroke. In light of the possible protective effects of light to moderate drinking, the American Diabetes Association has suggested that persons who choose to drink may be told that they can do so in moderation, which translates into one drink daily for women and two for men.[3] Health care providers should not encourage non-drinkers to begin drinking to reduce their risk of heart disease, because it is difficult to predict who will develop problem drinking or alcohol dependence. Finally, teenagers and young people should not be encouraged to drink alcohol for preventive purposes, because all of the studies demonstrating this effect were done in middle aged and older people at much higher risk of heart disease.

Contraindications to alcohol

Alcohol should be completely avoided by patients with neuropathy or cardiomyopathy, as alcohol alone can cause both conditions as well as potentially exacerbate them in patients with diabetes as the primary cause. There is no evidence linking alcohol use and nephropathy or retinopathy independent of effects of drinking on glycemic and blood pressure control.[20] Women who are pregnant or contemplating pregnancy should abstain from alcohol because of the risk of fetal alcohol syndrome, which consists of mental retardation and characteristic facial dysmorphism. Persons with a personal or family history of alcohol dependence or abuse should avoid alcohol. Patients who use metformin should drink very moderately if at all, because of the risk of lactic acidosis in patients with liver dysfunction who use metformin. Patients with diabetes should never drink and drive; the presence of any amount of alcohol on a breathalyzer test or noticeable on the patient's breath may result in serious hypoglycemia being mistaken for alcohol intoxication by law enforcement personnel,

which may result in delayed treatment and death. Patients with Type 1 diabetes have not been shown to obtain the cardiovascular benefits of moderate drinking from alcohol consumption and are more likely to experience hypoglycemia as a consequence; thus these patients should consume alcohol with caution, if at all.

Counseling and management in clinical practice

Health care providers should routinely query patients about alcohol consumption. Several simple screening questionnaires, with reasonably good sensitivity and specificity may be used for the purpose. The CAGE questionnaire (Table 5.2) is widely used, has been validated in numerous populations, and is easy to remember. Persons who are identified as problem drinkers or potential problem drinkers may be referred to treatment programs and self-help groups such as Alcoholics Anonymous. Although relapse is frequent, such

Have you ever felt you should cut down on your drinking?

Have people annoyed you by criticizing your drinking?

Have you ever felt bad or guilty about your drinking?

Have you ever had a drink first thing in the morning to steady your nerves or to get rid of a hangover (eye opener)?

Table 5.2
CAGE questionnaire. Reproduced from Mayfield et al.[29]

programs do succeed in many patients. Children and adolescents should be asked about drinking and offered anticipatory guidance to help them to develop strategies for resisting peer pressure to consume alcohol. Adults who have chosen to drink in moderation should be informed of the risks and benefits and any contraindications. Women of childbearing potential should be counseled about the potential effects of alcohol on the developing fetus; women with diabetes contemplating pregnancy should receive preconception care, i.e. a program of intensive glycemic control, which has been shown to improve outcomes for children of mothers with diabetes.[21]

Tobacco

Epidemiology

Tobacco is the leading preventable cause of death in most Western countries, Japan and China, although obesity is rapidly overtaking tobacco in the USA, as the prevalence of smoking has decreased while that of obesity has increased in recent decades. There are over 1 billion smokers worldwide. In the USA smoking causes over 400,000 deaths annually and accounts for about half of all deaths in smokers. Although there have been decreases in smoking in recent decades in response to public health efforts and changing attitudes toward smoking, about 25% of the adult population still smokes in the USA. Worldwide, it is estimated that smoking caused about 4 million deaths in 1998 and this figure is expected to increase rapidly, especially in the developing world.[4] People with diabetes have smoking patterns similar to the rest of the population. Unlike alcohol, there are no significant health benefits from smoking in any amount. Any small benefits such as a possible slight decrease in

the incidence of estrogen-dependent cancers is greatly outweighed by the harmful effects, and this is especially true of patients with diabetes. People with diabetes who smoke are not only subject to the same hazards of smoking that are seen in the general population, such as lung, oral pharyngeal, laryngeal, esophageal and bladder cancers, an increase in cardiovascular disease, and chronic obstructive lung disease, but also at greater risk for both micro- and macrovascular complications specific to diabetes. Recent studies also demonstrate a link between smoking and the development of diabetes.

Smoking and diabetes etiology

Smoking has been shown to increase the incidence of diabetes in several cohort studies. The magnitude of this effect is moderate; smoking is estimated to increase the incidence of diabetes by 1.5–3-fold.[22,23] The mechanism of this effect is not known but may be that smoking contributes to upper body obesity, which is associated with the metabolic syndrome of central obesity, insulin resistance, glucose intolerance or overt diabetes, hypertension and dyslipidemia.

Smoking and diabetes management

Persons with an established diagnosis of diabetes may experience poor metabolic control as a result of insulin resistance as well as increases in growth hormone, arginine vasopressin and cortisol.[21] Smoking also raises systolic blood pressure and makes hypertension more difficult to control. Hypertension is a common co-morbidity of diabetes and increases the risk of a cardiovascular event $\times$ percent for each 10 mmHg rise in systolic blood pressure. Smoking cessation ameliorates these effects.

Smoking and diabetes complications

Smoking is one of the major risk factors for cardiovascular disease, as is diabetes. These effects are additive. Smoking has been shown to be associated with increases in death rates for participants with diabetes in the Multiple Risk Factor Intervention Trial, the Finnish Prospective study, and the Paris Policeman's study. Peripheral vascular disease is also increased and contributes to the development of foot ulcers and amputations.

Smoking is also associated with the development of diabetic microvasular complications. Microalbuminuria and nephropathy are increased both in Type 1 and Type 2 patients with diabetes who smoke. Smoking also increases the risk of neuropathy in patients with diabetes. Smoking has not been shown to increase the incidence of retinopathy.[21]

Intervention strategies

Tobacco use generally begins in adolescence. Therefore, prevention of the initiation of smoking is an important component of anticipatory guidance in all children and adolescents, but especially those with diabetes. Unfortunately, despite frequent contact with health care providers and a chronic illness that greatly amplifies the hazards of smoking, teenagers with diabetes are about as likely to start smoking as other young people. In recent years there has been an increase in the proportion of teenage girls who smoke, perhaps a reflection of the perception that smoking is an effective way to remain slim.

Smoking cessation programs can reduce the prevalence of smoking and should be recommended to patients who smoke. Pharmacological aids to smoking cessation may be helpful. The antidepressant bupropion (Zyban®,

Assessment of smoking status and history
- Systematic documentation of a history of tobacco use must be obtained from all adolescent and adult individuals with diabetes.

Counseling on smoking prevention and cessation.
- All health care providers should advise individuals with diabetes not to initiate smoking. This advice should be consistently repeated to prevent smoking and other tobacco use among children and adolescents with diabetes under age 21 years.
- Among smokers, cessation counseling must be completed as a routine component of diabetes care.
- Every smoker should be urged to quit in a clear, strong, and personalized manner that describes the added risks of smoking and diabetes.
- Every diabetic smoker should be asked if he or she is willing to quit at this time.

If no, initiate brief and motivational discussion regarding the need to stop using tobacco, the risks of continued use, and encouragement to quit, as well as support when ready.

If yes, assess preference for and initiate either minimal, brief, or intensive cessation counseling and offer pharmacological supplements as appropriate.

Effective systems for delivery of smoking cessation
- Training of all diabetes health care providers in the Agency for Health Care Policy and Research Guidelines regarding smoking should be implemented.
- Follow-up procedures designed to assess and promote quitting status must be arranged for all diabetic smokers.

Table 5.3
Recommendations regarding diabetes and smoking. Reproduced with permission from American Diabetes Association[30]

Burroughs Wellcome) and nicotine patches or gum can be useful for some patients and certainly are safer than smoking. It has been demonstrated in clinical trials that patients who are advised to stop smoking by a health professional are more likely to stop than are patients who are not so advised. Despite this, many smokers report that no health care provider has ever discussed smoking cessation with them.

The American Diabetes Association recommends smoking assessment and intervention to promote smoking cessation (Table 5.3). These recommendations are based on extensive evidence documenting the harm of smoking for diabetes and on research demonstrating success of interventions to increase rates of smoking cessation in the general population.

Caffeine

Caffeine is a stimulant found in various plants, including coffee, tea, and some soft drinks especially colas, and chocolate. So ubiquitous is the use of caffeine that it is difficult to imagine how the work of the world would ever be done without it! Little specific research exists on the effect of caffeine on diabetes. Used in moderation, coffee may cause some glucose intolerance, but the clinical effect of this is unclear. Caffeine has been shown in some small studies to increase the symptoms of hypoglycemia and to sensitize users to levels of hypoglycemia not normally causing symptoms. For this reason, its use has been proposed as an adjunct to the therapy of hypoglycemia unawareness, although this has not been rigorously studied in patients with this problem.[22-24] The American Diabetes Association suggests that caffeine up to the amount of three cups of coffee/day, or about 150 mg, is probably safe for most people.[1] Caffeine avoidance is recommended for persons with mood or anxiety disorders, which are aggravated by caffeine

consumption, and for people with cardiac arrhythmia. Persons wanting to eliminate caffeine should do so gradually to avoid withdrawal symptoms, chiefly headache.

Marijuana

Marijuana use is probably the most commonly used illicit drug worldwide. The active agent in marijuana, delta-tetrahydrocannabinol, is generally obtained by smoking the dried leaves and stems of the plant, as well as in other forms such as hashish. No specific metabolic effects of marijuana on glucose metabolism have been described. However, marijuana has nutritional effects, which may impact on the management of diabetes.[25] These include increased appetite, particularly for sweets, and disinhibition of eating behavior. Marijuana may also impair judgment and reasoning skills, resulting in non-compliance or errors in judgment. Some medical uses have been proposed for marijuana, but there is no literature establishing the usefulness or safety of marijuana or its derivatives in the management of patients with diabetes.

Cocaine and other stimulants
Epidemiology

Cocaine is a potent stimulant with sympathomimetic activity. During the 1980s and continuing into the present century, the USA has experienced an epidemic increase in the use of crack cocaine. Cocaine may be smoked, inhaled, or injected and is commonly combined with other substances, such as alcohol, heroin or marijuana. Small amounts of data are available describing the incidence of cocaine abuse in patients with diabetes; the incidence in the general population is approximately 0.25% but may be higher in some subgroups, such as the urban poor.

Amphetamines are stimulants with adverse effects similar to those seen with cocaine. 'Ecstasy' (3,4-methylenedioxymethamphetamine, or MDMA) is a stimulant that produces euphoria, users often use and purchase this drug at 'raves' where young people may dance all night. Hypoglycemia or diabetic ketoacidosis may result.[26] Other acute effects include hypertension, hyperthermia, rhabdomyolysis, hyponatremia, cerebral infarction, disseminated intravascular coagulopathy, cardiac arrhythmias, and hepatic and renal failure.

Cocaine and diabetes etiology

No information is available regarding cocaine as a risk factor for the development of diabetes.

Cocaine and diabetes management

Cocaine users may experience acute tachycardia and hypertension, which may result in angina, arrhythmia, myocardial infarction, stroke and sudden death. Pregnant women may experience fetal loss, still birth and miscarriage, and premature delivery as well as an increase in neuropsychiatric abnormalities in the offspring. Patients with diabetes are already at increased cardiovascular risk and may be more likely to develop these complications. Cocaine may also causes seizures, which could be confused with or obscure hypoglycemia.

Hypoglycemia may result from decreased food intake and high activity levels, or hyperglycemia may result from failure to use insulin or oral agents. The euphoric state induced by cocaine and the intensity of craving and drug-seeking behavior reduce the ability of the user to engage in even simple self-care tasks such as eating meals and are certainly not compatible with the complex task of diabetes self-management.

Cocaine users who inject the drug are subject to all of the complications of intravenous drug use, which are described in the section on narcotic abuse.

Intervention strategies

Inquiring about illegal drug use should be a routine part of the medical history for new patients and should be updated periodically. Cocaine use should be considered in the differential diagnosis of patients with unexplained episodes of tachycardia, chest pain or seizures. Children and adolescents should be made aware of the risks of using cocaine. Cocaine users should be referred to drug treatment programs whenever possible.

Narcotics

Prescription narcotics have many legitimate uses for patients with severe acute or chronic pain and those with terminal illness. Because of a deficient receptor, patients with diabetes may be relatively insensitive to opiates. Prescription narcotics, such as hydromorphone (Dilaudid®), meperidine (Demerol®) and oxycycodone (Percocet®, Oxycontin®) may be abused by patients for whom they are prescribed or may be diverted to others. Most adverse effects of illegal, injected narcotics as well as other injected drugs of abuse relate to lack of sterile injection procedures and the presence of bacterial, fungal, or viral contaminants, the presence of chemical contaminants, and the lack of dose standardization in illegally supplied drugs. Infectious complications include diseases such as HIV, hepatitis C and bacterial endocarditis, skin abscess and Fournier's gangrene or necrotizing fasciitis. Chemical contaminants may cause allergic or toxic injuries, and lack of dose standardization may result in overdose. Patients with poor glycemic control may be especially vulnerable to infection.

Of note is that hepatitis C, of which intravenous drug use is a major cause, predisposes to the development of Type 2 diabetes. This may explain part of the surge in Type 2 diabetes seen in the last 30 years, as hepatitis C has reached epidemic proportions in many parts of the world. Thus, intravenous drug use may indirectly play a role in the etiology of diabetes.[27]

A substantial proportion, 44% in one survey, of IVDUs report obtaining needles from people with diabetes.[28] Insulin users should dispose of used needles and syringes in tamper resistant containers. Patients with diabetes in a family or neighborhood setting where there are IVDUs may wish to purchase separately packaged syringes and needles to ensure that their supply will not be surreptitiously used by others, placing the patient at risk for hepatitis or HIV.

Sedative-hypnotics

Drugs in this class include benzodiazapines, barbiturates and other sedating drugs. Acute behavioral effects may resemble those of alcohol. These drugs are habit forming and should be prescribed with caution to patients lacking a solid indication for their use.

Miscellaneous agents: hallucinogens, designer drugs, and phencyclidine

Hallucinogens such as LSD or mescaline cause visual and auditory distortions and hallucinations and may greatly affect the perception of the passage of time. The principal danger for diabetes patients is a lapse in self-care management and monitoring.

Numerous 'designer' drugs, in addition to 'Ecstasy', which is an amphetamine, have appeared on the drug scene in recent years. These include gamma-hydroxybutyrate, a sedative-hypnotic, and flunitrazepam, a benzodiazapine. Little is known about specific effects of these agents in patients with diabetes.

Summary

Patients with diabetes should be routinely asked about use of alcohol, tobacco, and recreational drugs. Patients, especially adolescents and young adults, should be warned of the consequences of recreational drug use on glycemic control, diabetes complications, and most importantly on the ability of users to participate in appropriate diabetes self-management activities. Patients who drink alcohol should be urged to do so in moderation and always with meals. Patients who smoke should be counseled about quitting at every scheduled diabetes visit and offered participation in programs for smoking cessation and pharmacological treatment. Users of illicit drugs should be referred to substance abuse programs and closely followed for their diabetes.

References

1. Jacobson AM, Hauser ST, Willett JB et al. Psychological adjustment to IDDM: 10 year follow-up of an onset cohort of child and adolescent patients. Diabetes Care 1997; 20: 811–18.
2. Glasgow AM, Tynan D, Schwartz R et al. Alcohol and drug use in teenagers with diabetes mellitus. J Adolesc Health 1991; 12: 11–14.
3. Franz MJ, Bantle JP, Beebe CA et al. Evidence-

based nutrition principles and recommendations for the treatment and prevention of diabetes and related complications (Technical Review). Diabetes Care 2002; 25: 148–98.

4. World Health Organization: http://www.who.int/whr/2001/main/en/chapter2/002e2.htm.

5. Centers for Disease Control: http://www.cdc.gov/nchs/fastats/alcohol.htm.

6. Ajani UA, Hennekens CH, Spelsberg A, Manson JE. Alcohol consumption and risk of Type 2 diabetes mellitus among US male physicians. Arch Intern Med 2000; 160: 1025–30.

7. Tsumura K, Hayashi T, Suematsu C et al. Daily alcohol consumption and the risk of Type 2 diabetes in Japanese men: the Osaka Health Study. Diabetes Care 1999; 22: 1432–7.

8. Wei M, Gibbons LW, Mitchell TL et al. Alcohol intake and incidence of type 2 diabetes in men. Diabetes Care 2000; 23: 18–22.

9. Bell RA, Mayer-Davis Elizabeth, Martin M et al. Association between alcohol consumption and insulin sensitivity and cardiovascular disease risk factors. Diabetes Care 2000; 23: 1630–6.

10. Vidal J, Ferrer JP, Esmatjes E et al. Diabetes mellitus in patients with liver cirrhosis. Diabetes Res Clin Pract 1994; 25: 19.

11. Yki-Jarvinen H, Nikkila EA. Ethanol decreases glucose utilization in healthy man. J Clin Endocrinol Metab 1985; 61: 941–5.

12. Turner BC, Jenkins E, Kerr D et al. The effect of evening alcohol consumption on next-morning glucose control in Type 1 diabetes. Diabetes Care 2001; 24: 1883–93.

13. Arky RA, Veverbrand E, Abramson EA. Irreversible hypoglycemia: a complication of alcohol and insulin. JAMA 1968; 206: 575–8.

14. Arauz-Pacheco C, Parrott MA, Raskin P. The treatment of hypertension in adult patients with diabetes (Technical Review). Diabetes Care 2002; 25: 134–47.

15. White JR, Campbell RK. Dangerous and common drug interactions in patients with diabetes mellitus. Endocrinol Metab Clin North Am 2000; 29: 789–802.

16. Hwang SW, Bugeja AL. Barriers to appropriate diabetes management among homeless people in Toronto. Can Med Assoc J 2000;163: 172–2.

17. Rimm EB, Klatsky A, Grobbee Stumpfer MJ. Review of moderate alcohol consumption and reduced risk of coronary heart disease: is the effect due to beer, wine, or spirits? BMJ 1996; 312: 731–6.

18. Ter Braak EW, Appelman AM, van de Laak M et al. Clinical characteristics of diabetic patients with and without severe hypoglycemia. Diabetes Care 2000; 23: 1467–71.

19. Levitt NS, Adams G, Salmon J et al. The prevalence and severity of microvascular complications in pancreatic diabetes and IDDM. Diabetes Care 1995;18: 971–4.

20. American Diabetes Association. Preconception care of women with diabetes (Position Paper). Diabetes Care 2002; 25: S82–S84.

21. Haire-Joshu D, Glasgow RE, Tibbs TL. Smoking and diabetes (Technical Review) Diabetes Care 1999; 22: 1887–98.

22. Kerr D, Sherwin RS, Pavalkis F et al. Effect of caffeine in the recognition of and responses to hypoglycemia in humans. Ann Intern Med 1993; 119: 799–804.

23. Rimm EB, Chan J, Stampfer MJ et al. Prospective study of cigarette smoking, alcohol use, and the risk of diabetes in men. BMJ 1995; 310: 555–59.

24. Keijzers B, De Galan BE, Tack, CJ, Smits P. Caffeine can decrease insulin sensitivity in humans. Diabetes Care 2002; 25: 364–9.

25. Mohs ME, Watson RR, Leonard-Green T. Nutritional effects of marijuana, heroin, cocaine, and nicotine. J Am Diet Assoc 1990; 90: 1261–7.

26. Seymour HR, Gilman D. Severe ketoacidosis complicated by 'ecstasy' ingestion and prolonged exercise. Diabet Med 1996; 13: 908–9.

27. Knobler H, Schattner A. Association of hepatitis C and diabetes mellitus. Ann Intern Med 2001; 135: 141.

28. Latkin CA, Forman VL. Patterns of needle acquisition and sociobehavioral correlates of needle exchange program attendance in Baltimore, Maryland, U.S.A. J Acquir Immun Defic Syndr 2001; 27: 398–404.

29. Mayfield D, McLeod G, Hall P. The CAGE questionnaire: validation of a new alcoholism instrument. Am J Psych 1974; 131: 1121–3.

30. American Diabetes Association. Smoking and diabetes (position paper). Diabetes Care 2002; 25: 580–1.

6

The St Vincent Declaration: experience gained for better outcome of cardiovascular, eye and kidney complications in the future

Massimo Massi Benedetti, Joyce Akwe Akwi, Piero Ferolla, Marco Orsini Federici

The St Vincent Declaration: the background

Quality of care has a fundamental role in determining disease outcomes in terms of physical and psychosocial well-being, especially for chronic disorders.[1] Poor quality of care can produce reduction of health, waste of resources and inequities.

Several experiences, in the past years, have shown a wide variation of care provided throughout Europe; moreover in some cases the quality of health care was far from set standards and recognized goals. This was mainly due to an incorrect use of available resources, related in the majority of cases to a lack of programmatic activities and clear health care policies.

In the 1980s, WHO Europe identified the necessity to emphasize the need for providing better health care by raising the performances of all partners involved in the health care process. This was reflected in the document 'European strategy for Health for All',[2] which identified appropriate technologies and interventions with the novelty of particular attention being directed at the patient's perspectives and the use of resources.

Diabetes is a major and growing chronic disease with a strong impact in terms of health and costs, both at an individual and social level. In spite of medical progress, a large number of people with diabetes still suffer from the consequences of the disease as a result of low quality of care received and social inequalities.[3]

In the late 1980s, medical experts and policy makers became progressively aware of two major events related to diabetes: first, the increasing prevalence of the inadequate social and political consideration given to diabetes and to a scarce participation of patients in the management of their condition, which very often generates a quality of care well below the desirable level; second, the consciousness that available knowledge and technologies can greatly ameliorate the condition and that their systematic application, supported by national governments and health care decision makers, produces a better quality of care and consequently a better quality of life for people suffering from the disease.

The St Vincent Declaration: the story

In October 1989 a meeting was convened in St Vincent (Italy) to discuss how to try to implement these considerations.[4] The meeting was organized under the auspices of the Regional

Offices of the World Health Organization and the International Diabetes Federation (IDF) and involved diabetes experts, and representatives of governments and patients' organizations from a number of European countries.

The immediate outcome of the meeting was the St Vincent Declaration (SVD), a document containing goals and targets for the improvement of the quality of life of people with diabetes.

The St Vincent Declaration: goals and targets

The SVD established two general goals for children and adults with diabetes:

1. Sustained improvement in health experiences and a life approaching normal expectations in quality and quantity.
2. Prevention and cure of diabetes and of its complications by intensifying research efforts.

A series of specific targets was also identified in order to reach these two general goals. They can be synthesized into the following points:

- Elaborate, initiate and evaluate comprehensive programmes for detection and control of diabetes and of its complications with self-care and community support as major components.
- Raise awareness in the population and among health care professionals of the present opportunities and the future needs for prevention of the complications of diabetes.
- Organize training and teaching in diabetes management and care for people of all ages with diabetes, and for their families, friends, working associates and the health care team.

- Ensure that care for children with diabetes is provided by individuals and teams specialized both in the management of diabetes and of children, and that families with a diabetic child get the necessary social, economic and emotional support.
- Reinforce existing centres of excellence in diabetes care, education and research.
- Create new centres where the need and potential exist.
- Promote independence, equity and self-sufficiency for all people with diabetes: children, adolescents, those in the working years of life and the elderly.
- Remove hindrances to the fullest possible integration of the diabetic person into society.
- Implement effective measures for the prevention of costly complications.
- Establish monitoring and control systems using state of the art information technology for quality assurance of diabetes health care provision and for laboratory and technical procedures in diabetes diagnosis, treatment and self-management.
- Promote European and international collaboration in programmes of diabetes research and development through national, regional and WHO agencies, and in active partnership with diabetes organizations.
- Take urgent action in the spirit of the WHO programme, 'Health for All', to establish joint machinery between WHO and IDF, European regions, and to initiate, accelerate and facilitate the implementation of these recommendations.

In particular the following very specific targets were fixed for the fight against diabetic complications:

(1) Reduce new blindness due to diabetes by one-third or more.

(2) Reduce numbers of people entering end-stage diabetic renal failure by at least one-third.

(3) Reduce by one-half the rate of limb amputations for diabetic gangrene.

(4) Cut morbidity and mortality from coronary heart disease in the diabetic by vigorous programmes of risk factor reduction.

(5) Achieve pregnancy outcome in the diabetic woman that approximates that of the non-diabetic woman.

SVD as a novelty

The SVD represented a point of novelty in the approach to diabetes care.

First, the recognition of the importance of participation by the 'diabetic patient' in disease management and in co-operating with health care professionals for his/her own care. Also emphasized is the role of the associations in influencing the health care policy according to specific needs and in providing support to other people suffering from the same disease, thus refusing the concept of handicap that is sometimes associated with diabetes.

Second, the document acknowledged the crucial importance of a formal recognition of the disease by governments with an adequate allocation of resources and the formulation of specific plans for prevention, identification and treatment of diabetes and its complications at local, national and European levels.

Finally the document strongly referred to the, at that time, new principles of the quality in health care delivery and to the need for their systematic and appropriate monitoring as the focal points for continuous improvement.

SVD and the reduction of diabetic complications: what has been achieved

Since October 1989, several actions have been undertaken at different levels throughout Europe for the implementation of quality of care programmes according to the SVD with the final aim of reducing the burden and complications of diabetes. Fifty-one governments have nominated liaison persons for formal relationships between the national communities and the overall SVD movement, and 46 have created National Diabetes Task Forces with the mission to develop and implement national and local diabetes programmes. In 37 European countries (72%), a national diabetes programme was designed and officially endorsed by national government.[5]

It was clear from the beginning that the major obstacle to the achievement of the desired results was the lack of information about the real entity of the problem. A survey based on questionnaires sent to the liaison persons indicated that data could be available in 55 % of the countries as regards blindness due to diabetes, in 60% end-stage renal disease leading to kidney transplantation and in 50 % amputations above ankle.[6] Some of the countries also produced various national data on the impact of the disease in terms of late complications.[6]

SVD and diabetic complications: working tools

A number of SVD Working Groups were created with the remit to elaborate guidelines for better care. As a result of their activity, the Steering Committee of the SVD edited in 1992 the St Vincent Declaration Action Programme, representing a plan for the practical implementation of the Declaration.[7] The document was accompanied by a series of guidelines for various aspects of diabetes care with particular attention to late complications, including a protocol for the screening of diabetic retinopathy, and guidelines for the prevention of renal failure, foot ulcers and amputations and coronary artery disease. An updated version of each of these guidelines was generated three years later in the SVD Action Programme Implementation Document.[8]

The protocol for the screening of diabetic retinopathy in Europe was approved by experts representing 30 diabetes and ophthalmic societies across Europe. The protocol addressed the following basilar questions for an effective retinopathy screening programme:

(1) Which method for fundus examination should be used?
(2) Who should do the screening?
(3) When to screen?
(4) How to collect data?

The aim of the protocol was the definition of a reliable screening tool able to identify early lesions and the most appropriate use of the resources in order to guarantee the same opportunities for access to eye examination to all subjects in different areas. A Diabetic Retinopathy Screening Card was generated for data collection and a specific computer programme, the Save Eyes in Europe (SEE) programme, was developed for the management of the screening protocol.

The guidelines for the prevention of renal failure were subdivided into indications for screening and indications for treatment. The section regarding screening provided guidance on the best procedures for the detection of microalbuminuria or persistent proteinuria. The second part provided clear indications for treatment of kidney disease according to the stage of progression.

The guidelines for the prevention of foot ulcers and amputations provided suggestions for the screening and diagnostic procedures, the follow-up of people at risk and for care of overt lesions. Particular attention was given to the definition of the team of professionals involved in foot care and to the fundamental role of education in the prevention of the onset or the progression of the lesions.

The guidelines on cardiovascular disease and stroke contained indications for primary and secondary prevention. Particular attention was paid to the control of the risk factors for macrovascular disease and to the target levels for each risk factor. The need for an adaptation of the guidelines according to local environmental differences was highly recommended.

SVD and diabetic complications: examples of activities

The SVD recommendations generated several initiatives for local implementation, some of which focused mainly on organizational and educational aspects, while others aimed more at clinical elements.

Eye complications

The SVD implementation in the Stockholm County Initiative comprised both organizational and educational aspects with an educational programme combined with a campaign for the screening of diabetic eye disease and the evaluation of a monitoring system for new blindness due to diabetes.[9] The educational programme was divided into two sections. The first aimed at increasing awareness and competence of health care professionals, people with diabetes, administrators and politicians, highlighting the effectiveness of preventative measures. The second was a two-week continuous medical educational programme for professionals working in the primary health care centres. The campaign for the screening of eye disease was conducted through a mobile photo-screening service, which contacts all diabetic patients from hospital in-patient registers followed by an immediate referral to the ophthalmologist in case of people at risk. Data collection covered the period 1981–1995 while the screening was performed from 1990 to 1995.[10] Results showed progressive decrease of blindness incidence from 1.2/100,000 population in the period 1981–1985 to 0.63 and 0.33/100,000 people in the periods 1986–1990 and 1991–1995 respectively. The final reduction was about one-third with respect to the basal level, indicating the achievement of the SVD target for diabetic retinopathy.

A prerequisite for planning effective treatment strategies is the availability of facilities. A study was conducted in 1991 in the UK to determine which treatment facilities were available and how treatment was provided.[11] A questionnaire was distributed to all ophthalmologists operating in England and Wales. The answers demonstrated that the screening facilities were inadequate for a large number of people and that there was a wide variation in care provided, especially in waiting times for first visit and treatment in different centres.

A similar experience was repeated in 1996 to evaluate the possible changes;[12] data confirmed a wide variation of care provided for screening, from 25% of cases in some centres to 90% in others. These results showed that the first step in the reduction of complications should be a coordinated effort both for screening and treatment.

The Liverpool Diabetic Eye Study in 1995 aimed at evaluating different community-based screening methods for the detection of sight threatening diabetic eye disease.[13] The study compared the sensitivity and specificity of community based photography with mydriasis and of direct ophthalmoscopy with reference standard of slit lamp biomicroscopy by a professional expert on retinal disease. The results indicated that photography had higher sensitivity than direct ophthalmoscopy, while the specificity was higher for the second method. Taking into consideration the fact that sensitivity is more important than specificity for a screening procedure, the photography seemed to be more effective for this purpose. Therefore it was concluded that fundus photography was the primary choice for an effective community-based screening programme according to the SVD recommendations.

In the early 1990s a practical community screening programme was conducted in 12 centres in the UK using the mobile retinal camera.[14] The screening was performed by different non-specialized professionals. During the study period, 64,905 screening tests were carried out and as a result, 2400 subjects were referred to ophthalmologists and 512 needed laser therapy. A progressive reduction in sight threatening retinopathy incidence was noticed over the years due to the detection of early lesions through the screening initiative.

A similar study was conducted in Sweden in the area of Lund with an observation period of 5 years from 1987 to 1992.[15] After 5 years the incidence rates of blindness were 0.5% in Type 1 and 0.6% in Type 2 diabetic patients. Most of the cases of blindness were observed in those people who had severe retinopathy at baseline, while just a small minority was observed in people with normal fundus examination at the time of the screening. This was due to an earlier referral to the ophthalmologist in case of initial lesions with the possibility of adequate and effective treatment.

A more recent survey was carried out in Germany with data on new cases of blindness collected from 1990 to 1998.[16] The study showed a reduction in the incident rate of 3% for each year of observation.

All these results showed that screening is an effective measure for reducing eye complications in accordance with the suggestions of the SVD specific guidelines.

Kidney complications

The PROSIT Project (PROteinuria Screening and Intervention Project) was launched in Germany as part of the national implementation of the SVD.[17] The project focused on the identification procedures for facilitating the screening of diabetic nephropathy. One of the major achievements of the project was the validation of self-testing for microalbuminuria. The study showed that the available self-test methods have high sensitivity and specificity and thus could be effectively used for screening. The combination of the effectiveness of the test and the low price creates the conditions for widespread screening for diabetic nephropathy. The need for action was highlighted in a preliminary experience within the same project showing that in Germany only a minority of people suffering from diabetes were screened annually for diabetic nephropathy.

An analysis of quality of care in the field of diabetic kidney disease was carried out in the UK in 1995 through a questionnaire regarding the adherence to the available guidelines for the screening of microalbuminuria.[18] The screening was performed by 69% of the clinicians involved in the survey, 74% of whom followed the guidelines in Type 1 and only 39% in Type 2 diabetes. The observation indicated that even if the screening was accessible in an acceptable ratio, the standardization of procedures was far from desired.

Poor attention to the indications about the screening of nephropathy was also highlighted in a survey on patterns of care in Italy.[19] The

study conducted in 1996 demonstrated that early indicators of risk for kidney failure were not measured in more than 33% of patients.

A recent study was conducted in 20 European countries to evaluate the compliance to guidelines on first referral to nephrologists.[20] While the SVD guidelines suggest that the first referral to nephrologists should be required when serum creatinine is higher than 150 µmol/l, only 30% of Type 1 and 22% of Type 2 diabetic patients had first referral according to guidelines. Moreover 50% of those who were placed on the replacement therapy had the first referral within 3 months prior to replacement. The results highlighted the scarce standardization of care and the negative impact on outcomes.

Diabetic amputations

The Danish Amputation Register Study Group analyzed the incidence of major lower limb amputations from 1982 to 1993.[21] In total, 2848 cases were collected and there was a progressive reduction of incidence, with a total of 40% reduction by 1993.

Different results were found in a German experience during the period 1990–1998.[22] In fact the analysis of the incidence rates during the observation period did not demonstrate significant reduction in incident cases between years.

In Sweden the incidence of amputations was evaluated from 1960 to 1990.[9] A total number of 1281 amputations were registered; a progressive reduction of about 20 cases per year was noticed, which was far from the 50% reduction in the SVD targets, clearly indicating the need for more effective intervention programmes on the diabetic foot.

Amongst the activities carried out within the regional Umbria Diabetes project in Italy, a survey on diabetes-related amputations highlighted that 1283 non-traumatic amputations were performed in the Umbria region from 1991 to 1998. No significant changes were observed in the overall incidence rate during the observational period; however, the ratio between major amputations (above the ankle) and minor amputations (below the ankle) was significantly reduced.[23]

SVD: *methodological problems in the evaluation of the impact*

More recently at the SVD meeting which took place in Istanbul in October 1999 on the occasion of the tenth anniversary of the SVD, a report was presented based on the information provided by the SVD national liaison personnel and on published information. The report indicated that reduction of blindness was obtained in three countries, the same number of countries experienced a reduction of cardiovascular disease and of end-stage renal disease; a reduction in major amputations was reported in six countries; five countries reported a reduction in hospitalization due to late complications of diabetes and two countries reported a reduction in health care expenditure related to diabetes.[6]

However one of the major issues in the SVD-related projects is the difficulty of scientifically documenting the evidence of the outcomes due to the intrinsic characteristics of such activities, which means that the results are usually produced as reports from health care implementation initiatives. In fact in population-based interventions, randomization and control groups are not applicable, making it difficult to compare the effectiveness of the action programmes. Moreover the factors that influence the outcome are not strictly identifiable, and unpredictable environmental varia-

tions might intervene in long-term, large-scale initiatives, such as political changes, variability of available resources, prevailing educational and cultural standards, conflicts, etc. This has been particularly true in Europe in the last decade.

By definition, the initiatives for the improvement of health and to a greater extent for the improvement of the quality of life of a given population are carried out in an unstable environment to which they need to adapt. In fact, generally speaking, determinants much stronger than the health care issues influence the evolution of the overall environment.

Other factors that make difficult the documentation of the outcomes are represented in many cases by the lack of precise and well-defined health care plans of action that are substituted by health care policies producing scattered initiatives; and also by the difficulty in coordinating multidisciplinary initiatives characterized by multifocal decisional power also residing outside the specific health care domain. Moreover it is difficult to define the role of the SVD movement in ongoing activities that might or might not have taken advantage of the SVD climate.

Another difficulty created in demonstrating the real impact of the SVD is related to the inappropriate request of evidence based on methodologies usually adopted for scientific protocols, for example randomized, double blind, placebo control group comparison. For the reasons already mentioned such methodologies are inapplicable to SVD-like activities that require, instead, specific methodologies able to provide solid evidence for interventions in evolving unstable environments. Some of them already exist, but more research is still required for adapting and validating such analytical procedures to diabetology.

A further element of difficulty is represented by the absence of baseline data collected according to appropriate epidemiological procedures in the geographical areas where the interventions are performed. In fact the statistical analysis of the effect of a given project cannot be referred to theoretical data derived from epidemiological information collected in remote places although with similar characteristics. On the other hand the collection of baseline data according to traditional epidemiological procedures can require unbearable costs in terms of resources and time.

The data collected in the quality development (QD) process have been frequently used for providing the evidence that should have been produced according to accepted epidemiological analysis. In fact the information required for the QD is gathered according to procedures designed for satisfying that specific process and not for epidemiological purposes.

SVD achievements: a platform for further development

The most relevant achievements of the SVD, representing a platform for further evolution of the interventions in favour of the improvement of the health and quality of life of people with diabetes in Europe, are represented by the consolidated awareness of the need for, and the feasibility of broad partnership, the promotion of appropriate approaches for the planning of interventions, the identification and implementation of specific methodologies for quality development, and the need to define and apply correct methods for producing evidence.[24]

The explicit and clear definition of the mission, the high level aims and the practical targets for the improvement of the lives of people with diabetes present in the SVD have been a great advantage for the definition of roles and responsibilities and as a consequence have facilitated synergies and collaboration and reduced the level of conflicts at international, national, regional and local levels. Under such circumstances the feasibility of long-term strategic planning of interventions with the contribution of all the possible interested parties has been proven: parties such as institutions, professionals, people with diabetes, and third parties such as industries, foundations and service institutions.

In many European countries this has produced national plans for diabetes endorsed and adopted by the governments, the impact of which, however, is extremely difficult to quantify owing to the complexity and variability of the different environments.

The promotion of defined and structured methodologies for the development of the quality of care has been one of the major focuses of the SVD movement and at present, although not extensively applied, are more deeply rooted in the cultural background of the diabetological community than in any other medical discipline throughout Europe. The benchmarking and external comparison, the quality circles, are well-known procedures, whose applicability in diabetes care has been experienced in many initiatives. Within the Diabcare project the indicators for diabetes care have been identified mostly in terms of outcomes (final and intermediate) and processes.[25] Instruments for data collection have been proposed, such as the Basic Information Sheet and various systems for data transmission like the Diabcare Programme and the Diabcare Fax solution within the Diabcare Quality Network (Qnet). In some countries, for example France,[26] Portugal,[27] Germany,[28] The Netherlands,[29] Italy,[30] Spain,[31] broad initiatives have proven the feasibility and the effectiveness of large-scale data collection and benchmarking for the improvement of quality of diabetes care.

However, as already mentioned, the information provided by such initiatives cannot be compared with the knowledge deriving from the major clinical trials, for example the DCCT[32] and the UKPDS,[33] or more specifically regarding the cardiovascular diseases such as the Scandinavian Simvastatin Survival Study,[34] the Helsinki Heart Study,[35] the Bezafibrate Infarction Prevention Study,[36] the HOPE Study,[37] the Appropriate Blood Pressure Control in Diabetes Study,[38] the FACET Study,[39] the DIGAMI Study,[40] etc. that have been designed for different purposes; the latter have been designed for producing knowledge, while the others have been designed to implement the available knowledge in order to improve the quality of life of the people with these conditions.

SVD: *the future*

A step forward to reconcile these two methodologies is represented by the progressive development and implementation of diabetes registries. Once in place they provide reliable population-based epidemiological data that are continuously updated, allowing monitoring of ongoing phenomena. The platform produced by the networks and installed for the registries supports the implementation of standards of care and facilitates a widespread adoption of shared care. A number of proposals are flourishing around the world; in Europe, especially relevant and advanced projects have been developed in a number of countries, such as the UK, Denmark, France, Germany, Italy, The Netherlands, Finland and Greece.[41]

While the technological aspects no longer represent a critical issue, owing to the fact that the available technology is far more advanced than necessary for the purpose, the most challenging topics are the regulatory issues, such as the ownership of data, confidentiality,

access rights, etc., and also the human, cultural and environmental barriers that need to be surmounted and that at present are responsible for the difficulties in the realization of large-scale experiences.[42]

The first decade of the SVD has demonstrated the feasibility and the possible effectiveness of new approaches to diabetes care and the importance of focusing on the real outcomes of the disease more than on the processes. It has also it has been demonstrated that local solutions to local problems need to be defined, taking advantage of others' experiences which must be tailored for the local needs according to the local environment: there are no general solutions available that can satisfy everybody's needs.

The experience gained has also demonstrated that available knowledge is poorly implemented, and this problem is not just found in the less advanced counties. Everywhere much better results could be obtained. The awareness of such widely accepted findings has created the cultural conditions for concrete initiatives aimed at large-scale prevention of end-stage diabetes complications. New instruments and methodologies that have been developed and are still under evolution are increasingly accepted and are so designed to integrate new knowledge when available. However, given the nature and the time scale for development and evolution of diabetes complications such as eye, kidney disease and CVD the real benefit of the SVD movement will require a sufficient length of time to be evident.

The St Vincent initiative is to be considered a cultural movement that has been successful in promoting, heavily supporting and facilitating the application of the new cultural frontiers for the global health of people with diabetes in Europe. This movement, initiated in Europe, successively spread throughout the world with sister initiatives such as the Declaration of the

Americas (DOTA), the Western Pacific Declaration (WPD) and others, which make it even more difficult to quantify the real benefit of the seed planted in St Vincent in 1989.

It is not inappropriate to claim that, in many countries worldwide, the effect of specific national action plans for diabetes produced a change in attitude of health care professionals, people with diabetes and health care stakeholders. This change is likely to reduce successfully the burden of diabetes by reducing blindness, end-stage renal failure, stroke and myocardial infarction in the years to come, which would not have been the case to such a large degree without the SVD movement.

References

1. WHO Regional Office for Europe. QualiCare: quality management in health care in the information age. Programme of quality of care and technologies. Copenhagen, December 1997.
2. WHO. Targets for health for all. World Health Organization, 1985.
3. The action programme for the implementation of the St Vincent Declaration for the improvement of diabetes health care. Jointly organized by the WHO/Europe and IDF/Europe. WHO icp/clr 055, 23 Oct 1990 (8438r).
4. World Health Organization (Europe) and International Diabetes Federation (Europe). Diabetes care and research in Europe: the St Vincent Declaration. Diabet Med 1990; 7: 360.
5. Background to St Vincent. The SVD Newsletter 1998; 13 Summer: 4.
6. Bergrem H, Kalo I, Staehr Johansen K. The St Vincent Declaration-Monitoring the St Vincent Declaration activities. The SVD Newsletter 10th Anniversary Issue 1999; 14 Autumn: 8.
7. Krans HMJ, Porta M, Keen H, Staehr Johansen K. Diabetes care research in Europe: St Vincent Declaration action programme. Copenhagen: WHO Office, 1995; EUR/ICT/CLR 055/3.
8. Krans HMJ, Porta M, Keen H, Staehr Johansen K. Diabetes care research in Europe: St Vincent Declaration action programme. Implementation

document. Giornale Italiano di Diabetologia 1995; 15: 1.
9. Rosenqvist U. Implementation of the St Vincent Declaration in Stockholm county, Sweden. Giornale Italiano di Diabetologia 1993; 13 Suppl: 75–6.
10. Backlund LB, Algvere PV, Rosenqvist U. New blindness in diabetes reduced by more than one-third in Stockholm County. Diabet Med 1997; 14: 732–40.
11. Kohner EM, Lavin M, Hamilton AM. The management of diabetic retinopathy. Giornale Italiano di Diabetologia 1993; 13 Suppl: 77–9.
12. Bagga P, Verma D, Walton C et al. Survey of diabetic retinopathy screening services in England and Wales. Diabet Med 1998; 15: 780–2.
13. Harding SP, Broadbent DM, Neoh C et al. Sensitivity and specificity of photography and direct ophthalmoscopy in screening for sight threatening eye disease: the Liverpool Diabetic Eye Study. BMJ 1995; 311: 1131–5.
14. Taylor R. Practical community screening for diabetic retinopathy using the mobile retinal camera: report of a 12 centre study. British Diabetic Association Mobile Retinal Screening Group. Diabet Med 1996; 13: 946–52.
15. Agardh E, Agardh CD, Hansson-Lundblad C. The five-year incidence of blindness after introducing a screening programme for early detection of treatable diabetic retinopathy. Diabet Med 1993; 10: 555–9.
16. Tautner C, Haastert B, Giani G, Berger M. Incidence of blindness in southern Germany between 1990 and 1998. Diabetologia 2001; 44: 147–50.
17. Piehlmeier W, Renner R, Kimmerling T et al. Evaluation of the Micral-Test S, a qualitative immunologic patient self-test for microalbuminuria: the PROSIT project. Proteinuria Screening and Intervention. Diabet Med 1998; 15: 883–5.
18. Gazis A, Page SR. Microalbuminuria screening in the UK: are we meeting European standards? Diabet Med 1996; 13: 764–7.
19. Nicolucci A, Scorpiglione N, Belfiglio M, Carinci F et al. Patterns of care of an Italian diabetic population. Diabet Med 1996; 14: 158–66.
20. Bergrem H. Quality of care for persons with diabetic nephropathy: timeliness of first referral to nephrologist. Diabetes Nutr Med 2002; 15: 109–15.

21. Ebskov B, Ebskov L. Major lower limb amputation in diabetic patients: development during 1982 to 1993. Diabetologia 1996; 39: 1607–10.

22. Trautner C, Haastert B, Spraul M et al. Unchanged incidence of lower-limb amputations in a German city, 1990–1998. Diabetes Care 2001; 24: 855–9.

23. Scionti L, Massi Benedetti M, on behalf of the Cooperative Study Group of the 'Progetto Umbria Diabete'. A 8-year population-based survey of non-traumatic lower extremity amputations in diabetic and non-diabetic patients in an Italian region. Diabetes 2001; 50 Suppl. 2: A228.

24. Bergrem H, Kalo I, Staehr Johansen K. The St Vincent Declaration – the main achievements. The SVD Newsletter 10th Anniversary Issue 1999; 14 Autumn: 8.

25. Piewernetz K, Home PD, Snorgaard O et al. Monitoring the targets of the St Vincent Declaration and the implementation of quality management in diabetes care: the DiabCare Initiative. Diabet Med 1993; 10: 371–7.

26. Attali J, Klinebreil L. The support of young students in the implementation of DiabCare Q-Net and the St Vincent declaration. The St Vincent Declaration Newsletter 1995; Suppl. 1: 27–8.

27. Selbmann HK, Pietsch-Breitfeld B. DiabCare Q-Net activities Germany. The St Vincent Declaration Newsletter 1995; Suppl. 1: 28–9.

28. DiabCare Q-Net NL, St Vincent goals into practice. Diabetes Nutr Metab 1997; 10 Suppl. 1: 59.

29. Massi Benedetti M, Norgiolini R, Capani F et al. The DiabCare Quality Network as an instrument for quality development in diabetes. Diabetes Nutr Metab 1997; 10 Suppl. 1: 68.

30. Brugues E, Bosch F, Corcoy R et al. Benefits of the combined operation of DiabCare Q-Net and Diabcard system: 'the Spanish experience'. Diabetes Nutr Metab 1997; 10 Suppl. 1: 64.

31. Piewernetz K, Almeida P, Bergem H et al. EU Project DiabCare Q-Net. 1996 report. Diabetes Nutr Metab 1997; 10 Suppl. 1: 63.

32. DCCT Research Group. The effect of intensive treatment of diabetes on the development and progression of long-term complications in insulin dependent diabetes mellitus. New Engl J Med 1993; 329: 977–86.

33. UK Prospective Diabetes Study Group. Intensive blood glucose control with sulphonylureas or insulin compared with conventional treatment and risk of complications in patients with Type 2 diabetes (UKPDS 33). Lancet 1998; 352: 837–53.

34. Pyorala K, Pedersen TR, Kjekshus J et al. Cholesterol lowering with Simvastatin improves prognosis of diabetic patients with coronary heart disease. A subgroup analysis of the Scandinavian Simvastatin Survival Study (4S). Diabetes Care 1997; 20: 614–20.

35. Koskinen P, Manttari M, Manninen V et al. Coronary heart disease incidence in NIDDM patients in the Helsinki Heart Study. Diabetes Care 1992; 15: 820–5.

36. Jonas M, Reicher-Reiss H, Boyko V et al. Usefulness of beta-blocker therapy in patients with non-insulin dependent diabetes mellitus and coronary artery disease. Bezafibrate Infarction Prevention (BIP) Study Group. Am J Cardiol 1996; 77: 1273–7.

37. Heart Outcomes Prevention Evaluation Study Investigators. Effects of ramipril on cardiovascular and microvascular outcomes in people with diabetes mellitus: results of the HOPE study and MICRO-HOPE substudy. Lancet 2000; 355: 253–9.

38. Estacio RO, Jeffers BW, Hiatt WR et al. The effect of nisoldipine as compared with enalapril on cardiovascular outcomes in patients with non-insulin-dependent diabetes and hypertension. N Engl J Med 1998; 338: 645–52.

39. Tatti P, Pahor M, Byington RP, Di Mauro P et al. Outcome results of the Fosinopril versus Amlodipine Cardiovascular Events Randomized Trial (FACET) in patients with hypertension and NIDDM. Diabetes Care 1998; 21: 597–603.

40. Malmberg K. Prospective randomised study of intensive insulin treatment on long term survival after acute myocardial infarction in patients with diabetes mellitus. DIGAMI (Diabetes Mellitus, Insulin Glucose Infusion in Acute Myocardial Infarction) Study Group. BMJ 1997; 314: 1512–15.

41. Diabetes 'Registers' Into the Millenium 7th Workshop of the DOIT EASD Study Group Gubbio, (PG-Italy), 12–14th May 2000; www.doit-easd.org/en/meetings.

42. Vaughan NJA. Confidentiality and diabetes registers. Diabetes Nutr Metab 2001; 14: 114–17.

7

Diabetes dyslipidaemia: novel treatment and prognosis in Type 1 and Type 2 diabetes
Daphne Owens, Gerald H Tomkin

Introduction

The two major problems facing diabetologists in this century are unfortunately no different from the problems that faced us in the last century. On the one hand we have to guide the patient to lead a normal life, and on the other hand we have to encourage the patient to pay meticulous attention to the control of diabetes so that the major complication of diabetes, which is arterial damage, can be prevented. The dyslipidaemia of diabetes affects the atherosclerotic process and therefore has been thought to be part of the pathogenesis of large vessel disease, but it must be remembered that small vessel disease alters renal function and disturbed renal function has major effects on lipoprotein metabolism.[1,2]

Macrovascular disease in diabetes

Hyperglycaemia and hypertension

Macrovascular disease is a major cause of the early mortality found not only in Type 2 diabetes but also in Type 1 diabetes. Indeed, since renal failure is now treatable by dialysis or transplantation, macrovascular disease has become an even greater problem for Type 1

diabetic patients.[3,4] Although there is excellent evidence that microvascular disease is related to glycaemic control the evidence that macrovascular disease has a similar relationship is less secure.[5,6] There is no doubt that many studies have demonstrated across the spectrum of blood sugar, even in non-diabetic patients, that there is a direct relationship between glycaemia and atherosclerosis.[7–10] However the normalization of hyperglycaemia has not been shown beyond doubt to improve the prognosis for people with either Type 1 or Type 2 diabetes from a cardio-vascular point of view.[5,8] There are some studies which do suggest that improvement in glycaemia does improve markers of arteriopathy in Type 1 diabetic patients,[11] and in secondary prevention, meticulous control of blood glucose has been shown to improve prognosis in Type 1 and Type 2 diabetes.[12] Hypertension very commonly accompanies Type 1 and Type 2 diabetes and perhaps the UKPDS study[13] was the most persuasive yet in demonstrating the benefit of lowering blood pressure to prevent atherosclerotic events. In Type 1 diabetes the evidence is also strongly persuasive if not as well defined.[14,15]

Hypercholesterolaemia

The role of hypercholesterolaemia in the development of atherosclerosis has been studied extensively in large epidemiological studies[16] and, with the advent of the statin group of drugs, the benefit of cholesterol lowering has been demonstrated.[17–20] In some studies statins have been shown to reduce the incidence of myocardial infarction (MI) to a greater extent in diabetic patients than in control subjects.[17] However not all studies have confirmed this.[18–20] Accumulating evidence suggests that statin drugs prevent atherosclerosis, not only by lowering cholesterol but also by mechanisms unrelated to dyslipidaemia.[21] These include increased lipoprotein sialylation[22] reduction in inflammatory cytokines and adhesion molecules,[23,24] C-reactive protein,[25,26] and fibrinogen.[27] Indeed, pravastatin has been shown to result in a 30% reduction in the hazard of becoming diabetic[28] and it has been postulated that this may be related to its ability to inhibit the acute phase response, since markers of inflammation predict diabetes,[29,30] heart disease[31] and atherosclerosis.[32] This is a persuasive hypothesis since a raised C-reactive protein has been shown to predict the development of diabetes. Thus, we cannot use the effect of statins on cholesterol lowering as evidence that hypercholesterolaemia is the major cause of atherosclerosis in diabetes.

In this chapter we will try to persuade the reader that the dyslipidaemia of diabetes is central to atherosclerosis and that meticulous attention to treatment at an early stage in Type 1 diabetes and in the pre-diabetic stage of Type 2 diabetes, will in future years prevent diabetic atherosclerotic heart disease.

Diabetes as a postprandial metabolic disorder

Diabetes is particularly a postprandial metabolic disorder and hypertriglyceridaemia is the major lipoprotein abnormality to be found.[33,34] It is therefore important to understand the physiology of lipoprotein metabolism and the shortcuts that are used in epidemiological studies. Most large studies fail to measure the postprandial metabolic disturbance that occurs in diabetes. This is particularly important when one considers the difference in turnover rates between chylomicron, very low density lipoprotein (VLDL) and low density lipoprotein (LDL) particles[35–41] and the further differences in lipoprotein turnover which occur in diabetes due to factors such as glycation.[42–45] The chylomicron is cleared in a matter of minutes after reaching the circulation from the intestine while LDL has a half-life of three to four days. Thus, it is impossible to make valid estimations from single measurements of the relative importance of the different lipoproteins to cardiovascular risk.

The chylomicron

The chylomicron is defined as an intestinally derived lipoprotein particle. It is characterized by apo B48 as its solubilizing protein,[46] there being only trace amounts of apo B100 produced in the human intestine.[47] The relevance of the chylomicron as an atherogenic particle has been disputed, but the very rapid turnover of the particle, and the finding of a specific apo B48 receptor on the macrophage[48] explains why the chylomicron is again becoming fashionable as a major potential atherogenic particle. Chylomicrons are synthesized in various sizes in the intestine and are delivered to the circulation via the lymph (Figure 7.1).[48,49] In human circulation ~10% of chylomicrons are floated with the VLDL fraction[50] and some authors suggest they are also present in intermediate density lipoprotein (IDL) and LDL in very low quantities,[51] although this has not been our finding. Chylomicron triglycerides are hydrolyzed by lipoprotein lipase in the capillar-

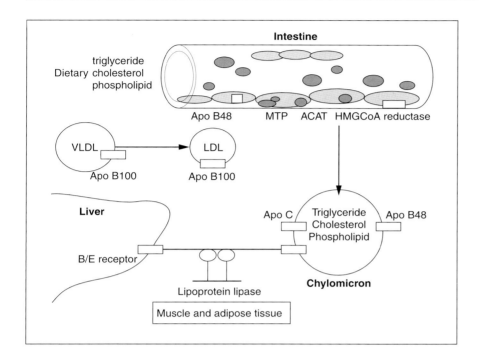

Figure 7.1
Assembly of the chylomicron in the intestine and VLDL in the liver.

ies of adipose tissue and muscle and the fatty acids are delivered to the cell for energy. The resultant chylomicron remnant particles are cleared by the liver. Insulin has been shown to regulate plasma apo B48 and triglyceride in the postprandial period in healthy individuals.[52] The term 'chylomicron' is confusing since the ultracentrifugation technique which separates lipoproteins according to size has demonstrated that the largest circulating particles are not pure chylomicrons but rather a mixture of both chylomicrons (the intestinally-derived apoB48–containing lipoprotein) and large VLDL which is an apo B100–containing lipoprotein originating from the liver (Figure 7.1). The distinction became important when Karpe et al.[53] described an independent relationship between apo B48 and carotid artery atherosclerosis progression in non-diabetic patients.

Very low density lipoprotein (VLDL)

VLDL production is suppressed by insulin and there is good evidence to confirm increased production of VLDL in diabetes.[54-57] Not only is VLDL production increased in diabetes but also clearance is delayed due to reduced lipoprotein lipase function in insulin-deficient or insulin-resistant states.[58] A recent paper using transgenic rabbits which over-expressed human lipoprotein lipase demonstrated as much as 80% decrease in plasma triglycerides and a 59% increase in plasma high density lipoprotein (HDL) in these animals.[59] LDL levels were significantly increased but, on a cholesterol-rich diet, the development of hypercholesterolaemia and atherosclerosis was dramatically suppressed. The part played by the increase in VLDL compared with the increase in chylomicrons has

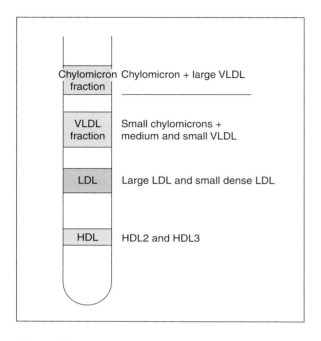

Figure 7.2
Lipoprotein isolation.

not been examined to any great extent due to the technical difficulties of separating and analyzing the lipid portion of apo B100 particles as compared to apo B48 particles (Figure 7.2). The chylomicron fraction isolated by ultracentrifugation contains ~50% apo B100 and 50% apo B48 particles and the VLDL fraction, which contains mainly apo B100 particles, also has ~10% apo B48 particles (Figure 7.2). However, it is apparent that both chylomicrons and VLDL are important in delivering cholesterol to the atherosclerotic plaque.[60,61] VLDL is also of major importance in determining the atherogenicity of LDL. VLDL regulates the cholesterol content of LDL and influences the size of the LDL particle. It has been shown that large VLDL, which has a high triglyceride content, is the precursor of small dense LDL, the particularly atherogenic form of LDL[40,41,62] (Figure 7.3).

In diabetes we have demonstrated that apo B48 is increased both in the chylomicron and

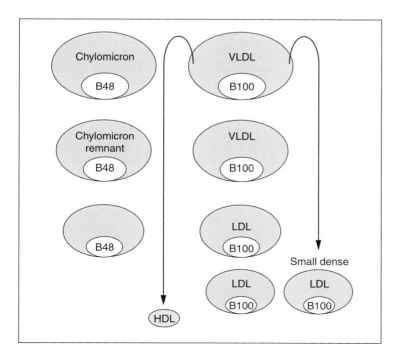

Figure 7.3
The lipoprotein cascade.

VLDL fractions[63,64] and we have shown that improvement in diabetic control significantly reduced postprandial apo B48 levels.[50] We found that whereas adding cholesterol to a meal in non-diabetic subjects did not alter their postprandial apo B48 levels in diabetic patients, cholesterol feeding significantly reduced the large postprandial chylomicron particles and caused a very large increase in the smaller apo B48-containing particles in the VLDL fraction.[63] This is of particular interest since Martins et al.[65] have suggested that the number of particles rather than the size determines their atherogenicity and the severity of coronary atherosclerosis in Type 2 diabetes has been related to the number of circulating triglyceride-rich lipoprotein particles.[66] It has also been shown that the large particles are cleared more slowly.[67] Experiments comparing apo E-deficient, apo B100-only mice, which would clear large particles very slowly, with LDL receptor-deficient, apo B100-only mice, which would clear small particles slowly, have demonstrated that although both animals had similar total cholesterol levels, the apo E-deficient mice had three to four-fold less atherosclerosis.[68] Because the apo E-containing particles are large triglyceride-rich particles, that study suggests that a large number of small apo B100-containing particles are more atherogenic than a lower number of large apo B100-containing particles.

Atherogenicity of the intestinally-derived lipoproteins

The atherogenicity of the apo B48 particles has been examined by Mero et al.[69] in diabetic patients with and without coronary artery disease (CAD). They found that the severity of the most significant coronary stenosis in angiography correlated with chylomicron AUC for apo B48. The authors concluded that postprandial change in small remnant particles may contribute to the severity of CAD in Type 2 diabetes. The mechanism by which apo B48-containing lipoproteins may be particularly atherogenic is poorly understood but it has been shown that remnant particles, (a mixture of apo B48 and apo B100 particles) were taken up by fibroblasts and arterial smooth muscle cells with greater affinity than LDL.[70] The discovery of the apo B48 receptor on the macrophage may be an explanation of preferential uptake of apo B48 particles into the atherosclerotic plaque.[47,71] It has been difficult to measure lipoprotein composition of the plaque and to show an increase in apo B48 in the plaque. Rapp et al.[72] isolated and characterized immunoreactive apolipoprotein B-containing lipoproteins from human atherosclerotic plaque and plasma. They extracted lipoproteins from plaques and isolated the lipoproteins from the extracts using anti-apoB immunoabsorption and separated the fractions by ultracentrifugation. The authors demonstrated that more than one-third of the total lipoprotein associated cholesterol in the extracts came from the VLDL and IDL fractions. However, they did not measure apo B48 and did not examine whether apo B48 differs from apo B100 in its ability to promote atherosclerosis. Veniant et al.[73] examined apo E-deficient mice and apo E-deficient mice that synthesized exclusively either apo B48 or apo B100. These authors showed that the susceptibility to atherosclerosis was dependent on cholesterol levels. Whether the animals had apo B48 or apo B100 did not seem to matter. Proctor and Mamo,[74,75] in elegant studies injected a large quantity of chylomicrons into eviscerated rabbits to generate remnant particles devoid of apo B100. Particles were re-isolated, a fluorescent label was attached to chylomicrons and injected into hepatectomized rabbits. Using confocal laser scanning microscopy, they demonstrated that chylomicron remnants migrate efficiently through the arterial wall resulting in substantial accumulation of remnants within the intimal area of the carotid arteries. The authors suggest that one source of artery wall cholesterol might be chylomicron remnants supporting the concept that atherogenesis is in part a postprandial phenomenon.

Low density lipoproteins

The Mediterranean diet

The Mediterranean-type diet has been associated with protection against atherosclerosis.[76] An oleic acid diet has been shown to improve blood glucose control and we have shown an improvement in insulin-mediated glucose uptake in the adipocyte of Type 2 diabetic patients on an oleic compared with a linoleic acid diet.[77] This improvement could be related to cell membrane fluidity.[78] We have recently shown that in Type 2 diabetic patients a change from a linoleic to an oleic acid diet reduced both fasting and postprandial chylomicron apo B48 and apo B100,[79] a possible mechanism for the effect of the Mediterranean diet in reducing atherosclerosis.

Atherogenic modifications of LDL

It is usually considered that LDL is the most important single lipoprotein in relation to delivering cholesterol to the atherosclerotic plaque since it carries the major cholesterol load around the body. This view may be changing with the realization that allowance should be made for the rather slow turnover of LDL (half-life two to three days) as compared with chylomicrons (half-life of minutes) and VLDL (half-life of hours).

It is probably the modification of LDL such as oxidation,[80,81] glycation[82] and desialy-lation[83–85] which makes it atherogenic. Modification of LDL allows it to be taken up by scavenger receptors.[86] This destroys the finely tuned cholesterol homoeostasis mechanism which applies when LDL is taken up by the native LDL receptor as described by Brown and Goldstein[87] (Figure 7.4). It has recently been shown that glycated LDL is taken up by fibroblasts, macrophages and endothelial cells in a lipoprotein lipase-mediated process and that uptake correlated with the degree of LDL glycation.[88] Glycated LDL is very susceptible to oxidation[82,89] and inhibition of glycation with pyridoxamine, an inhibitor of advanced glycation reactions, reduces LDL oxidation.[90] Oxidized LDL is probably highly atherogenic since, as well as promoting unregulated cellular cholesterol uptake, it stimulates cytokine and adhesion molecule expression,[91] which promote macrophage infiltration into the artery wall and plaque formation. LDL oxidation is a particular problem in diabetes due to the increase in free-radical formation.[92,93] Hyperglycaemia in diabetes leads to glycation of both the protein and lipid.[94,95] Hypercholesterolaemia is known to increase LDL oxidizability,[96] but we have shown increased susceptibility of LDL from diabetic patients to in vitro oxidation even when the patients were normolipidaemic.[97] Although there is a significant correlation between glycaemia and LDL oxidizability, and improvement in control will reduce oxidizability,[98] it is interesting to read that age also significantly predicts the susceptibility to oxidation.[99] Another factor which determines LDL oxidizability is the type of fatty acids in the LDL (Figure 7.5). Only fatty acids with two or more conjugated double bonds are susceptible to oxidation. We and others have shown an increase in linoleic acid in diabetic patients.[100–103] This may be related to the dietary advice given to diabetic patients or to a defect in the metabolism of linoleic acid

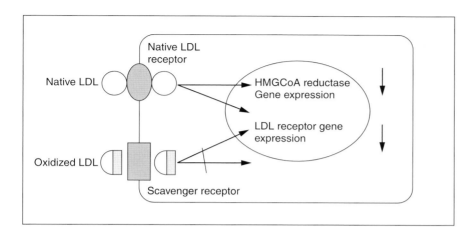

Figure 7.4
The LDL receptor.

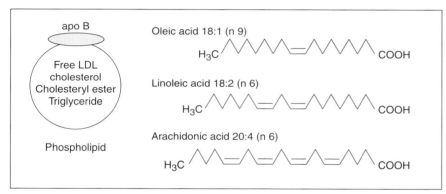

Figure 7.5
Principal fatty acids in LDL.

due to reduced activity of the insulin-sensitive desaturase enzymes.[104,105]

Small dense LDL

Small dense LDL, which is thought to be particularly atherogenic, is more susceptible to oxidation.[106] It is associated with hypertriglyceridaemia and particularly with elevated levels of large triglyceride-rich VLDL[60] and more recently with remnant lipoprotein cholesterol levels.[107] Lahdenpera et al. also confirmed the relationship between hypertriglyceridaemia and LDL particle size in diabetes.[108] Type 2 diabetes and insulin resistance does not seem to have any direct effect on LDL particle size, at least in mildly hypertriglyceridaemic subjects.[109] In Japanese men who have a low prevalence of coronary artery disease (CAD), Koba et al[110] found a high prevalence of small dense LDL with CAD irrespective of the presence of diabetes. A recent study comparing three subgroups of Type 2 diabetic patients, divided according to fasting plasma triglycerides, found that the relative proportion of cholesterol ester transferred from HDL to VLDL1 increased progressively with increase in plasma triglycerides.[111] Dense LDL acquired on average 45% of total cholesteryl ester transferred from HDL to LDL. The authors concluded that CETP contributes significantly to the formation of small dense LDL in Type 2 diabetes.

Antibodies to LDL and atherogenesis

This story is even more complex, since modified LDL become antigenic and the antibodies to modified LDL have been shown to cause deposition of cholesterol in the atherosclerotic plaque. We have demonstrated a relationship between polyunsaturated fatty acids and antibodies to oxidized LDL in diabetic patients and confirmed the previously described association between antibodies to oxidized LDL and CAD.[112,113] We have also shown that diabetic patients, even if they did not suffer from CAD, had raised levels of oxidized LDL antibodies, another possible mechanism for the predisposition of diabetic patients to atherosclerosis. A study of LDL receptor-deficient mice has provided further evidence for the relationship between circulating antibodies to oxidized LDL and the oxidized LDL content of atherosclerotic lesions.[114] Immunization of hypercholesterolaemic rabbits with oxidized LDL has been found to reduce lesion formation.[115] Zhou et al.[116] examined the mechanism by which immunization might protect against atherosclerosis and found that increased titres of T-cell dependent IgG antibodies correlated with decreased lesion formation. Thus, good control of diabetes has the potential to lessen considerably the atherogenicity of LDL in a number of ways.

HDL and reverse cholesterol transport

It has long been known that high HDL levels are protective against atherosclerosis,[117] although the curve is U shaped.[118] The total cholesterol/HDL cholesterol ratio is a useful determinant of risk, but not all studies have shown that high HDL is protective. The confusion probably relates to the rate of turnover of cholesterol within the HDL particle.[119] Thus, a low HDL, which is rapidly transporting cholesterol to the liver and to the apo B-containing lipoproteins, may be even more protective than a high HDL level with very slow cholesterol turnover. The story of HDL has fired the imagination of lipidologists since the discovery of the mechanism of Tangier disease. Tangier disease is a very rare hereditary disorder, which results in the accumulation of lipid in the reticuloendothelial system. It has been shown to be due to a mutation in a gene encoding the ATP cassette binding protein-1 (ABC1).[120–123] That gene has been named ABCA1 and its protein, the cholesterol efflux receptor protein (CERP). Marcil et al.[124] have demonstrated a defect in the ABCA1 gene in familial HDL deficiency which is related to defective cholesterol efflux. Elegant studies have described the mechanism by which cellular cholesterol migrates to the caveoli in the cell membrane, where CERP facilitates its transfer onto lipid depleted apo A1 or apo A1/A2 to form HDL2. The cholesterol is re-esterified by lecithin cholesterol acyltransferase (LCAT) and transferred by cholesteryl ester transfer protein (CETP) to triglyceride-rich lipoproteins in exchange for triglyceride.[125] The mechanism by which the majority of cholesterol in HDL is delivered to the liver has also been described. Apo A1 proteins, unlike apo B100, are able to discharge cholesterol in the liver and remain free to re-circulate as relatively lipid-free HDL3. The scavenger receptor B1 (SRB1) binds HDL with high affinity and this binding is essential for HDL-mediated cellular cholesterol efflux.[126,127] Overexpression of SR-B1 increases efflux of cholesterol from the cell to HDL particles but not to free apo A.[128] This receptor also binds to native and modified LDL and also to native HDL.[126,129]

HDL *as an antioxidant*

HDL has other functions, which are thought to be important in the anti-atherosclerotic process. The most important is perhaps the protection of LDL against oxidation through paraoxonase, an enzyme which is found tightly associated with apo A1 in the HDL particle and is in interstitial fluid associated with HDL.[130] The enzyme exerts its protective effect by hydrolyzing oxidized phospholipids.[131] Members of the pon gene family are pon-1, pon-2 and pon-3. There is interest in the pon-1 and pon-2 gene polymorphism in relation to atherosclerosis particularly in some ethnic groups.[132–134] Pon-1 and pon-2 have been shown to induce monocyte chemotaxis and binding to endothelial cells.[135] It is also of interest that pon-1 and pon-2 polymorphisms are associated with fasting glucose levels in diabetic subjects and the risk of CAD.[136,137] Pon-2 is not detectable in HDL or LDL but is expressed in both primary and immortalized human endothelial cells and human aortic smooth muscle cells. Thus, unlike pon-1 and pon-3, pon-2 exerts its antioxidant functions at the cellular level.[138] Apo A11 is the second major HDL protein accounting for 20% of HDL protein. In contrast to apo A1, apo A11 seems to be pro-atherogenic and is associated with an increase in plasma free fatty acids and triglycerides.[139] Apo A11 is also not associated with antioxidant function and inhibits reverse cholesterol transport.[140,141] Apo A11 locus has emerged as a candidate gene for diabetes since Apo A11 may also have a role in insulin resistance.[142–144]

Metabolic defects which cause hypercholesterolaemia

The story of cholesterol metabolism has revealed even more exciting information. The most frequent monogenic disease at present is familial hypercholesterolaemia due to a defect in the LDL receptor and very many mutations of the receptor have now been described.[145] Apo B gene defects are another common cause of hypercholesterolaemia.[146–148] A rare form of hypercholesterolaemia, in which neither parent may have elevated serum cholesterol, has been described as autosomal recessive hypercholesterolaemia (ARH).[149] In this syndrome, whose severity approaches the severity of familial hypercholesterolaemia (FH), obligate heterozygous parents of ARH, unlike the heterozygous parents of FH homozygotes, have normal plasma LDL. The defect in this condition has been traced to the ARH gene encoding the previously undescribed LDL receptor adaptor protein. Diabetes does not appear to play any part in the above three abnormalities. Recently the regulation of cholesterol absorption and excretion has been further unravelled through the investigation of the rare condition sitosterolaemia.[150] Normally sitosterol is not absorbed and indeed causes cholesterol malabsorption. This has resulted in the popularization of sitosterol-containing spreads which cause a 10% reduction in cholesterol while being very palatable. In sitosterolaemia, sitosterol is absorbed and incorporated into the LDL particle along with cholesterol. This results in an increase in atherosclerosis. Research into this rare condition has helped to clarify the mechanism of cholesterol homoeostasis. The gene which causes sitosterolaemia resides on chromosome 2p-21 and the gene products are ABC-G5 and ABC-G8.[151–153] These two proteins work together, probably as a heterodimer and perhaps with the help of ABC-A1 in the intestine, to promote the efflux of cholesterol from enterocytes back into the lumen. In the liver these proteins regulate excretion of cholesterol into the bile (Figure 7.6). This is presumably the mechanism which

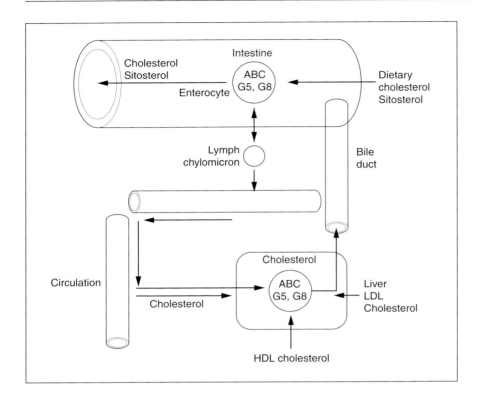

Figure 7.6
Sterol metabolism.

was so successful in allowing the man, immortalized in the *New England Journal of Medicine*, to continually eat 25 eggs a day and yet survive into his eighties without severe hypercholesterolaemia or atherosclerosis.[154] In experimental diabetes, intestinal cholesterol synthesis but not absorption is increased[155–157] and in humans cholesterol synthesis has also been shown to be increased.[158] The finding of increase in cholesterol in the lymph of diabetic animals[49,157] and the finding of increase in cholesterol in the triglyceride-rich lipoproteins in the early postprandial phase in diabetic patients suggests considerable disruption of the ABC system.

Treatments for diabetic dyslipidaemia

Hydroxymethylglutaryl co-enzymeA (HMGCoA) reductase and acyl-CoA: cholesterol acyltransferase (ACAT)

The mechanisms so far are presented so that the reader can more easily appreciate the new exciting areas of pharmacological research, focused on the development of new treatments for hyperlipidaemia, that are opening up. Cholesterol synthesis, the other important area to receive attention, has a history of longer duration but has perhaps received less publicity in recent years. The success of the HMGCoA reductase inhibitors focused attention on the importance of inhibition of cholesterol synthesis.[18,159] It became apparent that although the primary effect of HMGCoA reductase inhibitors was indeed the reduction of cholesterol synthesis, the very important secondary effect was the upregulation of the LDL receptor and it was this upregulation that was central to the clearance of LDL and the lowering of serum cholesterol.[160] It had been known for many years that cholesterol must be esterified before it can be packaged into the chylomicron in the intestine or into VLDL in the liver. The enzyme acyl-CoA:cholesterol acyltransferase (ACAT) which esterifies cholesterol was an obvious target, and early animal studies using ACAT inhibitors showed great promise.[161–162] A recent study has demonstrated that the combined effect of inhibiting both ACAT and HMGCoA reductase led to very impressive reduction in atherosclerotic lesion size in rabbits.[163] In the hypercholesterolaemic rabbit the drug has been shown to reduce macrophage cholesterol accumulation and expression of metalloproteinases, important enzymes in vascular remodelling and plaque destabilization. The drug may therefore have an exciting future, especially in diabetes.[164] It is only recently that ACAT inhibitors have been shown to be potentially successful in humans. Insull et al.[165] evaluated a new wholly synthetic ACAT inhibitor in patients with combined hyperlipidaemia and low HDL. These authors found no statistically significant differences in total cholesterol, HDL cholesterol or apo B between treated and untreated groups. On the other hand, there was a prompt and significant reduction in plasma VLDL triglyceride and cholesterol. It is interesting that in miniature pigs the ACAT inhibitor avasimbe reduced

both VLDL and LDL apo B concentrations primarily by decreasing apo B secretion.[166,167] We are not aware of any postprandial studies and it is possible that ACAT inhibition may be particularly valuable in reducing chylomicrons.

Microsomal triglyceride transfer protein (MTP)

MTP is very important in the regulation of chylomicron and VLDL formation.[168,169] There is a close relationship between ACAT and MTP, and certain flavonoids have been shown to inhibit apo B secretion by reducing the expression and activity of ACAT and MTP.[170] The MTP gene promoter contains a sterol and an insulin response element, so there has been interest in this gene in both hypercholesterolaemia and diabetes. Animal studies have demonstrated an increase in MTP expression and activity in the intestine and liver in diabetes and in insulin resistance.[48,171,172] A common polymorphism of the MTP gene promoter region has been demonstrated to lower plasma cholesterol in healthy men[173] and to protect against the steatosis of Type 2 diabetes as demonstrated by ultrasound and liver enzymes.[174] Alas, MTP inhibitors to date, although effective in reducing lipoprotein secretion, result in steatosis.

Postprandial hyperlipidaemia

In diabetes, the avenues towards improvement in dyslipidaemia all start in the postprandial phase. To date little attention has been paid to pharmacological manipulation of the postprandial lipoproteins in diabetes. However, we have demonstrated that cerevastatin significantly reduced postprandial apo B48 and apo B100 in Type 2 diabetic patients and, in particular, it decreased the amount of the larger, less dense particles.[64] This may be of importance because these particles stay longer in the circulation.[66]

The Diabetes Atherosclerosis Intervention Study (DAIS)[175] examined the role of fenofibrate on coronary atherosclerosis in Type 2 diabetes. The study demonstrated a significantly smaller increase in percentage diameter stenosis of coronary arteries on treatment when compared with placebo. The study strongly supports the concept that the postprandial phase is particularly important in the development of atherosclerosis. The relationship between postprandial hypertriglyceridaemia and endothelial function was examined in patients with CAD by Bae et al.[176] who showed that fenofibrate reduced superoxide anion formation, an index of oxidative stress. Although the authors were unable to show any change in endothelial function, the reduction in postprandial hypertriglyceridaemia may act through reduction in free-radical production.

Remnant lipoproteins

The remnant-like lipoprotein particle (isolated using immunoaffinity anti-apo A1/anti-apo B100 gel) has been used as a measurement of chylomicrons but it also includes a sub-population of apo E-rich, apo B100 lipoproteins in plasma.[177,178] Although it is not yet clear whether the measurement of these particles is a surrogate measurement of apo B48 particles.[179] They have been related to intima-media thickness of the carotid artery independently of LDL cholesterol and plasma triglycerides.[60] Karpe et al.[61] demonstrated a significant relationship between these particles and the occurrence of new lesions in vein grafts of patients who have had successful coronary bypass operations. Patients treated with gemfibrozil, another fibrate, were much less likely to present with a new lesion during the study period. Gemfibrozil reduced the median remnant-like protein cholesterol concentration by 34%. A mechanism to explain these results may be related to the ability of remnant-like lipoprotein particles to upregulate intercellular adhesion molecule-1 (ICAM-1), vascular adhesion molecule-1 (VCAM-1) and tissue factor, partly through a redox sensitive mechanism.[180] Measurement of the remnant-like lipoprotein particle may become an important tool in the evaluation of anti-atherogenic compounds for the protection against atherosclerosis in diabetic patients (Figure 7.7).

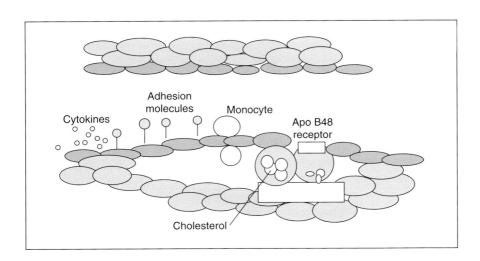

Figure 7.7
Atherosclerotic plaque.

Cytokines

Adhesion molecules

Monocyte

Apo B48 receptor

Cholesterol

Cholesterol absorption inhibitors

Sitosterol, a plant sterol as stated previously, when incorporated into margarine, causes significant cholesterol lowering. Drugs, which inhibit cholesterol absorption might have a place in the treatment of hypercholesterolaemia, particularly if they could be combined with an intestinal cholesterol synthesis inhibitor and/or chylomicron synthesis inhibitor. Gylling and Miettinen[181] demonstrated that stanol ester margarine which inhibits cholesterol absorption, when combined with Simvastatin treatment reduced cholesterol absorption and serum cholesterol more consistently in subjects with high rather than low baseline absorption of cholesterol. A cholesterol absorption inhibitor, ezetimibe, has been progressing through trials.[182] It is metabolized in the intestine, which is its site of action, and has been shown to reduce cholesterol absorption in rats by up to 90%. A recent paper examined the effect of ezetimibe on combined hypertriglyceridaemic and hypercholesteolaemic, obese hyperinsulinaemic hamsters.[182] Ezetimibe, although not affecting obesity, body weight or leptin, significantly decreased LDL cholesterol and completely eliminated the accumulation of cholesteryl and free cholesterol in the liver. In human studies of primary hypercholesterolaemia another cholesterol absorption inhibitor from the same company significantly reduced LDL cholesterol and apo B.[183,184]

Peroxisome proliferator activated receptors (PPARs)

The recognition of the role of PPARα in the regulation of fatty acid metabolism and the importance of PPARγ in insulin resistance has stimulated the search for drugs which may have effects on both PPAR systems. It has already been shown that the thiazolidinedione group of drugs which have major effects on PPARγ and insulin resistance have some PPARα effects and tend to lower triglyceride levels.[185,186] They have, however, been associated with weight gain. The retinoid X receptors (RXR) function as a heterodimer with PPARs. It is interesting to read that a synthetic RXR and PPARγ antagonist (HX531) decreased triglyceride content in white adipose tissue, skeletal muscle and liver.[187] The compound was shown to potentiate leptin's effect and ameliorate diet-induced obesity and Type 2 diabetes in a mouse model. This new information is exciting and opens up the potential for the development of successful antiobesity agents in the treatment of Type 2 diabetes.

The fibrates which are major PPARα agonists[188] also improve insulin resistance, at least to some extent.[189] Experiments using PPARα null mice have demonstrated a difference between male and female. The female, but not male mice displayed high serum apo B associated with VLDL and increased hepatic triglyceride secretion. The male PPARα null mice showed increased susceptibility to high fat diet in terms of apo B.[190] It has also been shown that PPARα deficiency is associated with protection against high fat diet-induced insulin resistance.[191] Both PPARα and PPARγ are expressed in fully differentiated human macrophages where they regulate genes implicated in the inflammatory response.[192,193] In primary human macrophages both PPARα and PPARγ activators induce the expression of the scavenger receptor CLA-1/SR-B1 which binds HDL with high affinity. Thus it is not clear whether activation of PPARγ in macrophages promotes or inhibits atherosclerosis. Chinetti et al.[194] have shown a regulatory role for PPARα and PPARγ in the first steps of the reverse cholesterol transport pathway through the activation of the ABC-A1 mediated cholesterol efflux in human macrophages. This suggests that, like the statins, further development of fibrates will result in compounds that will reverse the atherosclerotic process through mechanisms independent of triglyceride metabolism. Protection from obesity and insulin resistance is a major world topic for discussion with the increasing awareness of the huge increase in diabetes throughout the world.

Apolipoproteins C1, apo C11, and apo C111

Apo C1 is attached to chylomicrons, VLDL and HDL. It has an inhibitory action on VLDL uptake by hepatic receptors and postprandial accumulation of large apo C-1-rich cholesterol-rich VLDL has been shown in normolipidaemic patients with CAD.[195] Apo C1 transgenic mice exhibit elevated plasma concentrations of free fatty acids but are not associated with insulin resistance. Indeed in the *ob/ob* mice overexpression of apo C1 significantly improved insulin sensitivity. It has also been shown that apo C1 transgenic mice, when crossbred on the genetically obese *ob/ob* background were fully protected from the development of obesity.[196] Perhaps another avenue for treatment in the future? Apo C11 is a co-factor for lipoprotein lipase and increased plasma lipoprotein lipase activity has been associated with reduced susceptibility to atherosclerosis in apo E-deficient mice.[197] The development of drugs, which increase apo C11 may yield beneficial results. Apo C111 protects the chylomicron and VLDL particle from delipidation and VLDL turnover is accelerated in apo C111 knockout mice.[198] The fibrates reduce apo C111 through their action on PPARα thereby increasing VLDL turnover.[199,200] In diabetic animals, apo E is decreased on the chylomicron particle[49,201] and in diabetic patients apo E/particle is reduced in both the chylomicron and VLDL fractions.[79] This is one explanation for the

increase in VLDL in diabetes since apo E is the principal ligand for VLDL receptor uptake in the liver and removal from the circulation.[202–204] The development of drugs that increase apo E/particle could have major benefits, particularly in diabetes.

Antioxidants and diabetes control in atherosclerosis prevention

The importance of oxidation of LDL, particularly in diabetes in the genesis of atheroma, is an attractive theory but it is disappointing that antioxidants have not been proved to be of benefit in the reduction of atherosclerosis in human studies.[205–209] Since free-radical production is increased in diabetes, improvement in diabetes control should reduce the atherosclerotic burden and indeed, in secondary prevention studies improved outcome has been shown when intensive insulin therapy has been instituted.[13] However, it is disappointing that there is so little evidence that improvement in diabetic control will reduce macrovascular disease in diabetes, particularly when the reduction in microvascular disease is beyond doubt.[5–11] One presumes that the time scale to develop macrovascular disease as compared to microvascular disease is the major reason for failure. This is particularly obvious when one looks at the massive sizes of trials that were necessary in non-diabetic patients to show benefit from hypotensive therapy[210–212] or statin therapy.[18–21,159] One must also remember the great difficulties we have in normalizing blood glucose in the diabetic patient over a long period of time.[8,213] We all expect that the whole position of atherosclerosis in diabetes will dramatically change with the improvement in methods to control blood glucose through the use of islet cell transplantation or the artificial pancreas.[214]

Anti-inflammatory agents in atherosclerosis

The immune mechanism in the development of atherosclerosis[215–217] and the role of modified LDL, whether it be by glycation or oxidation[82] in raising antibodies against LDL, has presented us with a new mechanism to explain the atherosclerotic plaque development in diabetes.[115,116] Interventions to increase specific T-cell dependent IgG antibodies against oxidized LDL and oxidized phospholipids may yield useful results in the future. The role of inflammation in atherosclerosis, as well as the relationship between LDL antibody formation and the inflammatory response in the atherosclerotic plaque, have still to be elucidated. The part played by aspirin in these events, and the importance of chronic inflammation are under intensive investigation at present. C-reactive protein, an important marker of inflammation, has been shown to mediate LDL uptake by macrophages.[218] It independently predicts early carotid atherosclerosis.[31,219] The recent finding that C-reactive protein can be reduced by statins,[220] and that there is equal benefit in cardiovascular event protection from cholesterol lowering in those patients who have low CRP levels and from CRP lowering in those patients who already have low cholesterol levels,[26] will have major implications in the identification and treatment of patients in CAD prevention.

Metalloproteinases and plaque stability

The stability of the atherosclerotic plaque is of major importance in the prevention of cardiovascular events. We are only at the beginning of our understanding of how the macrophage may destabilize the plaque through the secretion of various metalloproteinases.[221,222]

However, in diabetes it may be of particular importance as it has been shown that certain extracellular matrix metalloproteinases are significantly increased in two rodent models of diabetes.[223] It is an exciting field of development, particularly since it has been shown that oxidized LDL stimulates metalloproteinase expression.[217] It has further been shown that metalloproteinase inhibitors induce plaque regression and prevent progression of vascular disease.[224] It is also exciting to learn that the ACAT inhibitor avasimbe limits macrophage accumulation and metalloproteinase expression.[164] HMGCoA reductase inhibitors have also been shown to inhibit metalloproteinase secretion by macrophages.[164,225,226]

HDL and lipid transfer

The smallest lipoprotein to be discussed is HDL, yet its influence on atherosclerosis is extremely important.[227] The levels of HDL are dependent on triglyceride levels to some extent. CETP is an important regulator of HDL through its transport of cholesterol to apo B-containing lipoproteins in exchange for triglyceride.[228] Phospholipid transfer protein (PLTP) also plays an important role in human HDL metabolism and both activity and mass have been shown to be higher in diabetic patients concomitant with hyperglycaemia.[229] The PLTP gene has been shown to be transcriptionally regulated by fenofibrate via the response elements for nuclear hormone receptors PPARs and farnesoid X-activated receptor.[230] It has also been shown that glucose regulates the mRNA levels of PLTP, ABC-A1 and SRB1 receptors.[229] The role of CETP and PLTP inhibitors has yet to be evaluated, particularly since levels of HDL are sometimes a poor predictor of atherosclerotic risk particularly in diabetes.[119,228] This may be because the level of HDL is dependent on HDL turnover and the load of cholesterol it is carry-

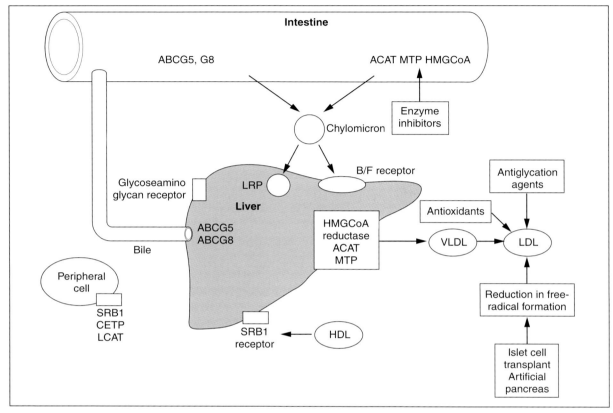

Figure 7.8
Possible sites for therapeutic intervention.

ing. High turnover of HDL therefore, which would be reflected by low HDL cholesterol, would be anti-atherogenic, whereas a high HDL with a low turnover would be pro-atherogenic.[231] This may be a reason to question the importance in atherogenesis terms of drugs, which lower LDL cholesterol but also lower HDL cholesterol.[227] Drugs which will affect ABC-A1 and therefore the efflux of cholesterol from the cell are obviously a prime target for pharmacologists. At the other end there are drugs which improve the SRB1 receptor and thus lower HDL cholesterol making lipid depleted HDL3 more available to the peripheral

tissues and may also have huge therapeutic benefits. A timely review by Tall et al.[228] entitled 'Is it time to modify the reverse cholesterol transport model?' suggests that lipoprotein researchers should place greater emphasis on the interaction of HDL and its apoproteins with cells and atheroma and devote less effort to pursuing the idea that it may be useful to increase cholesterol transport by increasing HDL. They suggest that successful interventions at the level of the foam cell, which could be mediated by ABC-A1 expression or by decreased HDL catabolism, may be the successful intervention pathway of the future (Figure 7.8).

Conclusion

Focus will now shift to the development of strategies based on new understanding of how cholesterol homoeostasis is maintained through the ABC-G1, G5 and G8, ABCA1 and SRB1 genes. In diabetes, it is tantalizing to realize how little we know about how diabetes per se damages the large vessel and how ineffective our strategy for lowering blood glucose is to inhibit atherosclerosis. It is certainly upsetting to have our cardiology colleagues suggest that they should take over the care of diabetic patients since they understand hypertension and dyslipidaemia and we as diabetologists have no idea of how to lower blood glucose in an effective way. Certainly papers are still being published demonstrating the decreased life expectancy of people with diabetes.[10,233] All the recent evidence suggests that the future will be less bleak for newly diagnosed people with diabetes as new methods of treatment come on stream. The diabetologist in the future will surely be able to defend his/her patients against intervention by cardiologists.

References

1. Baigent C, Burbury K, Wheeler D. Premature cardiovascular disease in chronic renal failure. Lancet 2000; 356: 147–52.
2. Shoji T, Emoto M, Kawagishi T et al. Atherogenic lipoprotein changes in diabetic nephropathy. Atherosclerosis 2001; 156: 425–33.
3. Laing SP, Swerdlow AJ, Stater SD et al. The British Diabetic Association Cohort Study 1. All cause mortality in patients with insulin-treated diabetes mellitus. Diabet Med 1999; 16: 459–65.
4. Laing SP, Swerdlow AJ, Stater SD et al. The British Diabetic Association Cohort Study 11. Cause specific mortality in patients with insulin-treated diabetes mellitus. Diabet Med 1999; 16: 466–71.
5. The Diabetes and Complications Trial Research Group. The effect of intensive treatment of diabetes on the development and progression of long-term complications in insulin-dependent diabetes mellitus. N Engl J Med 1993; 329: 977–86.
6. Diabetes Control and Complications Trial. Type 1 diabetic patients with good or poor metabolic control. Diabetes Care 2001; 24: 1275–9.
7. Meigs JB, Nathan DM, Wilson P et al. Metabolic risk factors worsen across the spectrum of non-diabetic glucose tolerance. Ann Intern Med 1998; 128: 524–33.
8. UK Prospective Diabetes Study (UKPDS) Group. Intensive blood-glucose control with sulphonylureas or insulin compared with conventional treatment and risk of complications in patients with Type 2 diabetes (UKPDS 33) Lancet 1998; 352: 837–53.
9. Epidemiology of Diabetes Interventions and Complications (EDIC) Research Group. Effect of intensive diabetes treatment on carotid artery wall thickness in the epidemiology of diabetes and complications. Diabetes 1999; 48: 383–90.
10. Fuller JH, Stevens LK, Lang S-L et al, and the WHO Multinational Study Group. Risk factors for cardiovascular mortality and morbidity: the WHO multinational study of vascular disease in diabetes. Diabetologia 2001; 44: S54–64.
11. Jensen-Urstad KJ, Richard PG, Rosfors JS et al. Early atherosclerosis is retarded by improved long-term blood glucose control in patients with IDDM. Diabetes 1996; 45: 1253–8.
12. Malmberg K, Norhammar A, Wedel H, Ryden L. Glycometabolic state at admission: important risk marker of mortality in conventionally treated patients with diabetes mellitus and acute myocardial infarction: long-term results from Diabetes and Insulin-Glucose Infusion in Acute Myocardial Infarction (DIGAMI) Study Circulation 1999; 99: 2626–32.
13. UK Prospective Diabetes Study (UKPDS) Group. Tight blood pressure control and the risk of macrovascular and microvascular complications in Type 2 diabetes. BMJ 1998; 317: 703–13.
14. Trocha AK, Schmidtke C, Didjurgeit U et al. Effects of intensified antihypertensive treatment in diabetic nephropathy; mortality and morbidity results of a prospective controlled 10-year study. J Hypertens 1999; 17: 1497–1503.

15. Orchard TJ, Forrest KY, Kuller LH, Becker DJ. Pittsburgh Epidemiology of Diabetes Complications Study. Lipid and blood pressure treatment goals for Type 1 diabetes: 10-year incidence data from the Pittsburgh Epidemiology of Diabetes Complications Study. Diabetes Care 2001; 24: 1053–9.

16. Castelli WP, Garrison RJ, Wilson PWF et al. Incidence of coronary heart disease and lipoprotein cholesterol levels: the Framingham Study. JAMA 1986; 256: 2835–8.

17. Pyorala K, Pedersen TR, Kjekshus J et al. The Scandinavian Simvastatin Survival Study (4S) Group. Cholesterol-lowering with simvastatin improves prognosis of diabetic patients with heart disease. Diabetes Care 1997; 20: 614–20.

18. Frick MH, Elo O, Haapa K et al. Helsinki Heart Study: Primary Prevention Trial with gemfibrozil in middle-aged men with dyslipidaemia. Safety of treatment, changes in risk factors and incidence of coronary heart disease. N Engl J Med 1986; 317: 1237–45.

19. Lewis SJ, Lemuel AM, Sacks F et al. Effect of pravastatin on cardiovascular events in older patients with myocardial infarction and cholesterol levels in average range. Results of the Cholesterol and Recurrent Events (CARE) Trial. Ann Intern Med 1998; 129: 681–9.

20. Ravnskov U, Anton C. Statins as the new aspirin. BMJ 2002; 324: 789.

21. Sparrow CP. Simvastatin has anti-inflammatory and antiatherosclerotic activities independent of plasma cholesterol lowering. Arterioscler Thromb Vasc Biol 2001; 21: 115–21.

22. Lindbohm N, Gylling H, Miettinen TE et al. Treatment increases the sialic acid content of LDL in hypercholesterolemic patients. Atherosclerosis 2000; 151: 545–50.

23. Romano M, Mezzetti A, Marulli C et al. Fluvastatin reduces soluble P-selectin and ICAM-1 levels in hypercholesterolemic patients: role of nitric oxide. J Invest Med 2000; 48: 183–9.

24. Kothe H, Dalhoff K, Rupp J et al. Hydroxymethylglutaryl coenzyme A reductase inhibitors modify the inflammatory response of human macrophages and endothelial cells infected with *Chlamydia pneumoniae*. Circulation 1999; 101: 1760–3.

25. Ridker PM, Rifai N, Clearfield M et al. for the Air Force/Texas Coronary Atherosclerosis Prevention Study Investigators. Measurement of C-reactive protein for the targeting of statin therapy in the primary prevention of acute coronary events. N Engl J Med 2001; 344: 1959–65.

26. Stein JD, Balis D, Grundy SM et al. Effect of hydroxymethyl glutaryl coenzyme A reductase inhibitor therapy on high sensitive C-reactive protein levels. Circulation 2001; 103: 1933–5.

27. Undas A, Brummel KE, Musial J et al. Simvastatin depresses blood clotting by inhibiting activation of prothrombin, factor V, and factor XIII and by enhancing factor Va inactivation. Circulation 2001; 103: 2248–53.

28. Freeman DJ, Norrie J, Sattar N et al. Pravastatin and the development of diabetes mellitus : evidence for a protective treatment effect in the West of Scotland Coronary Prevention Study. Circulation 2001; 103: 357–62.

29. Schmidt MI, Duncan BB, Sharrett AR et al. Markers of inflammation and prediction of diabetes mellitus in adults (Atherosclerosis Risk in Communities study) Lancet 1999; 353: 1649–52.

30. Freeman DJ, Norrie J, Caslake MJ et al. C-reactive protein is an independent predictor of risk for the development of diabetes in the West of Scotland Prevention Study. Diabetes 2002; 51: 1596–600.

31. Pradhan AD, Manson JE, Rifai N et al. C-reactive protein, interleukin 6, and risk of developing Type 2 diabetes mellitus. JAMA 2001; 286: 327–34.

32. Hashimoto H, Kitagawa K, Hougaku H et al. C-reactive protein is an independent predictor of the rate of increase in early carotid atherosclerosis. Circulation 2001; 104: 63–8.

33. Sniderman AD, Scantlebury T, Cianflone K. Hypertriglyceridaemic hyper-apo B: The unappreciated atherogenic dyslipoprotinaemia in Type 2 diabetes mellitus. Ann Intern Med 2001; 135: 447–59.

34. Tomkin GH, Owens D. ApoB lipoproteins, diabetes and atherosclerosis. Diabetes Metab Res Rev 2001; 17: 27–43.

35. Grundy SM, Mok HYI. Chylomicron clearance in normal and hyperlipidaemic man. Metabolism 1976; 25: 1225–39.

36. Welty FK, Lichtenstein AH, Barrett PHR et al. Effects of apo E genotype on apo B48 and apo B100 kinetics with stable isotopes in humans. Atheroscler Thromb Vasc Biol 2000; 20: 1807–10.

37. Welty FK, Lichtenstein AH, Barrett PH et al. Human apolipoprotein (Apo) B-48 and ApoB-100 kinetics with stable isotopes. Arterioscler, Thromb Vasc Biol 1999; 19: 2966–74.

38. Li X, Catalina F, Grundy AM, Patel S. Method to measure apolipoprotein B48 and B100 secretion rates in an individual mouse: evidence for a very rapid turnover of VLDL and preferential removal of B48 relative to B100–containing lipoproteins. J Lipid Res 1996; 37: 210–20.

39. Redgrave TG, Ly HL, Quintao CF et al. Clearance from plasma of triacylglycerol and cholesterol ester after intravenous injection of chylomicron-like lipid emulsions in rat and man. Biochem J 1993; 290: 843–7.

40. Caslake MJ, Packard CJ, Series JJ et al. Plasma triglycerides and low density lipoprotein metabolism. Eur J Clin Invest 1992; 22: 96–104.

41. Packard CJ, Demant T, Stewart JP et al. Apolipoprotein B metabolism and the distribution of VLDL and LDL subfractions. J Lipid Res 2000; 41: 305–18.

42. Kissebah AH, Alfarsi S, Evans DJ et al. Plasma low density lipoprotein transport kinetics in non-insulin-dependent diabetes mellitus. J Clin Invest 1983; 71: 655–67.

43. Howard B, Abbott WG, Beltz et al. Integrated study of low density lipoprotein metabolism and very low density lipoprotein metabolism in non-insulin-dependent diabetes. Metabolism 1987; 9: 870–7.

44. Phillips C, Madigan C, Owens D, Collins P, Tomkin GH. Defective chylomicron synthesis as a cause of delayed particle clearance in diabetes? Int J Exp Diab Res 2002; 3: 171–8.

45. Deegan P, Owens D, Collins P et al. Association between low-density lipoprotein composition and its metabolism in non-insulin-dependent diabetes mellitus. Metabolism Clin Exp 1999; 48: 118–24.

46. Phillips ML, Pullinger C, Kroes I et al. A single copy of apolipoprotein B48 is present on the human chylomicron remnant. J Lipid Res 1997; 38: 1170–7.

47. Hoeg JM, Sviridov DD, Tennyson GE et al. Both apolipoproteins B-48 and B-100 are synthesized and secreted by the human intestine. J Lipid Res 1990; 31: 1761–9.

48. Gianturco SH, Ramprasad MP, Song R et al. Apolipoprotein B48 or its apolipoprotein B100 equivalent mediates the binding of triglyceride-rich lipoproteins to their unique human monocyte-macrophage receptor. Arterioscler Thromb Vasc Biol 1998; 18: 968–76.

49. Gleeson A, Anderton K, Owens D et al. The role of microsomal triglyceride transfer protein and dietary cholesterol in chylomicron production in diabetes. Diabetologia 1999; 42: 944–9.

50. Phillips C, Murugasu G, Owens D et al. Improved metabolic control reduces the number of postprandial apolipoprotein B48-containing particles in Type 2 diabetes. Atherosclerosis 2000; 148: 283–91.

51. Lovegrove J, Isherwood SG, Jackson KG, et al. Quantification of apo B48 in triglycerol-rich lipoproteins by specific enzyme-linked immunosorbent assay. Biochem Biophys Acta 1996; 1301: 221–9.

52. Harbis A, Defoort C, Narbonne H et al. Acute hyperinsulinism modulates plasma apolipoprotein B-48 triglyceride-rich lipoproteins in healthy subjects during the postprandial period. Diabetes 2001; 50: 462–9.

53. Karpe F, Steiner G, Uffelman K et al. Postprandial lipoproteins and the progression of coronary atherosclerosis. Atherosclerosis 1994; 106: 83–97.

54. Cummings MH, Watts GF, Umpleby AM et al. Acute hyperinsulinaemia decreases the hepatic secretion of very low density lipoprotein apolipoprotein B100 in NIDDM. Diabetes 1995; 44: 1059–65.

55. Cummings MH, Watts GF, Umpleby AM et al. Increased hepatic secretion of very low density lipoprotein apolipoprotein B100 in NIDDM. Diabetologia 1995; 38: 955–67.

56. Bioletto S, Golay A, Munger R et al. Acute hyperinsulinemia and very-low-density and low-density lipoprotein subfractions in obese subjects. Am J Clin 2000; 71: 443–9.

57. Duvillard L, Pont F, Florentin E et al. Metabolic abnormalities of apolipoprotein B-containing lipoproteins in non-insulin-dependent diabetes: a stable isotope kinetic study. Eur Clin Invest 2000; 30: 685–94.

58. Goldberg IJ. Lipoprotein lipase and lipolysis: central roles in lipoprotein metabolism and atherogenesis. J Lipid Res 1996; 37: 693–707.

59. Fan J, Unoki H, Kojima N et al. Over expression of lipoprotein lipase in transgenic rabbits inhibits diet-induced hypercholesterolaemia and atherosclerosis. J Biol Chem 2001; 276: 40071–9.

60. Karpe F, Boquist S, Tang R et al. Remnant lipoproteins are related to intima-media thickness of the carotid artery independently of LDL cholesterol and plasma triglycerides. J Lipid Res 2001; 42: 17–21.

61. Karpe F, Taskinen MR, Nieminen MS et al. Remnant-like lipoprotein particle cholesterol concentration and progression of coronary and vein-graft atherosclerosis in response to gemfibrozil treatment. Atherosclerosis 2001; 157: 181–7.

62. Gaw A, Packard CJ, Lindsay GM et al. Overproduction of small, very low density lipoproteins (sf 20–60) on moderate hypercholesterolaemia: relationship between apolipoprotein B kinetics and plasma lipoproteins. J Lipid Res 1995; 36: 158–71.

63. Taggart C, Gibney J, Owens D et al. The role of dietary cholesterol in the regulation of postprandial apolipoprotein B48 levels in diabetes. Diabetes Med 1997; 14: 1051–8.

64. Battula SB, Fitzsimons O, Moreno S et al. Postprandial apolipoprotein B48 and B100–containing lipoproteins in Type 2 diabetes: do statins have a specific effect on triglyceride metabolism? Metabolism 2000; 49: 1–7.

65. Martins IJ, Mortimer B-C, Miller J, Redgrave TG. Effects of particle size and number on the plasma clearance of chylomicrons and remnants. J Lipid Res 1996; 37: 2696–705.

66. Tkac I, Kimball BP, Lewis G et al. The severity of coronary atherosclerosis in Type 2 diabetes mellitus is related to the number of circulating triglyceride-rich lipoprotein particles. Arterioscler Thromb Vasc Biol 1997; 17: 3633–8.

67. Rensen PC, Herijgers N, Netscher MH et al. Particle size determines the specificity of apo E-containing triglyceride-rich emulsions for LDL receptor versus hepatic remnant receptor in vivo. J Lipid Res 1997; 38: 1070–84.

68. Veniant MM, Sullivan MA, Kim SK et al. Defining the atherogenicity of large and small lipoproteins containing apolipoprotein B100. J Clin Invest 2000; 106: 1501–10.

69. Mero N, Malmstrom R, Steiner G et al. Postprandial metabolism of apolipoprotein B-48- and B-100-containing particles in Type 2 diabetes mellitus: relations to angiographically verified severity of coronary artery disease. Atherosclerosis 2000; 150: 167–77.

70. Proctor SD, Pabla CK, Mamo JC. Arterial intimal retention of pro-atherogenic lipoproteins in insulin deficient rabbits and rats. Atherosclerosis 2000; 149: 315–22.

71. Brown ML, Ramprasad PM, Umeda PK et al. A macrophage receptor for apo B48: cloning, expression and atherosclerosis. Proc Natl Acad Sci USA 2000; 97: 7488–93.

72. Rapp JH, Lespine A, Hamilton R et al. Triglyceride-rich lipoproteins iosolated by selected-affinity anti-apolipoprotein B immunsorption from human atherosclerotic plaque. Atheroscler Thromb Vasc Biol 1994; 14: 1767–74.

73. Veniant MM, Pierotti V, Newland D et al. Susceptibility to atherosclerosis in mice expressing exclusively apolipoprotein B48 or apolipoprotein B100. J Clin Invest 1997; 100: 180–8.

74. Mamo JCL, Proctor SD, Smith D. Retention of chylomicron remnants by arterial tissue; importance of an efficient clearance mechanism from plasma. Atherosclerosis 1998; 141: S63–S69.

75. Proctor SD, Mamo JCL. Retention of fluorescent-labeled chylomicron remnants within the intima of the arterial wall – evidence that plaque cholesterol may be derived from postprandial lipoproteins. Eur J Clin Invest 1998; 28: 497–503.

76. de Lorgeril M, Salen P, Martin JL et al. Mediterranean diet, traditional risk factors, and the rate of cardiovascular complications after myocardial infarction: final report of the Lyon Diet Heart Study. Circulation 1999; 99: 779–85.

77. Ryan M, McInerney D, Owens D et al. Diabetes and the Mediterranean diet: a beneficial effect of oleic acid on insulin sensitivity, adipocyte glucose transport and endothelium dependent vasoreactivity. QJM 2000; 93: 85–91.

78. Tong P, Thomas T, Berrish T et al. Cell membrane dynamics and insulin resistance in

non-insulin-dependent diabetes mellitus. Lancet 1995; 345: 357–8.

79. Madigan C, Ryan M, Owens D et al. Dietary unsaturated fatty acids in Type 2 diabetic patients. Higher levels of postprandial lipoproteins on a linoleic acid-rich sunflower oil diet compared with an oleic acid-rich olive oil diet. Diabetes Care 2000; 23: 1472–7.

80. Steinberg D, Parthasarathy S, Carew TE et al. Beyond Cholesterol: modifications of LDL which increase its atherogenicity. N Engl J Med 1989; 320: 915–23.

81. Wang X, Greilberger J, Ratschek M, Jurgens G. Oxidative modifications of LDL increases its binding to extracellular matrix from human aortic intima: influence of lesion development, lipoprotein lipase and calcium. J Path 2001; 195: 244–50.

82. Lyons TJ, Jenkins AJ. Lipoprotein glycation and its metabolic consequences Curr Opin Lipidol 1997; 8: 174–80.

83. Orekhov AN, Tertov VV, Mukhin DN. Desialylated low density lipoprotein – naturally occuring modified lipoprotein with atherogenic potential. Atherosclerosis 1991; 86: 153–61.

84. Lindbohm N, Gylling H, Miettinen TA. Sialic acid content of low density lipoprotein and its relation to lipid concentrations and metabolism of low density lipoprotein cholesterol. J Lipid Res 2000; 41: 1110–17.

85. Tertov VV, Kaplun VV, Sobenin IA, Orekhov AN. Low-density lipoprotein modification occurring in human plasma possible mechanism of in vivo lipoprotein desialylation as a primary step of atherogenic modification. Atherosclerosis 1998; 138: 183–95.

86. Boullier A, Gillotte KL, Horkko S et al. The binding of oxidized low density lipoprotein to mouse CD36 is mediated in part by oxidized phospholipids that are associated with both the lipid and protein moieties of the lipoprotein. J Biol Chem 2000; 275: 9163–9.

87. Brown MS, Goldstein JL. A receptor-mediated pathway for cholesterol homeostasis. Science 1986; 232: 34–47.

88. Zimmermann R, Panzenbock U, Wintersperger A et al. Lipoprotein lipase mediates the uptake of glycated LDL in fibroblasts, endothelial cells, and macrophages. Diabetes 2001; 50: 1643–53.

89. Moro E, Alessandrini P, Zambon C et al. Is glycation of low density lipoprotein in patients with Type 2 diabetes mellitus a LDL pre-oxidative condition? Diabetes Med 1999; 16: 663–9.

90. Onorato JM, Jenkins AJ, Thorpe SR, Baynes JW. Pyridoxamine, an inhibitor of advanced glycation reactions, also inhibits advanced lipoxidation reactions. Mechanism of action of pyridoxamine. J Biol Chem 2000; 275: 21177–84.

91. Takei A, Huang Y, Lopes-Virella MF. Expression of adhesion molecules by human endothelial cells exposed to oxidized low density lipoprotein. Influences of degree of oxidation and location of oxidized LDL. Atherosclerosis 2001; 154: 79–86.

92. Capes SE, Hunt D, Mamberg K, Gerstein HC. Stress, hyperglycaemia and increased risk of death after myocardial infarction in patients with and without diabetes. A systematic overview. Lancet 2000; 355: 773–8.

93. Marfella R, Quagliaro L, Nappo F et al. Acute hyperglycaemia induces an oxidative stress in healthy individuals. J Clin Invest 2001; 108: 635–63.

94. Brownlee M, Cerami A, Vlassara H. Advanced glycosylation end products in tissues and the biochemical basis of diabetic complications. N Engl J Med 1988; 318: 1315–21.

95. Vlassara G, Bucala R, Striker L. Pathological effects of advanced glycosylation: biochemical, biological and clinical implications for diabetes and aging. Lab Invest 1994; 70: 138–51.

96. Babiy AV, Gebicki JM, Sullivan DR, Willey K. Increased oxidisability of plasma lipoproteins in diabetic patients can be decreased by probucol therapy and is not due to glycation. Biochem Pharmacol 1992; 43: 995–1000.

97. Bowie A, Owens D, Collins P et al. Glycosylated low density lipoprotein is more sensitive to oxidation: implications for the diabetic patient? Atherosclerosis 1993; 102: 63–7.

98. Liguori A, Abete P, Hayden JM et al. Effect of glycaemic control and age on low density lipoprotein susceptibility to oxidation in diabetes mellitus Type 1. Eur Heart J 2001; 22: 2075–84.

99. Valabhji J, Elkeles RS. Type 1 diabetes and ageing: does oxidation mediate their association? Eur Heart J 2001; 22: 2045–7.

100. Dimitriadis E, Griffin M, Owens D et al. Oxidation of low density lipoprotein in non-insulin dependent diabetes: its relationship to fatty acid composition. Diabetologia 1995; 38: 1300–6.

101. Dimitriadis E, Griffin M, Owens D et al. Lipoprotein composition in NIDDM. The effect of dietary oleic acid on composition and oxidisability and function of low and high density lipoproteins. Diabetologia 1996; 39: 667–76.

102. Griffin M, Dimitriadis E, Lenehan K et al. Dietary monounsaturated fatty acids alter low density lipoprotein composition and function in Type 2 diabetes mellitus. QJM 1996; 89: 211–16.

103. Prescott J, Owens D, Collins P et al. The relationship between low density lipoprotein fatty acid composition and size in diabetes. Biochim Biophys Acta 1999; 1439: 110–16.

104. Horobin DF. Fatty acid metabolism in health and disease. The role of delta-6-desaturase. Am J Clin Nutr 1993; 57 Suppl: 732–75.

105. Storlien LH, Jenkins AB, Chisholm DJ et al. Influence of dietary fat composition on development of insulin resistance in rats: relationship to muscle triglyceride and omega-3 fatty acids in muscle phospholipid. Diabetes 1991; 40: 280–9.

106. Tribble DL, Holl LG, Wood PD, Krauss RM. Variation in oxidative susceptibility among six low density lipoprotein subfractions of differing density and particle size. Atherosclerosis 1992; 93: 189–99.

107. Deighan CJ, Caslake MJ, McConnell M et al. The atherogenic lipoprotein phenotype: small dense LDL and lipoprotein remnants in nephrotic range proteinuria. Atherosclerosis 2001; 157: 211–20.

108. Lahdenpera S, Syvanne M, Kahri J, Taskinen M-R. Regulation of low density lipoprotein particle size and distribution in NIDDM and coronary artery disease: importance of serum triglycerides. Diabetologia 1996; 39: 453–61.

109. Lahdenpera S, Sane T, Vourinen-Markkola H et al. LDL particle size in mildly hypertriglyceridaemic subjects; no relation to insulin resistance or diabetes. Atherosclerosis 1995; 113: 227–36.

110. Koba S, Hirano T, Yoshino G et al. Remarkably high prevalence of small dense low density lipoprotein in Japanese men with coronary artery disease, irrespective of the presence of diabetes. Atherosclerosis 2002; 160: 249–56.

111. Guerin M, LeGoff W, Lassel TS et al. Proatherogenic role of elevated CE transfer from HDL to VLDL1 and dense LDK in Type 2 diabetes. Impact of the degree of triglyceridaemia. Arterioscler Thromb Vasc Biol 2001; 21: 282–8.

112. Griffin M, McInerny D, Collins P et al. Autoantibodies to oxidized LDL are related to LDL fatty acid composition in diabetes. Diabet Med 1997; 14: 741–7.

113. Salonen JT, Yla-Herttuala S, Yamamoto R et al. Autoantibodies against oxidized low density lipoprotein predicting myocardial infarction. Atheroscler Thromb Vasc Biol 1997; 17: 3159–63.

114. Tsimikas S, Palinski W, Witztum JL. Circulating autoantibodies to oxidized LDL correlate with arterial accumulation and depletion of oxidized LDL in LDL receptor-deficient mice. Arterioscler Thromb Vasc Biol 2001; 21: 95–100.

115. Shaw PX, Horkko S, Tsimikas S et al. Human-derived anti-oxidized LDL autoantibody blocks uptake of oxidized LDL by macrophages and localizes to atherosclerotic lesions in vivo. Arterioscler Thromb Vasc Biol 2001; 21: 1333–9.

116. Zhou X, Caligiui G, Hamsen A et al. LDL immunisation induces T-cell-dependent antibody formation and protection against atherosclerosis. Arterioscler Thromb Vasc Biol 2001; 21: 108–14.

117. Gordon DJ, Probstfield JL, Garrison RJ et al High density lipoprotein cholesterol and cardiovascular disease: four prospective American studies. Circulation 1989; 79: 8–15.

118. de Backer G, de Bacquere D, Kornitzer M. Epidemiological aspects of high density lipoprotein cholesterol. Atherosclerosis 1998; 137 Suppl: S1–S6.

119. Bo S, Cavallo-Perin P, Gentile L et al. Low HDL-cholesterol: a component of the metabolic syndrome only in the presence of fasting hypertriglyceridemia in Type 2 diabetic patients. Diabetes Metab 2001; 27: 31–5.

120. Bodzioch M, Orso E Kluchen J et al. The gene encoding ATP-binding cassette transporter 1 is mutated in Tangier disease. Nat Genet 1999; 22: 347–51.

121. Brooks-Wilson A, Marciel M, Clee SM et al. mutations in ABC1 in Tangier disease and familial high density lipoprotein deficiency. Nat Genet 1999; 22: 336–45.

122. Remaley AT, Rust S, Rosier M et al. Human ATP-binding cassette transporter1 (ABC1), genomic organization and identification of the genetic defect in the original Tangier disease kindred. Proc Natl Acad Sci USA 1999; 96: 12685–90.

123. Rust S, Rosier M, Funke H et al. Tangier disease caused by mutations in the gene encoding ATP-binding cassette transporter1. Nat Genet 1999; 22: 352–5.

124. Marcil M, Brooks-Wilson A, Clee SM et al. Mutations in the ABC1 gene in familial HDL deficiency with defective cholesterol efflux. Lancet 1999; 354: 1341–6.

125. Santamarina-Fojo S, Remaley AT, Neufeld EB, Brewer HB Jr. Regulation and intracellular trafficking of the ABCA1 transporter. J Lipid Res 2001; 42: 1339–45.

126. Kreiger M. Charting the face of the good cholesterol identification and characterisation of high density lipoprotein receptor SR-B1. Annu Rev Biochem 1999; 63: 523–58.

127. Gu X, Kozarsky K, Krieger M. Scavenger receptor class B Type 1–mediated [3H]cholesterol efflux to high and low density lipoprotein is dependent on lipoprotein binding to the receptor. J Biol Chem 2000; 39: 29993–30001.

128. Arai T, Wang N, Bezouevski M et al. Decreased atherosclerosis in heterozygous low density lipoprotein receptor-deficient mice expressing the scavenger receptor BI transgene. J Biol Chem 1999; 274: 2366–71.

129. Acton S, Rigotti A, Landschulz KT et al. Identification of the scavenger receptor SRB1 as a lipoprotein receptor. Science 1996; 217: 518–20.

130. Mackness MI, Arrol S, Abbott C, Durrington PN. Protection of low density lipoprotein against oxidative modification by high density lipoprotein associated paraoxonase. Atherosclerosis 1993; 104: 129–35.

131. Navab M, Berlliner JA, Watson AD et al. The Yin and Yang of oxidation in the development of the fatty streak. Arterioscler Thromb Vasc Biol 1996; 16: 831–42.

132. Ruiz J, Blanche H, James R et al. A polymorphism of paraoxonase and coronary heart disease in Type 2 diabetes. Lancet 1995; 346: 869–72.

133. Serrato M, Marian AJ. A variant of human paraoxonase/arylesterase (HUMPONA) gene is a risk factor for coronary artery disease. J Clin Invest 1995; 96: 3005–8.

134. Zama T, Murata M, Matsubara Y et al. A varient of the human paraoxoinase (HUMPONA) gene polymorphism is associated with an increased risk for coronary artery disease in the Japanese. Arterioscler Thromb Vasc Biol 1997; 17: 3565–9.

135. Watson AD. Berliner JA. Hama SY et al. Protective effect of high density lipoprotein associated paraoxonase. Inhibition of the biological activity of minimally oxidized low density lipoprotein. J Clin Invest 1995; 96: 2882–91.

136. Mackness B, Durrington PN, Abuashia B et al. Low paraoxonase activity in type II diabetes mellitus complicated by retinopathy. Clin Sci 2000; 98: 355–63.

137. Sanghera DK, Aston CE, Saha N, Kamboh MI. DNA polymorphisms in two paraoxonase genes (PON1 and PON2; are associated with the risk of coronary heart disease. Am J Hum Genet 1998; 62: 36–44.

138. Ng CJ, Wadleigh DJ, Gangopadhyay A et al. Paraoxonase-2 is a ubiquitously expressed protein with antioxidant properties and is capable of preventing cell-mediated oxidative modification of low density lipoprotein. J Biol Chem 2001; 276: 44444–9.

139. Fielding CJ, Fielding PE. Molecular physiology of reverse cholesterol transport. J Lipid Res 1995; 36: 211–28.

140. Castro G, Nihoul LP, Dengremont C et al. Cholesterol efflux, lecithin-cholesterol acyltransferase activity, and pre-beta particle formation by serum from human apolipoprotein A-I and apolipoprotein A-I/apolipoprotein A-II transgenic mice consistent with the latter being less effective for reverse cholesterol transport. Biochemistry 1997; 36: 2243–9.

141. Hedrick CC, Castellani LW, Wong H, Lusis

AJ. In vivo interactions of apoA-II, apoA-I, and hepatic lipase contributing to HDL structure and antiatherogenic functions. J Lipid Res 2001; 42: 563–70.

142. Weng W, Breslow JL. Dramatically increased high density lipoprotein cholesterol, increased remnant clearance and hypersensitivity to insulin in apoprotein A11 knockout mice suggest a complex role for apoprotein A11 in atherosclerosis susceptibility. Proc Natl Acad Sci USA 1996; 93: 14788–94.

143. Castellani LW, Aimie M, Goto M et al. Studies with apolipoprotein A-II transgenic mice indicate a role for HDLs in adiposity and insulin resistance Diabetes 2001; 50: 643–51.

144. van't Hooft FM, Ruotolo G, Boquist et al. Human evidence that the apolipoprotein A-II gene is implicated in visceral fat accumulation and metabolism of triglyceride-rich lipoproteins Circulation 2001; 104: 1223–8.

145. Goldstein JL, Hobbs HH, Brown MS. In: Scriver CR, Beaudet AL, Sly WS, Valle D, eds. The Metabolic and Molecular Basis of Inherited Disease, New York: McGraw Hill, 2001.

146. Innerarity TL, Weisgraber KH, Arnold KS et al. Familial defective apolipoprotein B-100: low density lipoproteins with abnormal receptor binding. Proc Natl Acad Sci USA 1987; 84: 19–23.

147. Vega GL, Grundy SM. In vivo evidence for reduced binding of low density lipoproteins to receptors as a cause of primary moderate hypercholesterolemia. J Clin Invest 1986; 78: 1410–14.

148. Innerarity TL, Mahley RW, Weisgraber et al. Familial defective apo B100: a mutation of apo B that causes hypercholesterolaemia. J Lipid Res 1990; 31: 1337–49.

149. Garcia CK, Wilund K, Arca M et al. Autosomal recessive hypercholesterolemia caused by mutations in a putative LDL receptor adaptor protein. Science 2001; 292: 1394–8.

150. Berge KE, Tian H, Graf GA et al. Accumulation of dietary cholesterol in sitosterolaemia caused by mutations in adjacent ABC transporters. Science 2000; 290: 1771–7.

151. Lee MH, Lu H, Hazard S et al. Identification of a gene ABCG5 important in the regulation of dietary absorption. Nat Genet 2001; 27: 79–83.

152. Lee MH, Gordon D, Ott J et al. Fine mapping of a gene responsible for regulating dietary cholesterol absorption; founder effects underlie cases of phytosterolaemia in multiple communities. Eur J Hum Genet 2001; 9: 375–84.

153. Lu K, Lee MH, Hazard S et al. Two genes that map to the STSL locus cause sitosterolemia: genomic structure and spectrum of mutations involving sterolin-1 and sterolin-2, encoded by ABCG5 and ABCG8, respectively. Am J Human Genet 2001; 69: 278–90.

154. Kern F. Normal plasma cholesterol in an 88-year-old man who eats 25 eggs a day. Mechanisms of adaption, N Engl J Med 1991; 324: 896–9.

155. Feingold KR. Importance of small intestine in diabetic hypercholesterolaemia. Diabetes 1988; 38: 141–5.

156. Feingold KR, Wilson DE, Wood LC et al. Diabetes increases hepatic hydroxymethyl glutaryl coenzyme A reductase protein and mRNA levels in the small intestine. Metabolism 1994; 43: 450–4.

157. Gleeson A, Owens D, Collins P et al. The relationship between cholesterol absorption and intestinal cholesterol synthesis in the diabetic rat model. Int J Exp Diabetes Res 2000; 1: 203–10.

158. Gylling H, Miettinen TA. Cholesterol absorption, synthesis and LDL metabolism in NIDDM. Diabetes Care 1997; 20: 90–5.

159. Shepherd J, Cobb SM, Ford I et al. Prevention of coronary heart disease with pravastatin in men with hypercholesterolaemia. N Engl J Med 1995; 333: 1301–7.

160. Aguilar-Salinas CA, Barrett H, Schonfield G, Metabolic modes of action of the statins. Atherosclerosis 1998; 141: 203–7.

161. Suckling KE, Strange EF. Role of Acyl-coA: cholesterol acyltransferase in cellular cholesterol metabolism. J Lipid Res 1985; 26: 647–71.

162. Roth BD. ACAT inhibitors: evolution from cholesterol-absorption inhibitors to anti-atherogenic agents. Drug Discovery Today 1998; 3: 219.

163. Bocan TM, Krause BR, Rosebury WS et al.

The combined effect of inhibiting both ACAT and HMG-CoA reductase may directly induce atherosclerotic lesion regression. Atherosclerosis. 2001; 157: 97–105.

164. Bocan TM, Krause BR, Rosebury WS et al. The ACAT inhibitor avasimibe reduces macrophages and matrix metalloproteinase expression in atherosclerotic lesions of hypercholesterolemic rabbits. Arterioscler Thromb Vasc Biol 2000; 20: 70–9.

165. Insull Jr W, Koren M, Davignon J et al. Efficacy and short-term safety of a new ACAT inhibitor, avasimbe, on lipids, lipoproteins, and apolipoproteins, in patients with combined hyperlipidaemia. Atherosclerosis 2001; 157: 137–44.

166. Burnett JR, Wilcox LJ, Telford DE et al. Inhibition of ACAT by avasimibe decreases both VLDL and LDL apolipoprotein B production in miniature pigs. J Lipid Res 1999; 40: 1317–132.

167. Huff MW, Telford DE, Barrett PHR et al. Inhibition of hepatic ACAT decreases apo B secretion in miniature pigs fed a cholesterol free diet. Arteriosclerosis 1994; 14: 1498–1508.

168. Hui TY, Olivier LM, Kang S, Davis RA. Microsomal triglyceride transfer protein is essential for hepatic secretion of apoB-100 and apoB-48 but not triglyceride. J Lipid Res 2002; 43: 785–93.

169. Hussain MH. A proposed model for assembly of chylomicrons. Atherosclerosis 2000; 148: 1–15.

170. Wilcox LJ, Borradaile NM, de Dreu LE. Huff MW. Secretion of hepatocyte apoB is inhibited by the flavonoids, naringenin and hesperetin, via reduced activity and expression of ACAT2 and MTP. J Lipid Res 2001; 42: 725–34.

171. Phillips C, Anderton K, Bennett A et al. Intestinal rather than hepatic microsomal triglyceride transfer protein as a cause of postprandial dyslipidemia in diabetes. Metabolism 2002; 51: 847–52.

172. Phillips C, Owens D, Collins P, Tomkin GH. Microsomal triglyceride transfer protein: the role of insulin resistance in the regulation of chylomicron assembly Atherosclerosis 2002; 160: 355–60.

173. Ledmyr H, Karpe F, Lundahl B et al. Varients of the microsomal triglyceride transfer protein gene are associated with plasma cholesterol levels and body mass index. J Lipid Res. 2002: 43: 51–8.

174. Bernard S, Touzet S, Personne I et al. Association between microsomal triglyceride transfer protein gene polymorphism and biological features of liver steatosis in patients with Type 2 diabetes. Diabetologia 2000; 43: 995–9.

175. Anonymous. Effect of fenofibrate on progression of coronary-artery disease in Type 2 diabetes: the Diabetes Atherosclerosis Intervention Study, a randomised study. Lancet 2001; 357: 905–10.

176. Bae JH, Bassenge E, Lee HJ et al. Impact of postprandial hypertriglyceridemia on vascular responses in patients with coronary artery disease: effects of ACE-inhibitors and fibrates. Atherosclerosis 2001; 158: 165–71.

177. Nakajima K, Okazaki M, Tanaka A et al. Separation and determination of remnant-like particles in human serum using monoclonal antibodies to apo B and apo A1. J Clin Ligand Assay 1996; 19: 177–83.

178. Schreuder PC, Twickler TB, Wang T et al. Isolation of remnant particles by immunoseparation: a new approach for investigation of postprandial lipoprotein metabolism in normolipaemic subjects. Atherosclerosis 2001; 157: 145–50.

179. Campos E, Kotite L, Blanche P et al. Properties of triglyceride-rich and cholesterol-rich lipoproteins in the remnant-like particle fraction of human blood plasma. J Lipid Res 2002; 43: 365–74.

180. Doi, H, Kugiyama K, Oka H et al. Remnant lipoproteins induce proatherothrombogenic molecules in endothelial cells through a redox-sensitive mechanism. Circulation 2000; 102: 670–6.

181. Gylling H, Miettinen TA. Baseline intestinal absorption and synthesis of cholesterol regulate its response to hypercholesterolaemic treatments in coronary patients. Atherosclerosis 2002; 160: 477–81.

182. Van Heek M, Austin TM, Farley C et al. Ezetimibe, a potent cholesterol absorption inhibitor in obese hyperinsulinaemic hamsters. Diabetes 2001; 50: 1330–5.

183. Dujovne CA, Bays H, Davidson MH et al.

Reduction of LDL cholesterol in patients with primary hypercholesterolemia by SCH48461: results of a multicenter dose-ranging study. J Clin Pharmacol. 2001; 41: 70–8.

184. van Heek M, Farley C, Compton DS et al. Comparison of the activity and disposition of the novel cholesterol absorption inhibitor, SCH58235, and its glucuronide, SCH60663. Br J Pharm 2000; 129: 1748–54.

185. Sohda T, Mizuno K, Momose Y et al. Studies on antibiabetic agents 11. Novel thiazolodine-dione derivative as potent hypoglycaemic agents. J Med Chem 1992; 35: 2617–26.

186. Ikeda H, Taketomi S, Sugiyama Y et al. Effects of pioglitazone on glucose and lipid metabolism in normal and insulin resistant animals. Drug Res 1990; 40: 156–62.

187. Yamauchi T, Waki H, Kamon J et al. Inhibition of RXR and PPAR ameliorates diet-induced obesity and Type 2 diabetes. J Clin Invest 2001; 108: 1001–13.

188. Schoonjans K, Staels B, and Auwerx J. Role of the peroxisome proliferator-activated receptor (PPAR) in mediating the effects of fibrates and fatty acids on gene expression. J Lipid Res 1996; 37: 907–25.

189. Ye JM, Doyle PJ, Iglesias MA et al. Peroxisome proliferator-activated receptor (PPAR)-alpha activation lowers muscle lipids and improves insulin sensitivity in high fat-fed rats: comparison with PPAR-gamma activation. Diabetes 2001; 50: 411–17.

190. Lindén D, Alsterholm M, Wennbo H, Oscarsson J. PPARα deficiency increases secretion and serum levels of apolipoprotein B-containing lipoproteins. J Lipid Res 2001; 42: 1831–40.

191. Guerre-Millo M, Rouault C, Poulain P et al. PPARγ-null mice are protected from high-fat diet-induced insulin resistance. Diabetes 2001; 50: 2809–14.

192. Jiang C, Ting AT, Seed B. PPAR-gamma agonists inhibit production of monocyte inflammatory cytokines. Nature 1998; 391: 82–6.

193. Ricote M, Li AC, Willson TM et al. The peroxisome proliferator-activated receptor-gamma is a negative regulator of macrophage activation. Nature 1998; 391: 79–82.

194. Chinetti G, Lestavel S, Bocher V et al. PPAR-alpha and PPAR-gamma activators induce cholesterol removal from human macrophage foam cells through stimulation of the ABCA1 pathway. Nat Med 2001; 7: 53–8.

195. Björkegren J, Boquist S, Samnegård A et al. Accumulation of apolipoprotein C-I-rich and cholesterol-rich VLDL remnants during exaggerated postprandial triglyceridemia in normolipidemic patients with coronary artery disease. Circulation 2000; 101: 227–30.

196. Jong MC, van Dijk KW, Dahlmans VE et al. Reversal of hyperlipidaemia in apolipoprotein C1 transgenic mice by adenovirus-mediated gene delivery of the low-density-lipoprotein receptor, but not by the very-low-density-lipoprotein receptor. Biochem J 1999; 338: 281–7.

197. Clee SM, Bissada N, Miao F et al. Plasma and vessel wall lipoprotein lipase have different roles in atherosclerosis. J Lipid Res 2000; 41: 521–31.

198. Jong M, Rensen PC, Dahlmans VE et al. Apolipoprotein C-III deficiency accelerates triglyceride hydrolysis by lipoprotein lipase in wild-type and apoE knockout mice. Lipid Res 2001; 42: 1578–85.

199. Auwerx J, Schoonjans K, Fruchart JC. Staels B. Transcriptional control of triglyceride metabolism: fibrates and fatty acids change the expression of the LPL and apo C-III genes by activating the nuclear receptor PPAR. Atherosclerosis 1996; 124 Suppl: S29–37.

200. Haubenwallner D, Essenburg AD, Barnett BC et al. Hypolipidemic activity of select fibrates correlates to changes in hepatic apolipoprotein C-III expression: a potential physiologic basis for their mode of action. J Lipid Res 1995; 36: 2541–51.

201. Levy E, Shafrif E, Ziv E, Bar-On H. Composition, removal and metabolic fate of chylomicrons derived from diabetic rats. Biochim Biophys Acta 1983; 834: 376–85.

202. Bradley WA, Gianturco SH. Apo E is necessary and sufficient for the binding of large triglyceride-rich lipoproteins to the LDL receptor; apo B is unnecessary. J Lipid Res 1986; 27: 40–8.

203. Weisgraber KH. Apoprotein E: structure-function relationships. Adv Protein Chem 1994; 45: 249–302.

204. Mahley RW, Ji Z-S. Remnant lipoprotein metabolism: key pathway involving cell surface heparin sulphate proteoglycans and apolipoprotein E. J Lipid Res 1999; 40: 111–16.

205. Vionnet N, Hani El-H, Dupont S et al. Vitamin E and beta carotene on the incidence of primary nonfatal myocardial infarction and fatal coronary heart disease. Arch Intern Med 1998; 158: 668–75.

206. Evans RW, Shaten BJ, Day BW, Kuller LH. Prospective association between lipid soluble antioxidants and coronary heart disease in men. The Multiple Risk Factor Intervention Trial. Am Jf Epidemiol 1998; 147: 180–6.

207. Rapola JM, Virtamo J, Ripatti S et al. Randomized trial of alpha-tocopherol and beta-carotene supplements on incidence of major coronary events in men with previous myocardial infarction. Lancet 1997; 349: 1715–20.

208. Brown BG, Zhao X-Q, Chait A, et al. Simvastatin and niacin, antioxidant vitamins, or the combination for the prevention of coronary disease. N Engl J Med 2001; 345: 1583–92.

209. Anonymous. MRC/BHF Heart Protection Study of cholesterol-lowering therapy and of antioxidant vitamin supplementation in a wide range of patients at increased risk of coronary heart disease death: early safety and efficacy experience. Eur Heart J 1999; 20: 725–41.

210. Gerstein HC, Mann JFE, Yi, Q et al. for the HOPE Study Investigators. Albuminuria and risk of cardiovascular events, death, and heart failure in diabetic and nondiabetic individuals. JAMA 2001; 286: 421–6.

211. Heart Outcomes Prevention Evaluation Study Investigators. Effects of ramipril on cardio-vascular and microvascular outcomes in people with diabetes mellitus: results of the HOPE study and MICRO-HOPE substudy. Lancet 2000; 355: 253–9.

212. Heart Outcomes Prevention Evluation (HOPE) Study Investigators. The effects of an angiotensin-converting enzyme inhibitor (ramipril) on cardiovascular events in high risk patients. N Engl J Med 2000; 342: 145–53.

213. Stratton IM, Adler AI, Neil HA et al. Association of glycaemia with macrovascular and microvascular complications of Type 2 diabetes (UKPDS 35). BMJ 2000; 321: 405–12.

214. Shapiro AMJ, Lakey JRT, Korbutt GS et al. Islet transplantation in seven patients with Type 1 diabetes mellitus using a glucocorti-coid free immunosuppressive regimen. New Engl J Med 2000; 343: 230–238.

215. Ross R. Atherosclerosis – an inflammatory disease. N Engl J Med 1999; 340: 115–26.

216. Witztum JKL, Palinski W. Are immunological mechanisms relevant for the development of atherosclerosis? Clin Immunol 1999; 90: 153–6.

217. Huang Y, Jaffa A, Koskinen S et al. Oxidised-containing immune complexes induce Fc gamma receptor 1-mediated mitogen-activated protein kinase activation in THP-1 macrophages. Arterioscler Thromb Vasc Biol 1999; 19: 1600–7.

218. Zwaka TP, Hombach V, Torzewski J. C-reactive protein-mediated low density lipoprotein uptake by macrophages: implications for atherosclerosis. Circulation 2001; 103: 1194–7.

219. Ridker PM, Hennekens CH, Buring JE et al. C-reactive protein and other markers of inflamation in the prediction of cardiovascular disease in women N Engl J Med 2000; 432: 836–43.

220. Jialal MD, Stein D, Balis D et al. Effect of hydrxymethyl glutaryl coenzyme A reductase inhibitor therapy on high sensitive c-reactive protein levels. Circulation 2001; 103: 1933–5.

221. Libby P. Changing concepts of atherogenesis. J Intern Med 2000; 247: 349–58.

222. Rajavashisth TB, Xu XP, Jovinge S et al. Membrane Type 1 matrix metalloproteinase expression in human atherosclerotic plaques: evidence for activation by proinflammatory mediators. Circulation 1999; 99: 3103–9.

223. Uemura S, Matsushita H, Li W et al. Diabetes mellitus enhances vascular matrix metallopro-teinase activity: role of oxidative stress. Circ Res 2001; 88: 1291–8.

224. Cowan KN, Lloyd Jones P, Rabinovitch M. Elastase and matrix metalloproteinase inhibitors induce regression, and tenascin-C

antisense prevents progression, of vascular disease. J Clin Invest 2000; 105: 21–34.

225. Crisby M, Nordin-Fredriksson G, Shah PK et al. Pravastatin treatment increases collagen content and decreases lipid content, inflammation, metalloproteinases, and cell death in human carotid plaques: implications for plaque stabilization. Circulation 2001; 103: 926–33.

226. Bellosta S, Ferri N, Arnaboldi L et al. Pleiotropic effects of statins in atherosclerosis and diabetes. Diabetes Care 2000; 23 Suppl 2: B72–8.

227. Von Echardstein A, Assmann G. Prevention of coronary heart disease by raising high density lipoprotein cholesterol. Curr Opin Lipidol 2000; 11: 627–37.

228. Von Echardstein A, Nofer JR, Assmann G. High density lipoprotein and atherosclerosis. Role of cholesterol efflux and reverse cholesterol transport. Arterioscler Thromb Vasc Biol 2001; 21: 13–27.

229. Tu AY, Albers JJ. Glucose regulates transcription of human genes relevant to HDL metabolism. Diabetes 2001; 50: 1851–6.

230. Tu AY, Albers JJ. DNA sequences responsible for reduced promoter activity of human phospholipid transfer protein by fibrates. Biochem Biophys Res Commun 1999; 264; 802–7.

231. von Eckardstein A, Schulte H, Assmann G. Increased risk of myocardial infarction in men with both hypertriglyceridemia and elevated HDL cholesterol. Circulation 1999; 99: 1925.

232. Tall AR, Wang N, Mucksavage P. Is it time to modify the reverse cholesterol transport model? J Clin Invest 2001; 108: 1273–5.

233. Roper NA, Bilous RW, Kelly WF et al. Excess mortality in a population with diabetes and the impact of material deprivation: longitudinal population based study. BMJ 2001; 322: 1389–93.

8

Cardiovascular disease in Type 2 diabetes

Mogher Khamaisi, Isaiah Wexler, Itamar Raz

Introduction

Type 2 (non-insulin dependent) diabetes mellitus (DM) is one of the most serious public health problems facing both developed and developing countries. The incidence of Type 2 DM is reaching epidemic proportions as a result of changing socioeconomic conditions that contribute to increased nutritional intake and a sedentary lifestyle.[1,2] Increased awareness of Type 2 DM and stricter definitions of normoglycemia have contributed to the increasing number of documented cases of Type 2 DM.

The severe long-term complications associated with chronic hyperglycemia complicate the course of Type 2 DM, increase the cost of treatment, and take a heavy toll on quality of the patients' lives.[3,4] Of all the long-term complications, cardiovascular disease (CVD) is one of the most serious outcomes in terms of morbidity and mortality of Type 2 DM.[5] The onset of CVD complicates and even exacerbates other diabetic-related complications. In this chapter the epidemiology, pathophysiology, and treatment of diabetic CVD will be discussed. Special attention will be given to risk factors associated with diabetic CVD, the contribution of an altered metabolic environment to the severity of diabetic CVD and the implications of new diagnostic criteria for Type 2 DM for early identification of diabetics at risk for developing CVD.

Epidemiology of cardiovascular complications of Type 2 diabetes mellitus

Macrovascular disease, especially CVD accounts for most of the mortality in patients with Type 2 DM who have a much greater age-related risk for CVD than non-diabetics. The higher risk is due to the greater prevalence of cardiovascular risk factors among diabetics, including an abnormal lipoprotein profile, prothrombotic tendency, hypertension, and obesity. Additionally, the altered metabolic environment (i.e. hyperglycemia, hyperinsulinemia and insulin resistance) resulting from the diabetic state directly impacts on the cardiovascular status.[6–8] Cardiovascular events such as myocardial infarction (MI) are associated with a greater case fatality rate, and this has been attributed to altered myocardial energy metabolism, impaired cardiac remodeling after infarction, and a higher incidence of congestive heart failure in the first year after the infarction.[9–11]

Accelerated cardiovascular and cerebrovascular atherosclerosis is the major cause of mortality in patients with DM.[12,13] This was well documented in the Wisconsin Epidemiology Study of Diabetic Retinopathy (WESDR). The median follow-up in the WESDR was 10 years in the younger-onset group and 8.3 years in the older-onset group.[14] There were 122

(12.9%) and 655 (51.8%) deaths in each group respectively. In the older-onset group, 47.2% patients died from heart disease, and an additional 9% from cerebrovascular events.

Increased incidence of cardiovascular complications in diabetic patients of similar or even higher magnitude have been reported in other studies.[15,16] In the presence of diabetes, the death rate attributable to CVD is increased 1.5- to 4.5-fold, and all-cause mortality is increased 1.5- to 2.7-fold.[17,18]

In addition to its very high prevalence, diabetes-associated macrovascular disease develops earlier than microvascular disease at a stage when there is only impaired glucose tolerance (IGT) and plasma glucose levels are in the pre-diabetic range.[19,20] The Funagata Diabetes Study, which focused on the initial stages of abnormal glucose metabolism, indicated relatively early dissociation of the survival curves for individuals with IGT as compared to the matched controls with normal glucose tolerance.[21] After six years of follow-up, the study showed that cardiovascular mortality was higher in individuals with IGT as compared to those with normal glucose tolerance, and that these differences were evident as early as four years after the detection of IGT. This observation suggests that even very mild derangement of glucose homeostasis associated with the pre- or early diabetic state can adversely impact on the severity of the process leading to cardiovascular complications.

Several epidemiologic findings regarding CVD in Type 2 diabetes are of clinical significance. The prevalence of CVD varies according to ethnicity.[1] For example, Pima Indians have a high incidence of Type 2 DM but a relatively low rate of CVD[22] in contrast to Asian Indians who migrated to western countries manifesting a high incidence of CVD owing to factors associated with Type 2 DM, including hyperinsulinemia and abdominal obesity.[23] The

prevalence of CVD is increased even in newly diagnosed Type 2 diabetics, especially females, as compared to matched non-diabetic controls.[24,25] The increased rate may be due to a delay in the diagnosis of overt Type 2 diabetes, the long-term presence of IGT that precedes overt Type 2 diabetes, or a combination of both. As pointed out by Zimmet, many of the risk factors associated with the development of CVD are operative prior to the development of overt DM.[26] Factors such as glucose intolerance, an abnormal Body Mass Index and waist/hip ratio, hypertension, hyperuricemia, hypertriglyceridemia, insulin resistance and hyperinsulinemia are found in a higher proportion of subjects destined to develop Type 2 DM than in the background population.[1,27,28] The pathophysiologic processes responsible for CVD in these patients include factors associated with the diabetic state, e.g. hyperglycemia, dyslipidemia, and advanced glycosylation end products (AGE) as well as obesity and hypertension that precede the diabetic state.[29–31]

A key issue in many epidemiologic studies pertaining to heart disease and DM has been the identification of specific factors that are unique to diabetes. One of the early reports on the outcome of MI in diabetic patients originated from Sweden in 1985.[32] In this study, mortality and re-infarction rates were evaluated in a group of 73 diabetic patients (80% with Type 2 DM) with MI who were followed for five years. The only clinical differences between diabetics and non-diabetics were that the serum cholesterol level was lower and the blood pressure higher among the diabetics. During the course of follow-up, the cumulative death rate was 52% in diabetics and 25% in non-diabetics indicating that the higher prevalence of hypertension among diabetics might have been a contributory factor. In a recently published study by the United Kingdom Prospective Diabetes Study (UKPDS), 3055 white patients with a relatively new onset of Type 2 DM without evidence of coronary artery disease were followed for a median duration of 7.9 years. Of this group, 335 individuals developed coronary artery disease. The investigators identified five modifiable risks factors associated with the development of CVD in Type 2 DM subjects: high LDL, low HDL, hypertension, hyperglycemia, and smoking.[33]

Severity of cardiovascular disease in diabetics

As an entity, the CVD that occurs in Type 2 DM differs from that in the general population. Both the incidence and severity of circulatory disturbances among all diabetic patients in general, and Type 2 diabetics in particular, is worse than in the general population.[9,34] Review of the available reports in diabetic patients with MI reveals an early and late mortality that is extremely high when compared to non-diabetics.[9,35–40] The high impact of CVD is reflected by the high rate of mortality in diabetics who experience MI. As shown in several studies, case-fatality is increased by 25–100% in diabetic as opposed to non-diabetic patients admitted with MI.[9,36,53,54] Mortality remains high even after correction for other prognostic factors related to CVD outcome.[38,39]

Diabetics who develop coronary artery disease are more likely to suffer from cardiovascular complications including re-infarction and conduction abnormalities. In the Swedish study cited above, Ulvenstam et al. found that significantly higher numbers of diabetic patients (31 cases, 42%) suffered from re-infarction compared to non-diabetic subjects (371 cases, 30%).[32] In another study of 341 patients with MI the in-hospital mortality was higher in the diabetic group (25 versus 16%). Those with diabetes also had an increased cumulative one-year mortality rate (53 versus 28%). While there were no significant differences between groups with regard to re-infarction rates (41 versus 33%, NS), the prevalence rate of fatal re-infarction was higher in the diabetic group (30 versus 14%). This contributed to the overall increased mortality rate among diabetics in the re-infarction group (72 versus 44%).[41] In a more recent Swedish study, the five-year rate for re-infarction was 55 versus 22% for diabetics as compared to non-diabetics with the five-year mortality rate being 72% in diabetics compared to 50% in non-diabetics.[42]

Women with MI tend to have a poorer outcome than men. The Secondary Prevention Reinfarction Israeli Nifedipine Trial (SPRINT) showed that women with MI and diabetes had the worst outcome after 12 years of follow-up (adjusted hazard ratio of 1.46 for women with diabetes compared to 1.13 for non-diabetic women).[43]

The increased case-fatality rate of Type 2 DM patients with MI has been attributed to altered myocardial energy metabolism, impaired cardiac post-infarction remodeling and a higher incidence of congestive heart failure in the first year after the infarction.[11,44] In addition, increased mortality is partially related to the greater prevalence of cardiovascular risk factors among diabetics including abnormal lipoprotein profile, prothrombotic tendency, and hypertension. IGT pre-diabetic state prior to the development of overt Type 2 diabetes may also contribute to the later increase in cardiovascular mortality.[39] Despite the recent advances in thrombolytic therapy, mortality rates for diabetics with AMI continue to remain higher than for non-diabetics, this being attributed to the increased thrombotic tendencies among diabetics.[44]

Analysis of various independent prognostic variables indicated that diabetes itself doubles the risk of cardiovascular mortality when adjusted for age, type of treatment, and left ventricular functional status. The poor prognosis of diabetics with coronary heart disease was also reported by Yudkin and Oswald,[45] who followed 83 diabetic patients with MI. In this study diabetic patients had more frequent pump failure than non-diabetic individuals. Factors that correlated with poor outcome were elevated plasma glucose and higher peak levels of aspartate transaminase (age, duration of diabetes and HbA1c prior to the admission were not significant factors).[45]

The presence of microvascular complications also exacerbates the clinical course of patients with diabetic CVD. The outcome of patients with CVD is much worse in the presence of diabetic nephropathy. Studies in the Steno Diabetes Center documented that both the incidence of first MI and atherosclerotic complications are increased in patients with Type 2 DM and microalbuminuria.[46,47]

The presence of diabetes also impacts on the prognosis of those undergoing specific therapeutic interventions for ischemic heart disease (IHD). Diabetic patients with coronary heart disease undergoing a coronary bypass graft (CABG), have a worse prognosis than non-diabetics undergoing the same.[48–51] A significant risk factor for poor outcome related to the diabetic state is the presence of proteinuria. A recent study among diabetics undergoing isolated CABG found that the five-year mortality rate for non-proteinuric and proteinuric groups was 20.2% and 29.1%, respectively.[52]

Even more disquieting about CVD and diabetes is the fact that there has been a decline in the mortality associated with coronary artery disease in the general population during the past four decades, whereas no such trend exists for patients with diabetes.[55] This fact is even more alarming given that the number of individuals with Type 2 DM has been increasing dramatically.[1] As a result of the discrepancy between diabetics and non-diabetics, great emphasis has been placed on finding the particular factors associated with diabetes – either related to the metabolic state or treatment modalities – which contribute to the severity of CVD in diabetic patients.[56]

Cardiovascular risk factors in diabetics

All known non-glycemic risk factors for atherosclerotic vascular disease operate in diabetic patients. Among them, hypercholesterolemia, hypertriglyceridemia, smoking and high blood pressure are probably the most important. However, several factors unique to Type 2 DM, may confound the impact of these factors and may independently influence the atherosclerotic process, thereby increasing the morbidity and mortality in this group. These additional risk factors include abdominal obesity, plasminogen activator 1, fibrinogen, chronic inflammation, AGE and genetic susceptibility.

Serum total cholesterol is a powerful predictor of IHD morbidity and mortality in both non-diabetic and diabetic subjects.[57] However, the impact of hypercholesterolemia in diabetics is much greater, as they have a two to three times higher risk for IHD than their non-diabetic counterparts for the same level of total serum cholesterol.[58-61] Besides total cholesterol, elevated triglycerides, high LDL-cholesterol, and low HDL-cholesterol have also been shown to increase independently cardiovascular mortality in diabetics.[29]

In addition, reduction in serum lipids, especially cholesterol, improves the outcome for diabetics as a group. In the Scandinavian Simvastatin Survival Study 202 diabetic patients with evidence of IHD were treated with a variety of modalities.[57] Lowering cholesterol HMG-CoA reductase inhibitors reduced the risk of a major IHD event, as well as the risk for any other atherosclerotic event. Similarly, subgroup analysis of the Helsinki Heart Study, a five-year IHD primary prevention trial using gemfibrozil, provided additional evidence for the benefit of lipid-lowering agents for both non-diabetics and diabetics.[62]

In another study of non-diabetic and diabetic patients who underwent CABG, the mortality risk, incidence of MI, and subsequent need for CABG or percutaneous transluminal coronary angioplasty were assessed.[63] Patients were randomized to more aggressive and less aggressive lipid-lowering treatment arms with or without anti-coagulants. Composite end-point analysis indicated that patients with DM who are not aggressively treated have a significantly higher CVD risk compared with either non-diabetics with similar non-aggressive treatment or aggressively treated diabetics.

The role of hypertension as a factor in the increased mortality among Type 2 diabetics has been extensively investigated. Not only is the prevalence of hypertension in Type 2 diabetes high, but hypertension develops early in the course of the disease. The prevalence of hypertension is already twice as high in patients with IGT than in normal controls.[64] The association of hypertension with Type 2 DM is ominous; mortality is higher by a factor of 4–7 in hypertensive Type 2 DM patients when compared to normotensive non-diabetic matched controls.[65,66]

The UKPDS strongly demonstrated the link between hypertension and the high risk for cardiovascular complications in Type 2 DM.[67] Decreasing blood pressure by use of β-blocking agents or angiotensin converting enzyme (ACE) inhibitors resulted in a significant reduction in mortality and/or MI. The Heart Outcome Prevention Evaluation (HOPE) study provided strong evidence that treatment with ACE-inhibitors reduced risk for cardiovascular death by 37% and MI by 22%.[68] Specifically, the ACE treatment was more effective in reducing the mortality and morbidity than a beta-blocker regimen.[69] Thus, the cardiovascular benefit of ACE inhibitor was greater than that attributable to its effect in decreasing blood pressure.

Few clinicians realize that IGT and insulin resistance are linked with about a two-fold higher risk of CVD and enhanced atherosclerosis. Although this is prominent in elderly Type 2 men,[70] insulin resistance syndrome predicts the risk of CVD also in middle-aged men as detected in the Helsinki Policemen Study.[71] Another group of patients with insulin-resistance syndrome was found with chronic complications including a higher prevalence of CHD (53 versus 21%), as well as micro- and macroalbuminuria.[72] In this respect, it is of special interest to emphasize that a rapid progression of albuminuria was found to be an independent predictor of cardiovascular mortality.[73] Among the factors influencing this relationship may be the association of insulin resistance and IGT with low HDL levels, hypertriglyceridemia, hypertension and increased blood coagulability. Because of the connection between CVD and insulin resistance syndrome prior to frank DM, it is necessary to start an early preventive treatment of the impending macrovascular disease by clinical screening, lifestyle change and drug intervention in young persons, since IGT is not a strictly age-progressing condition and may be arrested before complications set in.[74]

Role of hyperglycemia in the pathogenesis of diabetic cardiovascular complications

The relationship between hyperglycemia and macrovascular disease is complex, and it is often difficult to isolate the effect of hyper-glycemia on the cardiovascular system from other risk factors. Studies done in the 1970s and 1980s aiming to define the relationship between hyperglycemia and vascular events yielded conflicting results.[53,75,76] One problem associated with these studies was their cross-sectional design and the parameters used for determining the existence of hyperglycemia just prior to the MI event. Moreover, as a result of methodological problems it was unclear whether the severity of MI was related to pronounced hyperglycemia or vice versa. However, these studies demonstrated the existence of a link between hyperglycemia and macrovascular disease in both non-diabetic and diabetic patients. Some reports in patients with MI indicated that plasma glucose levels at admission to the coronary care unit correlated strongly with mortality regardless of whether or not the patient had diabetes.[77] In addition, Van den Berghe et al. have shown that inten-sive insulin therapy maintaining the blood glucose below 6.1 mmol/l reduces morbidity and mortality.[78] It was suggested in other studies that hospital fatality rates are improved in patients with optimal control, judged by blood glucose levels measured just before the infarct.[39]

Recent studies provide a stronger indication that hyperglycemia is an important and independent risk factor for CVD in patients with Type 2 DM.[5,8,14,20,79,80] The UKPDS report on the results of a large prospective observa-tional study of 4585 patients who were either randomized to intensive glycemic control inter-ventions or conventional treatment, showed that for every 1% decrease in HbA1c, there was a 14% reduction in risk for MI.[81]

Large prospective epidemiologic studies, by including comprehensive multivariate analyses of all major risk factors, have provided a much more accurate evaluation of the cardiovascular risk associated with hyperglycemia. In these studies, it has become clear that there are many temporal aspects of hyperglycemia, and that to truly understand the relationship between hyperglycemia and CVD, it is necessary to analyze independently the subcomponents of hyperglycemia. Specifically, the pathogenic effects of fasting, postprandial, and total glycemic exposure have to be separately assessed. Similarly, the different forms of CVD that were previously lumped together as 'diabetic cardiovascular complications', need to be broken down into subgroups that include chronic progressive atherosclerotic disease, MI, and sudden cardiovascular death so as to better define the causative role of hyperglycemia. Refining the definitions of hyperglycemia and cardiovascular disease has allowed for a detailed analysis of the relationship between the two, and has facilitated the development of better and rational treatment strategies for the diabetic patient.

The role of postprandial hyperglycemia has recently come under scrutiny in terms of being a significant factor in the development of diabetic CVD.[82] Early studies such as the Whitehall Study had shown that IGT in non-diabetics was associated with increased cardio-vascular and coronary artery disease mortality.[84] The Diabetes Intervention Study, a multicenter trial conducted in East Germany showed that patients with better postprandial glucose levels (<8 mmol/l) had a lower incidence of MI and cardiovascular death.[85] The DECODE (Diabetes Epidemiology Collaborative Analysis Of Diagnostic Criteria in Europe) study presented a systematic evalu-ation of the predictive value of hyperglycemia with regard to mortality in either non-diabetics, those with borderline abnormalities in blood glucose, or those with diabetes based on the American Diabetes Association's revised criteria for the diagnosis of DM.[86] The results of this study showed that postprandial blood glucose fluctuations after the 75 g glucose challenge are an independent predictor of mortality.

Association of insulin levels with CVD

The role of insulin as a factor in diabetic CVD is an important issue for Type 2 DM patients who may be hyperinsulinemic as a result of insulin resistance or be receiving significant quantities as part of enhanced glycemic control protocols. Clearly, increasing dosages of insulin can cause obesity, which is a risk factor for CVD. A different issue is whether insulin, a growth factor, is atherogenic. Accumulated evidence indicates that increased levels of insulin, proinsulin or its partial split products are associated with enhanced plasminogen activator inhibitor-1 activity which causes attenuation of the fibrinolytic response leading to increased thrombosis. Insulin resistance has also been associated with hyperlipidemia, and several studies have shown that carotid intimal-medial thickness, a marker for atherosclerotic disease, is increased in individuals with hyper-insulinemia.

On the other hand, in several large epidemiologic studies insulin, as a treatment modality, does not appear to confer additional risk for CVD. Savage et al.[87] did not find an increased incidence of CVD in patients receiving insulin in place of oral hypoglycemic agents. The same finding was also noted in the recently completed UKPDS. Additional support for the lack of a relationship between insulin levels and atherosclerosis is based on a study of a large series of insulinoma patients, in whom there were no signs of unusual progressive atherosclerosis despite the very high levels of sustained hyperinsulinemia.[88]

In conclusion, hyperglycemia (both fasting and postprandial) and possible hyperinsulinemia play a role in the development of cardiovascular complications in diabetic patients. There is a possibility that some additional, poorly defined diabetes-specific risk factors have importance in the pathogenesis of vascular disease. Another important consideration, especially with regard to developing health initiatives to improve treatment of Type 2 DM. Absolute reduction in risk, depends not only on the percentage reduction of a specific risk factor but also on the prevalence of the risk factor. For instance, even if the intensive treatment of hypertension and dyslipidemia yields a greater reduction in the relative risk in individuals with these specific risk factors, the total number of patients benefitting from therapy is lower compared with those benefitting from intensive treatment of hyperglycemia even though the reduction of relative risk is less.

The impact of revised diagnostic criteria for DM

A reflection of this issue is the recent alterations of the diagnostic criteria for DM issued by the American Diabetes Association (ADA) and the World Health Organization (WHO).[89,90] The revised criteria changed both the levels of glucose at which DM is diagnosed and the preferred methodology for diagnosis. Both organizations have lowered the threshold for fasting plasma glucose to 7.0 mmol/l or greater for the diagnosis of DM. The ADA diagnostic criteria place great emphasis on fasting plasma glucose, and have de-emphasized the importance of the oral glucose tolerance test (OGTT). The WHO, in contrast, still recommends using the OGTT in diagnosing DM. It has been shown in many, but not all, reports that the concordance between the fasting glucose criterion of ADA and the OGTT definition of WHO is often low and that different subsets of subjects are diagnosed as diabetic by the two sets of criteria.

The DECODE study provides some insight to this problem.[86] According to the DECODE report, which compared the prevalence of DM based on either the ADA criterion of a fasting plasma glucose of ≥7 mmol/l or the WHO criterion of a two-hour postprandial plasma glucose of >11.1 mmol/l. If fasting glucose alone is used as a diagnostic criterion, then 31% of diabetic subjects with a non-diabetic fasting glucose, but a high two-hour glucose would not be diagnosed.

Another problem with diagnostic criteria revolves around the issue of individuals without overt DM, but abnormal glucose metabolism. The ADA established a category of individuals with impaired fasting glucose (IFG) (6.1–6.9 mmol/l) whereas the WHO uses a two-hour postprandial plasma glucose of between 7.8 and 11.1 mmol/l as a definition for IGT. Several questions have been raised regarding differences between IGT and IFG:

(1) Is the pathogenesis of IGT and IFG identical?
(2) Is the phenotype associated with IGT different from that of IFG?
(3) Is the conversion rate from IFG or IGT to overt DM identical?
(4) Do these subtypes have different cardiovascular risk profiles and mortality rates?
(5) What are the implications for treatment of patients with either IGT or IFG?

Not all of these issues have been answered, but some studies have shed light on the issues of phenotypic characteristics, cardiovascular risk distribution, and outcomes of IGT and IFG with regard to the role of hyperglycemia and insulin resistance in conferring the risk for macrovascular disease.

The Funagata Diabetes Study investigators evaluated risk for overall and cardiovascular mortality in a cohort of individuals in Japan, in various categories of abnormal carbohydrate metabolism including IGT, IFG and overt DM. Individuals with either IGT or frank diabetes were at significantly higher risk for death from cardiovascular causes than non-diabetics and those with IFG. As expected, the highest risk was found among those with fully expressed DM. Those with IFG did not differ from non-diabetics in terms of mortality. The survival rate was lower among individuals with IGT beginning at six years after diagnosis, and the cardiovascular mortality was significantly higher beginning four years after the diagnosis. The increase in mortality, especially cardiovascular, underscores the importance of postprandial hyperglycemia as a risk factor, and lends credence to the claim that elevated postprandial blood glucose, as determined by OGTT, has important prognostic significance.

A number of other epidemiological reports reinforce the thesis that postprandial glucose is a risk factor for mortality. In the Chicago Heart Study investigators reported that cardiovascular mortality was significantly increased in men with asymptomatic postchallenge hyperglycemia (>11.1 mmol/l one hour after a 50 g OGTT).[30] Data from the Rancho Bernardo cohort suggest that older women with isolated postchallenge hyperglycemia, i.e. two-hour postchallenge glucose >11.1 mmol/l, but FPG <7.0 mmol/l, have a cardiovascular mortality rate 2.6 times that of age-matched euglycemic control subjects. Meta-analysis of association between glycemia and CVD also indicates higher cardiovascular risk with increases in one-hour/two-hour and fasting glucose levels.[91,92] Again, the strongest predictors are fasting and two-hour postprandial blood glucose levels, suggesting that even mild blood glucose elevation is a major variable in the development of macrovascular disease.

Several possible mechanisms that affect cardiovascular risk have been proposed as operating in patients with postprandial blood glucose oscillations, including QT interval prolongation, hypercoagulability, increased blood pressure, and postprandial elevation in lipid concentration. The results of the DECODE study show that postprandial blood glucose fluctuations after the 75 g glucose challenge predict an increased risk of death in an independent manner.

It has also been noted that individuals with IGT tend to have a certain phenotype that is not necessarily found in those with abnormalities in fasting glucose only. Results from the DECODE study indicate that patients with IGT have increased prevalence of obesity. Others have also observed that IGT patients are more obese, more insulin resistant, and have higher insulin levels than normal individuals.[2–7] Whether insulin secretion is impaired in individuals with IGT remains controversial because both lower and normal early and late insulin secretion responses have been reported.[1,2,6–11] Basal endogenous insulin output, indicating compensatory oversecretion, has also been found to be increased in individuals with IGT. This usually occurs late in the pre-diabetic stage suggesting that IGT is a more advanced stage than IFG in DM development.

The impact of therapeutic interventions for diabetic cardiovascular disease

Different interventions have been attempted to reduce cardiovascular mortality in Type 2 DM. Lifestyle changes such as cessation of smoking, weight reduction, low saturated fat diet and exercise are beneficial. Exercise is particularly valuable both as a primary prevention for Type 2 DM and because of its probable effects on dyslipidemia and glycemic control.[93] As discussed above, risk factors associated with increased cardiovascular mortality include dyslipidemia and hypertension, and therapeutic agents that correct these metabolic abnormalities have been shown to reduce cardiovascular mortality. In addition, hyperglycemia is associated with increased mortality, and it would be expected that reduction in average blood glucose would reduce cardiovascular mortality. The recently completed UKPDS study provides an indication that intensive glycemic control in Type 2 DM improves cardiovascular outcome. In this study, a reduction of 11% HbA1c was achieved in the intervention group with statistically borderline decrease in cardiovascular complications.[94] This is in contrast to other factors such as improved control of hyperlipidemia and hypertension in which there was a clear-cut advantage in terms of cardiovascular mortality.[95,96]

Aspirin has been found to be effective in secondary prevention of cardiovascular events in the general population, and is also effective in terms of primary prevention.[97,98] The Early Treatment Diabetic Retinopathy Study Research Group (ETDRS), which included diabetics with or without CVD, demonstrated a reduction in MI. Bleeding complications were not significant even in the presence of proliferative diabetic retinopathy.[99,100] The utility of aspirin to reduce the risk of CVD was also confirmed by the Israeli Bezafibrate Infarction Prevention Study Group, which showed that aspirin was more effective in reducing both cardiac and total mortality in diabetics than non-diabetics.[101] Presently, many authorities recommend the use of aspirin in diabetics with cardiovascular symptoms while others recommend it as primary prevention in all patients with diabetes.[102] However, a recent study indicates that aspirin, as a preventative therapy, is underutilized among diabetics.[103]

The use of beta-blockers for prevention of a second MI in patients with DM is well documented.[104–106] Retrospective analysis of the Bezafibrate Infarction Prevention Study demonstrated that there was a 44% reduction in the three-year mortality rate in patients receiving beta-blockers compared with those who were not.[107] A specific benefit of the beta-blockers is that these drugs have been shown to reduce the incidence of silent ischemia, which is increased in diabetic patients presumably due to cardiac autonomic neuropathy.[108]

Particular drug regimens may have an impact on cardiovascular morbidity and mortality, and their use in diabetics must be carefully assessed. A long-standing controversy revolves around the use of sulfonylurea drugs. In the 1970s, the University Group Diabetes Program (UGDP) reported that there was a high mortality rate associated with the use of these agents.[109] In the last decade, the effect of sulfonylureas on cardiac adenosine-5' triphosphate dependent potassium (K_{ATP}) channels has been investigated. It is thought that these agents may amplify ischemic changes in the myocardium by impairing ischemic preconditioning.[110,111] Garratt et al.,[112] found that sulfonylureas increased early mortality in diabetics undergoing direct angioplasty for acute myocardial infarction. Other studies, including the UKPDS, have not found increased mortality associated with the use of sulfonylureas.[94,113] As the conflict surrounding sulfonylureas has not been resolved, the use of these agents in diabetics at high risk for IHD should be weighed carefully. (See also Chapter 25.)

Frequently, patients with Type 2 DM and CVD (with or without diabetic nephropathy) require the use of either ACE-inhibitors or calcium channel blockers. ACE-inhibitors, because of their beneficial effect on the progression of nephropathy, are widely used in Type 2 DM with hypertension. These agents have a beneficial effect in terms of increasing survival among non-diabetic patients with congestive heart failure following acute MI. ACE-inhibitors reduce left ventricular mass, left ventricular hypertrophy, and left ventricular afterload.[114] These agents may be of particular benefit to diabetics who have a significantly increased rate of congestive heart failure especially after MI.[115] Subsets of patients with DM participating in large-scale trials of ACE-inhibitors do benefit from the use of ACE-inhibitors both in terms of improved left ventricular function, heart failure, and overall short- and long-term post-MI mortality. The HOPE study, discussed above, specifically studied diabetics and found that ramipril has a beneficial effect on both the incidence of myocardial infarction and the cardiovascular mortality rate.[68] Recently, this observation was supported by the LIFE study in 1195 diabetic patients.[128] This study compared long-term effects of losartan with atelenol in patients with hypertension and left ventricular hypertrophy on the frequency of cardiovascular morbidity and mortality and found that losartan was more effective, both in non-diabetic and diabetic patients.

Calcium channel blockers (CCBs) have been one of the most common drugs prescribed for hypertension. However, their role in DM is controversial. The Appropriate Blood Pressure Control in Diabetes (ABCD) trial, designed to determine the most effective means of intensively controlling blood pressure, was halted early after it was determined that patients with hypertension receiving nisoldipine (a dihydropyridine CCB) had an almost five-fold increase in fatal and non-fatal MI than those receiving ACE-inhibitors.[119] This was confirmed in the FACET (Fosinopril versus Amlodipine Cardiovascular Events Trial) in which Type 2 diabetic patients receiving amlodipine (a CCB) had an almost two-fold greater incidence in cardiovascular incidents including stroke and

MI than those receiving an ACE-inhibitor.[120] The increased cardiovascular mortality associated with CCBs may be due to the altered levels of cholesterol in contractile cell plasma membranes of diabetics leading to increased levels of CCBs in membranes causing cardiovascular toxicity.[122] It should be noted that there are other studies that do not show any deleterious effects associated with the use of CCBs[123,124] and recently the angiotensin receptor antagonist irbesartan was shown to reduce cardiovascular events in Type 2 diabetic patients treated for progressive nephropathy.[125]

As detailed above, patients with postprandial hyperglycemia or DM are at increased risk for CVD. This raises the question of whether intense intervention to lower blood glucose, especially postprandial hyperglycemia, during acute cardiac events may have a positive benefit on cardiovascular mortality. Data from prospective, randomized, interventional trials that examine the effect of treating hyperglycemia on cardiovascular outcomes of Type 2 DM are very limited. The results of the Diabetes Mellitus Insulin Glucose Infusion in Acute Myocardial Infarction study (DIGAMI) have shed some light on this issue. This was a prospective trial of 620 diabetic patients with MI who were randomized either to an acute treatment with glucose-insulin infusion followed by multidose s.c. insulin for at least three months, or to a control group, which was treated in most cases with diet and oral hypoglycemic medication. After 12 months 26.1% of patients in the control group died, in contrast to 18.6% of insulin-treated patients – a reduction of relative mortality of 29%. During the first year of treatment the number of fatal re-infarctions was also significantly reduced from 45% in the control group to 28% in the insulin group.[126] After a mean follow-up of 3.4 years there were 33% of deaths in the insulin group compared to 44% in the control group.[127] The question raised by this pivotal study is whether it was the reduction of hyperglycemia that contributed to the reduced mortality, or some other factor. In terms of overall glycemic control, there was only a modest reduction in HbA1c levels at both three months and one year (7.1 and 7.3% in the intensive group and 7.5 and 7.6% in the controls). It is therefore unlikely that the limited difference with regard to the overall metabolic status caused the significant improvement in mortality among MI patients. One possible explanation of the DIGAMI study results relates to potential iatrogenic effect of oral agents, as a very high proportion of patients in the control group were treated with sulfonylurea drugs. A second possibility is that while there were no significant differences in metabolic control between the two main groups (intervention versus control), there were substantial differences between specific subgroups. For example, subjects who were not on insulin treatment before the intervention and were at low risk for CVD, had a much more significant improvement in metabolic control when placed on an intensive insulin regimen. Finally, it is possible that better control of postprandial hyperglycemia as a result of the insulin therapy contributed to an improved outcome. However, there are not sufficient data from the DIGAMI study to support such a conclusion, and further investigation is necessary.

Prevention of progression of IGT and Type 2 diabetes by diet, exercise and pharmacological modalities and the relevance to CVD

It goes without saying that lack of physical activity, sedentary life, and obesity are prominent risk factors for IGT and its progression to overt DM with cardiovascular complications. It is well known that drastic change in lifestyle is difficult to achieve. But it should also be stressed that diet and exercise, even without marked loss in weight, are beneficial, particularly in high risk persons.

In the Malmo Feasibility Study (MFS) three groups were investigated: asymptomatic Type 2 patients, IGT subjects and controls.[128] Weight loss of 2.3–3.7% was achieved in the Type 2 group versus 0.5–1.7% in the control (IGT and no intervention groups). IGT was normalized in 50% of subjects by the end of the six-year period. Weight loss and exercise were separately beneficial but additive when taken together. As demonstrated elsewhere, exercise induces the translocation of the GLUT4 transporter in human skeletal muscle in diabetes and improves glucose uptake and thus reduces hyperglycemia.[129] Further innovative programs for changing the behavior and nutrition of IGT patients should be urgently devised.[130]

The oral antidiabetic agents should be considered not only in frank diabetes but in an attempt to avoid the lapse from IGT to diabetes. Reduction of glycemia and free fatty acids means reduction of peripheral gluco- and lipotoxicity, which bring about the insulin resistance. In case of IGT there is only limited glucose toxicity and the most appropriate drug for such individuals would be that which potentiates and/or sensitizes insulin action. Representatives of such a drug family are thiazolidinediones,[131–135] metformin and acarbose.[6] By preventing the progression from IGT to overt DM these drugs may minimize the incidence of CVD. The main mechanism of action of these agents is improving tissue insulin response and return to normalcy. These results emphasize that the real effort should be put into achieving reversal of IGT and prevention of Type 2 DM with CVD lesions.

Concluding remarks

Macrovascular complications are the main medical and economic problems associated with chronic hyperglycemia of Type 2 DM. Accelerated cardiovascular and cerebrovascular atherosclerosis is the major cause of mortality in patients with Type 2 DM. Case-fatality is increased by 25–100% in diabetics compared with non-diabetic subjects with MI, indicating that coronary artery disease has a much worse course in diabetes. All of the known general risk factors for atherosclerosis are operative or even exacerbated in diabetic patients, including hypercholesterolemia, hypertriglyceridemia, hypertension, abdominal obesity, smoking, and increased levels of plasminogen activator 1 and fibrinogen. Recent studies indicate that hyperglycemia is an important and independent risk factor for CVD in patients with Type 2 DM. Specifically, increased risk of CVD is directly related to both elevated one-hour and two-hour postprandial blood glucose averages as well as to fasting hyperglycemia. The DIGAMI and UKPDS studies suggest that improved blood glucose control reduces CVD risks. To reduce the rate of CVD among subjects with IGT and Type 2 DM, exercise and pharmacological treatment regimens should be applied so as to maximize glycemic control to ensure consistently lower postprandial and fasting glucose values.

References

1. Zimmet PZ, Alberti KG. The changing face of macrovascular disease in non-insulin-dependent diabetes mellitus: an epidemic in progress. Lancet 1997; 350: SI1–4.
2. King H, Aubert RE, Herman WH. Global burden of diabetes, 1995–2025: prevalence, numerical estimates, and projections. Diabetes Care 1998; 21: 1414–31.

3. Wake N, Katayama T, Kishikawa H et al. Cost-effectiveness of intensive insulin therapy for Type 2 diabetes: a 10-year follow-up of the Kumamoto study. Diabetes Res Clin Pract 2000; 48: 201–10.
4. Gray A, Raikou M, McGuire A et al. Cost effectiveness of an intensive blood glucose control policy in patients with Type 2 diabetes: economic analysis alongside randomised controlled trial (UKPDS 41). United Kingdom Prospective Diabetes Study Group. BMJ 2000; 320: 1373–8.
5. Laakso M. Hyperglycemia and cardiovascular disease in Type 2 diabetes. Diabetes 1999; 48: 937–42.
6. Harris MI, Eastman RC. Is there a glycemic threshold for mortality risk. Diabetes Care 1998; 21: 331–2.
7. Kekalainen P, Sarlund H, Pyorala K, Laakso M. Hyperinsulinemia cluster predicts the development of Type 2 diabetes independently of family history of diabetes. Diabetes Care 1999; 22: 86–92.
8. Laakso M, Kuusisto J. Epidemiological evidence for the association of hyperglycaemia and atherosclerotic vascular disease in non-insulin-dependent diabetes mellitus. Ann Med 1996; 28: 415–18.
9. Haffner SM, Lehto S, Ronnemaa T et al. Mortality from coronary heart disease in subjects with Type 2 diabetes and in non-diabetic subjects with and without prior myocardial infarction. N Engl J Med 1998; 339: 229–34.
10. Aronson D, Rayfield EJ, Chesebro JH. Mechanisms determining course and outcome of diabetic patients who have had acute myocardial infarction. Ann Intern Med 1997; 126: 296–306.
11. Jacoby RM, Nesto RW. Acute myocardial infarction in the diabetic patient: pathophysiology, clinical course and prognosis. J Am Coll Cardiol 1992; 20: 736–44.
12. Garcia MJ, McNamara PM, Gordon T, Kannel WB. Morbidity and mortality in diabetics in the Framingham population. Sixteen year follow-up study. Diabetes 1974; 23: 105–11.
13. Casiglia E, Zanette G, Mazza A et al. Cardiovascular mortality in non-insulin-dependent diabetes mellitus. A controlled study among 683 diabetics and 683 age- and sex-matched normal subjects. Eur J Epidemiol 2000; 677–84.
14. Klein R. Hyperglycemia and microvascular and macrovascular disease in diabetes. Diabetes Care 1995; 18: 258–68.
15. Barrett-Connor EL, Cohn BA et al. Why is diabetes mellitus a stronger risk factor for fatal ischemic heart disease in women than in men? The Rancho Bernardo Study. JAMA 1991; 265: 627–31.
16. Kleinman JC, Donahue RP, Harris MI et al. Mortality among diabetics in a national sample. Am J Epidemiol 1988; 128: 389–401.
17. Wingard DL, Barrett-Connors E. Heart disease and diabetes. In: Harris M, ed. Diabetes in America. Bethesda: National Institutes of Health, 1995: 429–56.
18. Geiss L, Herman WH, Smith PJ. Mortality in non-insulin-dependent diabetes. In: Harris M, ed. Diabetes in America. Bethesda: National Institutes of Health, 1995: 233–55.
19. Haffner SM. Cardiovascular risk factors and the prediabetic syndrome. Ann Med 1996; 28: 363–70.
20. Haffner SM. The importance of hyperglycemia in the nonfasting state to the development of cardiovascular disease. Endocr Rev 1998; 19: 583–92.
21. Tominaga M, Eguchi H, Manaka H et al. Impaired glucose tolerance is a risk factor for cardiovascular disease, but not impaired fasting glucose. The Funagata Diabetes Study. Diabetes Care 1999; 22: 920–4.
22. Nelson RG, Sievers ML, Knowler WC et al. Low incidence of fatal coronary heart disease in Pima Indians despite high prevalence of non-insulin-dependent diabetes. Circulation 1990; 81: 987–95.
23. McKeigue PM, Miller GJ, Marmot MG. Coronary heart disease in south Asians overseas: a review. J Clin Epidemiol 1989; 42: 597–609.
24. Manson JE, Colditz GA, Stampfer MJ et al. A prospective study of maturity-onset diabetes mellitus and risk of coronary heart disease and stroke in women. Arch Intern Med 1991; 151: 1141–7.
25. Kuusisto J, Mykkanen L, Pyorala K, Laakso M. NIDDM and its metabolic control predict

coronary heart disease in elderly subjects. Diabetes 1994; 43: 960–7.

26. Zimmet PZ. Hyperinsulinemia – how innocent a bystander? Diabetes Care 1993; 16: 56–70.

27. Saad MF, Knowler WC, Pettitt DJ et al. Insulin and hypertension. Relationship to obesity and glucose intolerance in Pima Indians. Diabetes 1990; 39: 1430–5.

28. Rewers M, Hamman RF. Risk factors for non-insulin-dependent diabetes. In: Harris M, ed. Diabetes in America. Bethesda: National Institutes of Health, 1995: 179–220.

29. Lehto S, Ronnemaa T, Haffner SM et al. Dyslipidemia and hyperglycemia predict coronary heart disease events in middle-aged patients with NIDDM. Diabetes 1997; 46: 1354–9.

30. Lowe LP, Liu K, Greenland P et al. Diabetes, asymptomatic hyperglycemia, and 22–year mortality in black and white men. Diabetes Care 1997; 20: 163–9.

31. Feener EP, King GL. Vascular dysfunction in diabetes mellitus. Lancet 1997; 350: SI9–13.

32. Ulvenstam G, Aberg A, Bergstrand R et al. Long-term prognosis after myocardial infarction in men with diabetes. Diabetes 1985; 34: 787–92.

33. Turner RC, Millns H, Neil HA et al. Risk factors for coronary artery disease in non-insulin dependent diabetes mellitus: United Kingdom Prospective Diabetes Study (UKPDS: 23). BMJ 1998; 316: 823–8.

34. Miettinen H, Lehto S, Salomaa V et al. Impact of diabetes on mortality after the first myocardial infarction. The FINMONICA Myocardial Infarction Register Study Group. Diabetes Care 1998; 21: 69–75.

35. Partamian JO, Bradley RF. Acute myocardial infarction in 258 cases of diabetes. Immediate mortality and five-year survival. N Engl J Med 1965; 273: 455–61.

36. Soler NG, Pentecost BL, Bennett MA et al. Coronary care for myocardial infarction in diabetics. Lancet 1974; 1: 475–7.

37. Smith JW, Marcus FI, Serokman R. Prognosis of patients with diabetes mellitus after acute myocardial infarction. Am J Cardiol 1984; 54: 718–21.

38. Henning R, Lundman T. Swedish Co-operative CCU Study. A study of 2008 patients with acute myocardial infarction from 12 Swedish hospitals with coronary care unit. Part I. A description of the early stage. Part II. The short-term prognosis. Acta Med Scand Suppl 1975; 586: 1–35.

39. Rytter L, Troelsen S, Beck-Nielsen H. Pre-valence and mortality of acute myocardial infarction in patients with diabetes. Diabetes Care 1985; 8: 230–4.

40. Schernthaner G. Cardiovascular mortality and morbidity in type-2 diabetes mellitus. Diabetes Res Clin Pract 1996; 31: S3–13.

41. Malmberg K, Ryden L. Myocardial infarction in patients with diabetes mellitus. Eur Heart J 1988; 9: 259–64.

42. Herlitz J, Bang A, Karlson BW. Mortality, place and mode of death and reinfarction during a period of 5 years after acute myocardial infarction in diabetic and non-diabetic patients. Cardiology 1996; 87: 423–8.

43. Benderly M, Behar S, Reicher-Reiss H et al. Long-term prognosis of women after myocardial infarction. SPRINT Study Group. Secondary Prevention Reinfarction Israeli Nifedipine Trial. Am J Epidemiol 1997; 146: 153–60.

44. Aronson D, Rayfield EJ, Chesebro JH. Mechanisms determining course and outcome of diabetic patients who have had acute myocardial infarction. Ann Intern Med 1997; 126: 296–306.

45. Yudkin JS, Oswald GA. Determinants of hospital admission and case fatality in diabetic patients with myocardial infarction. Diabetes Care 1988; 11: 351–8.

46. Jensen JS, Feldt-Rasmussen B, Borch-Johnsen K et al. Microalbuminuria and its relation to cardiovascular disease and risk factors. A population-based study of 1254 hypertensive individuals. J Hum Hypertens 1997; 11: 727–32.

47. Jensen JS, Borch-Johnsen K, Feldt-Rasmussen B et al. Urinary albumin excretion and history of acute myocardial infarction in a cross-sectional population study of 2,613 individuals. J Cardiovasc Risk 1997; 4: 121–5.

48. Johnson WD, Pedraza PM, Kayser KL. Coronary artery surgery in diabetics: 261 consecutive patients followed four to seven years. Am Heart J 1982; 104: 823–7.

49. Herlitz J, Wognsen GB, Emanuelsson H et al. Mortality and morbidity in diabetic and non-diabetic patients during a 2-year period after coronary artery bypass grafting. Diabetes Care 1996; 19: 698–703.

50. Cohen Y, Raz I, Merin G, Mozes B. Comparison of factors associated with 30-day mortality after coronary artery bypass grafting in patients with versus without diabetes mellitus. Israeli Coronary Artery Bypass (ISCAB) Study Consortium. Am J Cardiol 1998; 81: 7–11.

51. Thourani VH, Weintraub WS, Stein B et al. Influence of diabetes mellitus on early and late outcome after coronary artery bypass grafting. Ann Thorac Surg 1999; 67: 1045–52.

52. Marso SP, Ellis SG, Gurm HS et al. Proteinuria is a key determinant of death in patients with diabetes after isolated coronary artery bypass grafting. Am Heart J 2000; 139: 939–44.

53. Gwilt DJ, Petri M, Lewis PW et al. Myocardial infarct size and mortality in diabetic patients. Br Heart J 1985; 54: 466–72.

54. Lehto S, Pyorala K, Miettinen H et al. Myocardial infarct size and mortality in patients with non insulin dependent diabetes mellitus. J Intern Med 1994; 236: 291–7.

55. Gu K, Cowie CC, Harris MI. Diabetes and decline in heart disease mortality in US adults. JAMA 1999; 281: 1291–7.

56. Haffner SM. Coronary heart disease in patients with diabetes. N Engl J Med 2000; 342: 1040–2.

57. Pyorala K, Pedersen TR, Kjekshus J et al. Cholesterol lowering with simvastatin improves prognosis of diabetic patients with coronary heart disease. A subgroup analysis of the Scandinavian Simvastatin Survival Study (4S). Diabetes Care 1997; 20: 614–20.

58. Kannel WB, McGee DL. Diabetes and cardiovascular risk factors: the Framingham study. Circulation 1979; 59: 8–13.

59. Rosengren A, Welin L, Tsipogianni A, Wilhelmsen L. Impact of cardiovascular risk factors on coronary heart disease and mortality among middle aged diabetic men: a general population study. BMJ 1989; 299: 1127–31.

60. Stamler J, Vaccaro O, Neaton JD, Wentworth D. Diabetes, other risk factors, and 12-yr cardiovascular mortality for men screened in the Multiple Risk Factor Intervention Trial. Diabetes Care 1993; 16: 434–44.

61. Vaccaro O, Stamler J, Neaton JD. Sixteen-year coronary mortality in black and white men with diabetes screened for the Multiple Risk Factor Intervention Trial (MRFIT). Int J Epidemiol 1998; 27: 636–41.

62. Koskinen P, Manttari M, Manninen V et al. Coronary heart disease incidence in NIDDM patients in the Helsinki Heart Study. Diabetes Care 1992; 15: 820–5.

63. Hoogwerf BJ, Waness A, Cressman M et al. Effects of aggressive cholesterol lowering and low-dose anticoagulation on clinical and angiographic outcomes in patients with diabetes: the Post Coronary Artery Bypass Graft Trial. Diabetes 1999; 48: 1289–94.

64. Harris MI. Impaired glucose tolerance in the U.S. population. Diabetes Care 1989; 12: 464–74.

65. The Hypertension in Diabetes Study Group. Hypertension in diabetes study (HDS): increased risk of cardiovascular complications in hypertensive Type 2 diabetic patients. J Hypertens 1993; 11: 319–25.

66. Sawicki PT, Heise T, Berger M. Antihypertensive treatment and mortality in diabetic patients. What is the evidence? Acta Paediatr Scand 1997; 40: S134–7.

67. Adler AI, Stratton IM, Neil HA et al. Association of systolic blood pressure with macrovascular and microvascular complications of Type 2 diabetes (UKPDS 36): prospective observational study. BMJ 2000; 321: 412–19.

68. Heart Outcomes Prevention Evaluation Study Investigators. Effects of ramipril on cardiovascular and microvascular outcomes in people with diabetes mellitus: results of the HOPE study and MICRO-HOPE substudy. Lancet 2000; 355: 253–9

69. Niskanen L, Hedner T, Hansson T et al. Reduced cardiovascular morbidity and mortality in hypertensive diabetic patients on first line therapy with an ACE inhibitor compared with a diuretic/beta-blocker-based treatment regimen: a subanalysis of the captopril prevention project. Diabetes Care 2001; 24: 2091–6.

70. Kuusisto J, Lempiainen P, Mykkanen L, Laakso M. Insulin resistance syndrome predicts coronary heart disease events in elderly Type 2

diabetic men. Diabetes Carre 2001; 24: 1629–33.

71. Pyorala M, Miettinen H, Halonen P et al. Insulin resistance syndrome predicts the risk of coronary heart disease and stroke in healthy middle-aged men: the 22-year follow-up results of the Helsinki Policement Study. Arterioscler Thromb Vasc Biol 2000; 20: 538–44.

72. Isomaa B, Henricsson M, Almgren P et al. The metabolic syndrome influences the risk of chronic complications in patients with type II diabetes. Diabetologia 2001; 44: 1148–54.

73. Spoelstra-De Man AM, Brouwer CB, Stehouwer CD, Smulders YM. Rapid progression of albumin excretion is an independent predictor of cardiovascular mortality in patients with Type 2 diabetes and microalbuminuria. Diabetes Care 2001; 24: 2097–101.

74. Tuomilehto J, Lindstrom J, Eriksson JG et al. Prevention of Type 2 diabetes mellitus by changes in lifestyle among subjects with impaired glucose tolerance. New Engl J Med 2001; 344: 1343–50.

75. Bornfeldt KE, Arnqvist HJ, Capron L. In vivo proliferation of rat vascular smooth muscle in relation to diabetes mellitus insulin-like growth factor I and insulin. Diabetologia 1992; 35: 104–8.

76. Yudkin JS, Oswald GA. Hyperglycaemia, diabetes and myocardial infarction. Diabet Med 1987; 4: 13–18.

77. Oswald GA, Corcoran S, Yudkin JS. Prevalence and risks of hyperglycaemia and undiagnosed diabetes in patients with acute myocardial infarction. Lancet 1984; 1: 1264–7.

78. Van den Berghe G, Wontess P, Weekers F et al. Intensive insulin therapy in the critically ill patients. N Engl J Med 2001; 345: 1359–67.

79. Lehto S, Ronnemaa T, Haffner SM et al. Dyslipidemia and hyperglycemia predict coronary heart disease events in middle-aged patients with NIDDM. Diabetes 1997; 46: 1354–9.

80. Uusitupa MI, Niskanen LK. Hyperglycemia and cardiovascular risk in NIDDM. Diabetes Care 1995; 18: 884–5.

81. Stratton IM, Adler AI, Neil HA et al. Association of glycaemia with macrovascular and microvascular complications of Type 2 diabetes (UKPDS 35): prospective observational study. BMJ 2000; 321: 405–12.

82. Monnier L. Is postprandial glucose a neglected cardiovascular risk factor in Type 2 diabetes? Eur J Clin Invest 2000; 30: 3–11.

84. Balkau B, Shipley M, Jarrett RJ et al. High blood glucose concentration is a risk factor for mortality in middle-aged nondiabetic men. 20-year follow-up in the Whitehall Study, the Paris Prospective Study, and the Helsinki Policemen Study. Diabetes Care 1998; 21: 360–7.

85. Hanefeld M, Fischer S, Julius U et al. Risk factors for myocardial infarction and death in newly detected NIDDM: the Diabetes Intervention Study, 11-year follow-up. Diabetologia 1996; 39: 1577–83.

86. Glucose tolerance and mortality: comparison of WHO and American Diabetes Association diagnostic criteria. The DECODE study group. European Diabetes Epidemiology Group. Diabetes epidemiology: collaborative analysis of diagnostic criteria in Europe. Lancet 1999; 354: 617–21.

87. Savage S, Estacio RO, Jeffers B, Schrier RW. Increased complications in noninsulin-dependent diabetic patients treated with insulin versus oral hypoglycemic agents: a population study. Proc Assoc Am Phys 1997; 109: 181–9.

88. Leonetti F, Iozzo P, Giaccari A et al. Absence of clinically overt atherosclerotic vascular disease and adverse changes in cardiovascular risk factors in 70 patients with insulinoma. J Endocrinol Invest 1993; 16: 875–80.

89. Puavilai G, Chanprasertyotin S, Sriphrapradaeng A. Diagnostic criteria for diabetes mellitus and other categories of glucose intolerance: 1997 criteria by the Expert Committee on the Diagnosis and Classification of Diabetes Mellitus (ADA), 1998 WHO consultation criteria, and 1985 WHO criteria. World Health Organization. Diabetes Res Clin Pract 1999; 44: 21–6.

90. Report of the Expert Committee on the Diagnosis and Classification of Diabetes Mellitus. Diabetes Care 1997; 20: 1183–97.

91. Laakso M, Lehto S. Epidemiology of risk factors for cardiovascular disease in diabetes and impaired glucose tolerance. Atherosclerosis 1998; 137: S65–S73.

92. Haffner SM. Epidemiological studies on the effects of hyperglycemia and improvement of glycemic control on macrovascular events in Type 2 diabetes. Diabetes Care 1999; 22: C54–6.

93. Tuomilehto J, Lindstrom J, Eriksson JG et al.

Prevention of Type 2 diabetes mellitus by changes in lifestyle among subjects with impaired glucose tolerance. N Engl J Med 2001; 344: 1343–50.

94. UK Prospective Diabetes Study Group. Intensive blood-glucose control with sulphonylureas or insulin compared with conventional treatment and risk of complications in patients with Type 2 diabetes (UKPDS 33) UK Prospective Diabetes Study (UKPDS) Group. Lancet 1998; 352: 837–53.

95. UK Prospective Diabetes Study Group. Tight blood pressure control and risk of macrovascular and microvascular complications in Type 2 diabetes: UKPDS 38. BMJ 1998; 317: 703–13.

96. Turner RC, Millns H, Neil HA et al. Risk factors for coronary artery disease in non-insulin dependent diabetes mellitus: United Kingdom Prospective Diabetes Study (UKPDS: 23). BMJ 1998; 316: 823–8.

97. Antiplatelet Trialists' Collaboration. Collaborative overview of randomized trials of anti-platelet therapy I: prevention of death, myocardial infarction, and stroke by prolonged anti-platelet therapy in various categories of patients. BMJ 1994; 308: 81–106.

98. Physicians' Health Study Group. Final report on the aspirin component of the ongoing Physicians' Health Study. Steering Committee of the Physicians' Health Study Research Group. N Engl J Med 1989; 321: 129–35.

99. ETDRS Investigators. Aspirin effects on mortality and morbidity in patients with diabetes mellitus. Early Treatment Diabetic Retinopathy Study report 14. JAMA 1992; 268: 1292–300.

100. Early Treatment Diabetic Retinopathy Study Research Group. Effects of aspirin treatment on diabetic retinopathy. ETDRS report number 8. Ophthalmology 1991; 98: 757–65.

101. Harpaz D, Gottlieb S, Graff E et al. Effects of aspirin treatment on survival in non-insulin-dependent diabetic patients with coronary artery disease. Israeli Bezafibrate Infarction Prevention Study Group. Am J Med 1998; 105: 494–9.

102. American Diabetes Association. Aspirin therapy in diabetes. Diabetes Care 1997; 20: 1772–3.

103. Rolka DB, Fagot-Campagna A, Narayan KM. Aspirin use among adults with diabetes: estimates from the Third National Health and Nutrition Examination Survey. Diabetes Care 2001; 24: 197–201.

104. Gundersen T, Kjekshus J. Timolol treatment after myocardial infarction in diabetic patients. Diabetes Care 1983; 285–90.

105. Kjekshus J, Gilpin E, Cali G et al. Diabetic patients and beta-blockers after acute myocardial infarction. Eur Heart J 1990; 11: 43–50.

106. Malmberg K, Ryden L, Hamsten A et al. Mortality prediction in diabetic patients with myocardial infarction: experiences from the DIGAMI study. Cardiovasc Res 1997; 34: 248–53.

107. Jonas M, Reicher-Reiss H, Boyko V et al. Usefulness of beta-blocker therapy in patients with non-insulin-dependent diabetes mellitus and coronary artery disease. Bezafibrate Infarction Prevention (BIP) Study Group. Am J Cardiol 1996; 77: 1273–7.

108. Webster MW, Scott RS. What cardiologists need to know about diabetes. Lancet 1997; 350: SI23–8.

109. Meinert CL, Knatterud GL, Prout TE, Klimt CR. A study of the effects of hypoglycemic agents on vascular complications in patients with adult-onset diabetes. II. Mortality results. Diabetes 1970; 19: 789–830.

110. Wascher TC. Sulfonylureas and cardiovascular mortality in diabetes: a class effect? Circulation 1998; 97: 1427–8.

111. Brady PA, Terzic A. The sulfonylurea controversy: more questions from the heart. J Am Coll Cardiol 1998; 31: 950–6.

112. Garratt KN, Brady PA, Hassinger NL et al. Sulfonylurea drugs increase early mortality in patients with diabetes mellitus after direct angioplasty for acute myocardial infarction. J Am Coll Cardiol 1999; 33: 119–24.

113. Klamann A, Sarfert P, Launhardt V et al. Myocardial infarction in diabetic vs non-diabetic subjects. Survival and infarct size following therapy with sulfonylureas (glibenclamide). Eur Heart J 2000; 21: 220–9.

114. Brown NJ, Vaughan DE. Angiotensin-converting enzyme inhibitors. Circulation 1998; 97: 1411–20.

115. Zuanetti G, Latini R. Impact of pharmacological treatment on mortality after myocardial

infarction in diabetic patients. J Diabetes Complications 1997; 11: 131–6.

116. Shindler DM, Kostis JB, Yusuf S et al. Diabetes mellitus, a predictor of morbidity and mortality in the Studies of Left Ventricular Dysfunction (SOLVD) Trials and Registry. Am J Cardiol 1996; 77: 1017–20.

117. Zuanetti G, Latini R, Maggioni AP et al. Effect of the ACE inhibitor lisinopril on mortality in diabetic patients with acute myocardial infarction: data from the GISSI-3 study. Circulation 1997; 96: 4239–45.

118. Lindholm LH, Ibsen H, Dahlof B et al. Cardiovascular morbidity and mortality in patients with diabetes in the Losartan Intervention For Endpoint reduction in hypertension study (LIFE): a randomised trial against atenolol. Lancet 2002; 359: 1004–10.

119. Estacio RO, Jeffers BW, Hiatt WR et al. The effect of nisoldipine as compared with enalapril on cardiovascular outcomes in patients with non-insulin-dependent diabetes and hypertension. N Engl J Med 1998; 338: 645–52.

120. Tatti P, Pahor M, Byington RP et al. Outcome results of the Fosinopril versus Amlodipine Cardiovascular Events Randomized Trial (FACET) in patients with hypertension and NIDDM. Diabetes Care 1998; 21: 597–603.

122. Mason RP, Mason PE. Calcium antagonists and cardiovascular risk in diabetes. A review of the evidence. Diabetes Care 1999; 22: 1206–8.

123. Verdecchia P, Schillaci G, Reboldi G et al. Calcium antagonists and cardiovascular risk in patients with hypertension and Type 2 diabetes mellitus: evidence from the PIUMA Study. Progetto Ipertensione Umbria Monitoraggio Ambulatoriale. Diabetes Nutr Metab 1999; 12: 292–9.

124. Tuomilehto J, Rastenyte D, Birkenhager WH et al. Effects of calcium-channel blockade in older patients with diabetes and systolic hypertension. Systolic Hypertension in Europe Trial Investigators. N Engl J Med 1999; 340: 677–84.

125. Lewis EJ, Hunsicker LG, Clarke WR et al. Renoprotective effect of the angiotensin-receptor antagonist irbesartan in patients with nephropathy due to Type 2 diabetes. N Engl J Med 2001; 345: 851–60.

126. Malmberg K, Ryden L, Hamsten A et al. Effects of insulin treatment on cause-specific one-year mortality and morbidity in diabetic patients with acute myocardial infarction. DIGAMI Study Group. Diabetes Insulin-Glucose in Acute Myocardial Infarction. Eur Heart J 1996; 17: 1337–44.

127. Malmberg K. Prospective randomised study of intensive insulin treatment on long term survival after acute myocardial infarction in patients with diabetes mellitus. DIGAMI (Diabetes Mellitus, Insulin Glucose Infusion in Acute Myocardial Infarction) Study Group. BMJ 1997; 314: 1512–15.

128. Eriksson KF, Lindgarde F. Prevention of Type 2 (non-insulin dependent) diabetes by diet and physical exercise: the 6-year Malmo Feasibility Study. Diabetologia 1991; 34: 891–8.

129. Kennedy JW, Hirshman MF, Gervino EV et al. Acute exercise induces GLUT4 translocation in skeletal muscle of normal human subjects and subjects with Type 2 diabetes. Diabetes 1999; 48: 1192–7.

130. Yale J-F. Prevention of Type 2 diabetes. Intl J Clin Pract 2001; 113; 35–9.

131. Antonucci T, Whitcomb R, Mclain R et al. Impaired glucose tolerance is normalized by treatment with the tghiazolinedione troglitazone. Diabetes Care 1997; 20: 185–93.

132. Barnett A. The thazolinedones: a new class of antidiabetic agents. Hosp Med 2000; 61: 185–8.

133. Nolan JJ, Jones NP, Partwardhan R, Deacon LF. Rosiglitazone taken once daily provides effective glycaemic control in patients with Type 2 diabetes mellitus. Diabet Med 2000; 17: 287–94.

134. Horton ES, Clinkingbeard C, Gatlin M et al. Nateglimide alone and in combination with metformin improves glycemic control by reducing mealtime glucose levels in Type 2 diabetes. Diabetes Care 2000; 23: 1660–5.

135. Chiassen SS et al. for the STOP–NIDDM Trial Research Group. Acarbose for prevention of type 2 diabetes mellitus: the STOP–NIDDM randomised trial. Lancet 2002; 359: 2072–7.

136. Barzilay JI, Jones CL, Davis BR et al. Baseline characteristics of the diabetic participants in the antihypertensive and lipid-lowering treatment to prevent heart attack trial (ALLHAT). ALLHAT Collaborative Research Group. Diabetes Care 2001; 24: 654–8.

9

Fight to prevent end-stage renal disease
Julia Lewis, Edmund J Lewis

It is projected that by the year 2025 there will be 300 million patients worldwide with Type 2 diabetes.[1] Without effective intervention, approximately 40% of these patients will develop renal disease. Currently, there are few therapeutic interventions of demonstrated benefit. These include glycemic control, control of hypertension, and the use of angiotensin II receptor blockers.

Glycemic control

The Diabetes Control and Complications Trial (DCCT) has shown a clear benefit of intensive glycemic control in preventing the development of microalbuminuria in patients with Type 1 diabetes.[2] Microalbuminuria serves as a marker for early diabetic nephropathy. Hence the DCCT results imply that the onset of the renal lesion of Type 1 diabetes can be significantly delayed and possibly prevented. Although intensive blood sugar control is of benefit in patients with Type 1 diabetes, the applicability of these findings in patients with Type 2 diabetes is unknown. Certainly, numerous cross-sectional studies and epidemiologic studies have demonstrated that poorer blood sugar control is associated with an increased incidence of diabetic nephropathy in patients with Type 2 diabetes.[3]

In a prospective trial, in 110 patients with Type 2 diabetes, Ohkubo demonstrated that patients randomized to a multiple insulin injection treatment (MIT) compared with a conventional insulin injection treatment (CIT) and followed every six months over a six-year period, had better blood sugar control and better renal outcomes.[4] However, the sample size in this study was small, and the applicability of these findings to non-Asian racial groups is unknown.

In the recently reported United Kingdom Prospective Diabetes Study (UKPDS), 3867 newly diagnosed patients with Type 2 diabetes were randomized to conventional diet therapy with a goal fasting blood glucose of <15.0 mmol/l or to intensive treatment with sulfonylureas or insulin and a goal fasting blood glucose <6.0 mmol/l.[5] Of the 1131 patients randomized to conventional diet treatment, 702 of these patients also received therapy with either sulfonylureas or insulin. The UKPDS had a complex design with many changes in the protocol over the 14 years patients were recruited into this study during the median follow-up of 11 years. There was an average median follow-up HbAlc of 7.0% in the intensive therapy group compared with 7.9% in the conventional group. The UKPDS was unable to demonstrate a benefit with intensive blood glucose control for any diabetes-related death or all-cause mortality or macrovascular outcomes. However, associated with this improvement in blood sugar control, the intensive treatment group did have a substantial 25% reduction in the risk of diabetic microvascular endpoints ($p = 0.0099$). The diabetic microvascular end points included renal outcomes. Most of the reported reduction was due to fewer patients requiring retinal photocoagulation. However, intensive blood sugar control led to a reduction in the risk for the development of albuminuria. The magnitude of this risk reduction and its statistical significance depended on the years of follow-up. After 9–15 years of follow-up, there was an approximately 30% risk reduction in albuminuria in the intensive blood sugar group. There was no significant benefit in patients with only six years of follow-up.

Similarly, with the renal outcomes of doubling in plasma creatinine and a doubling of plasma urea, biochemical markers which imply halving of the glomerular filtration rate, risk reductions and statistical significance varied with the years of follow-up. However, overall there appears to be a beneficial effect of intensive blood sugar control on these renal outcomes as well. It is important to note that in the UKPDS, plasma creatinine was measured at six months, one year, and annually thereafter, and urinary albumin was similarly measured only yearly. These infrequent measurements of renal outcomes decreased the sensitivity of the study to assess potential beneficial effects of treatment on renal outcomes.

The UKPDS study was a complex trial and was not primarily intended to examine renal outcomes. The patients enrolled in the UKPDS were patients with newly diagnosed diabetes and, even in the time course of this trial, it would have been anticipated that few patients would have had significant renal outcomes. It is important to note that the separation in HbAlc in the patients with Type 2 diabetes enrolled into the UKPDS study was only 0.9% as compared to 2% in patients enrolled in the Type 1 DCCT trial. This small separation in mean HbAlc in the UKPDS may have decreased the ability to assess the efficacy of more intensive blood sugar control on renal outcomes. Despite all these constraints, the UKPDS data supports a beneficial effect of intensive blood sugar control, primarily on reducing urinary albumin excretion, in patients with Type 2 diabetes.

In aggregate, looking at the epidemiologic, cross-sectional and prospective follow-up studies done in patients with Type 2 diabetes suggesting an association between blood sugar control and the development of poor renal outcomes, the strong data from the DCCT supporting the benefits of intensive blood sugar control in preventing renal outcomes in patients with Type 1 diabetes, and now the results of the UKPDS, one can recommend tight blood sugar control for the patient with Type 2 diabetes to help prevent the development and progression of diabetic nephropathy.

Blood pressure control

Many studies in patients with Type 1 diabetes have demonstrated the clear benefit of blood pressure control on the rate of progression of renal disease.[6,7,8] Early studies examining the rate of decline in renal function in patients before and after blood pressure control showed a marked decrease in the rate of decline in renal function after blood pressure control in individual patients. In a more recent study of 129 patients with Type 1 diabetes and diabetic nephropathy, patients were randomly assigned to a mean arterial blood pressure goal of <92 mmHg or to a mean arterial blood pressure goal of 100–107 mmHg. All patients received varying doses of ramipril as the primary therapeutic antihypertensive agent. All patients were followed for a minimum of two years. The patients randomized to the <92 mmHg mean arterial blood pressure goal had a significant decrease in their urinary total protein excretion compared with the 100–107 mmHg group (p = 0.02). In patients with Type 1 diabetes and diabetic nephropathy, the mean arterial blood pressure goal should be 92 mmHg or less for optimal renoprotection if renoprotection is defined as including decreased proteinuria.

Multiple epidemiologic and cross-sectional studies have demonstrated that small sustained increases in blood pressure increase the risk of kidney failure.[9] Patients with hypertension have 22 times the risk of end-stage renal disease as do patients with normal blood pressure.[10] In an analysis of multiple long-term (>3 yrs) follow-up studies in patients with Type 2 diabetes and diabetic nephropathy, it was demonstrated that patients who achieved lower blood pressures had a slower rate of decline in renal function.[11] The patients in these studies were not randomized to different blood pressure goals and these analyses were based on achieved blood pressures. However, the rate of decline in renal function appeared to be a continuous function of these achieved arterial blood pressure levels.

In the Aggressive Blood Pressure Control in Diabetes (ABCD) study, there were 480 normotensive patients with Type 2 diabetes who were randomized to moderate (diastolic 80–90 mmHg) versus intensive (diastolic decrease of 10 mmHg) blood pressure control. The patients in the moderate group received placebo whereas the patients in the intensive group were randomized to receive either nisoldipine or enalapril in a blinded manner. Mean blood pressure in the intensive group was 128/75 mmHg versus 137/81 mmHg in the moderate group (p = 0.0001). Over a five-year follow-up period, intensive blood pressure control slowed the progression to incipient and overt diabetic nephropathy. The progression

from normal albumin excretion to microalbuminuria was decreased (p = 0.012) as well as the progression from microalbuminuria to overt albuminuria (p = 0.028). There was however no statistically significant difference in alteration in renal function as measured by creatinine clearance between the groups. There was no difference in outcome between patients on enalapril versus nisoldipine.[12,13]

The recent UKPDS had embedded within it a study designed to determine whether tight blood pressure control reduced morbidity and mortality in hypertensive patients with Type 2 diabetes.[14] A total of 758 patients were allocated to tight blood pressure control with the goal of <150/85 mmHg, and 390 patients were allocated to less tight control of blood pressure aiming initially for a target of <200/105 mmHg, which was in the course of the study modified to a target of <180/105 mmHg. During the course of the study, the mean difference in systolic blood pressure was 10 mmHg and for diastolic blood pressure, 5 mmHg between the two groups. Reductions in risk in the group assigned to tighter control of blood pressure compared with that assigned to less tight control were 24% in diabetes-related end points, 32% in deaths related to diabetes, 44% in strokes and 37% in microvascular end points. Approximately 17% of patients at baseline had microalbuminuria (urinary albumin concentrations >50 mg/l) and 3.5% proteinuria (urinary albumin concentrations >300 mg/l). After six years of follow-up, there was a significant reduction in microalbuminuria in the tight blood pressure control group compared with the conventional treatment group (20.3% versus 28.5%, p <0.009). However, in the nine-year follow-up, this beneficial effect was not apparent, with the reduction in urinary albumin concentrations being 28.8% and 33.1% respectively in the tight and conventional blood pressure groups

F/U time	Microalbuminuria (%)		Risk reduction (%)	P value
	Tight	Less tight		
6 years	20.3	28.5	29	$p < 0.009$
9 years	28.8	33.3	13.5	$p = 0.33$

Table 9.1
UKPDS hypertension study renal outcomes[14]

Notes: Baseline microalbuminuria 17% ($n = 185$ patients)
Baseline proteinuria 3.5% ($n = 40$ patients)

($p = 0.33$). (Table 9.1). This discrepancy may be due to the smaller sample size in the nine-year follow-up group. There was no significant difference in plasma creatinine concentration or in the proportion of patients who had a two-fold increase in creatinine concentration between the two groups.

Overall, the evidence supports blood pressure control as an important intervention in slowing the progression of diabetic nephropathy in patients with Type 2 diabetes. The precise level of blood pressure control which would provide maximum benefit for the patient with Type 2 diabetic nephropathy has not been determined by clinical studies. Systolic hypertension can be extremely difficult to treat in this older population of patients who tend to have advanced vascular disease. Currently, there have been no reports of a 'J curve' phenomenon, indicating increased mortality and morbidity associated with more intense efforts at blood pressure lowering. However, orthostatic hypertension is a practical concern in this patient population which tends to have peripheral autonomic neuropathy. In light of current information, one can support the recommended goals of 135 mmHg systolic and 85 mmHg diastolic blood pressures. However, these recommendations must be individualized according to the medical condition of any given patient.

Agents that inhibit the renin–angiotensin system

As will be discussed below, in stark contrast to the strong evidence supporting the use of ACE-inhibitors to slow the progression of Type 1 diabetic nephropathy, there is a meager amount of data addressing the effect of these agents in Type 2 diabetes. However, three recent large clinical trials have concluded that angiotensin II receptor blockers prevent the progression of early (microalbuminuria) and late (proteinuria) diabetic nephropathy in patients with Type 2 diabetes. In the Irbesartan and Diabetic Nephropathy Trial (IDNT), 1715 hypertensive patients with Type 2 diabetes and ≥900 mg of urinary protein excretion were enrolled.[15] The baseline serum creatinine concentration was required to be between 1.0 and 3.0 mg/dl in women and 1.2 and 3.0 mg/dl in men. The patients were randomized to receive either irbesartan (300 mg daily), amlodipine (10 mg daily) or placebo. The target blood pressure was 135/85 mmHg or less in all groups. Other antihypertensives, excluding calcium channel blockers, angiotensin converting enzyme (ACE)-inhibitors or angiotensin II receptor blockers, were used to achieve these blood pressure goals. The primary outcome was time to a composite end point of doubling of the baseline serum creatinine concentration, the

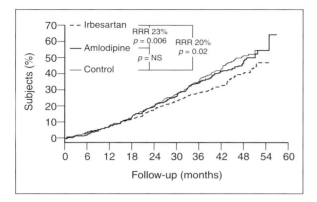

Figure 9.1
Kaplan-Meier curve of the percentage (doubling of serum creatinine, end-stage renal disease or death) in the irbesartan trial in patients with Type 2 diabetes and proteinuria and renal insufficiency (modified from ref. 15).

development of end-stage renal disease, or death from any cause. The mean duration of follow-up was 2.6 years. Treatment with irbesartan was associated with a risk of the primary composite end point, which was 20% lower than that in the placebo group ($p = 0.02$) and 23% lower than that in the amlodipine group ($p = 0.006$) (Figure 9.1). The risk of a doubling of the serum creatinine concentration was 33% lower in the irbesartan group than in the placebo group ($p = 0.003$) and 37% lower in the irbesartan group than the amlodipine group (p <0.001). Treatment with irbesartan was also associated with a relative risk of end-stage renal disease that was 23% lower than in both other groups ($p = 0.07$ for both comparisons). There was no difference in the rate of death from all causes. Proteinuria was reduced on average by 33% in the irbesartan group as compared with 6% in the amlodipine group and 10% in the placebo group. Thus the angiotensin II receptor blocker irbesartan was demonstrated to be renoprotective, that is it

was effective in protecting against the progression of nephropathy due to Type 2 diabetes and this protection was independent of the reduction in blood pressure.

In a second study, 1513 patients with Type 2 diabetes and ≥500 mg of urinary protein excretion were randomized to receive either losartan (50–100 mg once daily) or placebo. Treatment with losartan was associated with the risk reduction of the primary end point which was identical to the primary composite end point in the irbesartan trial. This was 16% lower than that in the placebo group ($p = 0.02$). The risk of doubling of serum creatinine concentration was 25% lower in the losartan group than in the placebo group ($p = 0.006$) and there was a risk reduction for end-stage renal disease of 28% ($p = 0.002$) (Table 9.2). There was no effect on the rate of death from all causes. The level of proteinuria declined by 35% with losartan compared with placebo (p <0.001).

In summary, these two studies in essentially identical patient populations and with similar clinical protocols, clearly demonstrate a beneficial effect of inhibition of the renal angiotensin system with angiotensin II receptor blockers on slowing the progression of renal disease in patients with Type 2 diabetes, proteinuria, and declining renal function (Table 9.2). In both studies, few adverse outcomes were noted in association with the use of angiotensin II receptor blockers. These significant improvements in renal outcomes were beyond what could be attributed to blood pressure control alone and demonstrate a specific beneficial effect of this class of agents preserving renal function in patients with Type 2 diabetes, proteinuria and declining renal function.

In the IDNT, one-third of the patients were randomized to receive the calcium channel blocker amlodipine. There was no demonstrated beneficial effect of amlodipine on renal outcomes. However, the patients randomized

Data	Irbesartan study	Losartan study
Sample size	1715	1513
Baseline age	59	60
Baseline median albuminuria	1.9 gm/day	1.25 gm/gmCr
Baseline serum creatinine	1.7 mg/dl	1.9 mg/dl
Risk reduction:		
composite outcome	20%	16%
Risk reduction:		
doubling of serum creatinine	26%	21%
Risk reduction:		
end-stage renal disease	23%	28%

Table 9.2
Angiotensin II receptor blockers in diabetic nephropathy

to amlodipine had outcomes similar to those patients randomized to placebo. All the patients in the trial were receiving additional antihypertensive agents (on average 2–3 other antihypertensives) in addition to the study drug. Hence amlodipine was observed to be an effective antihypertensive agent in this patient population. Despite earlier studies in small numbers of patients, which demonstrated amlodipine causing increased urinary protein excretion implying a potential danger to long-term renal outcomes, urinary protein excretion decreased in the IDNT patients randomized to amlodipine. This result could be due to improved overall blood pressure control in the IDNT. Thus, despite previous reports, this agent appears to be a safe antihypertensive agent in the Type 2 diabetic nephropathy population, although it is not, in itself, renoprotective.

In the losartan trial in diabetic nephropathy, patients were allowed to receive other antihypertensive agents, including a variety of calcium channel blockers, in addition to their randomized study drug.[16] There was no demonstrable detrimental effect on the beneficial effects of losartan due to the addition of a calcium channel blocker agent to the patients'

regimen. Data from these two studies, in combination, suggest that calcium channel blockers do not appear to be specifically beneficial to the kidney but not harmful either compared with other antihypertensive agents.

A second study was done using irbesartan to examine the potential benefits of angiotensin II receptor blockers in patients with Type 2 diabetes, microalbuminuria and well-preserved renal function. A total of 590 hypertensive patients with Type 2 diabetes and microalbuminuria were randomly assigned to irbesartan, either 150 mg daily or 300 mg daily or placebo.[17] The patients were followed for two years. The primary outcome was time to the onset of persistent proteinuria >200 mg/min or at least 30% higher than the baseline level. The relative risk reduction was 39% for irbesartan 150 mg versus the control group ($p = 0.08$) and 70% for irbesartan 300 mg versus the control group ($p < 0.001$) (Figure 9.2). A secondary end point in the irbesartan microalbuminuria trial was change in overnight urinary albumin excretion rate. Albumin excretion rate was reduced in the two irbesartan groups throughout the study (−24% and −38% in 24 months, compared with baseline in the irbesartan 150 mg and 300 mg groups, respectively).

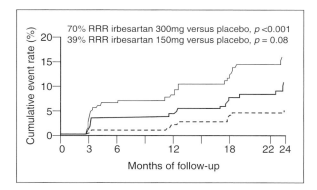

Figure 9.2
Incidence of progression to diabetic nephropathy in the irbesartan trial in patients with Type 2 diabetes and microalbuminuria.

Albumin excretion rate remained unchanged in the control group (−2% in 24 months compared with baseline). Creatinine clearance remained in the normal range in all three groups throughout the study as expected in these patients with early diabetic nephropathy manifested by microalbuminuria. Thus importantly, this study demonstrated that in both patients with established diabetic nephropathy with overt proteinuria and declining renal function and in patients with Type 2 diabetes and early nephropathy as manifested by microalbuminuria, inhibition of the renal angiotensin system with angiotensin II receptor blockers slows the progression of renal disease dramatically. These three studies clearly demonstrated that patients with Type 2 diabetes and nephropathy manifested by either microalbuminuria or proteinuria and declining renal function should be treated with angiotensin II receptor blockers as their 'kidney medicine', independent of their blood pressure.

An important question is whether or not ACE-inhibitors have a beneficial effect similar to angiotensin II receptor blockers in patients with Type 2 diabetes and diabetic nephropathy. The question of whether inhibition of the renal effects of angiotensin II by ACE inhibition and by angiotensin receptor blockade are clinically equivalent has practical ramifications. Clearly these are two distinct classes of drugs with known differences in pharmacologic effect. One of the best known examples of these differences is the ability of ACE-inhibitors to slow the enzymatic catabolism of bradykinin. Angiotensin receptor blockers (ARBs), on the other hand specifically block angiotensin II binding to Type 1 angiotensin receptors, but not Type 2, with the implication of possible beneficial effects of angiotensin II binding to the latter class of receptors. In a practical sense, based on the proven effectiveness of ACE-inhibitors in Type 1 diabetic nephropathy, many patients are receiving these agents. This therapeutic pattern has been reinforced by the HOPE study, which demonstrated improved cardiovascular outcomes in patients with Type 2 diabetes when treated with the ACE-inhibitor ramipril, and the micro HOPE report, which indicated that ramipril decreased protein excretion in patients with microalbuminuria. It is therefore not surprising that there is reticence on the part of some physicians to replace ACE-inhibitor therapy with angiotensin receptor blockers. It must be stated, however, that while the current evidence for the use of angiotensin receptor blockers in Type 2 diabetic nephropathy is robust, clear evidence for equivalent therapeutic effect of ACE inhibition in the patient population is correspondingly weak.

Australian investigators randomized 24 patients with Type 2 diabetes, hypertension and microalbuminuria to either the angiotensin converting enzyme inhibitor perindopril or the calcium channel blocker nifedipine.[18] Twelve months of treatment with either agent, significantly reduced urinary albumin excretion and preserved renal function, suggesting equivalent beneficial effects from blood pressure control with either ACE-inhibitors or calcium channel blockers. In the UKPDS, the group randomized to tight blood pressure control was also randomized to either receive atenolol, a beta-blocker or captopril, an ACE-inhibitor.[19] Blood pressure lowering with captopril or atenolol was similarly effective in reducing the incidence of diabetic complications, including renal complications, in this study.[19] These results contrast with the renoprotective effect of irbesartan and losartan when compared with standard antihypertensive therapy in the IDNT and RENAAL (Reduction in Endpoints in NIDDM with the AII Antagonist Losartan) trials.

In the GISEN (Gruppo Italiano di Studii Epidemiologici in Nefrologia) group study, 352 patients with proteinuria and chronic renal insufficiency were randomized to either ramipril or placebo.[20] This study demonstrated a dramatic beneficial effect of randomization to ramipril for the group as a whole. However, in the 27 patients with Type 2 diabetes and diabetic nephropathy in this trial, there was a statistically significant decrement in renal function in those patients randomized to ramipril when compared with patients in the control group. Clearly this is subgroup analysis in a small sample of patients.

In contrast to the above, the data in a multi-center, randomized study by Ravid and co-workers, 94 patients with Type 2 diabetes and microalbuminuria were randomized to the ACE-inhibitor enalapril 10 mg/day or placebo and followed for five years.[21] More patients in the placebo group received long acting nifedipine for blood pressure control compared with the enalapril group. Compared to placebo, enalapril decreased the number of patients who progressed from microalbuminuria to proteinuria. Renal function measured by reciprocal creatinine was also better preserved in patients receiving enalapril.

Thus, given the data regarding ACE-inhibitors as having a beneficial effect in patients with nephropathy secondary to Type 1 diabetes,[22] one might hypothesize that inhibition of the renin–angiotensin system with either ACE-inhibitors or angiotensin II receptor blockers would benefit patients with Type 1 or Type 2 diabetes and diabetic nephropathy. However, as noted above, the beneficial effects of ACE inhibition have not been established in patients with Type 2 diabetes and diabetic nephropathy. The beneficial effects of angiotensin II receptor antagonists in patients with Type 2 diabetes and nephropathy have been conclusively demonstrated in three large clinical trials.

Other therapeutic interventions

Dyslipidemia has been demonstrated to cause a more rapid loss of renal function in animal models of renal disease. Dyslipidemia is a strong risk factor for the development of diabetic nephropathy and for a more rapid progression to end-stage renal disease in large epidemiologic studies in humans with Type 2 diabetes.[23–25] In a small, randomized study in 34 patients with Type 2 diabetes, proteinuria and chronic renal insufficiency, the patients randomized to receive a cholesterol lowering agent (a statin) had a slower rate of decline in renal function compared with those randomized to receive placebo.[26] Although clearly the study has too small a sample size to draw firm conclusions about the beneficial effects of cholesterol lowering agents on renal function, it is certainly a hypothesis-generating study that suggests a larger clinical trial should be conducted.

The Modification of Diet in Renal Disease (MDRD) study which enrolled 840 patients with chronic renal insufficiency (only 26 patients with Type 2 diabetes) was unable to demonstrate a clear benefit of a low protein diet on the rate of progression of renal disease by its intention to treat design.[27] Two studies in patients with Type 2 diabetes, one conducted in Japan and the other in Canada, were able to demonstrate beneficial effects of low protein diets in patients with Type 2 diabetes and nephropathy. However, the number of patients receiving these diets was less than 30 in each study.[28,29] Thus low protein diets remain of unproven benefit in patients with Type 2 diabetes and diabetic nephropathy. Owing to the complexity of conducting trials in patients randomized to different diets, it is unlikely that this hypothesis will be further tested.

Multiple epidemiologic studies have shown a clear association between smoking and the development and progression of diabetic nephropathy.[30] For ethical reasons, there will never be a randomized trial to test this hypothesis. However, given the overall risks of smoking, it would be prudent to recommend to patients with Type 2 diabetes and diabetic nephropathy that quitting smoking may also benefit their kidneys.

Potential risks of therapy

The clear benefit of drugs which interrupt the renin–angiotensin–aldosterone system in Type 1 and Type 2 diabetic nephropathy must be measured in the context of potential risks to the patient. Certainly, and particularly in the Type 2 diabetes population, the effect of these agents on potassium metabolism deserves examination. While neither irbesartan nor losartan were associated with any apparent sudden deaths due to hyperkalemia, it must be emphasized that unsurprisingly, both of these agents were associated with significantly more hyperkalemia than occurred in the respective control groups in these studies. These findings

emphasize the need for careful monitoring of patients with Type 2 diabetes for evidence of elevation of the serum potassium. The use of furosemide, or other loop diuretic agents, in this patient population is valuable in order to increase renal potassium excretion. Neither the IDNT, not the RENAAL studies, encompassing a total of over 1250 patients receiving ARBs, observed the occurrence of acute renal failure associated with bilateral renal artery stenosis. While serious vascular disease would be anticipated in this patient population, the phenomenon of acute renal failure due to angiotensin II inhibition would appear to be rare. Nevertheless, monitoring of the serum creatinine during the initial weeks of ARB or ACE-inhibitor therapy would appear judicious.

Summary

The devastating complication of end-stage renal disease in patients with Type 2 diabetes and diabetic nephropathy can be delayed with blood sugar control, blood pressure control, and most importantly, the use of angiotensin II receptor blockers. Clearly, however, new avenues of intervention will have to be developed to halt the development or progression of this complication of Type 2 diabetes.

References

1. The World Health Report 1997: Concurring, suffering, enriching humanity. Geneva, Switzerland, 1997.
2. Diabetes Control and Complications Trial Research Group. Effect of intensive therapy on the development and progression of diabetic nephropathy in the Diabetes Control and Complications Trial. Kidney Int 1995; 47: 1703–20.
3. Gilbert RE, Tsalamadris C, Bach LA et al. Long-term glycemic control and the rate of

progression of early diabetic kidney disease. Kidney Int 1993; 44: 8585–859.

4. Ohkubo Y, Kishikawa H, Araki E et al. Intensive insulin therapy prevents the progression of diabetic microvascular complications in Japanese patients with non-insulin-dependent diabetes mellitus: a randomized prospective 6-year study. Diabetes Res Clin Pract 1995; 28: 103–17.

5. UK Prospective Diabetes Study (UKPDS) Group. Intensive blood-glucose control with sulphonylureas or insulin compared with conventional treatment and risk of complications in patients with Type 2 diabetes (UKPDS 33). Lancet 1998; 352: 837–53.

6. Mogensen CE. Long-term antihypertensive treatment inhibiting progression of diabetic nephropathy. BMJ 1982; 285: 685–8.

7. Parving HH, Andersen AR, Smidt UM et al. Effect of antihypertensive treatment on kidney function in diabetic nephropathy. BMJ 1987; 294: 1443–7.
Bjorck S, Nyberg G, Mulec H et al. Beneficial effects of angiotensin converting enzyme inhibition on renal function in patients with diabetic nephropathy. BMJ 1986; 293: 471–4.

8. Lewis JB, Berl T, Bain RP, Lewis EJ. Effect of intensive blood pressure control on the course of type I diabetic nephropathy. Am J Kidney Dis 1999; 34: 809–17.

9. Ritz E, Stefanski A. Diabetic nephropathy in type II diabetes. Am J Kidney Dis 1996; 27: 167–94.

10. Klag MJ, Whelton PK, Randall BL et al. Blood pressure and end-stage renal disease in men. N Engl J Med 1996; 334: 13–18.

11. Bakris GL. Progression of diabetic nephropathy. A focus on arterial pressure level and methods of reduction. Diabetes Res Clin Pract 1998; 39 Suppl: S35–S42.

12. Estacio RO, Jeffers BW, Gifford N, Schrier RW. Effect of blood pressure control on diabetic microvascular complications in patients with hypertension and Type 2 diabetes. Diabetes Care 2000; 23: B54–B64.

13. Schrier RW, Estacio RO, Esler A, Mehler P. Effects of aggressive blood pressure control in normotensive Type 2 diabetic patients on albuminuria, retinopathy and strokes. Kidney Int 2002; 61: 1086–97.

14. UK Prospective Diabetes Study Group. Tight blood pressure control and risk of macrovascular and microvascular complications in Type 2 diabetes: UKPDS 38. BMJ 1998; 517: 709–12.

15. Lewis EJ, Hunsicker LG, Clarke WR et al. Renoprotective effect of the angiotensin-receptor antagonist irbesartan in patients with nephropathy due to Type 2 diabetes. N Engl J Med 2001; 345: 851–60.

16. Brenner BM, Cooper ME, de Zeeuw D et al. Effects of losartan on renal and cardiovascular outcomes in patients with Type 2 diabetes and nephropathy. N Engl J Med 2001; 345: 861–9.

17. Parving HH, Lehnert H, Brochner-Mortensen J et al. The effect of irbesartan on the development of diabetic nephropathy in patients with Type 2 diabetes. N Engl J Med 2001; 345: 870–8.

18. Melbourne Diabetic Nephropathy Study Group. Comparison between perindopril and nifedipine in hypertensive and normotensive diabetic patients with microalbuminuria. BMJ 1991; 302: 210–16.

19. UK Prospective Diabetes Study Group. Efficacy of atenolol and captopril in reducing risk of macrovascular and microvascular complications in Type 2 diabetes: UKPDS 39. BMJ 1998; 317: 713–20.

20. The GISEN Group. Randomised placebo-controlled trial of effect of ramipril on decline in glomerular filtration rate and risk of terminal renal failure in proteinuric, non-diabetic nephropathy. Lancet 1997; 349: 1857–63.

21. Ravid M, Savin H, Jutrin I et al. Long-term stabilizing effect of angiotensin-converting enzyme inhibition on plasma creatinine and on proteinuria in normotensive type II diabetic patients. Ann Intern Med 1993; 118: 577–81.

22. Lewis EJ, Hunsicker LG, Bain RP, Rohde RD. The effects of angiotensin-converting-enzyme inhibition on diabetic nephropathy. N Engl J Med 1993; 329: 1456–62.

23. Nelson RG, Knowler WC, Pettitt DJ et al. Incidence and determinants of elevated urinary albumin excretion in Pima Indians with NIDDM. Diabetes Care 1995; 18: 182–7.

24. UK Prospective Diabetes Study Group. Urinary albumin excretion over 3 years in diet-treated Type 2 (non-insulin-dependent) diabetic patients, and association with hypertension,

hyperglycaemia and hypertriglyceridaemia. Diabetologia 1993; 36: 1021–9.

25. Fried LF, Orchard TJ, Kassiske BL. Effect of lipid reduction on the progression of renal disease: a meta analysis. Kidney Int 2001; 59: 260–9.

26. Lam KSL, Cheng IKP, Janus Ed, Pang RWC. Cholesterol-lowering therapy may retard the progression of diabetic nephropathy. Diabetologia 1995; 38: 604–9.

27. Klahr S, Levey AS, Beck GJ et al. The effects of dietary protein restriction and blood-pressure control on the progression of chronic renal disease. N Engl J Med 1994; 330: 877–84.

28. Pomerleau J, Verdy M, Garrel DR, Nadeau MH. Effect of protein intake on glycaemic control and renal function in Type 2 (non-insulin-dependent) diabetes mellitus. Diabetologia 1993; 36: 829–34.

29. Shichiri M, Nishio Y, Ogura M, Marumo F. Effect of protein, very-low-phosphorus diet on diabetic renal insufficiency with proteinuria. Am J Kidney Dis 1991; 18: 26–32.

30. Ritz E, Ogata H, Orth SR. Smoking: a factor promoting onset and progression of diabetic nephropathy. Diabetes Metab 2000; 26 Suppl 4: 54–63.

10

New modalities in diagnosis and prevention of vision loss in diabetic retinopathy: outlook for the future

Robert N Frank

Introduction

Despite the availability of effective treatments, and the widespread recognition of the importance of excellent blood glucose control, diabetic retinopathy remains an important cause of vision loss in the USA. This is almost certainly true in other Western countries, but because of the absence of adequate epidemiologic data, there is little knowledge of the impact of this disease on vision in populations elsewhere in the world. In a 1995 publication, Klein and Klein stated: 'Diabetes, particularly diabetic retinopathy, is the leading cause of new cases of blindness in people age 20–74 years in the United States. Approximately 8% of those who are legally blind are reported to have diabetes as the etiology, and it is estimated that more than 12% of new cases of blindness are attributable to diabetes. Twelve percent of insulin-dependent persons with diabetes for 30 or more years are blind. Persons who have diabetic retinopathy are 29 times more likely to be blind than nondiabetic persons.'[1] In an editorial written a few years earlier, Ferris[2] had presented a somewhat more optimistic picture. He pointed out that effective intervention by laser photocoagulation at a sufficiently early stage could reduce the incidence of severe vision loss (visual acuity less than 5/200 – equivalent to 6/240 or 0.025 on the metric or decimal scales) to less than 5%. However, these commendable results do not reflect the more somber facts that present-day laser and surgical interventions do not salvage vision in all diabetic patients, and that laser treatment for diabetic macular edema in particular can prevent or slow progression of vision loss from that disorder, but produces visual improvement of one line or better on the vision chart in only about 20% of treated patients.[3]

Approaches to prevention and treatment

Growth hormone antagonists

The first attempt to treat diabetic retinopathy derived from the observation, now nearly 50 years ago, of spontaneous regression of proliferative retinopathy in a young woman following hemorrhagic infarction of the pituitary as a consequence of pregnancy.[4] Ablation of the pituitary by surgery or radiation was therefore introduced as an effective treatment for proliferative diabetic retinopathy, and was moderately widely used.[5] Morbidity and mortality were high, however, and the procedure has fallen into disuse following the demonstration of the high efficacy of retinal laser photocoagulation. Since the realization that the efficacy of pituitary ablation probably results from the loss of growth hormone secretion and the resultant loss of stimulation of production of insulin-like growth factor-1 (IGF-1), which may itself promote retinal neovascularization,[6-8] or may be a required permissive factor that allows other growth factors to stimulate retinal new vessel growth,[9] there has been a renewal of interest in medical approaches to the inhibition of IGF-1 secretion or action. Recently, Grant et al.[10] reported that administration of maximally tolerated doses of octreotide, a somatostatin analog, to a small group of patients with severe non-proliferative or early proliferative diabetic retinopathy significantly reduced the risk of progression to proliferative disease by comparison with a group of control patients in a randomized, controlled clinical trial of 15 months' duration. In another study, a small group of patients with early proliferative retinopathy were treated with the growth hormone receptor blocker pegvisomant for three months.[11] In that trial, no regression of the retinopathy was seen. Differences in design between these two studies are, first, their duration; second, the end points (progression to 'high risk' proliferative retinopathy in the octreotide trial; photographic evidence of regression of retinopathy in the pegvisomant trial); and third, the relative efficacy of the drugs at the doses employed. In the octreotide trial, maximally tolerated doses of the drug were used and these reduced serum IGF-1 levels to 25% of baseline. In the pegvisomant trial, IGF-1 levels were reduced to 50% of baseline. In successful surgical or radiation-induced pituitary ablation, growth hormone (and, therefore, presumably IGF-1) levels were reduced to zero. Combination therapy with octreotide and pegvisomant together has never been attempted, to determine if there is an additive or even synergistic effect due to the different mechanisms of action of the two drugs. Such treatment might reduce IGF-1 levels to a much greater degree than one drug alone, with a resultant more efficacious reduction in proliferative retinopathy, and this regimen should also greatly decrease the risk of drug toxicity.

Photocoagulation

The current standard of care for treatment, both of proliferative diabetic retinopathy and of diabetic macular edema, is retinal laser photocoagulation. The initial photocoagulation instrument was the xenon arc, which produced an intense beam of white light.[12] The intent was to coagulate abnormal blood vessels by the heat produced by the xenon beam within the vascular lumina and in nearby pigmented tissues, such as the retinal pigment epithelium and choroid. This instrument required a fairly prolonged exposure (of the order of 1 sec) to produce a burn and, because it was composed of white light, could only produce a rather large focal point on the retina. Therefore, it was hazardous for treatment around the macula. Subsequent work by Aiello et al.,[13] based on observations that eyes with extensive retinal scarring from injuries or disease processes rarely developed severe diabetic retinopathy, indicated that 'pan-retinal' photocoagulation produced by placing many smaller burns around the mid-peripheral retina, avoiding the macula, can produce extensive iatrogenic scarring that has little effect on central vision. Such treatment will cause regression of new blood vessels in proliferative diabetic retinopathy, even when these vessels are not treated directly. In fact, the original protocol which these investigators used could not treat the new vessels directly because the instrument they employed was the ruby laser, which produces a red light beam that is transmitted through the blood column of the retinal vessels and cannot coagulate them. It is unclear why this procedure is effective, but the most widely cited current hypotheses are that retinal new vessels develop as a response to tissue hypoxia from the diabetic vascular disease, and such extensive laser treatment reduces retinal metabolism and therefore the stimulus to neovascularization. A second possibility is that the extensive laser treatment breaks down the blood–tissue barrier that exists in the retinal pigment epithelium between the choroidal capillaries and the neural retina, allowing for greater diffusion of oxygen and other nutrients to the retina.

The efficacy of pan-retinal photocoagulation for prevention of severe vision loss resulting from proliferative diabetic retinopathy was demonstrated in the Diabetic Retinopathy Study (DRS), a large randomized, controlled clinical trial conducted in the USA beginning in 1972.[14,15] Progression from good vision (≥20/100, equivalent to 6/30 or 0.2) to severe vision loss was reduced by approximately 50% by such treatment over a five-year follow-up, by comparison with fellow eyes that were not laser treated. In the DRS, treatment was applied either with the xenon arc photocoagulator or with the newer, argon laser which produces blue–green and green wavelengths that can be focused to as small as 50 μm on the retina (the usual burn size for pan-retinal treatment is 500 μm) and can produce a substantial burn in 0.05–0.1 sec. Pan-retinal laser photocoagulation is usually done with a total of approximately 1500–2000 laser burns placed in a closely packed pattern throughout the mid-peripheral retina, sparing the macula (Figure 10.1a), although if this does not produce regression of the proliferative retinopathy (Figure 10.1b,c), additional laser treatment may be applied.

Laser photocoagulation is also effective for treatment of diabetic macular edema, that is, swelling of the central retinal tissues due to leakage from the blood vessels in the macular region. When this involves the fovea at the center of the macula, visual acuity may be substantially reduced. The Early Treatment Diabetic Retinopathy Study (ETDRS) was a randomized, controlled clinical trial that took place between 1980–91 and evaluated the efficacy of several different protocols for applying argon laser treatment to the macula and/or mid-peripheral retina for diabetic macular edema and for 'pre-proliferative' retinopathy; that is, moderately severe to severe retinopathy that had not progressed to the stage of actual new blood vessel formation. In treating diabetic macular edema, focal laser treatment, using spot sizes of 50–100 μm, is applied to areas of vascular leakage which are usually identified by intravenous fluorescein angiography. Alternatively, for macular edema with 'diffuse' fluorescein leakage and no focal areas of vascular abnormality, 'grid' laser can be placed surrounding the center of the macula with several rows of 50–100 μm burns in a staggered pattern, leaving a space at least equal to one burn diameter between each laser application (Figure 10.2a–d). The ETDRS found that, for edema that involves the center of the macula or that threatens the center (at least part of which is located within 500 μm, or approximately one-half optic disc diameter or the center) – so-called 'clinically significant' macular edema – focal or grid laser treatment can produce regression of the macular edema and prevent progression of visual loss, defined here as a doubling of the visual angle (worsening, say, from 20/20 to 20/40, or 20/50 to 20/100 acuity) by about 50% over a five-year follow-up by comparison with untreated eyes.[3,16] Although focal treatment for diabetic macular edema can prevent vision loss, it only infrequently results in improved vision: only 20% of eyes receiving focal treatment in the ETDRS improved their visual acuity by as little

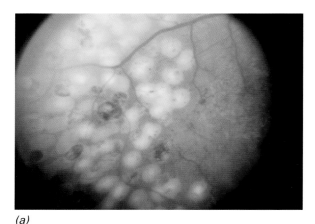

(a)

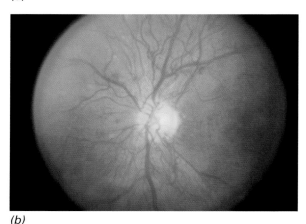

(b)

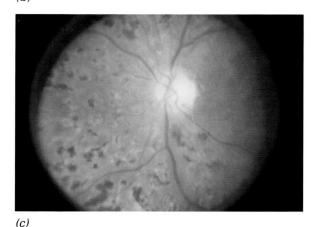

(c)

Figure 10.1

Pan-retinal photocoagulation for proliferative diabetic retinopathy. (a) View just temporal to the right macula of a patient immediately following laser treatment. The multiple round, white marks are the acute laser burns with surrounding retinal edema. This photograph shows the spacing of the treatment burns, which typically have a diameter of 500 μm (slightly less than one-half the diameter of the optic nerve head). The untreated area to the right is the temporal portion of the macula, showing blot hemorrhages and some fine, tortuous vascular abnormalities. The pigmented spots are old laser treatment marks. (b) Photograph of the left optic nerve head and surrounding retina of a 32-year-old woman with a 15-year history of Type 1 diabetes. An extensive frond of new vessels surrounds the optic nerve head, constituting a 'high risk' finding for progression to severe vision loss in three to five years, according to the Diabetic Retinopathy Study (DRS) criteria; (c) The same patient as in (b), six months after she had received pan-retinal laser treatment. Note the extensive pigmented laser scars. The new vessels have regressed completely and the retinal veins are markedly reduced in caliber. A slightly curved, white fibrous band representing the fibrous tissue that surrounded the now regressed new vessels extends superiorly and inferiorly at the temporal (left) margin of the optic nerve head. Since every individual has a unique retinal vascular pattern, one can determine that (b) and (c) are of the same person because, except for the reduction in caliber of the veins and the absence of new vessels in (c), the vascular pattern in the two photographs is constant.

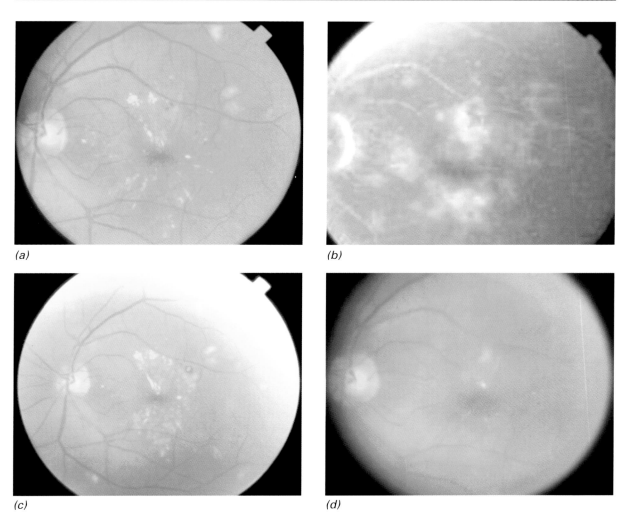

(a)

(b)

(c)

(d)

Figure 10.2
Diabetic macular edema. Vision in the left eye of this 62-year-old man with a 15-year history of Type 2 diabetes was 20/200; (a) Pre-treatment color photograph. Multiple 'hard' lipid exudates and a few blot hemorrhages surround the center of the macula (dark area at the center of the photograph). At the upper left, a few 'cotton wool spots' can also be seen. By stereo ophthalmoscopic viewing or optical coherence tomography (see Figure 10.5), the macular retina demonstrates considerable thickening; (b) Late arteriovenous phase photograph during a fluorescein angiographic sequence, showing diffuse fluorescein dye leakage from abnormal vessels in the left macula. The areas of dye leakage can be used as a guide for the placement of laser treatment; (c) Color photograph of the left macular region immediately following laser treatment. The laser burns (white spots) generally cover the pattern of abnormal dye leakage. Because the leakage was relatively diffuse, the laser burns are placed more in a 'grid' than in a 'focal' pattern; (d) Color photograph of the same eye nine months following laser treatment. Note the substantial regression of the lipid deposits and other lesions. The laser burns are scarcely visible. The retinal thickening had largely disappeared. However, the patient's vision had not improved. This is a typical result following laser treatment for diabetic macular edema, which generally stops or slows central vision loss but produces an improvement of vision in only about 20% of eyes according to ETDRS results.

as one line on the vision chart.[3] Treatment of eyes with macular edema using pan-retinal photocoagulation initially, however, may be harmful, leading to an initial reduction of visual acuity and no reduction in the macular edema.[16] Therefore, eyes with macular edema that require pan-retinal treatment for proliferative retinopathy should receive the focal laser treatment first with a delay of four to six weeks before applying the pan-retinal photocoagulation, unless the appearance of the proliferative retinopathy is extremely threatening.

Vitrectomy

For many years, surgical entry into the vitreous cavity of the eye was considered extremely hazardous. The pioneering work of Machemer,[17] using specialized instruments designed for the purpose, demonstrated that surgical manipulations within the vitreous cavity could be carried out safely. Initially, the procedure was performed for the removal of non-clearing vitreous hemorrhages due to proliferative diabetic retinopathy and other retinal vascular diseases, but it was later extended to the removal of proliferative membranes and the repair of complex, tractional retinal detachments due to diabetic retinopathy.[18] Vitrectomy surgery has been used for diseases other than diabetic retinopathy including the removal of intraocular foreign bodies, the diagnosis and treatment of severe intraocular infections, and the repair of retinal 'giant tears', to name a few. However, the major disease entity for which vitrectomy techniques are used is diabetic retinopathy. A clinical trial, the Diabetic Retinopathy Vitrectomy Study (DRVS) sponsored, as were the earlier DRS and ETDRS, by the US National Eye Institute, demonstrated the efficacy of early vitrectomy for salvaging vision after vitreous hemorrhages caused by proliferative diabetic retinopathy,[19]

and for protecting central vision when threatened by fibrous traction membranes.[20]

Medical therapies

Glycemic control

The most obvious, and over the years since the discovery of insulin, most highly debated, strategy for preventing retinopathy and other complications of diabetes, is to attempt to control blood glucose levels in diabetic patients as closely as possible within the physiological range. Two very large and rigorous randomized, controlled clinical trials, the Diabetes Control and Complications Trial (DCCT) in the United States and Canada[21] and the United Kingdom Prospective Diabetes Study (UKPDS) in the United Kingdom,[22] unequivocally demonstrated for Type 1 and Type 2 diabetes, respectively, that 'tight' blood glucose control significantly reduces the incidence and progression of diabetic retinopathy and other microvascular complications of diabetes. Additionally, the UKPDS demonstrated, at least for Type 2 diabetes, that better control of blood pressure also reduced the incidence and severity of diabetic retinopathy, regardless of whether the initial antihypertensive agent used was a beta-blocker or an angiotensin convertase (ACE) inhibitor.[23] This is of importance because a number of retrospective analyses over the years suggested that blood pressure control was of value for the prevention of diabetic retinopathy, and one recent controlled clinical trial suggested that ACE-inhibitors were effective in this regard.[24]

The DCCT and its follow-up, the Epidemiology of Diabetes Interventions and Complications study (EDIC)[25] had several other interesting findings. The DCCT had divided its subjects, all of whom had Type 1 diabetes, into a 'primary prevention' group which had no photographic evidence of retinopathy at the beginning of the study, and a 'secondary intervention' group which had evidence of mild to moderate non-proliferative retinopathy at the outset. In each group, individuals who were randomized to 'tight' blood glucose control had better retinopathy outcomes at the end of the trial, but also in each group, individuals on 'tight' control showed no improvement over the 'standard' control subjects for approximately two and a half years into the study. Additionally, in the 'secondary intervention' group, approximately 5–10% of the individuals placed on 'tight' control showed a transient worsening of their retinopathy by comparison with individuals on 'standard' control over this initial two and a half-year period.[21] Although a cause for this 'early worsening' has not been found definitively, it has been the subject of considerable discussion and speculation.[6,25,26]

A second interesting finding is that, four years after the conclusion of the DCCT, blood glucose control had improved substantially in the previous 'standard control' group, from an average glycated hemoglobin level of 9.1% to a subsequent level of 8.2%, while blood glucose control in the 'tight control' group had worsened from an average of 7.2% to 7.9%, that is, nearly equal to that of the 'standard control' group. Nevertheless, individuals in the 'tight control' group continued to show markedly diminished retinopathy development and progression by comparison with those in the original 'standard control' group.[27] This prolongation of the effects of initial good (or poor) blood glucose control is analogous to results reported earlier in dogs with initial poorly controlled diabetes[28] or with diet-induced galactosemia,[29] which produces a retinopathy virtually identical to that of diabetes in these animals. After two and a half years of poorly controlled diabetes or galactosemia, one eye of each animal was removed and showed no histologic evidence of retinopathy. The diabetic animals were then tightly controlled with insulin, and the galactosemic animals were returned to a normal diet. The animals were killed two and a half years later and, despite their return to normoglycemia, substantial retinopathy had developed in both the insulin-treated diabetic and the previously galactosemic dogs. These results from long-term studies in both humans and animals clearly indicate that the level of glycemic control produces 'a phenomenon with a memory', as Lorenzi and her colleagues once termed a biochemical phenomenon they had observed in cultured cells that was prolonged after exposure to high glucose.[30] The biochemical mechanism by which this 'memory' is exerted, however, has not been established, but it seems likely to play a major role in the pathogenesis of diabetic retinopathy and, perhaps, other complications of diabetes.

Finally, although the DCCT clearly established the importance of 'tight' glycemic control for the prevention of diabetic retinopathy, the study also showed that severe retinopathy did tend to cluster in certain multiplex families with diabetes.[31] This suggests that there are genetic determinants of severe retinopathy that are especially susceptible to hyperglycemia.

Aspirin, aldose reductase inhibitors

Aspirin (625 mg/day) was tested in the ETDRS under the hypothesis that its inhibition of platelet aggregation might improve perfusion in small blood vessels and, hence, prevent the development of retinopathy. This therapy was unsuccessful,[32] although the anticoagulant effect of aspirin also did not increase the incidence of vitreous hemorrhages, indicating that, for diabetic patients with retinopathy who require aspirin for other medical reasons, their retinopathy is not a contraindication. More recently, based on experiments with diabetic dogs, Kern[33] has suggested that aspirin therapy initiated at the time of first diagnosis of diabetes, rather than when moderate retinopathy is present as in the ETDRS, might be beneficial. While a clinical trial of this hypothesis might be of value, it would be extremely prolonged and expensive, and seems unlikely of accomplishment at this time.

The 'sorbitol pathway', consisting of the enzymes aldose reductase and sorbitol dehydrogenase, has been an important hypothesis for the pathogenesis of complications of diabetes, and in particular retinopathy, since the work of Pirie and van Heyningen in the late 1950s and then of Kinoshita and colleagues beginning in the following decade.[34] This hypothesis suggested that sorbitol, the sugar alcohol of glucose, accumulates in susceptible cells in diabetes as a result of the action of aldose reductase, producing damaging effects. Several variations on this hypothesis have also been proposed, involving a role of myo-inositol,[35] and the production of a 'pseudohypoxia' by accumulation of NADPH through excessive sorbitol pathway activity.[36] The ability of aldose reductase inhibitors (ARIs) to prevent retinopathy in diabetic, or galactosemic, experimental animals has been controversial.[37-40] (The aldohexose galactose is an even better substrate for aldose reductase than is glucose, and its sugar alcohol is not oxidized to the corresponding keto-sugar by sorbitol dehydrogenase. Animals fed high galactose diets are easier to maintain for long durations than are insulin-requiring diabetic animals and they develop a diabetic-like retinopathy.[37-41] Hence, experimental galactosemia is considered an excellent experimental system for studying this presumed pathogenetic mechanism for diabetic retinopathy.) However, two clinical trials of ARIs in humans with diabetic retinopathy have been unsuccessful (see ref. 42 for the trial of Pfizer's Sorbinil; results of Wyeth-Ayerst's trial of Tolrestat are unpublished). A recent study in short-term diabetic or galactosemic rats, using a new magnetic resonance imaging method for evaluating retinal oxygenation, showed that a powerful, new ARI (WAY-509 or minalrestat, Wyeth-Ayerst) prevents the oxygenation defect in the retinas of these animals.[43] This is consistent with our own finding that this agent prevents retinopathy in long-term galactosemic rats,[38] and suggests that WAY-509 might be of value for a clinical trial in humans since its ability to cross the blood–retinal barrier and to inhibit aldose reductase is superior to previous agents that have been clinically tested without success.

Aminoguanidine and non-enzymatic glycation

Non-enzymatic glycation of proteins with the subsequent formation of crosslinked, 'advanced glycation end products' (AGE proteins) was proposed some years ago as a possible pathogenetic mechanism for the complications of diabetes, including retinopathy.[44] Subsequently, these authors suggested that aminoguanidine could act as a therapeutic agent to prevent the formation of AGEs.[45] A clinical trial of aminoguanidine for diabetic nephropathy was negative (unpublished), and this agent will likely not be tested for its effects on retinopathy. We reported that aminoguanidine had no effect in preventing retinopathy in galactosemic rats.[38] Kern and Engerman confirmed this observation in galactosemic dogs, but also found that aminoguanidine did prevent retinopathy in diabetic animals.[33]

Antioxidants

Antioxidant therapy has been proposed for the treatment of a large variety of conditions, including cancer, atherosclerosis, diabetes and the complications thereof, and aging.[46-49] It is possible that at least some of the agents described above, including ARIs and amino-guanidine, might also act as antioxidants. Vitamin E, a well known antioxidant (but which can also act as a protein kinase C inhibitor), has been reported to improve the decreased blood flow seen in the retinal circulation of diabetic animals.[50] Other studies have demonstrated that different antioxidants can improve various metabolic abnormalities in the retina of diabetic animals, and in cultured retinal cells maintained in high glucose media.[51,52] Kowluru et al.[51] also reported that antioxidant therapy could prevent some of the morphologic lesions of retinopathy in diabetic or galactosemic rats.

Antivascular endothelial growth factor (anti-VEGF) therapies

Vascular endothelial growth factor (VEGF) a polypeptide that exists in several forms produced by alternative splicing of a single gene, produces both vascular endothelial cell proliferation which presumably leads to diabetic retinal neovascularization,[53] and increased vascular permeability, which may result in diabetic macular edema.[54] It appears to be upregulated as a result of hypoxia[55,56] (which is known to occur in the retina in diabetes), and it is upregulated in the retina of diabetic patients before retinopathy can be demonstrated histologically.[57,58] VEGF has recently been the focus of very intense interest with regard to the understanding of the pathogenesis of diabetic retinopathy and the development of new therapies. Such therapeutic approaches, which thus far have been applied only in experimental models of proliferative retinopathy in non-diabetic animals, include the intraocular (into the vitreous cavity) injection of anti-VEGF antibodies,[59] the injection of chimeric molecules in which a portion of a VEGF receptor was conjugated to a portion of an immunoglobulin molecule,[60] and the

intravitreal injection of 'anti-sense' strands of VEGF cDNA.[61] Such therapies have not yet been attempted in humans with diabetic retinopathy, although consideration is being given to similar approaches.

Pigment epithelium-derived factor (PEDF)

Although it is produced in many tissues, this molecule is especially prominent in the retinal pigment epithelium (RPE), where preliminary evidence suggests that it is secreted from the apical plasma membrane of these cells.[62] PEDF was initially recognized as a factor that enhanced the differentiation of neurons,[63] but recent data indicate that it markedly suppresses neovascularization.[64-66] These facts probably account for the normal absence of blood vessels in the outer layers of the vertebrate retina, and the fact that retinal neovascularization is nearly always directed toward the vitreous. There is some data to suggest that, in the RPE of diabetic subjects, PEDF secretion is diminished, which, together with the upregulation of VEGF, may enhance the tendency to develop new vessels.[67,68] Enhancing PEDF production in order to suppress neovascularization and also, perhaps, to maintain or enhance the differentiation of retinal neurons, would therefore appear to be of benefit in the prevention and treatment of diabetic retinopathy and other retinal and choroidal vascular diseases.

Protein kinase C (PKC) inhibitors

The protein kinases are a very large family of phosphorylating enzymes. The PKCs are a branch of this family that utilize specific co-factors and are important in activating specific enzymes and membrane receptors. PKCs are upregulated by diacylglycerol (DAG), whose concentration is increased by the hyperglycemia of diabetes.[69] There is evidence that PKC activity upregulates VEGF production.[70]

In turn, VEGF interaction with its cell membrane receptors increases intracellular PKC activity, which then appears to stimulate intracellular processes in vascular endothelial cells, leading to blood–retinal barrier breakdown and endothelial cell proliferation.[71] Because the members of the PKC family are so ubiquitous, generalized PKC inhibition might be harmful. However, because the β isoform of PKC is prominent in the retina, specific PKCβ inhibition would appear to be a safe approach to prevention and therapy of diabetic retinopathy. In animal models, there is some evidence that PKCβ inhibition prevents pathologic retinal neovascularization,[72] and can prevent retinal vascular leakage in experimental diabetes.[73] Clinical trials of an orally administered PKCβ inhibitor in human subjects with diabetic retinopathy are now in progress.

Diagnostic approaches

Fluorescein and indocyanine green angiography

Two types of fluorescent dyes, which are easily administered intravenously, have been in use for several years for the better evaluation of pathophysiological processes in retinal and choroidal vascular diseases. Of these, sodium fluorescein has been in longest use (since the 1960s) and has the most value for diabetic retinopathy (Figures 10.2b and 10.3). Fluorescein is a small molecule (MW 327 daltons) that is loosely (ca. 67%) bound to plasma proteins. It readily leaks through breaks in the blood–retinal barrier. Fluorescein is excited by blue light and fluoresces in green wavelengths, and filter pairs have been developed for its use in film or, increasingly, digital angiography. Because of the heightened contrast in black and white images, fluorescein angiography reveals microaneurysms more

prominently than does ophthalmoscopy or color photography (Figure 10.3b). It also demonstrates blood–retinal barrier breakdown in, and even prior to, the development of macular edema, as well as retinal neovascularization (which, however, is usually easy to see by ophthalmoscopy or color photography) and areas of capillary non-perfusion which indicate areas of ischemia and presumed hypoxia which are considered to be major factors in the pathogenesis of retinal neovascularization (Figure 10.3c).

Indocyanine green angiography (ICGA) uses a dye that is excited by, and fluoresces in, the near-infrared range. For this reason, indocyanine green fluorescence in the choroidal circulation is readily visible through the melanin pigment of the RPE and choroid, which blocks the visible wavelengths of fluorescein fluorescence. Choroidal vascular abnormalities are therefore more readily seen with ICGA than with fluorescein angiography. However, although some investigators have described a choroidal angiopathy in diabetic human eyes,[74] this has not yet been widely studied or considered of major clinical or pathogenetic importance in clinical or experimental diabetic retinopathy.

Ocular ultrasound

Ultrasonic visualization of structures in the posterior ocular globe or in the orbit is important when they cannot be seen by the unaided eye, by ophthalmoscopy, or by diagnostic techniques that use wavelengths in the visible spectrum. Ocular ultrasound using so-called B-scan methodology is therefore of use in diabetes as a way of visualizing, for example, tractional retinal detachments resulting from advanced proliferative retinopathy when the ophthalmoscopic view of the retina is obscured by dense vitreous hemorrhage, cataract, or corneal opacity (Figure 10.4).

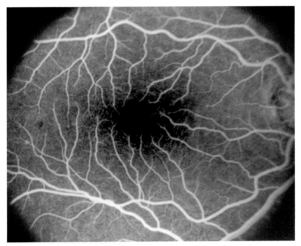

(a)

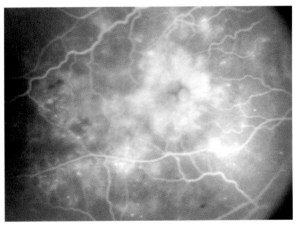

(b)

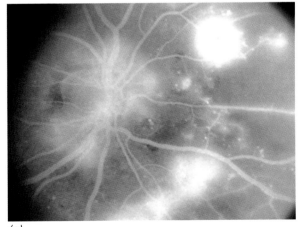

(c)

Figure 10.3

Fluorescein angiography. (a) Mid-arteriovenous phase photograph of the right macular region of a normal 25-year-old man. A portion of the optic nerve head is seen at 3 o'clock at the right border of the photograph. The central, round, completely dark area is the 'foveal avascular zone', since the foveal retina consists of the photoreceptor layer only with the inner layers of the retina swept to the side. There are normally no blood vessels in the outermost retinal layers. Surrounding the fovea one can see blood vessels of all sizes, including even the fine capillaries that are well demonstrated in angiographic studies of individuals with clear ocular media. Larger vessels are clearly seen. Note, in particular, the large venule stretching from the 4 o'clock to the 5 o'clock meridian at the lower right of the frame. This vessel demonstrates 'laminar flow', typical of the retinal venous system. There is a dark central stripe (the column of blood cells) and two flanking fluorescent columns, representing the surrounding plasma. (b) A late phase angiographic frame of the right macular region of a 54-year-old woman with a 10-year history of Type 2 diabetes. There is diffuse dye leakage surrounding the center of the macula. Directly in the center are three round, fluorescent 'blebs' divided by a dark Y-shaped figure. These represent cyst-like spaces between the axons of Henle's fiber layer in the fovea. This pattern is, therefore, called 'cystoid macular edema' or 'CME'. Multiple white dots at the outermost parts of the pattern represent microaneurysms. (c) Late phase angiographic view of the optic nerve head and region nasal to it in the right eye of a 45-year-old man with a 15-year history of Type 2 diabetes. Note the diffuse dye leakage from the optic nerve head and the multiple areas of very intense, diffuse leakage to the right of and below the optic nerve head. These represent new vessel formation (neovascularization) on, and partially surrounding, the optic nerve head. To the right of the neovascular formations, note that the angiographic pattern looks empty, with no small vessels apparent between the large arterioles and venules. This demonstrates the 'capillary non-perfusion' that frequently occurs in diabetic retinopathy. When the capillaries no longer function, the inner layers of the retina (which are supplied by the retinal circulation) become relatively hypoxic. Retinal hypoxia is thought to be a major stimulus to neovascularization, as demonstrated here by the fact that the new vessels are arising directly at the edge of the hypoxic zones of the retina.

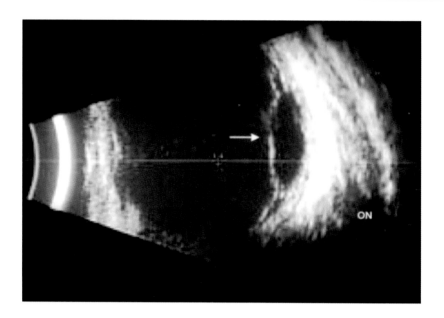

Figure 10.4
B-scan ultrasound image of the left eye of a patient with diabetic retinopathy in whom ocular media opacities prevented visualization of the retina by ophthalmoscopy. A traction detachment of the posterior retina is visible (white arrow). The optic nerve (ON) is visible as a dark shadow indenting the scleral outline.

Electroretinography

The electroretinogram (ERG) is a mass potential recorded from retinal neurons. The amplitudes and latencies of its component parts are indications of the relative health of various populations of retinal neurons and glial cells. Extensive destruction of retinal neurons, for example by pan-retinal laser photocoagulation, reduces the amplitudes of the ERG potentials.[75] There has been a great deal of study of the so-called 'oscillatory potentials' on the b-wave of the ERG.[76] Reduction in these potentials, in diabetic patients with little or no demonstrable retinopathy, has been claimed to be an adverse prognostic sign. In most clinical practices at present, however, this test is rarely used.

Optical coherence tomography (OCT)

OCT is a non-invasive technique that uses a pair of relatively low intensity helium-neon laser beams that are focused on the posterior retina. The coherence of their reflected beams from retinal and choroidal structures is measured by a Michelson interferometer and produces a series of anatomical cross-sections of the retina and choroid.[77] These images can be used to interpret anatomic abnormalities of the retina, and can also be used to make quantitative measurements of retinal thickness, with much greater accuracy than can be estimated visually using stereoscopic ophthalmoscopy or by stereoscopic retinal photography (Figure 10.5). OCT can be used to demonstrate diabetic macular edema and to follow its progression or regression over time following therapeutic procedures, such as laser photocoagulation.[78] This technique, which is now commercially available, is of great value for the demonstration of diabetic macular edema and other abnormalities of the central retina, and also should be useful in clinical trials of agents designed for the treatment of macular edema. An advanced OCT procedure using a different laser and electronics has recently been described.[79] This procedure gives retinal cross-sectional images that reproduce

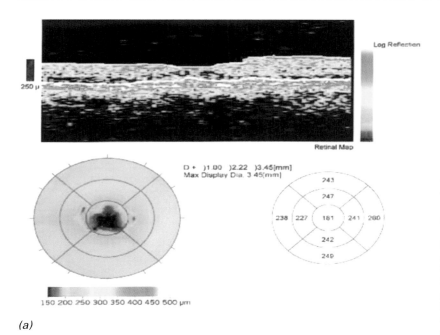

(a)

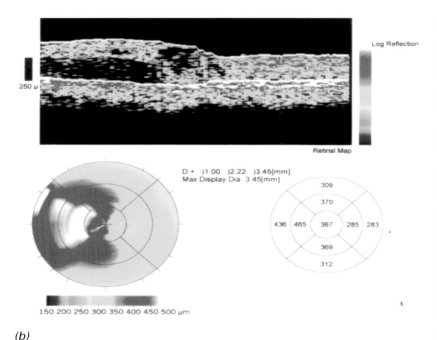

(b)

Figure 10.5

Optical coherence tomography (OCT). (a) OCT images of the macula of the normal eye of a 58-year-old, non-diabetic man. Visual acuity was 20/20 (6/6, or 1.0). A single OCT scan through the fovea is shown at the top. Note the depression, representing the foveal pit. The vitreous is dark and there are various colors representing the degree of reflectance (see color scale at the right of the figure). The roughly horizontal white line between the retina and vitreous is arbitrarily drawn by the software to represent the retina–vitreous junction, as is the white line that represents the junction between the retinal pigment epithelium/choroid and the neural retina. The software calculates retinal thickness, in microns, by calculating the vertical distance between these two lines at various points. The round color map at the lower left illustrates the thickness of the macular retina using the color scale beneath the map. The numerical map to the right of the color map gives the mean thickness, in microns, of the enclosed areas. (b) OCT scan of the left macula of a 64-year-old diabetic woman with 'clinically significant' diabetic macular edema, according to the definitions of the Early Treatment Diabetic Retinopathy Study (i.e. retinal thickening less than 500 μm of the center of the macula). In the cross-sectional view at the top, note the fluid-filled spaces indicating intraretinal edema. The foveal depression is absent. Both the color map and the thickness map demonstrate the considerable increase in retinal thickness compared to the normal image in (a) above. (The OCT scans were performed by Mauricio Pons, MD.)

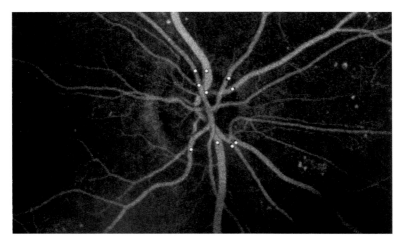

Figure 10.6

Retinal blood flow measurements in the eye of a normal human subject by videoangiography using a scanning laser ophthalmoscope. This is a single frame image of the optic nerve and radiating retinal arteries and veins following injection of fluorescein dye. The white dots indicate measurement sites, arbitrarily selected. Using sequential images, the change with time of the fluorescence intensity at these sites is measured. (Image courtesy of Mauricio Pons, MD.)

the anatomy of the retina with astonishing fidelity, resembling '*in vivo* biopsies'. Its potential ability to advance retinal diagnosis and the cellular anatomy of diabetic retinopathy and other retinal diseases, once the equipment becomes commercially available, is most exciting. A similar method, called the 'Retinal Thickness Analyzer' (RTA) has also been described.[80] It does not have the capability of giving 'maps' of retinal thickness across the macular region.

Retinal blood flow measurements: laser Doppler and scanning laser ophthalmoscopy

Several methods have been described for measuring retinal blood flow. There have been claims that retinal blood flow is accelerated in early diabetes,[81] and that it is diminished.[82] The laser Doppler technique measures the velocity of columns of red blood cells moving through a major retinal arteriole or venule at right angles to the laser beam.[83] Disadvantages of the method are, first, that it cannot be used to measure blood velocity through very small vessels, such as capillaries, and second, that it

can only measure the velocity through a single vessel at a time.

Fluorescein videoangiography measures the advancement of a fluorescein column through the retinal vessels using a real time digital videoangiogram. Digital subtraction of the dye front (or any other part of the dye column of an arbitrary fluorescence intensity) in sequential images allows one to measure the speed of the fluorescein dye in any vessel one chooses in an angiographic sequence (Figures 10.6 and 10.7). With adequate resolution and magnification, for example, in younger subjects with clear ocular media, one should even be able to measure flow through capillaries, though in practice this is difficult with most subjects. This method has been used in diabetic rats[82] and in human diabetic subjects,[84] and has been reported to show that treatment with a PKCβ inhibitor normalizes the reduced blood flow caused by diabetes. A disadvantage of the technique, however, is that it measures flow of the plasma column (in which the fluorescein dye is located) rather than of the cells, and thus may not accurately measure true blood flow, or

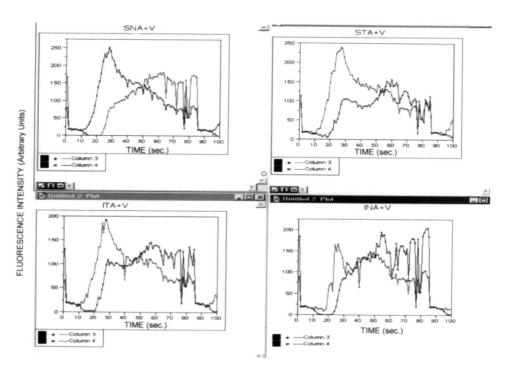

Figure 10.7
Retinal blood flow measurements in the eye of a normal human subject by videoangiography using a scanning laser ophthalmoscope. Top left: the superonasal artery and vein (SNA+V); top right: the superotemporal artery and vein (STA+V); bottom left: the inferotemporal artery and vein (ITA+V); bottom right: the inferonasal artery and vein (INA+V). In all of the graphs, the rise in arterial fluorescence precedes that of the vein, as expected. These curves allow one to measure plasma flow in all four pairs of vessels in the posterior pole of the human eye simultaneously. (Study performed by Mauricio Pons, MD, New York Eye and Ear Infirmary.)

at least the availability of oxygen complexed to red blood cells to the retinal tissue.

Novel functional magnetic resonance imaging measurements of retinal oxygenation

Retinal oxygenation is considered an important prognostic factor for the development of retinal neovascularization in diabetic retinopathy and other diseases. The ability to assess retinal oxygenation is therefore most important both for research in diabetic humans and in experi-

mentally diabetic animals, and for assessing needs for prevention of retinopathy in human diabetic patients. A newly developed, non-invasive technique using functional magnetic resonance imaging (fMRI) may be able to fulfill this need. The method does not directly measure the partial pressure of oxygen (PO_2) in the retina. Rather, digital subtraction of retinal MRI images is performed when the subject is breathing room air, and when the subject is breathing a high oxygen content gas (e.g. 100% O_2). This

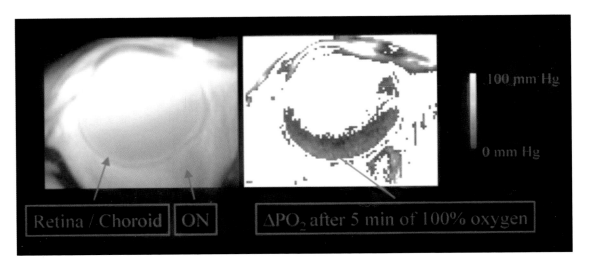

Figure 10.8

Measurement of retinal oxygenation in retinas of rats, using functional magnetic resonance imaging (fMRI). (Left) Representative T_1 weighted images (pixel size 0.39 × 0.39 mm²). The white line in the posterior region of the eye represents the retina/choroid complex. (Right) ΔPO_2 parameter map illustrating the signal intensity enhancement during 5 min of oxygen breathing. Note that only signal changes in the avascular vitreous can be unambiguously assigned to oxygen. The enhancement of optic nerve represents both oxygen and perfusion changes and so data interpretation over this region is not clear. (The images in this figure are courtesy of Bruce Berkowitz, PhD, Department of Anatomy and Cell Biology, Wayne State University School of Medicine.)

produces a measurement of the 'ΔPO_2', whose magnitude accurately measures the retinal oxygenation response.[85] Alternatively, the subject can breathe carbogen (95% O_2, 5% CO_2), which permits more vasodilation as opposed to the considerable vasoconstriction produced by pure O_2, and which therefore may allow more accurate measurements. The fMRI method is highly sensitive and currently has an in-plane spatial resolution of 390 μm² (human) and 50 μm² (rats and mice) (Figure 10.8).[43,86] Although the bulk of the studies to date have been in animal experiments breathing carbogen, the first 'proof-of-concept' studies in normal human volunteers inhaling 100% oxygen have been published.[86] These data are expected to lead to the development of a non-invasive clini-

cal tool to evaluate the risk for retinopathy development and progression and to measure therapeutic effectiveness.

Conclusion: outlook for the future

This chapter has described the progress to date in the treatment of diabetic retinopathy, and has provided information of advanced diagnostic techniques that are useful both for research and for prevention of the disease or its progression in human diabetic subjects. A variety of new therapeutic approaches are also being tested. Studies of the pathogenesis, evaluation, and treatment of diabetic retinopathy remain among the most active and fruitful areas in ophthalmic and endocrinologic research at the present time. Among the problems that are at the forefront of current research are methods, largely pharmacologic, to prevent the onset and progression of diabetic retinopathy, and not only to prevent progression, but also to restore central vision that has been lost from diabetic macular edema. The outlook for future progress is extremely bright.

References

1. Klein R, Klein BEK. Vision disorders in diabetes. In: National Diabetes Data Group, Diabetes in America, 2nd ed. US National Institutes of Health, National Institute of Diabetes and Digestive and Kidney Diseases, NIH Publication No. 95–1468, Washington, DC: US Government Printing Office; 1995: 293–338.

2. Ferris FL III. How effective are treatments for diabetic retinopathy? JAMA 1993; 269: 1290–1.

3. The Early Treatment Diabetic Retinopathy Study Research Group. Photocoagulation for diabetic macular edema, Early Treatment Diabetic Retinopathy Study report no. 1. Arch Ophthalmol 1985; 103: 1796–806.

4. Poulsen JE. The Houssay phenomenon in man: recovery from retinopathy in a case of diabetes with Simmond's disease. Diabetes 1953; 2: 7–12.

5. Lundbaek K, Malmros R, Andersen HC et al. Hypophysectomy for diabetic angiopathy: a controlled clinical trial. In: Goldberg MF, Fine SL, eds. Symposium on the Treatment of Diabetic Retinopathy. US Public Health Service Publication No. 1890. Washington, DC: US Government Printing Office; 1968: 291–311.

6. Chantelau E, Kohner EM. Why some cases of retinopathy worsen when diabetic control improves. BMJ 1997; 315: 1105–6.

7. Daneman D, Drash AL, Lobes LA et al. Progressive retinopathy with improved control in diabetic dwarfism (Mauriac's syndrome). Diabetes Care 1981; 4: 360–5.

8. Thrailkill KM, Quattrin T, Baker L et al. Cotherapy with recombinant human insulin-like growth factor I and insulin improves glycemic control in Type 1 diabetes. RhIGF-I in IDDM Study Group. Diabetes Care 1999; 22: 585–92.

9. Smith LEH, Kopchick JJ, Chen W et al. Essential role of growth hormone in ischemia-induced retinal neovascularization. Science, 1997; 276: 1706–9.

10. Grant MB, Mames RN, Fitzgerald C et al. The efficacy of octreotide in the therapy of severe nonproliferative and early proliferative diabetic retinopathy: a randomized controlled study. Diabetes Care 2000; 23: 504–9.

11. Growth Hormone Antagonist for Proliferative Diabetic Retinopathy Study Group. A growth hormone receptor blocker does not cause regression of proliferative diabetic retinopathy. Ophthalmology 2001; 108: 2266–72.

12. Meyer-Schwickerath G. Light Coagulation, St. Louis: CV Mosby, 1968.

13. Aiello LM, Beetham WP, Balodimos MC et al. Ruby laser photocoagulation in treatment of diabetic proliferating retinopathy: preliminary report. In: Goldberg MF, and Fine SL, eds. Symposium on the Treatment of Diabetic Retinopathy, US Public Health Service Publication No. 1890, Washington, DC: US Government Printing Office, 1968: 437–64.

14. The Diabetic Retinopathy Study Research Group. Preliminary report on effects of photo-coagulation therapy. Am J Ophthalmol 1976; 81: 383–96.

15. Diabetic Retinopathy Study Research Group. Photocoagulation treatment of proliferative diabetic retinopathy: clinical application of Diabetic Retinopathy Study (DRS) findings, DRS report number 8. Ophthalmology 1981; 88: 583–600.

16. Early Treatment Diabetic Retinopathy Study Research Group. Early photocoagulation for diabetic retinopathy. ETDRS Report Number 9. Ophthalmology1991; 98 Suppl: 766–85.

17. Machemer R, Buettner H, Norton EW, Parel JM. Vitrectomy: a pars plana approach. Trans Am Acad Ophthalmol Otolaryngol 1971; 75: 813–20.

18. Thompson JT, de Bustros S, Michels RG, Rice TA. Results and prognostic factors in vitrectomy for diabetic traction-rhegmatogenous

retinal detachment. Arch Ophthalmol 1987; 105: 503–7.

19. The Diabetic Retinopathy Vitrectomy Study Research Group. Early vitrectomy for severe vitreous hemorrhage in diabetic retinopathy. Two-year results of a randomized trial. Diabetic Retinopathy Vitrectomy Study report 2. Arch Ophthalmol 1985; 103: 1644–52.

20. The Diabetic Retinopathy Vitrectomy Study Research Group. Early vitrectomy for severe proliferative diabetic retinopathy in eyes with useful vision. Clinical application of results of a randomized trial – Diabetic Retinopathy Vitrectomy Study Report 4. Ophthalmology 1988; 95: 1321–34.

21. DCCT Research Group. The effect of intensive treatment of diabetes in the development and progression of long-term complications in insulin-dependent diabetes. N Engl J Med 1993; 329: 977–86.

22. UK Prospective Diabetes Study (UKPDS) Group. Intensive blood-glucose control with sulphonylureas or insulin compared with conventional treatment and risk of complications in patients with Type 2 diabetes (UKPDS 33). Lancet 1998; 352: 837–53.

23. UK Prospective Diabetes Study Group. Tight blood pressure control and risk of macrovascular and microvascular complications in Type 2 diabetes: UKPDS 38. BMJ 1998; 317: 703–13.

24. Chaturvedi N, Sjolie AK, Stephenson JM et al. Effect of lisinopril on progression of retinopathy in normotensive people with Type 1 diabetes. The EUCLID Study Group. EURO-DIAB Controlled Trial of Lisinopril in Insulin-Dependent Diabetes Mellitus. Lancet 1998; 351: 28–31.

25. Diabetes Control and Complications Trial (DCCT) Research Group. Early worsening of diabetic retinopathy in the Diabetes Control and Complications Trial. Arch Ophthalmol 1998; 116: 874–86.

26. Lu M, Amano S, Miyamoto K et al. Insulin-induced vascular endothelial growth factor expression in retina. Invest Ophthalmol Vis Sci 1999; 40: 3281–6.

27. Diabetes Control and Complications Trial/ Epidemiology of Diabetes Interventions and Complications Research Group. Retinopathy and nephropathy in patients with Type 1 diabetes for four years after a trial of intensive therapy. N Engl J Med 2000; 342: 381–9.

28. Engerman RL, Kern TS. Progression of incipient diabetic retinopathy during good glycemic control. Diabetes 1987; 36: 808–12.

29. Engerman RL, Kern TS. Retinopathy in galactosemic dogs continues to progress after cessation of galactosemia. Arch Ophthalmol 1994; 113: 355–8.

30. Roy S, Sala R, Cagliero E, Lorenzi M. Overexpression of fibronectin induced by diabetes or high glucose: phenomenon with a memory. Proc Natl Acad Sci USA 1990; 87: 404–8.

31. DCCT Research Group. Clustering of long-term complications in families with diabetes in the diabetes control and complications trial. Diabetes 1997; 46: 1829–39.

32. Early Treatment Diabetic Retinopathy Study Research Group. Effects of aspirin treatment on diabetic retinopathy. ETDRS Report Number 8. Ophthalmology 1991; 98: 757–65.

33. Kern TS, Engerman RL. Pharmacological inhibition of diabetic retinopathy: aminoguanidine and aspirin. Diabetes 2001; 50: 1636–42.

34. Kinoshita JH. Cataracts in galactosemia. Invest Ophthalmol 1965; 4: 786–99.

35. Greene DA, Lattimer SA, Sima AA. Sorbitol, phosphoinositides, and sodium-potassium-ATPase in the pathogenesis of diabetic complications. N Engl J Med 1987; 316: 599–606.

36. Williamson JR, Chang K, Franzos M et al. Hyperglycemic pseudohypoxia and diabetic complications. Diabetes 1993; 42: 801–13.

37. Robison WG Jr, Nagata M, Laver N et al. Diabetic-like retinopathy in rats prevented with an aldose reductase inhibitor. Invest Ophthalmol Vis Sci 1989; 30: 2285–92.

38. Frank RN, Amin R, Kennedy A, Hohman TC. An aldose reductase inhibitor and aminoguanidine prevent vascular endothelial growth factor expression in rats with long-term galactosemia. Arch Ophthalmol 1997; 115: 136–47.

39. Engerman, RL and Kern TS. Aldose reductase inhibition fails to prevent retinopathy in diabetic and galactosemic dogs. Diabetes 1993; 42: 820–5.

40. Kador, PF, Akagi, Y, Takahashi, Y et al. Prevention of retinal vessel changes associated with diabetic retinopathy in galactose-fed dogs

by aldose reductase inhibitors. Arch Ophthalmol 1990; 108: 1301–9.

41. Engerman RL, Kern TS. Experimental galactosemia produces diabetic-like retinopathy. Diabetes 1984; 33: 97–100.

42. Sorbinil Retinopathy Trial Research Group. A randomized trial of sorbinil, an aldose reductase inhibitor, in diabetic retinopathy. Arch Ophthalmol 1990; 108: 1234–44.

43. Berkowitz BA, Ito Y, Kern TS et al. Correction of the subnormal superior hemiretinal ΔPO_2 predicts therapeutic efficacy in experimental diabetic retinopathy. Invest Ophthalmol Vis Sci, in press.

44. Brownlee M, Cerami A. The biochemistry of the complications of diabetes mellitus. Annu Rev Biochem 1981; 50: 385–432.

45. Brownlee M, Vlassara H, Kooney A et al. Aminoguanidine prevents diabetes-induced arterial wall protein cross-linking. Science 1986; 232: 1629–32.

46. Bertone ER, Hankinson SE, Newcomb PA et al. A population-based case–control study of carotenoid and vitamin A intake and ovarian cancer (United States). Cancer Causes Control 2001; 12: 83–90.

47. Tardif JC. Insights into oxidative stress and atherosclerosis. Can J Cardiol 2000; 16 (Suppl. D): 2D-4D.

48. Rosen P, Nawroth PP, King G et al. The role of oxidative stress in the onset and progression of diabetes and its complications: a summary of a Congress Series sponsored by UNESCO-MCBN, the American Diabetes Association and the German Diabetes Society. Diabetes Metab Res Rev 2001; 17: 189–212.

49. Lindsay DG. Diet and ageing: the possible relation to reactive oxygen species. J Nutr Health Aging 1999; 3: 84–91.

50. Kunisaki M, Bursell SE, Clermont AC et al. Vitamin E prevents diabetes-induced abnormal retinal blood flow via the diacylglycerol-protein kinase C pathway. Am J Physiol 1995; 269 (2 Pt 1): E239–46.

51. Kowluru RA, Tang J, Kern TS. Abnormalities of retinal metabolism in diabetes and experimental galactosemia. VII. Effect of long-term administration of antioxidants on the development of retinopathy. Diabetes 2001; 50: 1938–42.

52. Obrosova IG, Minchenko AG, Marinescu V et

al. Antioxidants attenuate early up regulation of retinal vascular endothelial growth factor in streptozotocin-diabetic rats. Diabetologia 2001; 44: 1102–10.

53. Malecaze F, Clamens S, Simorre-Pinatel V et al. Detection of vascular endothelial growth factor messenger RNA and vascular endothelial growth factor-like activity in proliferative diabetic retinopathy. Arch Ophthalmol 1994; 112: 1476–82.

54. Mathews MK, Merges C, McLeod DS, Lutty GA. Vascular endothelial growth factor and vascular permeability changes in human diabetic retinopathy. Invest Ophthalmol Vis Sci 1997; 38: 2729–41.

55. Pe'er J, Shweiki D, Itin A et al. Hypoxia-induced expression of vascular endothelial growth factor (VEGF) by retinal cells is a common factor in neovascularization. Lab Invest 1995; 72: 638–45.

56. Aiello LP, Northrup JM, Keyt BA et al. Hypoxic regulation of vascular endothelial growth factor in retinal cells. Arch Ophthalmol 1995; 113: 1538–44.

57. Amin RH, Frank RN, Kennedy A et al. Vascular endothelial growth factor is present in glial cells of the retina and optic nerve of human subjects with nonproliferative diabetic retinopathy. Invest Ophthalmol Vis Sci 1997; 38: 36–47.

58. Lutty GA, McLeod DS, Merges C et al. Localization of vascular endothelial growth factor in human retina and choroid. Arch Ophthalmol 1996; 114: 971–7.

59. Adamis AP, Shima DT, Tolentino MJ et al. Inhibition of vascular endothelial growth factor prevents retinal ischemia-associated iris neovascularization in a nonhuman primate. Arch Ophthalmol 1996; 114: 66–71.

60. Aiello LP, Pierce EA, Foley ED et al. Suppression of retinal neovascularization in vivo by inhibition of vascular endothelial growth factor (VEGF) using soluble VEGF-receptor chimeric proteins. Proc Natl Acad Sci USA 1995; 92: 10457–61.

61. Robinson GS, Pierce EA, Rook SL et al. Oligodeoxynucleotides inhibit retinal neovascularization in a murine model of proliferative retinopathy. Proc Natl Acad Sci USA 1996; 93: 4851–6.

62. Becerra SP, Wu YQ, Montuenga L et al. Pigment epithelium-derived factor (PEDF) in the monkey eye: apical secretion from the retinal pigment epithelium (Abstract). Invest Ophthalmol Vis Sci 2001; 42: S772.

63. Steele FR, Chader GJ, Johnson LV, Tombran-Tink J. Pigment epithelium-derived factor: neurotrophic activity and identification as a member of the serine protease inhibitor gene family. Proc Natl Acad Sci USA 1993; 90: 1526–30.

64. Dawson DW, Volpert OV, Gillis P et al. Pigment epithelium-derived factor: a potent inhibitor of angiogenesis. Science 1999; 285: 245–8.

65. Stellmach V, Crawford SE, Zhou W, Bouck N. Prevention of ischemia-induced retinopathy by the natural ocular antiangiogenic agent pigment epithelium-derived factor. Proc Natl Acad Sci USA 2001; 98: 2593–7.

66. Mori K, Duh E, Gehlbach P et al. Pigment epithelium-derived factor inhibits retinal and choroidal neovascularization. J Cell Physiol 2001; 188: 253–63.

67. Ogata N, Tombran-Tink J, Nishikawa M et al. Pigment epithelium-derived factor in the vitreous is low in diabetic retinopathy and high in rhegmatogenous retinal detachment. Am J Ophthalmol 2001; 132: 378–82.

68. Gao G, Li Y, Zhang D et al. Unbalanced expression of VEGF and PEDF in ischemia-induced retinal neovascularization. FEBS Lett 2001; 489: 270–6.

69. Xia P, Inoguchi T, Kern T et al. Characterization of the mechanism for the chronic activation of diacylglycerol-protein kinase C pathway in diabetes and hypergalactosemia. Diabetes 1994; 43: 1122–9.

70. Williams B, Gallacher B, Patel H, Orme C. Glucose-induced protein kinase C activation regulates vascular permeability factor mRNA expression and peptide production by human vascular smooth muscle cells in vitro. Diabetes 1997; 46: 1497–1503.

71. Xia P, Aiello LP, Ishii H et al. Characterization of vascular endothelial growth factor's effect on the activation of protein kinase C, its isoforms, and endothelial cell growth. J Clin Invest 1996; 98: 2018–26.

72. Danis RP, Bingaman DP, Jrousek M, Yang Y. Inhibition of intraocular neovascularization due to retinal ischemia in pigs by PKCβ inhibition with LY333531. Invest Ophthalmol Vis Sci 1998; 39: 171–9.

73. Aiello LP, Bursell SE, Clermont A et al. Vascular endothelial growth factor-induced retinal permeability is mediated by protein kinase C in vivo and suppressed by an orally effective beta-isoform-selective inhibitor. Diabetes 1997; 46: 1473–80.

74. Fukushima I, McLeod DS, Lutty GA. Intrachoroidal microvascular abnormality: a previously unrecognized form of choroidal neovascularization. Am J Ophthalmol 1997; 124: 473–87.

75. Frank RN. Visual fields and electroretinography following extensive photocoagulation. Arch Ophthalmol 1975; 93: 591–8.

76. Bresnick GH, Palta M. Predicting progression to severe proliferative diabetic retinopathy. Arch Ophthalmol 1987; 105: 810–14.

77. Huang D, Swanson EA, Lin CP et al. Optical coherence tomography. Science 1991; 254: 1178–81.

78. Rivellese M, George A, Sulkes D et al. Optical coherence tomography after laser photocoagulation for clinically significant macular edema. Ophthalmic Surg Lasers 2000; 31: 192–7.

79. Drexler W, Morgner U, Ghanta RK et al. Ultrahigh-resolution ophthalmic optical coherence tomography. Nat Med 2001; 7: 502–7.

80. Zeimer R, Shahidi M, Mori M et al. A new method for rapid mapping of the retinal thickness at the posterior pole. Invest Ophthalmol Vis Sci 1996; 37: 1994–2001.

81. Grunwald JE, Riva CE, Martin DB et al. Effect of an insulin-induced decrease in blood glucose on the human diabetic retinal circulation, Ophthalmology 1987; 94: 1614–20.

82. Ishii H, Jirousek MR, Koya D et al. Amelioration of vascular dysfunctions in diabetic rats by an oral PKC beta inhibitor. Science 1996; 272: 728–31.

83. Grunwald JE, Riva CE, Sinclair SH et al. Laser Doppler velocimetry study of retinal circulation in diabetes mellitus. Arch Ophthalmol 1986; 104: 991–6.

84. Aiello LP, Bursell SE, Devries T et al. Amelioration of abnormal retinal hemodynamics by a protein kinase C b selective inhibitor

(LY333531) in patients with diabetes: results of a Phase 1 safety and pharmacodynamic clinical trial (Abstract). Invest Ophthalmol Vis Sci 1999; 40: S912.

85. Berkowitz BA. Adult and newborn rat inner retinal oxygenation during carbogen and 100% oxygen breathing. Comparison using magnetic resonance imaging delta pO2 mapping. Invest Ophthalmol Vis Sci 1996; 37: 2089–98.

86. Berkowitz BA, McDonald C, Ito Y et al. Measuring the human retinal oxygenation response to a hyperoxic challenge using MRI: eliminating blinking artifacts and demonstrating proof of concept. Magn Reson Med 2001; 46: 412–16.

11

Advances in the treatment of the diabetic foot

Edward B Jude, Samson O Oyibo, Andrew JM Boulton

Introduction

Diabetic foot problems, which account for more hospital admissions than any of the other long-term complications of diabetes, are associated with increasing morbidity and mortality in diabetic patients.[1] They tend to occur in about 20% of the diabetic population,[2] and the costs of services (direct and indirect) that are associated with the management of the diabetic foot are phenomenal.[3-5] Diabetic foot problems are responsible for more than two-thirds of all non-traumatic lower limb amputations.[6]

The diabetic foot encompasses a number of foot pathologies, including diabetic peripheral neuropathy, Charcot's neuroarthropathy, lower extremity arterial disease, foot ulceration and infection. Diabetic foot problems continue to provide a challenge for health care professionals, as far as prevention and treatment are concerned.[7]

In this chapter we outline the management of the diabetic foot. We discuss the epidemiology, diagnoses and treatment of the various diabetic foot problems, highlighting some of the recent treatment advances.

Peripheral neuropathy

Peripheral neuropathy is a common long-term complication of diabetes mellitus with the distal sensory type being the most common form. A large UK study revealed that symptomatic neuropathy was present in 28.5% of 6500 diabetic patients.[8] Similarly, a European multicentre study reported a 28% prevalence rate in Type 1 diabetic patients.[9]

The Diabetes Control and Complications Trial[10] and other long-term trials[11,12] have demonstrated that strict glycaemic control influences the onset and progression of diabetic neuropathy. However, the exact mechanism by which hyperglycaemia causes nerve damage remains a subject of debate. Current metabolic theories include adverse alterations in the polyol pathway, abnormalities in myo-inositol metabolism, detrimental effect of advanced glycation end product formation, oxidative stress, abnormal fatty acid metabolism, neuro-autoimmune factors and defective neurotrophic support.[13] Vascular theories comprise neuro-vascular disease, arterio-venous shunting at the level of the epineurial vasculature, and endoneurial hypoxia.[14]

The clinical presentation ranges from severely painful ('positive') symptoms at one extreme, to the completely painless ('negative') symptoms at the other. Positive symptoms include burning pain, paraesthesiae, shooting, stabbing and lancinating pain, hyperaesthesiae and allodynia. Negative symptoms are usually 'numbness' and 'deadness' in the feet. Many patients find the positive symptoms difficult to describe, but most report them to be extremely

Test	Right foot	Left foot
Vibration sense (big toe) Present = 0 Reduced/absent = 1		
Pin-prick sense (big toe) Present = 0 Reduced/absent = 1		
Temperature sense (dorsum of foot) Present = 0 Reduced/absent = 1		
Ankle jerk Present = 0 Present on reinforcement = 1 Absent = 2		
Total score		

Notes: The NDS is the sum of the total scores derived from both feet. An NDS of 3–4 is mild neuropathy, 5–7 is moderate and a score of 8–10 indicates severe neuropathy

Table 11.1
The Neuropathy Disability Score (NDS)

uncomfortable, distressing and prone to nocturnal exacerbation. Many patients at risk of neuropathic foot ulceration have no symptoms, and since neuropathy cannot be diagnosed by history alone, clinical examination of the feet is mandatory for all diabetic patients.

A simple examination using a tuning fork for vibration perception at the apex of the great toe and temperature sense on the dorsal aspect of the feet, a pin (neurotip) for pain sensation just proximal to the great toe nail, and a tendon hammer for the ankle reflex allows the use of a neuropathy disability score (NDS) for risk assessment (Table 11.1).[15] A score (from both feet) of 6/10 or more is indicative of significant neuropathy, and is associated with a seven-fold increased risk of future development of a foot ulcer.[16] Quantitative tests using a biothesiometer for vibration perception threshold, 10 g Semmes-Weinstein monofilament for pressure perception or the tactile circumferential discriminator[17] to assess large fibre function are simple, quick, inexpensive tests that can be carried out in a routine clinic setting. A vibration perception threshold (VPT) of more than 25 volts in the lower limb indicates increased risk of future foot ulceration.[18]

Management

The management of peripheral neuropathy, although largely symptomatic, entails the need for regular follow-up for the prevention and early detection of neuropathic sequelae, to which these patients are susceptible. The treatment of diabetic peripheral neuropathy is far from satisfactory. Probably the most important form of treatment is achieving near-normal glycaemic control, which has been shown to delay the onset and slow the progression of diabetic nerve damage.[19,20] Several studies have been performed to assess the ability of various agents to modify or reverse the nerve damage inflicted by diabetes, but these have been rewarded with less than adequate success.

Disease modifying agents

The use of various agents, e.g. aldose-reductase inhibitors, antioxidants, gamma-linolenic acid, ACE-inhibitors, nerve growth factors etc., have been studied in patients with diabetic neuropathy. The aldose-reductase inhibitors (ARI) can improve axonal transport, which is impaired in experimental diabetes and other toxic and metabolic neuropathies.[21] Early clinical trials in Japan reported that epalrestat produced improvement in subjects with symptomatic neuropathy,[22] and encouraging results have also been produced by another ARI tolrestat.[23] However, the consistent benefit of ARIs for the treatment of diabetic neuropathy is yet to be confirmed by larger randomized controlled clinical trials.

A randomized controlled trial using the antioxidant, alpha-lipoic acid has shown some improvement in neuropathic symptoms, when given intravenously.[24] These findings substantiate that i.v. treatment with alpha-lipoic acid using a dose of 600 mg/day over three weeks is superior to placebo in reducing symptoms of diabetic peripheral neuropathy, without causing significant adverse reactions. Oral preparations have also been tried, and preliminary data over two years indicate possible long-term improvement in motor and sensory nerve conduction in the lower limbs.[25]

Impaired conversion of linoleic acid to gamma-linolenic acid (GLA) has been demonstrated in animal diabetes and inferred from blood fatty acid profiles in human diabetes. This impairment could theoretically lead to defective nerve function because metabolites of GLA, e.g. prostacyclin, are important in nerve membrane structure, nerve blood flow, and nerve conduction.[26] In a small placebo-controlled clinical trial, GLA improved symptom scores and nerve fibre function in patients with diabetic neuropathy.[27]

ACE-inhibitors such as lisinopril and trandolapril have been shown to improve both nerve conduction velocity and quantitative sensory tests in subjects with mild diabetic neuropathy.[28,29] The mechanism of action is most likely through the improvement of neuronal microvascular supply. However, larger clinical trials are needed to confirm these potentially beneficial reports.

Although a preliminary clinical trial in humans suggests that nerve growth factor may be effective in the treatment of diabetic neuropathy,[30] subsequent larger trials have not confirmed these initial optimistic findings.

Despite various clinical trials, the disease-modifying potentials of these agents need to be confirmed in large double blind placebo-controlled trials.

Glycaemic control

Strict glycaemic control has been shown to improve the symptoms of painful diabetic neuropathy.[31] The reduction in the number of glycaemic excursions may play a pivotal role in the control of intermittent painful symptoms.[32] The potential benefit of continuous s.c. infusion therapy for the control of painful neuropathic symptoms is currently under investigation.

Drug therapy

Drugs commonly used for the treatment of neuropathic pain include antidepressants, anti-epileptics, and simple or opiate-related analgesics.[33] However, these agents are not free from untoward side effects. The following list shows some of the therapeutic agents that are commonly used:

(1) *Oral medication:*
   - Anti-epileptic drugs
     – Gabapentin 900–3600 mg daily
     – Carbamazepine up to 800 mg daily
   - Tricyclic antidepressant drugs
     – Imipramine 25–150 mg daily
     – Amitriptyline 25–150 mg daily
   - Tramadol 50–200 mg daily
(2) *Topical medication:*
   - Acupuncture therapy
   - Capsaicin cream
   - Opsite spray or dressing.

Lidocaine

The role of s.c. or i.v. lidocaine (lignocaine) in the management of neuropathic pain has been increasingly studied.[34] Several clinical trials, with small sample sizes, have demonstrated positive results when i.v. lidocaine (5 mg/kg body weight) was used for the treatment of painful diabetic neuropathy.[35,36] Larger randomized clinical trials are needed to evaluate its safety and efficacy.

Acupuncture therapy

Acupuncture therapy continues to be a safe and effective therapy for the long-term management of painful diabetic neuropathy, although its mechanism of action remains speculative.[37]

Electrical stimulation therapy

Recent data from the USA demonstrates the possible use of electrical therapy for the treatment of painful diabetic neuropathy.[38] The potential benefit of this exciting new therapy for the treatment of painful diabetic neuropathy is currently under investigation.

Vascular insufficiency

Peripheral arterial disease, especially associated with medial arterial calcification is commonly associated with diabetes mellitus.[39] In a cohort of patients with peripheral arterial disease, diabetic patients not only have worse disease, but also have a poorer outcome, when compared with non-diabetic patients.[40] Diabetic patients present late as the presence of neuropathy may mask symptoms of intermittent claudication and hence these patients do worse than their non-diabetic counterparts. Smoking, hypertension and hyperlipidaemia are important risk factors.[41] Peripheral arterial disease is also an important risk factor for lower extremity amputation in patients with chronic diabetic foot ulceration.[42]

Diabetic patients with peripheral arterial disease may not have the classical symptoms (claudication, rest pain) because of the presence of severe neuropathy. Palpation of the pedal pulses and/or the measurement of the ankle–brachial pressure index (ABPI) will assess the lower limb vascular supply: the absence of both pedal pulses and/or an ABPI <0.8 in the affected foot is clinical evidence of ischaemia. A non-invasive ultrasound vascular study will confirm severe vascular disease (ABPI <0.6). Falsely elevated readings (ABPI >1.2) may be produced by vascular calcification, and such results should be viewed with caution. If severe ischaemia is suspected, lower limb angiography is necessary to assess the need for angioplasty or vascular reconstructive surgery.

Management

Diabetic patients with intermittent claudication, ischaemic ulcers or gangrene need referral to a vascular surgeon. Cessation of smoking, strict glycaemic control, treatment of hypertension and dyslipidaemia, and the use of aspirin should be advised. However, some patients still require vascular reconstructive surgery (e.g. angioplasty, stent placement, arterial by-pass surgery, etc). The performance of more distal vessel reconstructive surgery is likely to improve the prognosis in those diabetic patients with severe distal vessel disease.

Diabetic foot ulceration

Various studies have reported the incidence of foot ulceration, ranging from 3–7% of the diabetic population.[43,44] As well as being a common reason for diabetic admissions, foot ulceration precedes >80% of diabetes-related amputation.[6]

The combination of diabetic neuropathy, foot deformity (Charcot foot, callus, bony prominence, etc.) and foot swelling contribute to an increased risk of foot ulceration caused by unperceived external trauma.[45] The presence of wound infection and ischaemia leads to chronic ulceration, and increases the predisposition to foot gangrene and resultant amputation.

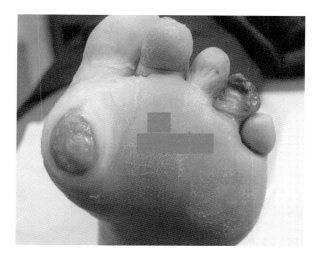

Figure 11.1
Diabetic foot ulcers.

The presentation of foot ulcers and patients' clinical characteristics vary considerably. Ulcers may be infected, ischaemic or both, and associated with local osteomyelitis. Since a majority of ulcers are painless, patients are likely to present late (Figure 11.1). However, some patients present with local foot gangrene only because of the smell, rather than the sight of the ulcer.

Stage	Grade			
	0	1	2	3
A	Pre- or post-ulcerative lesion completely epithelialized	Superficial ulcer, not involving tendon, capsule, or bone	Ulcer penetrating to tendon or capsule	Ulcer penetrating to bone or joint
B	With infection	With infection	With infection	With infection
C	With ischaemia	With ischaemia	With ischaemia	With ischaemia
D	With infection and ischaemia	With infection and ischaemia	With infection and ischaemia	With infection and ischaemia

Table 11.2
The University of Texas Diabetic Wound Classification System

Regular examination of both feet, looking for bony prominence, differences in temperature, foot pulses, dry skin, callus, bunions and overgrown toenails will help in early detection of pre-ulceration. Classification of foot ulcers is necessary for the prognosis and management.[46] The University of Texas Wound Classification system (Table 11.2) can be used to assess ulcer grade and stage.[47] This system, which grades ulcer depth on the horizontal axis and stages the presence of infection and ischaemia on the vertical axis, has been shown to predict outcome in terms of healing and amputations.[48] Ulcer size should also be documented to assess progress.[49] The ability to probe to bone in the presence of infection is a strong indicator of underlying osteomyelitis.[50]

Management

The treatment of superficial ulcers entails regular debridement and dressing, and relief of pressure around the ulcer, by using a total-contact plaster cast[51] or a Scotchcast boot (Figure 11.2).[52] Patients who wear these forms of offloading devices are less active on their feet, than patients who wear their regular shoes.[53] Deeper ulcers should have curetted specimens sent off for culture. If infection is suspected then broad-spectrum antibiotics, such as cephalexin, Augmentin (amoxycillin and clavulinic acid) or clindamycin can be used to cover most pathogens.[54]

Foot ulcers complicated by osteomyelitis usually require long-term treatment (up to six months) with clindamycin or Augmentin.[55] However recalcitrant osteomyelitis needs referral to an orthopaedic surgeon for debridement, sequestrectomy, or as a last resort, amputation (Figure 11.3).

Patients with neuroischaemic foot ulcers need proper vascular assessment, as these patients may require vascular reconstruction to

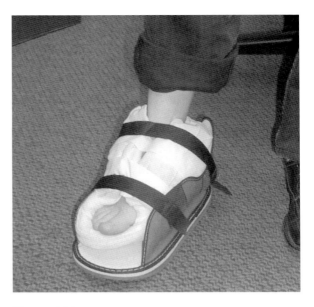

Figure 11.2
Scotchcast boot.

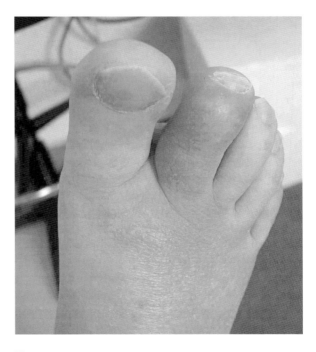

Figure 11.3
Osteomyelitis in second toe.

aid the healing of their ulcers, thus reducing the probability of requiring amputation. Foot gangrene requires urgent hospital admission, control of diabetes and infection, and amputation. Such patients are best managed on the surgical ward by a vascular surgeon.

New therapeutic approaches to foot ulcers

This section on new therapeutic approaches to diabetic foot problems will consider developments and innovations that have been reported in the past five years. Treatments that may potentially prevent the development of foot ulcerations, such as footwear and silicone injection, will be considered first. This will be followed by specific therapies for the management of patients with active foot ulcers.

Therapeutic footwear

The use of footwear is certainly not a new approach: examples of footwear worn by Roman soldiers can be seen at Hadrian's Wall museum in the north of England. It is well recognized that inappropriate footwear is an important component cause in the pathway to foot ulceration, as noted above. However, although it has been stated for many years that good footwear prevents the development of ulcers, controlled data in this area have been lacking until recently. In a systematic review of foot ulcer prevention in patients with Type 2 diabetes, Mason et al., found only one controlled study that had assessed the efficacy of therapeutic shoes to reduce the recurrence of foot ulcers.[56] Uccioli et al., in a randomized study of 69 patients with previous ulcerations, reported significantly fewer recurrent ulcers in those wearing therapeutic shoes rather than normal footwear.[57] This study therefore demonstrates the important health benefits derived from wearing appropriately designed footwear. A systematic approach to footwear, involving a multidisciplinary team is required to improve the long-term outcome of the diabetic foot.[58]

Injected liquid silicone

Important predictive factors for the development of foot ulceration include high plantar pressure, which usually occurs at sites with bony prominences such as the metatarsal heads, and the presence of callus, which acts as a foreign body ultimately causing ulceration.[59] Previous uncontrolled reports from the USA have suggested that the therapeutic use of liquid silicone injections in the foot to replace fat padding at callus sites, corns and localized painful areas led to a reduction in callus formation and foot ulcer occurrence.[60]

A recent randomized, controlled trial compared the effectiveness of injecting liquid silicone into the diabetic foot with a saline placebo.[61] Those patients who received silicone had significantly increased plantar tissue thickness at the injection sites and correspondingly, significantly decreased plantar pressures at 3, 6 and 12 months after the injection. These preliminary data suggest the potential efficacy of plantar silicone injections, which appear to be safe and without side effects. Further larger studies are now indicated.

Platelet-derived growth factors

Several controlled trials using Becaplermin, a recombinant human platelet-derived growth factor, have confirmed the efficacy of this topically applied agent in promoting healing of neuropathic foot ulcers. In a meta-analysis of four randomized controlled studies, Smiell et al., showed that active treatment with Becaplermin was associated with a significant increase in the probability of complete healing compared with placebo gel.[62] This topically applied growth factor is now licensed for use in many countries and has mainly been used in difficult to heal neuropathic ulcers that fail to respond to standard treatment such as offloading, treatment of infection and regular debridement. Its widespread use is somewhat limited by cost, however, when used selectively, it can accelerate the wound healing of neuropathic foot ulcers. During the conduct of these growth factor trials, the importance of extensive and regular sharp debridement was confirmed.[63] It was postulated that sharp debridement encouraged cellular migration and the release of cytokines and growth factors, needed for proper wound healing.

Skin graft

The recent development of living human skin equivalents, produced by tissue engineering techniques, has produced new possibilities for wound healing therapies for chronic ulcers such as those caused by venous disease and diabetic neuropathy. Graft skin is a bi-layered, cultured skin equivalent, which consists of human epidermis and a collagenous dermal layer containing human fibroblasts. In a recently presented study, Veves et al., evaluated the efficacy of graft skin in the management of chronic neuropathic diabetic foot ulcers.[64] Graft skin or standard treatment (saline moisturized gauze) was applied to more than 200 patients, who also received standard good wound care for the diabetic foot ulcer comprising sharp debridement and offloading. After 12 weeks of treatment, 56% of graft skin-treated patients achieved complete healing compared with 38% of the controls.

Dermagraft

Dermagraft is a three-dimensional, allogeneic, human neonatal dermal fibroblast culture grown on a degradable scaffold and cryopreserved. Recent clinical trials have demonstrated the efficacy of this compound in the healing of chronic diabetic foot ulcers.[65–67]

It appears, therefore, that treatments such as graft skin and possibly Dermagraft might be useful adjuncts to the treatment of diabetic neuropathic foot ulcers. However, it must be pointed out that both living skin equivalents and topically applied growth factors are expensive treatments and should not be seen as a replacement, but as an addition to good wound care that must always comprise adequate offloading and regular debridement.

Granulocyte colony stimulating factor

Neutrophil superoxide generation, a crucial part of neutrophil bactericidal activity, is impaired in diabetes. Granulocyte-colony stimulating factor (G-CSF) increases the release of neutrophils from the bone marrow and improves neutrophil function by increasing its superoxide production. In a placebo-controlled trial, i.v. G-CSF (Filgrastim) treatment was associated with improved clinical outcome of foot infection in diabetic patients, including fewer amputations, shorter hospital stay and faster healing of foot ulcers.[68]

Antibiotic-impregnated calcium sulphate pellets

Plaster of Paris was first used as a delivery vehicle for antiseptics in 1928, when antiseptic-impregnated calcium sulphate was inserted into infected defects in the long bones of canines.[69] Antibiotic-impregnated calcium sulphate pellets for deep, infected diabetic foot wounds, with or without osteomyelitis, have been used both in the UK and the USA with increasing anecdotal success.[70] These radio-opaque pellets once inserted into a wound, tend to dissolve completely over several weeks, eluting the majority of their antibiotic load over the first four weeks.[71] It appears that the use of antibiotic-impregnated calcium sulphate pellets might be another useful adjunct to treatment of infected diabetic foot ulcers. However, randomized controlled trials are needed to assess their efficacy.

Larval therapy

Larval therapy, that is the ability of maggots to cleanse wounds, control infection and promote healing, like footwear is hardly new. Indeed, an early reference to larval therapy was made during the Napoleonic wars when it was observed that wounds accidentally infested by maggots did not become infected and appeared to heal better. In recent years the use of sterile larvae (larvae of the green bottle fly) has been investigated with encouraging results, and they are becoming increasingly popular for infected and necrotic wounds.[72,73] It is thought that maggots remove dead tissue by secreting powerful enzymes that break down dead tissue into a liquid form, which is then ingested.[74] The mechanisms by which larvae prevent or combat infection are also complex but there is anecdotal evidence that these may help in combating antibiotic-resistant strains of bacteria. There is a growing clinical experience with larval therapy, suggesting that it is useful in the management of patients with necrotic, sloughy, and often neuroischaemic ulcers. Clearly, controlled trials are difficult in this area, but the use of this therapy is now quite widespread in diabetic foot care and also in branches of plastic surgery.

Low-intensity laser therapy

Various clinical studies indicate that laser therapy by low light doses may be a valuable method for treating diabetic foot ulcers.[75,76] Although the mechanism of action is still poorly understood, this form of therapy has been shown to accelerate wound healing, possibly by increasing microcirculatory blood flow in the affected area.[77] This use of nondestructive lasers for bio-stimulation, requires further research to assess its efficacy in the management of diabetic foot ulcers.

Topical hyperbaric oxygen therapy

Delayed wound healing in diabetic patients is associated with defective cellular and humoral immunity. In particular, decreased chemotaxis, decreased phagocytosis, impaired bacterial killing and abnormal leucocyte function have been observed, resulting in a reduced inflammatory reaction and defective wound healing.[78] Hyperbaric oxygen therapy can raise local tissue oxygen tensions, which can improve leucocyte function and inhibit or kill certain anaerobic bacteria. As an adjunct, it has been shown in small trials to improve the healing of diabetic foot ulcers.[79,80] However, larger randomized controlled trials are needed to assess the efficacy of hyperbaric oxygen therapy for chronic diabetic foot ulcers.

Retrograde venous perfusion

It is well known that severe peripheral arterial disease and possibly microangiopathy delays wound healing. Not only is there reduced oxygen tension, but also local tissue levels of the systemically administered therapeutic agents may be insufficient.

Retrograde venous perfusion techniques have been used as a research tool in conditions where arterial occlusive disease plays a major contributory role, such as myocardial ischaemia, stroke and peripheral arterial occlusive disease.[81–83] Recently the technique has been introduced into the management of diabetic foot ulcers.[84,85] Using the Bier's method of regional anaesthesia, various drugs, especially antibiotics, can be administered intravenously distal to an arterial block in legs with severe arterial insufficiency. It is assumed that ischaemic skin, while being cut off from arterial supply may still be reached by the venous route.

Charcot neuroarthropathy

Charcot neuroarthropathy is a rare, but devastating disorder, which typically affects the joints of the feet in patients with severe diabetic neuropathy. The incidence in diabetic patients range from 0.1 to 7.5%, but typical radiographic changes may be found in 10 to 16% of patients who have a history of neuropathic foot ulceration.[86,87]

The pathogenesis is associated with the coexistence of severe peripheral neuropathy and autonomic dysfunction. Trauma to the foot, usually trivial, appears to precipitate simultaneous bone destruction and remodelling. Previous studies have demonstrated increased vascularity and arteriovenous shunting in the affected bones.[88] This increased bone blood flow results in activation of osteoclasts and localized osteoporosis, which may precede the development of Charcot's neuroarthropathy.[89]

Management

Clinically, the patient presents with a warm, painless, swollen foot with or without a history of preceding trauma. Some patients may complain of discomfort, in the absence of pain, but the majority are symptom free. It is usually unilateral, but can be bilateral in about 10% of cases (Figure 11.4). The diagnosis is based on finding a hot, swollen, usually painless foot in a patient with diabetic neuropathy. There are usually distended veins over the affected feet. The presence of destructive bony changes and a typical disorganized joint can be seen on X ray (Figure 11.5). Occasionally, a white cell bone scan or magnetic resonance imaging may be required to differentiate this condition from osteomyelitis.

The treatment of Charcot foot is directed at reducing or limiting further destruction of the joints. Immobilization achieved using an air cast boot, total-contact cast or a Scotchcast boot and reduced weight bearing is still the mainstay of therapy for the acute Charcot foot.[90] Anti-inflammatory drugs such as

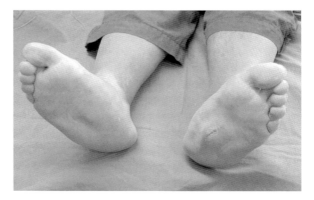

Figure 11.4
Bilateral Charcot foot.

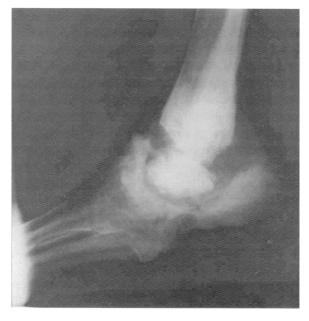

Figure 11.5
X ray showing a Charcot joint.

indomethacin may be prescribed, however, renal function should be monitored. Immobilization and rest should be continued during and after the active phase (evidenced by increased skin temperature >2°C over the active joint compared with the corresponding site of the uninvolved contralateral foot), following which special custom-fitted shoes with moulded insoles should be worn. Patients usually require immobilization for an average of six months before they can be prescribed special shoes.[91]

Recent studies have looked at the possibility of treating Charcot neuroarthropathy with radiotherapy and ultrasound. However, these studies showed no substantial benefit in this group of patients. Pharmacological management was initially considered in an open-labelled trial using Pamidronate infusion twice monthly over 12 weeks with the proviso that it reduces osteoclastic activity, which has been shown to be increased in active Charcot arthropathy patients. This study demonstrated a reduction in biochemical parameters (alkaline phosphatase) as well as clinical improvement (decrease in disease activity as measured by temperature difference between active and contralateral foot).[92] This was then followed by a double blind randomized controlled trial.

In this randomized trial, 39 patients were recruited to receive either placebo (normal saline) or pamidronate (90 mg) as a single intravenous infusion at baseline.[93] Disease activity (temperature difference), patients' symptoms and bone turnover markers were assessed at baseline and at each subsequent visit (10 in total) over the next 12 months. All patients received standard treatment of the affected foot, including immobilization and bed rest. Patients in both groups demonstrated a reduction in temperature and symptoms score over the next 12 months. There was a significant reduction in temperature the placebo and

active groups when compared with baseline. However, although there was a further reduction in temperature in the active group this did not reach statistical significance. Symptom scores were, however, significantly reduced in the active group when compared with the placebo group. There was also a significant reduction in the bone resorption marker (urinary deoxypyridinoline) and the bone formation marker (bone-specific alkaline phosphatase). This effect of pamidronate was limited and the bone markers returned towards baseline levels from 6–12 months after the infusion. However, larger studies are required to assess the appropriate dose, duration and frequency of treatment as well as other possible routes of administration as in recent years potent oral bisphosphonates have become available.

Surgical treatment of the Charcot foot is contraindicated during the acute stage, but may be helpful in the quiescent stage, when required to stabilize the joints of the foot or to remove bony deformities, which can precipitate foot ulceration.

Follow-up and education: the multidisciplinary approach to foot care

The real conundrum in the management of diabetic foot ulcers is not just healing them, but keeping them healed. Despite all efforts geared towards the treatment of the diabetic foot, these problems still recur. Litzelman et al. confirmed the value of a multidisciplinary approach to education and self-care for diabetic patients, in reducing the incidence of foot lesions in general practice.[94] A recent prospective study has also demonstrated the effectiveness of the multidisciplinary approach to diabetic foot care. Recurrence rates were considerably reduced by regular follow-up by a team of physicians, nurses and podiatrists, with re-education every three months and the provision of special footwear as required.[95]

Conclusions

Frequent examination of the diabetic foot, identifying risk factors and regular follow-up in a specialist foot clinic are important in the management of the 'diabetic foot'. Early diagnosis, wound care and pressure relief will help reduce amputations. It should be remembered that the new wound-healing therapies (e.g. growth factors, artificial skin) are no substitute for basic wound care, i.e. wound debridement, offloading, treating infections and re-vascularization. The importance of a multidisciplinary team approach to foot care in patients with diabetes foot problems cannot be overemphasized. This is the only way by which the aims of the St Vincent Declaration[96] can be achieved, i.e. to reduce the number of amputations resulting from diabetic foot gangrene by 50%.

References

1. Boyko EJ, Ahroni JH, Smith DG, Davignon D. Increased mortality associated with diabetic foot ulcer. Diabet Med 1996; 13: 967–72.
2. Morgan CL, Currie CJ, Stott NC et al. The prevalence of multiple diabetes-related complications. Diabet Med 2000; 17: 146–51.
3. Songer TJ. The economics of diabetes care. In: Alberti KGMM, DeFronzo RA, Keen H, Zimmet P, eds. International Textbook of Diabetes Mellitus. Chichester: Wiley, 1987: 1643–54.
4. Reiber GE. Diabetic foot care: financial implications and practical guidelines. Diabetes Care 1992; 15 Suppl. 1: 29–31.
5. Williams DRR, Airey M. The size of the problem: epidemiological and economic aspects of foot problems in diabetes. In: Boulton AJM, Connor H, Cavanagh PR, eds. The Foot in Diabetes, 3rd edn. Chichester: John Wiley & Son; 2000: 3–17.
6. Pecoraro RE, Reiber GE, Burgess EM. Pathways to diabetic limb amputation: basis for prevention. Diabetes Care 1990; 13: 513–21.
7. Oyibo SO, Abouaesha F, Connor H, Boulton AJM. The diabetic foot 2000. Diabet Med 2000; 17: 875–6.
8. Young MJ, Boulton AJM, McLeod AF et al. A multicentre study of the prevalence of diabetic peripheral neuropathy in the UK hospital clinic population. Diabetologia 1993; 36: 150–4.
9. Tesfaye S, Stevens LK, Stephenson JM et al. The prevalence of diabetic peripheral neuropathy and its relation to glycaemic control and potential risk factors: the EURODIAB IDDM complications study. Diabetologia 1996; 39: 1377–84.
10. DCCT research group. The effect of intensive treatment of diabetes on the development and progression of long-term complications in insulin-dependent diabetes mellitus. N Engl J Med 1993; 329: 977–86.
11. Ziegler D, Wiefels K, Dannehl K, Grie FA. Effects of one year of near-normoglycaemia on peripheral nerve function in Type 1 (insulin dependent) diabetic patients. Klin Wochenschr 1988; 66: 388–96.
12. Wang PH, Lau J, Chalmers TC. Meta-analysis of effects of intensive blood glucose control on the late diabetic complications of Type 1 diabetes. Lancet 1993; 341: 1306–9.
13. Cotter MA, Cameron NE. The aetiopathogenesis of diabetic neuropathy: metabolic theories. In: Boulton AJM, ed. Diabetic Neuropathy. Lancashire: Marius Press; 1997: 97–119.
14. Cotter MA, Cameron NE. The aetiopathogenesis of diabetic neuropathy: vascular theories. In: Boulton AJM, ed. Diabetic Neuropathy. Lancashire: Marius Press; 1997: 121–46.
15. Young MJ, Boulton AJM, Williams DRR et al. A multi-centre study of the prevalence of diabetic neuropathy in patients attending UK diabetic clinics. Diabetologia 1993; 36: 150–4.
16. Abbott CA, Carrington AL, Faragher B et al. Prospective risk factors for diabetic foot ulceration in a large population sample. Diabetes 1999; 48 Suppl. 1: A78.
17. Vileikyte L, Hutchings G, Hollis S et al. The tactile circumferential discriminator: a new,

simple screening device to identify diabetic patients at risk of foot ulceration. Diabetes Care 1997; 20: 623–6.

18. Young MJ, Breddy JL, Veves A et al. The prediction of diabetic foot ulceration using vibration perception thresholds. Diabetes Care 1994; 17: 557–61.

19. DCCT Research Group. The effect of intensive diabetes therapy on the development and progression of neuropathy. Ann Intern Med 1995; 122: 561–8.

20. Navarro X, Sutherland DE, Kennedy WR. Long-term effects of pancreatic transplantation on diabetic neuropathy. Ann Neurol 1997; 42: 727–36.

21. Sidenius P, Jakobsen J. Axonal transport in human and experimental diabetes. In: Dyck PJ, Thomas PK, Asbury AK et al., eds. Diabetic Neuropathy. Philadelphia: WB Saunders; 1987: 260–5.

22. Steele JW, Faulds F, Goa KL. Epalrestat. A review of its pharmacology and therapeutic potential in late-onset complications of diabetes mellitus. Drugs Aging 1993; 3: 532–55.

23. Boulton AJM, Levin SR, Comstock JP. A multi-centre trial of the aldose reductase inhibitor, tolrestat, in patients with symptomatic diabetic neuropathy. Diabetologia 1990; 33: 431–7.

24. Ziegler D, Hanefeld M, Ruhnau KJ et al. Treatment of symptomatic diabetic peripheral neuropathy with anti-oxidant alpha-lipoic acid: a 3-week multicentre randomised controlled trial (ALADIN Study). Diabetologia 1995; 38: 1425–33.

25. Ziegler D, Reljanovic M, Mehnert H et al. Alpha-lipoic acid in the treatment of diabetic polyneuropathy in Germany: current evidence from clinical trials. Exp Clin Endocrinol Diabetes 1999; 107: 421–30.

26. Horrobin DF. Essential fatty acids in the management of impaired nerve function in diabetes. Diabetes 1997; 46 Suppl. 1: S90–93.

27. Jamal GA, Carmichael H. The effect of gamma-linolenic acid on human diabetic peripheral neuropathy: a double-blind placebo-controlled trial. Diabet Med 1990; 7: 319–23.

28. Reja A, Tesfaye S, Harris N, Ward JD. Improvement in nerve conduction and quanti-tative sensory tests after treatment with lisino-pril. Diabet Med 1995; 12: 307–9.

29. Malik RA, Williams S, Abbott C et al. Effect of angiotensin-converting-enzyme (ACE) inhibitor trandolapril on human diabetic neuropathy: randomised double-blind controlled trial. Lancet 1998; 352: 1978–81.

30. Apfel SC, Schwartz S, Adornato BT et al. Efficacy and safety of recombinant human nerve growth factor in patients with diabetic polyneuropathy: a randomised controlled trial. rhNGF Clinical Investigator Group. JAMA 2000; 284: 2215–21.

31. Boulton AJ, Drury J, Clarke B, Ward JD. Continuous subcutaneous insulin infusion in the management of painful diabetic neuropathy. Diabetes Care 1982; 5: 386–90.

32. Oyibo SO, Prasad YDM, Jackson NJ et al. The relationship between blood glucose excursions and painful diabetic peripheral neuropathy: a pilot study. Diabet Med 2002; 19: 870–3.

33. Boulton AJM. Current and emerging treatments of diabetic neuropathies. Diabetes Rev 1999; 7: 379–86.

34. Edwards AD. The role of systemic lidocaine in neuropathic pain management. J Intraven Nurs 1999; 22: 273–9.

35. Kastrup J, Petersen P, Dejgard A et al. Intravenous lidocaine infusion – a new treat-ment of chronic painful diabetic neuropathy? Pain 1987; 28: 69–75.

36. Kastrup J, Bach FW, Petersen P et al. Lidocaine treatment of painful diabetic neuropathy and endogenous opioid peptides in plasma. Clin J Pain 1989; 5: 239–44.

37. Abuaisha BB, Costanzi JB, Boulton AJM. Acupuncture for the treatment of chronic painful peripheral diabetic neuropathy: a long-term study. Diabetes Res Clin Pract 1998; 39: 115–21.

38. Hamza MA, White PF, Craig WF et al. Percutaneous electrical nerve stimulation: a novel analgesic therapy for diabetic neuropathic pain. Diabetes Care 2000; 23: 365–70.

39. Young MJ, Adams JE, Anderson GF et al. Medial arterial calcification in the feet of diabetic patients and matched non-diabetic control subjects. Diabetologia 1993; 36: 615–21.

40. Jude EB, Oyibo SO, Chalmers N, Boulton AJM. Peripheral arterial disease in diabetic and non-diabetic patients: a comparison of severity and outcome. Diabetes Care 2001; 24: 1433–7.

41. Fowkes FG, Housley E, Riemersma RA et al. Smoking, lipids, glucose intolerance, and blood pressure as risk factors for peripheral atherosclerosis compared with ischemic heart disease in the Edingburgh Artery Study. Am J Epidemiol 1991; 135: 331–40.
42. Reiber GE, Pecoraro RE, Koepsell TD. Risk factors for amputation in patients with diabetes: a case–control study. Ann Intern Med 1992; 117: 97–105.
43. Kumar S, Ashe HA, Parnell LN et al. The prevalence of foot ulceration and its correlates in Type 2 diabetic patients: a population based study. Diabet Med 1994; 11: 480–4.
44. Abbott CA, Vileikyte L, Williamson SH et al. Multi-centre study of the incidence and predictive factors for diabetic foot ulceration. Diabetes Care 1998; 21: 1071–5.
45. Reiber GE, Vileikyte L, Boyko EJ et al. Causal pathways for incident lower-extremity ulcers in patients with diabetes from two settings. Diabetes Care 1999; 22: 157–62.
46. Jeffcoate WJ, Macfarlane RM, Fletcher EM. The description and classification of diabetic foot lesions. Diabet Med 1993; 10: 676–9.
47. Lavery LA, Armstrong DG, Harkless LB. Classification of diabetic foot wounds. J Foot Ankle Surg 1996; 35: 528–31.
48. Oyibo SO, Jude EB, Tarawneh I et al. Comparison of two diabetic foot ulcer classification systems: the Wagner and the University of Texas Systems. Diabetes Care 2001; 24: 84–8.
49. Oyibo SO, Jude EB, Tarawneh I et al. The effects of ulcer size and site, patient's age, gender and type and duration of diabetes on the outcome of diabetic foot ulcers. Diabet Med 2001; 18: 133–8.
50. Grayson ML, Gibbons GW, Balogh K et al. Probing to bone in infected pedal ulcers: a clinical sign of underlying osteomyelitis in diabetic patients. JAMA 1995; 273: 721–3.
51. Mueller MJ, Diamond JE, Sinacore DR et al. Total contact casting in treatment of diabetic plantar ulcers. Controlled clinical trial. Diabetes Care 1989; 12: 384–8.
52. Burden AC, Jones R, Jones GR et al. Use of 'Scotchcast boot' in treating diabetic foot ulcers. BMJ 1983; 286: 1555–7.
53. Armstrong DG, Nguyen HC, Lavery LA et al. Offloading the diabetic foot wound: a randomised clinical trial. Diabetes Care 2001; 24: 1019–22.
54. Lipsky BA, Pecoraro RE, Larson SA et al. Outpatient management of uncomplicated lower-extremity infections in diabetic patients. Arch Intern Med 1990; 150: 790–7.
55. Venkatesan P, Lawn S, Macfarlane RM et al. Conservative management of osteomyelitis in the feet of diabetic patients. Diabet Med 1997; 14: 487–90.
56. Mason J, O'Keeffe C, McIntosh A et al. A systematic review of foot ulcers in patients with Type 2 diabetes: prevention. Diabet Med 1999; 16: 801–62.
57. Uccioli L, Aldeghi A, Faglia E et al. Manufactured shoes in the prevention of diabetic footwear. Diabetes Care 1995; 18: 1376–8.
58. Dahmen R, Haspels R, Koomen B et al. Therapeutic footwear for the neuropathic foot: an algorithm. Diabetes Care 2001; 24: 705–9.
59. Murray HJ, Young MJ, Hollis S, Boulton AJM. The association between callus formation, high pressures and neuropathy in diabetic foot ulceration. Diabet Med 1996; 13: 979–82.
60. Balkin SW, Kaplan L. Injectable silicone and the diabetic foot: a 25-year report. Foot 1991; 2: 83–8.
61. van Schie CHM, Whalley A, Vileikyte L et al. Efficacy of injected liquid silicone in the diabetic foot to reduce risk factors for foot ulceration. Diabetes Care 2000; 23: 634–8.
62. Smiell J, Wieman TJ, Steed DL et al. Efficacy and safety of Becaplermin (recombinant human platelet-derived growth factor-BB) in patients with non-healing lower extremity diabetic ulcers: a combined analysis of four randomised controlled studies. Wound Rep Regen 1999; 7: 335–46.
63. Steed DL, Donohoe D, Webster NW et al. Effect of extensive debridement and treatment on the healing of diabetic foot ulcers. J Am Coll Surg 1996; 183: 61–4.
64. Veves A, Falanga V, Armstrong DG et al. Graftskin, a human skin equivalent, is effective in the management of noninfected neuropathic diabetic foot ulcers: prospective randomised multicentre clinical trial. Diabetes Care 2001; 24: 290–5.
65. Gentzkow G, Iwasaki SD, Hershon KS et al. Use of Dermagraft, a cultured human dermis to

treat diabetic foot ulcers. Diabetes Care 1996; 19: 350–4.

66. Mansbridge J, Liu K, Patch R et al. Three-dimensional fibroblast culture implant for the treatment of diabetic foot ulcers: metabolic activity and therapeutic range. Tissue Eng 1998; 4: 403–14.

67. Mansbrige JN, Liu K, Pinney RE et al. Growth factors secreted by fibroblasts: role in healing diabetic foot ulcers. Diabetes Obes Metab 1999; 1: 265–79.

68. Gough A, Clapperton M, Rolando N et al. Randomised placebo-controlled trial of granulocyte-colony stimulating factor in diabetic foot infection. Lancet 1997; 350: 855–9.

69. Petrova A. Gipsfulung von Knochenhohlen bei Osteomyelitis. Zentral Ges Chir 1928; 43: 885.

70. Armstrong DG, Findlow A, Oyibo SO, Boulton AJM. The use of absorbable antibiotic-impregnated calcium sulphate pellets in the management of diabetic foot ulcers. Diabet Med 2001; 18: 941–2.

71. Mackey D, Varlet A, Debeaumont D. Antibiotic loaded plaster of Paris pellets: an in vitro study of a possible method of local antibiotic therapy in bone infection. Clin Orthop 1982; 167: 263–8.

72. Thomas S, Jones M, Shutler S, Jones S. Using larvae in modern wound management. J Wound Care 1996; 5: 60–9.

73. Thomas S. New drugs for diabetic foot ulcers: larval therapy. In: Boulton AJM, Connor H, Cavanagh PR, eds. The Foot in Diabetes, 3rd ed. Chichester: John Wiley & Son; 2000: 185–191.

74. Casu RE, Eisemann CH, Vuoclo T, Tellman RL. The major excretory/secretory protease from Lucilia cuprina larvae is also gut digestive protease. Int J Parasitol 1996; 26: 623–8.

75. Schindl A, Schindl M, Pernerstorfer-Schon H et al. Diabetic neuropathic foot ulcer: successful treatment by low-intensity laser therapy. Dermatology 1999; 198: 314–16.

76. Forney R, Mauro T. Using lasers in diabetic wound healing. Diabetes Technol Ther 1999; 1: 189–92.

77. Schindl A, Schindl M, Schon H et al. Low-intensity laser irradiation improves skin circulation in patients with diabetic microangiopathy. Diabetes Care 1998; 21: 580–4.

78. Nwomeh BC, Yager DR, Cohen IK. Physiology of the chronic wound. Clin Plastic Surg 1998; 25: 341–56.

79. Zamboni WA, Wong HP, Stephenson LL et al. Evaluation of hyperbaric oxygen for diabetic wounds: a prospective study. Undersea Hyperb Med 1997; 24: 175–9.

80. Bakker DJ. Hyperbaric oxygen therapy and the diabetic foot. Diabetes Metab Res Rev 2000; 16 (Suppl. 1): S55–S58.

81. Schultz LS, Ferguson RM, Pliam MB et al. Retrograde perfusion as a method for myocardial revascularisation. Eur Surg Res 1976; 8: 358–76.

82. Usui A, Hotta T, Hiroura M et al. Cerebral metabolism and function during normothermic retrograde cerebral perfusion. Cardiovasc Surg 1993; 1: 107–12.

83. Scheffler A, Friedrichs EA, Reiger H. Use of retrograde venous perfusion in patients with advanced peripheral arterial occlusive disease. Vasa 1991; 20: 274–9.

84. Siedel C, Richter UG, Buhler S, Hornstein OP. Drug therapy of the diabetic neuropathic foot ulcer: transvenous retrograde perfusion versus systemic regimen. Vasa 1991; 20: 388–93.

85. Buhler-Singer S, Hiller D, Boateng B et al. Disordered cutaneous microcirculation in the diabetic foot. Is modification by retrograde transvenous perfusion therapy possible? Hautarzt 1995; 46: 400–5.

86. Sanders LJ, Frykberg RG, Diabetic neuropathic osteoarthropathy: the Charcot foot. In: Frykberg RG, ed. The High Risk Foot in Diabetes Mellitus. New York: Churchill Livingstone; 1991: 297–338.

87. Cavanagh PR, Young MJ, Adams JE et al. Radiographic abnormalities in the feet of patients with diabetic neuropathy. Diabetes Care 1994; 17: 209–10.

88. Boulton AJM, Scarpello JH, Ward JD. Venous oxygenation in the diabetic foot: evidence of arteriovenous shunting? Diabetologia 1982; 22: 6–8.

89. Edmonds ME, Clarke MB, Newton S et al. Increased uptake of bone radiopharmaceutical in diabetic neuropathy. Q J Med 1985; 57: 843–55.

90. Jude EB, Boulton AJM. End stage complications of diabetic neuropathy. Diabetes Rev 1999; 7: 395–410.

91. Armstrong DG, Todd WF, Lavery LA et al. The natural history of acute Charcot's arthropathy in a diabetic foot specialty clinic. Diabet Med 1997; 14: 357–63.

92. Selby PL, Young MJ, Adams JE, Boulton AJM. Bisphosphonate: a new treatment for diabetic Charcot neuroarthropathy. Diabet Med 1994; 11: 14–20.

93. Jude EB, Page S, Donohue M et al. Pamidronate in diabetic Charcot neuroarthropathy: a randomised placebo-controlled trial. Diabetologia 2001; 44: 2032–7.

94. Litzelman DK, Slemenda CW, Langfeld CD et al. Reduction of lower extremity clinical abnormalities in patients with non-insulin dependent diabetes mellitus: a randomised controlled trial. Ann Intern Med 1993; 119: 36–41.

95. Dargis V, Pantelejeva O, Jonushaite A et al. Benefits of a multidisciplinary approach in the management of recurrent diabetic foot ulceration in Lithuania: a prospective study. Diabetes Care 1999; 22: 1428–31.

96. WHO/IDF Europe. Diabetes care and research in Europe: the St. Vincent declaration. Diabet Med 1990; 7: 360.

12

Sexual dysfunction in diabetes
Dan Ziegler

Epidemiology of erectile dysfunction

Male erectile dysfunction (ED), defined as 'the inability to achieve or maintain an erection sufficient for sexual intercourse',[1] is one of the most common sexual dysfunctions in men. ED is more common with advancing age, and since the aged population will increase, its prevalence will continue to rise.[2] Diabetes mellitus is the most frequent organic cause for ED, the onset of which starts about 15 years earlier in the diabetic than in the non-diabetic population. In the Massachusetts Male Aging Study (MMAS), the age-adjusted prevalence of minimal, moderate, or complete ED was 17%, 25%, and 10% among 1238 non-diabetic men and 8%, 30%, and 25% among 52 treated diabetic men, respectively.[3] Thus, although the number of diabetic subjects in the MMAS was low, this population-based study showed an increased prevalence, particularly of complete ED among men with diabetes. The crude incidence rate of ED in the MMAS was 26 cases/1000 man-years in 847 men aged 40–69 without ED at baseline who were followed for an average of 8.8 years.[4] Population projections for men in this age group suggest an estimate of 618,000 new cases of ED per year for the USA. The age-adjusted risk of ED was higher for men with lower education, diabetes, heart disease, and hypertension. The incidence rate of ED in diabetic men was increased two-fold, with 50 cases/1000 man-years.

In a population-based study from southern Wisconsin, the prevalence of ED among 365 Type 1 diabetic patients increased with age from 1.1% in those aged 21–30 years to 47.1% in those 43 years of age or older and with increasing duration of diabetes.[5] In a recent study from Italy including 9868 men with diabetes, 45.5% of those aged >59 years reported ED. Risk factors and clinical correlates included the following (OR [95%CI]): autonomic neuropathy (5.0 [3.9–6.4]), diabetic foot (4.0 [2.9–5.5]), peripheral neuropathy (3.3 [2.9–3.8]), peripheral arterial disease (2.8 [2.4–3.3]), nephropathy (2.3 [1.9–2.8]), poor glycaemic control (2.3 [2.0–2.6]), retinopathy (2.2 [2.0–2.4]), hypertension (2.1 [1.6–2.9]), and diabetes duration (2.0 [1.8–2.2]).[6] In another survey from Italy the combination of diabetes and hypertension was the major risk factor for ED, giving an OR (95%CI) of 8.1 (1.2–55.0) as compared with diabetes without hypertension 4.6 (1.6–13.7), hypertension without diabetes 1.4 (0.7–3.2), current smoking 1.7 (1.2–2.4), and ex-smoking 1.6 (1.1–2.3).[7] However, even when neuropathic complications are present, psychiatric illness such as generalized anxiety disorder or depression may be important contributors to ED in men with diabetes.[8] Thus, a psychogenic component must not be overlooked in many patients.

Physiology and pathophysiology

Penile erection is a neurovascular event modulated by psychological factors and hormonal status depending on appropriate trabecular smooth muscle and arterial relaxation in the corpus cavernosum. On sexual stimulation, nerve impulses cause the release of cholinergic and non-cholinergic non-adrenergic (NANC) neurotransmitters that mediate erectile function by relaxing the smooth muscle of the corpus cavernosum. A principal neural mediator of erection is nitric oxide (NO) which activates guanylate cyclase to form intracellular cyclic guanosine monophosphate (GMP), a potent second messenger for smooth muscle

relaxation (Figure 12.1). Cyclic GMP in turn activates a specific protein kinase, which phosphorylates certain proteins and ion channels, resulting in a drop in cytosolic calcium concentrations and relaxation of the smooth muscle. During the return to the flaccid state, cyclic GMP is hydrolyzed by phosphodiesterase type 5 (PDE5).[2,9] In the corpus cavernosum four PDE isoforms have been identified (types 2, 3, 4 and 5). PDE5 is the predominant isoform, the others do not appear to have an important role in erection.[9]

The pathogenesis of ED in diabetes is multifactorial as it may be linked to neuropathy, accelerated atherosclerosis, and alterations in the corporal erectile tissue. Such alterations may include smooth muscle degeneration, abnormal collagen deposition, and endothelial

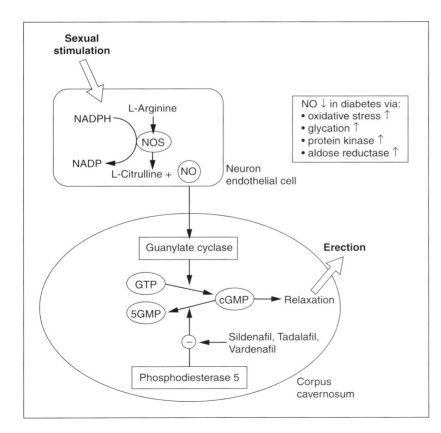

Figure 12.1
Mechanisms of erection mediated by cavernosal smooth muscle relaxation including the generation of nitric oxide (NO) by nitric oxide synthase (NOS), which is impaired in diabetes. Notes: ROS: reactive oxygen species, PKC: protein kinase C, AR: aldose reductase.

cell dysfunction.[10] If irreversible, these corporal degenerative changes can limit the success of any pharmacotherapy. Advanced glycation end products (AGEs) have been shown to quench NO and to be elevated in human diabetic penile tissue. It has been hypothesized that AGEs may mediate ED via upregulation of inducible nitric oxide synthase (iNOS) and downregulation of endothelial NOS (eNOS).[11] Furthermore, protein kinase C activation by diabetes may reduce NOS activity.[12]

In vivo studies of isolated corpus cavernosum tissue from diabetic men have shown functional impairment in neurogenic and endothelium-dependent relaxation of corpus cavernosum smooth muscle.[13] In diabetic rats, endothelium-dependent NO mediated relaxation to acetylcholine and NANC stimulation are reduced by 40% after 4–8 weeks.[14] These alterations were prevented by administration of the antioxidant α-lipoic acid, suggesting an involvement of increased oxidative stress. In contrast, endothelium-independent relaxation to the NO donor sodium nitroprusside is not impaired by diabetes.[14] Increased penile endothelial and total NOS activity was found after two to three months in diabetic rats.[15] After four to eight months, however, reduced penile total (endothelial and neuronal) NOS activity and neuronal NOS levels were observed in Type 1 and Type 2 diabetic rats.[16] Thus, diabetes-induced changes in NOS activity may be biphasic, with an initial increase followed by a decrease. Finally, an increased rate of apoptosis in corpus cavernosum was recently described in diabetic rats.[17]

Diagnosis of erectile dysfunction

A good clinical history and physical examination are the basis of assessment. It is important to establish the nature of the erectile problem and to distinguish it from other forms of sexual difficulty such as penile curvature or premature ejaculation. An interview with the partner is advisable and will confirm the problem but may also reveal other causes of the difficulties e.g. vaginal dryness. The relative importance of psychological and organic factors may be determined from the history. Drugs which may be associated with ED include tranquilizers (phenothiazines, benzodiazepines), antidepressants (tricyclics, selective serotonin reuptake inhibitors), and antihypertensives (β-blockers, vasodilators, central sympathomimetics, ganglion blockers, diuretics, ACE-inhibitors).[18] In most patients sophisticated investigation is not indicated. A three-step diagnostic approach follows:

Step 1: general sexual history;
  clinical examination; relevant laboratory parameters;
  information about treatment options.
Step 2: therapeutic trial with Sildenafil.
Step 3: intracavernous pharmacotesting: colour Doppler or duplex ultrasound of penile arteries.

A detailed history is most important, and for many patients examination can be limited to the regular monitoring of diabetes and its risk factors and complications as well as examination of the genitalia. Patients should be informed about the advantages and disadvantages of each treatment and given advice on treatment outcome and ease of use.[19]

Other sexual problems in men

Diminished or absent testicular pain has been described as an early sign of autonomic neuropathy. Retrograde ejaculation from the prostatic urethra into the bladder may occur occasionally and follows loss of sympathetic innervation of the internal sphincter which normally contracts during ejaculation. Complete loss of ejaculation probably indicates widespread pelvic sympathetic involvement and, like retrograde ejaculation, causes infertility which may be treated by insemination.[20]

Female sexual dysfunction

The scientific knowledge on sexual dysfunction in women with diabetes is rudimentary. Problems affecting sexuality in diabetic women are fatigue, changes in perimenstrual blood glucose control, vaginitis, decreased sexual desire, decreased vaginal lubrication, and an increased time to reach orgasm. Even minor episodes of depression which is twice more frequent than in men can result in a loss of libido. The degree to which these symptoms are related to autonomic neuropathy has also been examined in a few studies, with varying results. The examination for a diabetic woman with sexual dysfunction should include the duration of symptoms, psychological state, concomitant medications, presence of vaginitis, cystitis, and other infections, frequency of intercourse, blood pressure, BMI, retinal status, pelvic examination, presence of discharge, and glycemic control.[21]

General management	Control of risk factors and diabetes; sexual counseling	
Pharmacological treatment	First-line therapy	Dose range
	Sildenafil (Viagra®)	50–100 mg
	[Tadalafil]*	10–20 mg
	[Vardenafil]*	10–20 mg
	Apomorphine (Uprima®, Ixense®)**	2–4 mg s.l.
	Oral therapy inappropriate	
	Transurethral alprostadil (MUSE)	500–1000 µg
	Intracavernosal injection therapy:	
	Alprostadil (Caverject®)	5–20 µg
	Papaverine/phentolamine (Androskat®)	
	Thymoxamine (Erecnos®)	10–20 mg
	VIP/phentolamine (Invicorp®)	
	Papaverine/phentolamine/alprostadil (Trimix®)	
Surgery and mechanical treatments	Pharmacological therapy inappropriate	
	Vacuum devices	
	Arterial/venous surgery	
	Penile prostheses	

Notes:
*Market approval expected in 2003
**Only marginally effective in unselected diabetic patients

Table 12.1
Stepwise algorithm for treatment of erectile dysfunction

Management of erectile dysfunction

A stepwise therapeutic approach for ED is shown in Table 12.1. The initial management should advise the patient to reduce possible risk factors and to optimize glycemic control. However, no studies are available to show that improvement in glycemic control will exert a favorable effect on ED. In fact, a recent study could not demonstrate an effect of intensive diabetes therapy maintained for two years on ED in Type 2 diabetic men.[22] Even if the cause is organic, almost all men with ED will be affected psychologically. Sexual counseling is an important aspect of any treatment, and it is preferable to also involve the partner.

Oral agents

Most men consider this to be the treatment of choice. The oral treatment options and their mechansims of action are summarized as follows:

(1) *Central mechanism of action*
  - Yohimbine (α_2 adrenergic antagonist)
  - Apomorphine (dopamine receptor antagonist)
(2) *Peripheral mechanism of action*
  - Phentolamine (non-selective adrenergic antagonist)
  - Phosphodiesterase isoenzyme type 5 inhibitors:
    – sildenafil
    – tadalafil
    – vardenafil.

Central initiators

Yohimbine
Yohimbine was the first drug officially listed for this indication. Yohimbine acts via central alpha-2-receptor blockade and thus increases the centrally initiated efferences of the erectogenic axis. Although its effectivity is often debated due to insufficient historic data, it showed a significant effect in a recent double blind prospective study compared with placebo. Its side effect profile is benign, including palpitations, tremor, hypertension, and anxiety. The pro-erectile effect usually starts after about two weeks.[23] In a meta-analysis, yohimbine has been found to be more effective than placebo for all types of ED combined, but the effect was most prominent in non-organic ED.[24] Because of its marginal effect on organic ED, yohimbine cannot be generally recommended for treatment of ED in diabetic men.

Apomorphine (Uprima®, Ixense®)
Apomorphine is a potent emetic agent that acts via central dopaminergic (D1 or D2) receptors as well as central μ-, δ-, and κ-receptors. In the hypothalamus, it increases the centrally initiated efferences of the erectogenic axis thus improving the erectile response in a patient with erectile failure.[25] The mechanism of action for apomorphine is illustrated in Figure 12.2. In large multicenter studies, a pro-erectile effect with full erections was observed after sublingual doses of 2, 4 and 6 mg apomorphine with an acceptable and dose-dependent rate of nausea side effects. A dose-dependent efficacy (defined as erections allowing intercourse/attempts) of 48–66% versus 37% for placebo was observed. Similarly, side effects were also strongly dose-dependent: nausea was seen in 0.4 to 17% (versus 0.2–0.4% for placebo), hypotension in 0.7–4.8% and syncope in 0.7–2.1%. These side effects tended to disappear in frequency and intensity with increasing use of the medication in an individual patient. There was no effect of apomorphine on mood and desire.[26,27]

A four-week multicenter, crossover, placebo-controlled trial using the sublingual formulation of apomorphine (Uprima®) evaluated 90

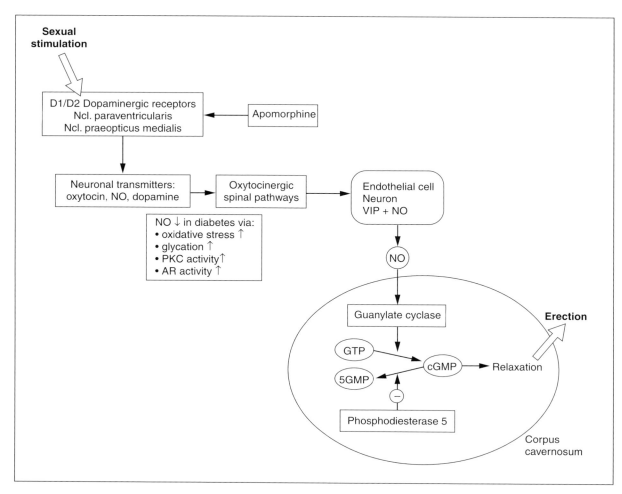

Figure 12.2
Mechanism of action for apomorphine.

diabetic patients on the 4 mg dose and 86 patients on the 5 mg dose. The percentages of attempts resulting in an erection firm enough for intercourse (primary end point) were 14.5 and 24.6% for placebo and 4 mg, respectively ($p = 0.02$) and 27.2 and 34.1% for placebo and 5 mg, respectively ($p = 0.18$). In the post-hoc combined analysis the corresponding rates were 20.4 and 28.9%, respectively ($p = 0.009$).

Thus, no dose response could be demonstrated in this trial. The Food and Drug Administration (FDA) concluded from these data that even though the 4 mg dose and the combined analysis showed statistical significance, the clinical significance is questionable due to the relatively modest benefits noted over placebo.[28] Indeed, the number needed to treat (NNT) for the 4 mg dose based on the aforementioned results is relatively high, i.e. ten patients need to be treated in order to achieve an erection firm enough for intercourse in one. The rates of nausea, the most prominent adverse effect of apomorphine, were 21.2%, 12.9% and 1.0% for 4 mg, 5 mg, and placebo, respectively. The corresponding rates of vomiting were 6.7%, 1.0% and 0%, respectively. Moreover, three syncopal events and three episodes of significant hypotension were reported in patients taking apomorphine.[28]

Peripheral conditioners

Phosphodiesterase 5 inhibitors

Sildenafil (Viagra®)

To understand the mode of action of sildenafil, a drug believed to act predominantly via PDE5 inhibition, the basic physiology is briefly explained: cAMP and cGMP are synthesized from the corresponding nucleoside triphosphates by their respective membrane-bound or -soluble adenylate or guanylate cyclases. cAMP and cGMP are inactivated by phosphodiesterases (PDE) by hydrolytic cleavage of the 3′-ribose-phosphate bond (see Figure 12.1). Because the distribution and functional role of PDE isoenzymes varies in different tissues, selective inhibitors have the potential to exert at least partially specific tissue effects. Currently, over 40 PDE-isoenzymes and -isoforms are known. In recent experiments by Küthe et al, expression of the following phosphodiesterase isoenzyme and isoform genes were detected in human cavernous tissue: PDE1A, PDE1B, PDE1C, PDE2, PDE3A, PDE4A, PDE4B, PDE4C, PDE4D, PDE5, PDE7, PDE8 and PDE9.[29] The functional assays reveal a predominant functional role for PDE3 and 5.[30] There was no difference in PDE-expression in diabetic compared with non-diabetic patients with erectile dysfunction.

Sildenafil acts as conditioner on the cavernous smooth muscle side by blocking PDE5. It is the first effective oral drug that has been approved for the treatment of ED and is generally regarded as a first-line treatment of ED of various causes including diabetes. Sildenafil is taken 60 min before anticipated sexual activity and its effects last approximately four hours. The drug is available in three doses (25, 50, or 100 mg). lt does not stimulate sexual desire and provoke an erection as such, but enhances the continued relaxation of the cavernous smooth muscle initiated by the release of endogenous nitric oxide with an improved quality of erection (Figure 12.1).

In a controlled, flexible-dose US multicenter trial including a mixed group of 268 Type 1 and Type 2 diabetic men, the rates of those with improved erections after 12 weeks of treatment with 25–100 mg sildenafil were 56% as compared with 10% in the placebo group.[31] In a 12-week European multicenter trial including 219 Type 2 diabetic men the response rate was even higher achieving 64.6% on sildenafil versus 10.5% on placebo.[32] The estimated percentages of intercourse attempts that were successful significantly improved from baseline to end of treatment in patients receiving sildenafil (14.4% to 58.8%) compared with those receiving placebo (13.2% to 14.4%). Three-quarters of the patients required the 100 mg sildenafil dose. The response rates were independent of the baseline HbA1c levels and number of chronic complications, suggesting that sildenafil is effective in improving ED even in cases with poor glycemic control and in the presence of angiopathy and neuropathy. In a combined analysis of 11 controlled trials of sildenafil (25–100 mg) the percentages of the maximum score for the six questions in the erectile function domain of the International Index of Erectile Function (IIEF) were 61.3% among 69 Type 1 and 60.8% among 399 Type 1 diabetic men on sildenafil as compared to 39.3% among 452 diabetic men on placebo.[33]

Side effects consist mainly of headache (18%), facial flushing (15%), and dyspepsia (2%). A mild and transient disturbance of color vision and also increased sensitivity to light or blurred vision has been found in 4.5% of diabetic men.[32] Concerns have been expressed regarding an increased number of deaths associated with sildenafil as compared with other treatments for ED.[34] However, after an average follow-up of six months the Prescription Event Monitoring (PEM) Study including 5601 sildenafil users from England showed an expected mortality rate of 28.9 per 1000/year for ischemic heart disease (IHD)/myocardial infarctions (MI). The comparison rate in the general population of England in 1998 was 73.9 per 1000/year.[35] The prevalence of diabetes in the cohort was 15%, which is similar to the rate of 16% included in the clinical trials of sildenafil, but much higher than the rate of 3.3% of men with diabetes in England in 1998. Although these results are reassuring, further follow-up of this study and other pharmaco-epidemiological research is needed for confirmation. In men with severe stenosis of at least one coronary artery, acute administration of sildenafil (100 mg) did not result in adverse hemodynamic effects on coronary blood flow or vascular resistance, but coronary flow reserve was improved.[36]

Apart from its effect on ED, favorable effects of sildenafil have recently been reported in pilot studies of various disorders, including primary pulmonary hypertension, achalasia, and endothelial dysfunction. The endothelium modulates the actual and demand vascular tone, the antithrombotic and antiadhesive properties of the vessel wall, vascular wall architecture, and vascular permeability. Endothelial dysfunction is regarded as an early key event in the development of atherosclerosis which is accelerated in diabetes. It has recently been demonstrated that erectile and endothelial dysfunction are associated in Type 2 diabetic patients. Plasma concentrations of markers for endothelial dysfunction such as soluble thrombomodulin, P-selectin, and intercellular cell adhesion molecules-1 (ICAM-1) were significantly elevated in Type 2 diabetic patients with ED compared to those without ED and were inversely related to the IIEF.[37] Endothelium-dependent flow-mediated dilatation (FMD) induced by 5 min occlusion of the brachial artery measured by ultrasound imaging is a reliable index of endothelial function that is impaired in diabetic patients. In a recent controlled crossover trial acute (25 mg) and chronic (25 mg/day for two weeks) administration of sildenafil (25 mg) improved endothelial function as compared with placebo in Type 2 diabetic patients, suggesting that PDE-5 inhibition may exert favorable cardiovascular effects.[38] Likewise, in patients with heart failure who frequently show endothelial dysfunction, the latter was improved after single-dose administration of 25 and 50 mg sildenafil, respectively.[39] These findings require further confirmation in larger studies.

According to the recommendations of the American Heart Association, sildenafil is contraindicated in men taking nitrates due to the risk of hypotension and those with severe cardiovascular disease. Before sildenafil is prescribed, treadmill testing may be indicated in men with heart disease to assess the risk of cardiac ischemia during sexual intercourse. Initial monitoring of blood pressure after the administration of sildenafil may be indicated in men with congestive heart disease with low borderline blood pressure and low volume status and men being treated with complicated, multidrug antihypertensive regimens.[40] Because sildenafil treatment is costly and ED is not a life-threatening illness, the appropriateness of insurance coverage for sildenafil has been questioned. However, recent cost-effectiveness studies using cost per quality-adjusted life-year (QALY) gained as outcome measures have shown that sildenafil treatment compared favorably with intracavernosal injection therapy[41] or with accepted therapies for other medical conditions.[42]

Tadalafil (Cialis®)

In a 12-week multicenter trial including 216 diabetic men (Type 2, 91%), but excluding sildenafil non-responders, the rates of men with improved erections were 64% with 20 mg tadalafil, 56% with 10 mg tadalafil, and 25% on placebo.[43] Both tadalafil 10 mg and 20 mg were superior to placebo in improving penetration ability (IIEF question 3) and ability to maintain an erection during intercourse. Thus, although non-responders to sildenafil were excluded, the effect of tadalafil was not superior to that of sildenafil. Treatment-related adverse events (>5%) on 20 mg, 10 mg, and placebo were dyspepsia (8.3, 11.0 and 0%) and headache (6.9, 8.2 and 1.4%).

Vardenafil (Nuviva®)

In a recent large 12-week multicenter trial including 439 diabetic men (Type 2, 88%) that excluded sildenafil non-responders, the rates of men with improved erections were 72% with 20 mg vardenafil, 57% with 10 mg vardenafil, and 13% with placebo.[44] Both vardenafil 10 mg and 20 mg were superior to placebo in improving the IIEF erectile function domain score (questions 1–5, 15). Similar to tadalafil, despite the exclusion of non-responders to sildenafil the effect of vardenafil was comparable to that reported previously for sildenafil. Treatment-related adverse events (>5%) on 20 mg, 10 mg, and placebo were headache (10, 9 and 2%), flushing (10, 9 and <1%), and headache (6, 3 and 0%).

Phentolamine (Vasomax®)

The non-selective alpha-blocking agent phentolamine was evaluated for a possible beneficial effect on the erectile behavior. In prospective, randomized, double blind studies, a beneficial effect of orally administered fast-resolving phentolamine on the erectile capacity of men with erectile dysfunction was shown. These beneficial effects were more pronounced in elderly men. The side effect profile of this drug, introduced decades ago for other indications, seems to be safe, with stuffy nose and some hypotension being the most frequent complaints. However, published data are minimal so that a thorough evaluation is not possible at the present time.[45]

Vacuum devices

These have the merit of being non-invasive and may be effective in all men. They create a vacuum around the penis and blood is drawn into the corporal spaces. A band is slipped off the plastic cylinder around the base of the penis to maintain penile tumescence without rigidity in the crura. The disadvantages are that they require some degree of dexterity in handling them, and some time spent in application of the device. They should only be used for 30 min at a time, and require the willing cooperation of the partner. There are few side effects, although there is some degree of discomfort and the penis feels cold. Ejaculation is usually blocked and some men find that this makes orgasm less satisfactory. Bruising can occur in 10–15% of men. Vacuum devices are particularly useful in older men in stable relationships and when other treatment options are ineffective. They may also be used to augment the result of pharmacotherapy. Some men find that the constrictive ring is a useful aid in itself for maintaining the erection without the use of a vacuum device.[18] However, the long-term dropout rates among users of vacuum constriction devices are relatively high. A recent study showed an overall drop-out rate over three years for the ErecAid® system of 65%, i.e. 100% in men with mild ED, 56% in those with moderate ED, and 70% in those with complete ED. The main reasons for stopping use were that the device was ineffective (57%), too cumbersome (24%), and too painful (20%).[46]

Transurethral alprostadil

Alprostadil was first licensed for the treatment of erectile dysfunction by intracavernous injection. Alprostadil, the synthetic preparation of the naturally occurring prostaglandin E1 acts by initiating the erection. In contrast to sildenafil, it initiates the relaxation of cavernous smooth muscle to bring about erection. This drug has been incorporated into a pellet that can be given by intraurethral application: MUSE (Medical Urethral System for Erection). Patients need to be instructed in the use of MUSE which is introduced into the urethra with a disposable applicator. The patient first passes urine to act as a lubricant to facilitate the passage of the applicator and the absorption of the drug. Absorption of the drug is also facilitated by the patient rolling his penis between the palms of his hands. Some patients find that a constrictive ring around the base of the penis enhances the efficacy. The erection takes about ten minutes to develop and the dose range varies between 125 and 1000 µg although the majority of patients require 500 or 1000 µg. The use of MUSE is contraindicated without a condom when the partner is pregnant or likely to conceive.[18]

In the US and European multicenter trials, about 65% of men with different causes of ED who tried MUSE had erections sufficient for intercourse during in-clinic testing.[47,48] About one-half of the treatments at home were successful, but the drop-out rate after 15 months was 75%, the main reason being lack of efficacy.[48] The most common side effects are penile pain (30%), urethral burning (12%) or minor urethral bleeding (5%).[49] Systemic side effects (such as hypotension or even syncope) were usually uncommon but help to highlight the role of the physician in administering the first supervised dose. Disappointing results have recently been reported in a study conducted in a urology practice setting, in which an adequate rigidity score was achieved in only 13 and 30% of the patients using 500 and 1000 µg, respectively. Pain, discomfort, or burning in the penis were observed in 18%, but orthostatic hypotension (defined as a decrease in systolic/diastolic blood pressure by 20/10 mmHg or orthostatic symptoms) was present in 41% of the patients. The discontinuation rate was very high, achieving 81% after 2–3 months.[50]

Intracavernosal injection therapy

Intracavernosal therapy requires some specialist knowledge and the ability to treat priapism should it occur. Many specialists used to regard this as the standard treatment and use it for both diagnostic and therapeutic reasons although its role as first-line therapy has been replaced by less invasive treatment modalities. Patients need to be taught how to perform self-injection and the dose needs to be chosen carefully to avoid prolonged erections or priapism. Some patients find it helpful to use one of the many autoinjector devices available. The erection occurs after ten minutes and may be enhanced by sexual stimulation. The incidence of complications varies with the different pharmacological agents. Some pain is not uncommon but long-term problems are limited to priapism or penile fibrosis.

Alprostadil is the most widely used agent.[51,52] It is effective in more than 80% of patients with different etiologies of ED and has a low incidence of side effects. In a recent comparative study of intracavernosal versus intraurethral administration of alprostadil, the rates of erections sufficient for sexual intercourse were 82.5 versus 53.0%, respectively.[52] Patient and partner satisfaction was higher with intracavernosal injection, and more patients preferred this therapy. Penile pain occurs in 15–50% of patients but is often not troublesome. The dose range is 5–20 µg but some physicians will increase it further or use a combination with papaverine and phentolamine. Priapism occurs in about 1% of patients. The cumulative incidence of penile fibrosis was 11.7% after a period of four years, and the risk of irreversible fibrotic alterations was 5%.[53] About half of the cases with fibrosis resolved spontaneously. Other less frequently used agents include thymoxamine (moxisylyte hydrocholoride [Erecnos®]), papaverine/phentolamine mixtures, (Androskat®), papaverine/phentolamine/ alprostadil mixtures (Trimix®), and VIP/phentolamine (Invicorp®).

Penile prostheses and surgery

This type of treatment is carried out only after careful patient selection and a trial of the less invasive options. There are a number of different devices ranging from the simple malleable prosthesis to more complex hydraulic prostheses. The choice of prosthesis is very much dependent upon the wishes of the patient and is often cost-related. A prosthesis does not restore a normal erection but makes the penis rigid enough for sexual intercourse. The hydraulic prostheses have the advantage of flaccidity and are now mechanically reliable with revision rates of less than 5% per annum. Infection remains a major complication in approximately 3–5% of cases with different

causes of ED and usually leads to removal of the device.[18]

Arterial reconstruction is associated with complication rates of more than 30% and remains an experimental procedure which cannot be generally recommended to diabetic patients with ED.

References

1. NIH consensus development panel on impotence. Impotence. JAMA 1993; 270: 83–90.
2. Wagner G, Saenz de Tejada I. Update on male erectile dysfunction. BMJ 1998; 316: 678–82.
3. Feldman HA, Goldstein I, Hatzichristou DG et al. Impotence and its medical and psychosocial correlates: results of the Massachusetts Male Ageing Study. J Urol 1994; 151: 54–61.
4. Johannes CB, Araujo AB, Feldman HA et al. Incidence of erectile dysfunction in men 40 to 69 years old: longitudinal results from the Massachusetts Male Aging Study. J Urol 2000; 163: 460–3.
5. Klein R, Klein BE, Lee KE et al. Prevalence of self-reported erectile dysfunction in people with long-term IDDM. Diabetes Care 1996; 19: 135–41.
6. Fedele D, Coscelli C, Santeusanio F et al. Erectile dysfunction in diabetic subjects in Italy. Diabetes Care 1998; 21: 1973–7.
7. Parazzini F, Menchini FF, Bortolotti A et al. Frequency and determinants of erectile dysfunction in Italy. Eur Urol 2000; 37: 43–9.
8. Lustman PJ, Clouse RE. Relationship of psychiatric illness to impotence in men with diabetes. Diabetes Care 1990; 13: 893–5.
9. Lue TF. Erectile dysfunction. N Engl J Med 2000; 342: 1802–13.
10. Saenz de Tejada I, Goldstein I. Diabetic penile neuropathy. Urol Clin North Am 1988; 15: 17–22.
11. Seftel AD, Vaziri ND, Ni Z et al. Advanced glycation end products in human penis: elevation in diabetic tissue, site of deposition, and possible effect through iNOS or eNOS. Urology 1997; 50: 1016–26.
12. Hirata K, Kuroda R, Sakoda T et al. Inhibition

of endothelial nitric oxide synthase activity by protein kinase C. Hypertension 1995; 25: 180–5.

13. Saenz de Tejada I, Goldstein I et al. Impaired neurogenic and endothelium-mediated relaxation of penile smooth muscle from diabetic men with impotence. N Engl J Med 1989; 320: 1025–30.

14. Keegan A, Cotter MA, Cameron NE. Effects of diabetes and treatment with the antioxidant α-lipoic acid on endothelial and neurogenic responses of corpus cavernosum in rats. Diabetologia 1999; 42: 343–50.

15. Elabbady AA, Gagnon C, Hassouna MM et al. Diabetes mellitus increases nitric oxide synthase in penises but not in major pelvic ganglia of rats. Br J Urol 1995; 76: 196–202.

16. Vernet D, Cai L, Garban H et al. Reduction of penile nitric oxide synthase in diabetic BB/WORdp (type I) and BBZ/WORdp (type II) rats with erectile dysfunction. Endocrinology 1995; 136: 5709–17.

17. Alici B, Gumustas MK, Ozkara H et al. Apoptosis in the erectile tissues of diabetic and healthy rats. Br J Urol Int 2000; 85: 326–9.

18. European Society for Impotence Research. Erectile Dysfunction: A Physicians' Guide to the Management of Erectile Dysfunction, 1998.

19. Ralph D, McNicholas T. UK management guidelines for erectile dysfunction. BMJ 2000; 321: 499–503.

20. Ewing DJ, Clarke BF. Diabetic autonomic neuropathy: present insights and future prospects. Diabetes Care 1986; 9: 648–65.

21. Jovanovic L. Sex and the woman with diabetes: desire versus dysfunction. IDF Bulletin 1998; 43: 23–8.

22. Azad N, Emanuele NV, Abraira C et al. The effects of intensive glycemic control on neuropathy in the VA Cooperative Study on Type II diabetes mellitus. J Diabetes Complications 2000; 13: 307–13.

23. Vogt HJ, Brandl P, Kockott G et al. Double-blind, placebo-controlled safety and efficacy trial with yohimbine hydrochloride in the treatment of nonorganic erectile dysfunction. Int J Impot Res 1997; 9: 155–61.

24. Ernst E, Pittler MH. Yohimbine for erectile dysfunction: a systematic review and meta-analysis of randomized clinical trials. J Urol 1998; 159: 433–6.

25. Rampin O, Bernabe J, Guilano F. Spinal control of penile erection. World J Urol 1997; 15: 2–13.

26. Padma-Nathan H, Auerbach S, Lewis R et al. Efficacy and safety of apomorphine versus placebo for male erectile dysfunction. J Urol 1999; 161: 821.

27. Lewis R, Agre K, Rudd D. Efficacy of Apomorphine versus placebo for erectile dysfunction in patients with hypertension. J Urol 1999; 161: 822.

28. Reproductive Health Drugs Advisory Committee. Urology Subcommittee. FDA briefing package, 2000; April 10: 42–110.

29. Küthe A, Wiedentoth A, Stief C et al. Identification of 13 PDE isoforms in human cavernous tissue. Eur Urol 1999; 35: 404.

30. Taher A, Stief CG, Raida M et al. Cyclic nucleotide phosphodiesterase activity in human cavernous smooth muscle and the effect of various selective inhibitors. Int J Impot Res 1992, 4 Suppl. 2: 11.

31. Rendell MS, Rajfer J, Wicker PA, Smith MD. Sildenafil for treatment of erectile dysfunction in men with diabetes: a randomized controlled trial. Sildenafil Diabetes Study Group [see comments]. JAMA 1999; 281: 421–6.

32. Boulton AJM, Selam J-L, Sweeney M, Ziegler D. Sildenafil citrate for the treatment of erectile dysfunction in men with type II diabetes mellitus. Diabetologia 2001; 44: 1296–301.

33. Sellam R, Ziegler D, Boulton AJM. Sildenafil citrate is effective and well tolerated for the treatment of erectile dysfunction in men with Type 1 or Type 2 diabetes mellitus. Diabetologia 2000; 43, Suppl 1: A253 (Abstract).

34. Mitka M. Some men who take Viagra die – Why? JAMA 2000; 283: 590–3.

35. Shakir SAW, Wilton LV, Boshier A et al. Cardiovascular events in users of sildenafil: results from first phase of prescription event monitoring in England. BMJ 2001; 322: 651–2.

36. Herrmann HC, Chang G, Klugherz BD, Mahoney PD. Hemodynamic effects of sildenafil in men with severe coronary artery disease. N Engl J Med 2000; 342: 1622–6.

37. De Angelis L, Marfella MA, Siniscalchi M et al. Erectile and endothelial dysfunction in Type II diabetes: a possible link. Diabetologia 2001; 44: 1155–60.

38. Desouza C, Parulkar A, Lumpkin D et al. Acute and prolonged effects of sildenafil on brachial artery flow-mediated dilatation in Type 2 diabetes. Diabetes Care 2002; 25: 1336–9.

39. Katz SD, Balidemaj K, Homma S et al. Acute type 5 phosphodiesterase inhibition with sildenafil enhances flow mediated vasodilation in patients with chronic heart failure. J Am Coll Cardiol 2000; 36: 845–51.

40. Cheitlin MD, Hutter AM, Brindis RG et al. Use of sildenafil (Viagra) in patients with cardiovascular disease. Circulation 1999; 99: 168–77.

41. Stolk EA, Busschbach JJ, Caffa M et al. Cost utility analysis of sildenafil compared with papaverine-phentolamine injections. BMJ 2000; 320: 1165–8.

42. Smith KJ, Roberts MS. The cost-effectiveness of sildenafil. Ann Intern Med 2000; 132: 933–7.

43. Saenz de Tejada I, Emmick J, Anglin G et al. The effect of as-needed tadalafil (IC351) treatment of erectile dysfunction in men with diabetes. Int J Impot Res 2001; 13, Suppl 4: S46.

44. Goldstein I. Vardenafil demonstrates improved erectile function in diabetic men with erectile dysfunction. 4th Congress of the European Society for Sexual and Impotence Research (ESSIR), Rome, Oct 2001.

45. Becker AJ, Stief CG, Machtens S et al. Oral phentolamine as treatment for erectile dysfunction. J Urol 1998; 159: 1214–16.

46. Dutta TC, Eid JF. Vacuum constriction devices for erectile dysfunction: a long-term, prospective study of patients with mild, moderate, and severe dysfunction. Urology 1999; 54: 891–3.

47. Padma-Nathan H, Hellstrom WJ, Kaiser FE et al. Treatment of men with erectile dysfunction with transurethral alprostadil. Medicated Urethral System for Erection (MUSE) Study Group. N Engl J Med 1997; 336: 1–7.

48. Porst H. Transurethrale Alprostadilapplikation mit MUSE™ (medicated urethral system for erection). Urologe [A] 1998; 37: 410–16.

49. Spivack AP, Peterson CA, Cowley C et al. VIVUS-MUSE Study Group. Long-term safety profile of transurethral alprostadil for the treatment of erectile dysfunction. J Urol 1997; 157 Suppl: 203 (Abstract).

50. Fulgham PF, Cochran JS, Denman JL et al. Disappointing initial results with transurethral alprostadil for erectile dysfunction in a urology practice setting. J Urol 1998; 160: 2041–6.

51. Linet OI, Ogrinc FG. Efficacy and safety of intracavernosal alprostadil in men with erectile dysfunction. The Alprostadil Study Group. N Engl J Med 1996; 334: 873–7.

52. Shabsigh R, Padma-Nathan H, Gittleman M et al. Intracavernous alprostadil alfadex is more efficacious, better tolerated, and preferred over intraurethral alprostadil plus optional actis: a comparative, randomized, crossover, multicenter study. Urology 2000; 55: 109–13.

53. Porst H, Buvat J, Meuleman EJH et al. Final results of a prospective multi-center study with self-injection therapy with PGE1 after 4 years of follow-up. Int J Impot Res 1996; 6: 151, D118.

13

Malformations in diabetic pregnancy: prevalence, pathogenesis and prevention

Rosa Corcoy, Alberto de Leiva

Prevalence

Nowadays, congenital malformations (CM) are unquestionably recognized as associated with diabetes mellitus (DM), their reduction is one of the main aims of prepregnancy care and their rate a key indicator of the quality of treatment in diabetic pregnancy. However, the increased prevalence of CM in diabetic pregnancy was only recognized in 1964 with the report of Molsted-Pedersen et al.[1] (Table 13.1). Afterwards, with the exception of Farquhar,[2] most authors reporting the rates of congenital malformations in infants of women with Type 1 pregestational DM have consistently found a higher prevalence in infants of diabetic mothers, whatever the country of origin or the study design.[1,3–13]

In Type 2 DM, the rate of CM has been described either as similar or higher than in Type 1 DM[2,14–17] and less frequently as lower.[5] In papers where data for Type 1 DM are lacking, the rate of CM in offspring of women with Type 2 DM is distinctly high[18,19] although in the paper by Towner et al.[19] the prevalence was biased because only women not participating in a prepregnancy program were included.

As for gestational DM, the findings of an increased prevalence of CM are less uniform. There are papers describing a prevalence similar to that of the control population.[4,8,12] There is also a significant number of publications reporting an increased prevalence.[10,11,20,21] It is nevertheless remarkable to find reports of increased prevalence of CM in infants of prediabetic women that nearly antedate those in overt DM.[22,23]

Types of malformation
Unspecific teratogenicity

Although the risk varies with the type of malformation as reported in different publications, Type 1 DM increases the risk of CM affecting most organ systems.[3,7,11,24–26] Most individual defects are considered neither sensitive nor predictive of DM,[9] which is considered to be a non-specific teratogen because it is associated with a wide range of malformations.[25] This view is in agreement with the study by Martínez-Frías in which an increased risk of CM was observed for 8 out of 16 CM analyzed[26] (Table 13.2).

Most frequent versus most specific malformations

The most frequent types of CM in infants of mothers with pregestational DM are those affecting the heart and central nervous system.[3,24,26] For example, in one study,[26] 21% of malformed infants had congenital heart

Table 13.1

Reference	Control (%)	Gestational DM (%)	Type 1 DM (%)	Type 2 DM (%)	Pregestational DM #(%)
Molsted-Pedersen et al.[1]	1.2				5.2[d]
Farquhar[2]			8.9	8.0	
Kucera[3]	1.65		4.8[b]		
Chung and Myvianthopoulous[4]	8.34 White mothers / 8.45 Black mothers	NS / NS			17.94, White mothers[d] / 13.64, Black mothers[d]
Day and Insley[5]	6.0		15.0	9.1	12
Soler et al.[6]	1.7				6.4[d]
Jervell et al.[7]	2.95				4.35[d]; RR 1.5
Amankwah et al.[20]	2.2*	5.1[a]			
Heckbert et al.[8]	1.3	2.4; OR 2.1			7.6[d]; OR 7.6
Khoury et al.[9]			OR 7.9[b]		
Hod et al.[10]	1.8	3.0[a]			6.8[d]
Serirat et al.[21]	0.6*	2.1[a]			
Omori et al.[14]			0%	5.8%[f]	
Janssen et al.[11]	2.4	2.7; OR 1.3[a]			7.2; OR 4.0[d]
Botta et al.[15]			3.7	1.4 oral agents –[f] / 11.6 oral agents +⎫⎬⎭[f]	
Kinalska et al.[16]			9.6	22.2	
Aberg et al.[12]		OR 1.06			OR 1.95[d]
Suhonen et al.[13]	1.36		4.23[b]		

Notes: NS: not significant; * Documented normal glucose tolerance; # Independent figures for Type 1 and Type 2 not available; [a] Significant versus control population; [b] Significant versus control population; [c] Significant versus control population; [d] Significant versus control population; [e] Significant versus conventional group; [f] Significant versus Type 1.

Table 13.1

Risk of major congenital malformations in infants of diabetic mothers. Figures are either prevalence (%) or OR according to the results expression in the original study

Table 13.2
Types of major malformation in infants of diabetic mothers. Risk versus control population (RR/OR)

Reference	Gestational DM	Type 1 DM
Kucera*[3] (calculated in Mills[27])	Not assessed	Caudal regression (RR 252) Situs inversus (RR 84) Ureter duplex (RR 23) Renal agenesis (RR 6) Cardiac anomalies (RR 4) Anencephalus (RR 3)
Pedersen#[24]	Not assessed	Cardiovascular (RR 7.5) Central nervous system (RR 8.5) Skeletal (RR 1.8) Other (RR 2.1)
Jervell et al.#[7]		Cardiovascular (RR 5.0) Central nervous system (RR 4.8) Cleft palate/lip (RR 1.0) All other (RR 1.0)
Becerra et al.*[25]	(Insulin-treated) Conus arteriosus defects (RR 76.0, 6.8–843.9) Transposition of great vessels (RR 57.1, 5.4–98.9) Patent ductus arteriosus (RR 48.9, 4.5–532.3) Ventricular septal defects (RR 32.6, 2.5–434.4)	Limb reduction deformities (RR 50.4, 6.3, 399.9) Vertebral anomalies (RR 42.3, 5.1–350.6) Cleft palate (RR 23.7, 3.1–183.1) Cardiovascular system (RR 18.0, 3.9–82.5) Central nervous system (RR 15.5, 3.3–73.8)
Martínez-Frías*[26]	Not assessed	(Type 1 + Type 2 DM) Upper + lower spine/ribs developmental field defect (OR 66, p <0.001) Caudal dysgenesis (OR 53, p <0.001) Lower spine developmental field defect (OR 39.3, p <0.001) Upper spine/ribs developmental field defect (OR 26.3, p <0.001) Lower limb deficiencies (OR 5.5, p = 0.002) Renal and urinary defects (OR 3.8, p <0.001) Central nervous system (OR 2.9, p <0.001) Congenital heart disease (OR 2.8, p <0.001)
Janssen et al.*[11]	Not significant	(Type 1 + Type 2) Skeletal (OR 4.4, 2.6–7.3) Cleft lip/palate (OR 7.7, 3.0–20.8) Heart malformations (OR 6.2, 3.3–11.7)
Martínez-Frías et al.*[28]	Holoprosencephaly (OR 3.27, 1.29–7.77) Upper/lower spine/rib defects (OR 2.90, 1.14–6.88) Renal/urinary defects (OR 1.81, 1.15–2.83)	Not assessed
Moore et al.*[31]	Sex chromosome aneuploidy (RR 7.7, 2.8–21.1)	

Notes: * Significance is provided. OR/RR is given for malformations with increased risk; # No information on significance is provided disease and 18.4% had central nervous system malformations. As these malformations are among the most frequent in infants of non-diabetic mothers, the most specific malformations for established DM (those with the highest prevalence odds ratio (OR) in diabetic versus non-diabetic mothers) are spine/rib defects and caudal dysgenesis.[26]

Teratogenic period

Using a developmental approach, the information on the type of CM was used by Mills in 1979 to deduce that anomalies described in infants of diabetic mothers occurred before the eigth week of gestation: caudal regression syndrome at 3 post-ovulatory weeks, neural tube defects at 4, situs inversus at 4, renal/ureteral anomalies at 5, cardiac anomalies at 5–6 and anal/rectal atresia at 6.[27] The fact that these infants also have more blastogenic (36.8 versus 10.3%) and midline anomalies (48.7 versus 21.1%) supports the same conclusion.[26]

Type of CM according to the type of DM

There are no major differences in the defects affecting the offspring of mothers with Type 1 or Type 2 DM.[26] In gestational DM, Martínez-Frías et al.[28] described an increased risk for 3 of 20 malformations studied (holoprosencephaly, spine/rib defects and renal/urinary defects). This means that these are the most specific anomalies in infants of diabetic mothers but not the most frequent, which in decreasing order are CM affecting genital, central nervous, renal/urinary and cardiovascular systems and cleft lip. Two additional reports indicate that anomalies match those of diabetic embryopathy.[29,30] Recently, an association between gestational DM and sex chromosome aneuploidy, mainly Klinefelter syndrome, has been described with prevalence ratio adjusted for confounders of 7.7.[31]

Multiple malformations (Table 13.3)

All authors agree on an increased prevalence of multiple CM in infants of diabetic mothers,

Reference	Type of DM	Percentage of newborns with multiple congenital malformations		Percentage of multiple congenital malformations in malformed infants	
		Control women	Diabetic women	Control women	Diabetic women
Molsted-Pedersen et al.[1]	Pregestational	0.2	1.6	16.7	30.8
Chung and Myrianthopoulos[4]	Pregestational	2.15	6.7	25.6	39.2
Soler et al.[6]	Pregestational				24.6
Pedersen et al.[24]	Pregestational	0.4	2.1	13.4	25.9
Khoury et al.[9]	Type 1 DM				1/3
Martínez-Frías et al.[26]	Pregestational			23.19	53.95
Janssen et al.[11]	Pregestational			5.95	14.46

Table 13.3
Multiple congenital malformations in infants of diabetic mothers (%)

both as overall prevalence and as percentage within malformed infants. Roughly, about 30% of malformed newborns of diabetic mothers have multiple malformations, a figure nearly two-fold that of control women (see Table 13.3). In the words of Janssen et al., the association with established DM is greater for neonates with multiple (OR 7.8, 3.3–18.1) rather than with single malformations (OR 2.9, 2.1–3.9).[11]

Lethality (Table 13.4)

The next characteristic of CM in diabetic pregnancy is their lethality. Not only has the prevalence of lethal CM been reported to be higher than in control women, but also their contribution to perinatal mortality in infants of diabetic mothers is increasing.[1,2,6,24,32–45] Soler et al. stated that increased attention was being directed to the incidence of CM because of the falling perinatal mortality.[6] Although we can see in Table 13.4 exceptions to the rule that high perinatal mortality is accompanied by a low contribution of CM and vice versa, the rule is always maintained within a series. In a specific center, when a decrease in perinatal mortality is achieved, the contribution of CM increases. We can cite the data of Olofsson et al.[35] as a paradigm. During a span of 20 years, perinatal mortality decreased from 68.6% to 3.4% whereas the contribution of CM to perinatal mortality increased from 18.2% to 75%.[35]

Clinical predictors
Genetics

The possibility that the origin of CM is related to the maternal genes of DM was rejected by the demonstration that infants of diabetic

fathers did not have an increased risk of CM in several studies, e.g. the Collaborative Perinatal Project and Pima Indians Study.[4,46]

Hyperglycemia

The first observation associating HbA1c with CM was made by Leslie et al.[47] Although no precise figures on HbA1c were reported, 'three out of five pregnant diabetics whose HbA1c was greater than that of well controlled diabetics gave birth to children with fatal CM. No abnormalities were detected in children born to mothers with an HbA1 level within the range of well controlled diabetics.' After this initial report, more elaborate investigations appeared, clearly demonstrating a positive association between HbA1c and the prevalence of CM.[13,48–56] The relationship of metabolic control with minor anomalies has been studied by fewer authors, and with some exceptions,[57] most authors report a positive association[49,55,56] (Table 13.5).

As regards the question about which level of HbA1c is safe, most publications indicate: 'lower than 4–6 SD over the mean of the control group' or, according to the American Diabetes Association's (ADA) Clinical Practice Recommendations 2002, 'up to 1% above normal'.[58] Nevertheless, the rates of CM continue to decrease at lower HbA1c values within the above-mentioned range.[13,52,53] So the final ADA recommendation is that 'the general goal for glycemic management in the preconception period and during the first trimester should be to obtain the lowest HbA1c level possible without undue risk of hypoglycemia in the mother'.[58]

Ketone bodies

Malins stated that 'ketoacidosis commonly leads to the death of the fetus, but there are no

| Reference | Type of DM | Perinatal mortality (%) | Prevalence of lethal CM (%) | | Mortality accounted for CM in infants of diabetic mothers (%) |
			Control mothers	Diabetic mothers	
Driscoll et al.[32]	Pregestational		0.3	2.1	16.8
Molsted-Pedersen et al.[1]	Pregestational				
Farquhar[2]	Pregestational	21.0		1.5	7.2
Soler et al.[6]	Pregestational	14.1 19.2 in 1950–1954 12.0 in 1970–1974		3.8	26.0 22.0 in 1950–1954 50.0 in 1970–1974
Pedersen[24]	Pregestational	5.9 7.4 in 1970–1972 4.6 in 1973–1975			48.0 41.0 in 1970–1972 58.0 in 1973–1975
Teramo et al.[33]	Pregestational	6.3 18.5 in 1970–1971 1.5 in 1975–1977		2.1	33.3 30.0 in 1970–1971 50.0 in 1975–1977
Lemons[34]	Pregestational			1.4	22.6
Olofsson et al.[35]	Pregestational	25.7 68.6 in 1960–1966 12.5 in 1967–1973 3.4 in 1974–1980		4.2	62.0 18.2 in 1960–1966 50.0 in 1967–1973 75.0 in 1974–1980
McFarland and Hemaya[36]	Pregestational + gestational	5.72 10.0 in 1978–1980 3.2 in 1981–1983			47.1 45.5 in 1978–1980 50.0 in 1981–1983
Drury[37]	Pregestational	4.5		1.75	38.5
Klebe et al.[38]	Pregestational	3.5		1.16	33.0
Small et al.[39]	Type 1	1.6		1.6	100.0
Martin et al.[40]	Pregestational	7.5 12.2 in 1970–1975 5.7 in 1976–1980 3.9 in 1981–1985		1.14	22.6 16.7 in 1970–1975 12.5 in 1976–1980 60.0 in 1981–1985
Nielsen and Nielsen[41]	Pregestational	4.3		0.4	9.0
Casson et al.[42]	Type 1	4.2		1.9	46.7
Brown et al.[43]	Type 1	6.25		3.75	60.0
Cundy et al.[44]	Type 1/Type 2	1.25/3.9		0.625/0.781	50/20
Gabbe et al.[45]	Type 1	1.7		0.0	0.0

Table 13.4
Lethality of congenital malformations in infants of diabetic mothers

| Reference | Degree of HbA1c elevation in SD above the mean (% major congenital malformations) | | | |
	Normal HbA1c	Moderate	High	Very high
Miller et al.[48]		< 7 (0)	7–9.8 (13.5)	> = 10 (21.7)
Ylinen et al.[49]		< 6 (3.2)	6–9.8 (8.1)	> = 10 (23.5)
Reid et al.[50]		< 6 (3.4)	6–9.9 (11.4)	> = 10 (24.0)
Key et al.[51]		< 3.8 (4.4)	5.8–9.4 (30.8)	> = 9.5 (100.0)
Miodovnik et al.[52]	<2 (0)	2.1–4 (6.7)	> 4 (8.7)	
Mills et al.[53]	≤2 (0.8)	> 2.1 (5.2)		
Greene et al.[54]		< 6 (3.0)	6–12 (4.9)	> = 12.0 (39.3)
Hanson et al.[55]		< 6 (0.7)	6–7.9 (6.5)	> = 8.0 (16.1)
Rosenn et al.[56]		< 4 (4.2)	4–9.9 (6.5)	> = 10.0 (25.0)
Suhonen et al.[13]	<2 (2.1)	2.1–5.9 (4.1)	6.0–9.9 (3.2)	> = 10.0 (5.2)

Table 13.5
Glycemic control and major congenital malformations in infants of diabetic mothers (%)

records of deformities which might be attributed to such an event in early pregnancy'.[59] A relationship between CM and diabetic ketoacidosis (or its absence) has not been reported since. The first trimester β-hydroxybutyrate levels in women with Type 1 diabetes have been reported to be moderately elevated. Surprisingly, they were found, both in diabetic and control mothers, to be lower rather than higher in cases with a malformed infant or pregnancy loss.[60] This has been attributed to the reasonably good control in diabetic women and to β-hydroxybutyrate levels 20–40-fold lower than those causing malformations in embryo culture.

Vasculopathy

The rate of CM has been associated with the severity of White class,[6,38] but there are exceptions.[5] Jorgen Pedersen suggested that, as malformations did not recur in subsequent,

well controlled pregnancies, the reason was the difficulty of achieving normal metabolic compensation in these women.[61] However, in studies where a multivariate analysis has been performed, divergent results have been reported: vasculopathy and early first trimester poor glycemic control were found to be independent predictors of CM,[52] vasculopathy did not improve prediction over that provided by HbA1c[55] or hyperglycemia increased the risk of fetal malformations when associated with maternal diabetes of longer duration and/or with vascular complications.[62]

Hypoglycemia

As to the possibility of hypoglycemia as a pathogenic factor of CM, insulin shock therapy has been associated with developmental abnormalities when administered in early pregnancy. In a review of published cases, Impastato et al.[63] described fetal damage in six out of 19 women

receiving insulin shock therapy (two malformations). Such incidence was higher than that of
the control population and associated with
gestational age at the administration of insulin
shock (six cases of fetal damage in nine treatments before the fourteenth week versus none
in ten later treatments). Nevertheless, the
relationship is less clear in diabetic mothers. For
example, Molsted-Pedersen et al. reported that
of 55 mothers with malformed infants, 8 had
an insulin coma but none in the first trimester.[1]
On the other hand, none of the 20 women with
an insulin coma in the first trimester had a
malformed infant (Pedersen, cited in[1]). In fact
one of the first clues towards the importance of
tight metabolic control in reducing the rate of
CM came from the observation that the
frequency of hypoglycemia during pregnancy
was four-fold higher in diabetic mothers of
infants born without CM than in those born
with congenital heart disease.[64] Reassuringly,
the more frequent and probably unavoidable
mild hypoglycemic episodes that occur when
optimization of blood glucose is undertaken,
have been reported not to be associated with
CM; in women in the preconception group the
rate of CM was 1.2% versus 14.3% in the
postconception group while in the first group,
hypoglycemic episodes (≤3.3 mmol/l) took place
in 58.3% of the first eight weeks of
pregnancy.[65]

Insulin/obesity

Despite the extensive information on insulin
teratogenicity derived from experimental
studies, the clinical experience is scarce. Only in
a recent paper dealing with the relationship
between obesity and CM in the general population, was hyperinsulinemia found to be an
independent predictor of CM even when
corrected for obesity.[66] Since 1969, obesity has
consistently been associated with CM in the
general population[67] with dose-response
relationship.[68,69] Such a relationship has been
demonstrated for different types of CM as
defects in the neural tube[68] and cardiovascular
system.[69] The mechanisms have not been elucidated. One of the suggestions is that obesity is
acting through hyperinsulinemia. The association between obesity and CM in diabetic
patients has been analyzed on very few
occasions but found to be positive: in a series
of mothers with overt DM/gestational DM and
no overall increase in CM, the obese subgroup
had an increase in risk (OR 0.98 in BMI <28,
3.1OR in BMI ≥28).[70]

Oral agents

Sulfonylureas are included in the FDA C class
for pregnancy use. In 1991, an impressive
increase in the rate of CM was reported in
newborns of Type 2 diabetic mothers exposed
to oral hypoglycemic drugs (mainly sulfonylureas) during embryogenesis (50% major and
minor CM versus 15% in the control group).[18]
Subsequent studies have been conflicting, refut-
ing[19,71] or confirming[15] the relationship.
Metformin is a drug within the FDA B category
for pregnancy, but it is not considered by the
ADA as a therapeutic option for Type 2
diabetes during pregnancy.[58] Nevertheless, it
has been used by several groups reporting a
suboptimal pregnancy outcome, which could
be attributed to suboptimal metabolic control,
but not to an increased rate of CM.[72,73] In
addition, in the context of recent controlled
trials, metformin has been shown to improve
ovulation in women with polycystic ovary
syndrome.[74] When intake has been continued
during pregnancy, the rate of abortions[75] and
gestational diabetes mellitus[76] were reduced
without increase in CM. Although caution is

needed, these results encourage further (controlled) trials of metformin.

Experimental teratogens (Table 13.6)

Vulnerable period

Embryos are vulnerable to diabetic teratogenicity in specific periods of development: gastrulation and neurulation,[77] equivalent to the fourth to seventh weeks of gestational age in humans and even in preimplantation stages.[78] In diabetic rats, an early insult has a carry-over effect with blastocysts remaining functionally affected and developing less well than control embryos when cultured under the same conditions.[79] Morphologic recovery of mouse embryos following a teratogenic exposure to ketosis has also been reported.[80]

- Hyperglycemia
- Hyperketonemia
- Hyperaminoacidemia
- Hyperosmolality
- Synergism between the former
- Hypoglycemia
- Insulin
  - deficiency
  - excess
- Somatomedin inhibitors
- Genetic susceptibility
- Period susceptibility
- Mediators:
  - inadequate glucose transporter down-regulation
  - tumor necrosis factor
  - zinc depletion
  - myo-inositol depletion
  - arachidonic acid depletion
  - PGE2 depletion
  - free oxygen radicals
  - abnormal DNA synthesis/structure
  - abnormal yolk sac function
- Oral agents
  - phenformin
  - tolbutamide/chlorpropamide

Table 13.6
Teratogens in experimental models that can be relevant in diabetic pregnancy

Insulin

Exogenous insulin can reduce the risk of CM in offspring of diabetic rats,[81] but not when added to diabetic serum *in vitro*.[82] However, insulin itself can be a teratogen. Teratogenicity of insulin in vertebrates was established already in 1945 in a chick model and it was clear that insulin was not acting through a metabolic pathway but affecting gene expression and enzyme function.[83,84] It was first believed that insulin during early development was acting through IGF-I receptor,[85] but later it became clear that insulin acts through its own receptor and at a time when IGF-I receptor is undetectable.[86] In mammals, receptors for insulin are expressed as early as the morula stage of preimplantation development and even at the eight-cell stage,[87] making possible an insulin effect very early on. A normal insulin range is required since insulin deficiency is also teratogenic.[88]

Genes

The fact that the teratogenic insult in diabetic pregnancy is metabolic and not dependent on the genetic background predisposing to diabetes is confirmed by the increased rate of CM in animal models of chemically-induced DM in the absence of a genetic predisposition.[89] However, though the teratogen is exogenous, the susceptibility depends on genetic predisposition: it is different in two strains of Sprague-Dawley rats and intermediate in hybrids.[90]

Hyperglycemia, hyperketonemia and hyperaminoacidemia

Hyperglycemia was the first fuel excess tested and demonstrated to be a teratogen,[91] later confirmed by a large number of papers. Next came ketones[92] and α-ketoisocaproic acid.[93] Generally, a dose-dependent effect has been demonstrated together with the requirement of doses higher than those in diabetic serum. This fact, together with the finding that there is synergism between different fuels in causing teratogenicity[92,93] has led to the conclusion that diabetes teratogenicity is multifactorial.

Osmolality

In initial experiments on the teratogenicity of hyperglycemia, the influence of hyperosmolality was also tested and shown to contribute; it was not teratogenic per se but exacerbated the malformations produced by hyperglycemia.[91]

Hypoglycemia

Hypoglycemia is teratogenic both in vitro[82] and in vivo.[94,95] However as in the case of hyperglycemia, there are specific periods of susceptibility, with teratogenesis being demonstrated in early[94] but not in late neurulation.[95]

Somatomedin inhibitor

Somatomedin inhibitors are present in serum of diabetic animals and were shown to be teratogenic when added to the growth medium for mouse embryos in whole embryo culture during the period of neurulation and craniofacial development.[96] Somatomedin is involved in the mechanism of yolk sac dysfunction.[97]

Mediators

Partial downregulation of GLUT-1
In a situation where exposure to hyperglycemia is deleterious, the late and partial downregulation of GLUT-1 in rat embryos and yolk sac implies a lack of protection against high ambient glucose.[98]

Zinc depletion
Zinc depletion is teratogenic[99] and has been proposed as a mediator of diabetic teratogenicity since maternal DM induces fetal zinc deficiency.[100] Low-zinc diets amplify teratogenicity in diabetic animals.[101] However, maternal supplementation with zinc does not improve fetal zinc deficiency or decrease CM.[101]

Tumor necrosis factor alpha
TNFα is one of the substances suggested as a mediator of diabetic teratogenesis: uterine epithelium cells from diabetic animals produce more TNF than those of control animals and the addition of anti-TNFα antibodies to the culture medium decreases the embryotoxic effects of diabetic serum.[102]

Myo-inositol depletion
Depletion of myo-inositol mediates diabetic teratogenesis:

(1) Addition of glucose to culture serum in vitro, reduces the myo-inositol content of embryos[103] and is associated with an increased CM rate.[104]
(2) Dietary[105] and in vitro[104] supplementation of myo-inositol is able to reverse the embryonic deficiency and the rate of malformations.

Nevertheless, beneficial effects of metabolic improvement of maternal diabetes by insulin treatment are greater than those achieved by correction of myo-inositol depletion.[105]

Arachidonic acid and prostaglandin E2 depletion

The depletion in myo-inositol induces a derangement in the metabolism of arachidonic acid and prostaglandin. A reduction in the frequency of neural tube defects has been demostrated with arachidonic acid supplementation both *in vivo*[106] and *in vitro*.[107] In its turn, reduced arachidonic acid leads to a decrease in prostaglandin production, which is the next teratogenic mediator; whereas the beneficial effects of myo-inositol supplementation on hyperglycemia-induced teratogenesis are prevented by cyclo-oxygenase inhibitors,[108] the supplementation of prostaglandin E2 is protective.[109]

Oxygen radicals

The same group that has pointed out the differences in genetic susceptibility to diabetic teratogenesis also demonstrated that genetic liability was associated with differences in erythrocyte catalase locus (higher catalase activities in CM-resistant strains).[110] Oxygen radical scavengers have been shown to decrease the malformations induced by glucose and non-glucose substrates *in vitro* (catalase, superoxide dismutase, glutathion peroxidase in glucose-induced malformations; superoxide dismutase in glucose, pyruvate, hydroxybutyrate and ketoisocaproic-induced malformations; N-acetylcysteine in glucose-induced malformations)[111,92,112] and by maternal diabetes *in vivo* (vitamin C and E in diabetic rats).[112,113] Since high doses of antioxidant agents are required, combined treatments (vitamin C + vitamin E) have been tested and demonstrated to be effective, but without a synergistic effect.[114]

Oxygen radicals can interfere with the prostaglandin mechanism[116] so that deranged prostaglandin metabolism would be a second step to both depletion of myo-inositol and increased oxidative stress. Interestingly, free-radical mediated oxidative DNA damage has been reported to be at least partly responsible for the teratogenicity of various agents such as ethanol,[117] phenytoin[118] or thalidomide.[119] The role of oxygen radicals in diabetic teratogenesis would add to the demonstration that mitochondrial superoxide production is involved in three pathways of hyperglycemic damage.[120]

DNA/chromosomal abnormalities

DNA synthesis has been shown to be reduced by teratogens operating in diabetic pregnancy through different mechanisms: both hypoglycemia[121] and increased ketone bodies[122] can reduce the availability of ribose molecules required for DNA synthesis and β-hydroxybutyrate can limit *de novo* pyrimidine biosynthesis.[80] In addition, embryos from diabetic mice have been described to bear more chromosomal abnormalities[123,124] and be more prone to mutations.[125]

Yolk sac abnormalities

Morphologic[126] and functional[127] abnormalities in the yolk sac have been described in post-implantation rat embryos exposed to hyperglycemia and to somatomedin inhibitors.[97] This is relevant to the rat model of diabetic teratogenesis because these experimental animals begin neural tube development at this stage, but it may not be applicable to human pregnancy.

Oral agents

In mouse embryos *in vitro*, teratogenesis has been elicited by incubation with serum from tolbutamide-treated animals or from control animals with added tolbutamide. Tolbutamide concentrations were similar to those in human serum and the malformation rate did not improve with glucose supplementation.[128] A

Reference	Percentage of major congenital malformations in infants of diabetic mothers		P
	Prepregnancy care	No prepregnancy care	
Steel et al.[135]	2.3	9.52	ns
Fuhrmann et al.[136]	3.6	3.2	ns
Fuhrmann et al.[137]	1.8	4.3	ns
Goldman et al.[138]	0	0	ns
Jensen et al.[139]	0	0	ns
Rowe et al.[140]	0	28.6	ns
Mills et al.[141]	2.1	4.5	ns
Steel et al.[141]	1.4	10.4	<0.05
Kitzmiller et al.[65]	1.2	10.9	<0.05
Rosenn et al.[143]	0.0	1.4	ns
Willhoite et al.[144]	1.6	6.6	ns
Diabetes Control and Complications Trial[145]	2.5	4.0	ns
García-Patterson et al.[146]	3.7	8.6	ns
Dunne et al.[147]	0	0	ns
Hermann et al.[148]	4.8	14.1	ns

Table 13.7
Prepregnancy care and major congenital malformations in infants of diabetic mothers (%)

direct embryotoxic effect at concentrations close to the therapeutic range has also been established for tolbutamide and chlorpropamide.[129,130]

Phenformin was reported to induce neural tube closure defects, craniofacial hypoplasia and reduction in size of first vertebral arches in mouse embryos in culture.[131] Metformin was not teratogenic.[131] In another report, toxic effects of metformin on mouse embryo were seen at high concentrations never achieved *in vivo*.[132]

Prevention

Prepregnancy care (Table 13.7)

Prepregnancy care is usually associated with pregestational DM and even more specifically with Type 1 DM. Nevertheless, one of the first papers on the subject deals with gestational DM: a decreased rate of CM was observed (retrospectively) in pre-diabetic women receiving diet therapy and tolbutamide able to normalize the glucose tolerance test.[133] Only in 1976 was a prepregnancy clinic for insulin-dependent diabetics initiated in Edinburgh[134] and in 1982 the first outcomes were reported.[135] In all reports[65,135-148] the rate of CM in women receiving prepregnancy care has been lower than for those who did not receive it. However, the difference was only significant in 2 of the 15 studies described in Table 13.7. Not surprisingly, a recent meta-analysis estimated the RR of CM in recipients of prepregnancy care as 0.36 of non-recipients (2.1% versus 6.5% absolute rate of CM).[149]

Obviously, prepregnancy care implies extra cost at a stage when only standard DM care costs apply for women not enrolled. Nevertheless, clear benefits from the economic point of view have been consistently demonstrated by including preconception, prenatal and postnatal cost.[148,150]

Despite the benefits of prepregnancy care (decreased CM, decreased cost and the option to improve the status of late complications of DM), the rate of attendance in preconception programs is low, and ranges from 20%[151] to 75%.[152] Intriguingly, diabetic women have been reported to plan pregnancy less often than their non-diabetic counterparts[153] and even less often when severe complications, e.g. diabetic nephropathy, occur.[154]

Other interventions

A randomized study showed that 4 mg of folic acid supplementation before conception prevented 71% of neural tube defects in women with an affected offspring in former pregnancy.[155] Additional evidence suggested that lower doses of folic acid were also effective, not only in preventing recurrences but as a primary prevention.[156] Even though pregnant diabetic women do not have a derangement in folate metabolism,[157] as women with pregestational DM have an increased risk of neural tube defects, they are included in the subgroups recommended for folic acid administration for prevention of first occurrence of neural tube defects.[158] Nevertheless, this issue is not mentioned in other recommendations.[58] Folic acid supplementation was recommended in only one of the studies included in the above-mentioned meta-analysis of prepregnancy care[149] and was taken by only 51% of pregnant diabetic women in a case series.[159] Specific data

on folate effectiveness in prevention of CM in women with DM are lacking, and this is relevant because folate benefit is decreased in some circumstances (obesity, college-education, Hispanic women).[69,160] Reassuringly, in a post-hoc analysis, the authors of prepregnancy care meta-analysis highlighted that the risk of CM was the lowest in the center that described the periconceptional use of folic acid for those who attended the prepregnancy care.[149]

While promoting the best possible prepregnancy care, the next logical step would be the performance of clinical trials testing the usefulness of maternal folate and antioxidant therapy in diabetic pregnancy.[161] Nevertheless, caution is required when supplementing with pharmacological doses of vitamins because these antioxidant agents can turn pro-oxidant with increasing concentrations.[162,163]

References

1. Molsted-Pedersen L, Tygstrup I, Pedersen J. Congenital malformations in newborn infants of diabetic women. Lancet 1964; 1: 1124–6.
2. Farquhar JW. Prognosis for babies born to diabetic mothers in Edinburgh. Arch Dis Child 1969; 44: 36–47.
3. Kucera J. Rate and type of congenital anomalies among offspring of diabetic women. J Reprod Med 1971; 7: 61–70.
4. Chung CS, Myrianthopoulos NC. Factors affecting risks of congenital malformations. II. Effect of maternal diabetes on congenital malformations. Birth Defects Orig Artic Ser 1975; 11: 23–38.
5. Day R, Insley J. Maternal diabetes and congenital malformations. Arch Dis Child 1976; 51: 935–8.
6. Soler NG, Walsh CH, Malins JM. Congenital malformations in infants of diabetic mothers. QJM 1976; 178: 303–13.
7. Jervell J, Bjerkedal T, Moe N. Outcome of pregnancies in diabetic mothers in Norway 1967–1976. Diabetologia 1980; 18: 131–4.

8. Heckbert SR, Stephens CR, Daling JR. Diabetes in pregnancy: maternal and infant outcome. Paediatr Perinat Epidemiol 1988; 2: 314–26.

9. Khoury MJ, Becerra JE, Cordero JF, Erickson JD. Clinical-epidemiologic assessment of pattern of birth defects associated with human teratogens: application to diabetic embryopathy. Pediatrics 1989; 84: 658–65.

10. Hod M, Merlob P, Friedman S et al. Prevalence of congenital anomalies and neonatal complications in the offspring of diabetic mothers in Israel. Isr J Med Sci 1991; 27: 498–502.

11. Janssen PA, Rothman I, Schwartz SM. Congenital malformations in newborns of women with established and gestational diabetes in Washington State, 1984–1991. Paediatr Perinat Epidemiol 1996; 10: 52–63.

12. Aberg A, Westbom L, Kallen B. Congenital malformations among infants whose mothers had gestational diabetes or preexisting diabetes. Early Hum Develop 2001; 61: 85–95.

13. Suhonen L, Hiilesmaa V, Teramo K. Glycaemic control during early pregnancy and fetal malformations in women with Type 1 diabetes mellitus. Diabetologia 2001; 43: 79–82.

14. Omori Y, Minei S, Testuo T et al. Current status of pregnancy in diabetic women. A comparison of pregnancy in IDDM and NIDDM mothers. Diabetes Res Clin Pract 1994; 24 Suppl. S273–S278.

15. Botta RM. Congenital malformations in infants of 517 pregestational diabetic mothers. Ann Ist Super Sanita 1997; 33: 307–11.

16. Kinalska I, Kinalski M, Telejko B et al. Pregnancy complicated by Type I, Type II and gestational diabetes: experiences from the diabetic-obstetric center of Bialystock. Pol Arch Med Wewn 1999; 102: 1039–45.

17. Brydon P, Smith T, Proffitt M et al. Pregnancy outcome in women with Type 2 diabetes mellitus needs to be addressed. Int J Clin Pract 2000; 54: 418–19.

18. Piacquadio K, Hollingsworth D, Murphy M. Effects of in-utero exposure to oral hypoglycaemic drugs. Lancet 1991; 338: 866–9.

19. Towner D, Kjos SL, Leung B et al. Congenital malformations in pregnancies complicated by NIDDM. Diabetes Care 1995; 18: 1446–51.

20. Amankwah KS, Kaufmann R, Roller RW et al. Incidence of congenital abnormalities in infants of gestational diabetic mothers. J Perinat Med 1981; 9: 223–7.

21. Serirat S, Sunthornthepvaraul T, Deerochanawong C, Jinayon P. Gestational diabetes mellitus. J Med Assoc Thai 1992; 75: 315–19.

22. Hagbard L. The 'prediabetic' period from an obstetric point of view. Acta Obstet Gynecol Scand 1958; 37: 497–518.

23. Navarrete VN, Rojas CE, Alger CR, Paniagua HE. Subsequent diabetes in mothers delivered of a malformed infant. Lancet 1970; 2: 993–5.

24. Pedersen J. The Pregnant Diabetic and Her Newborn. Copenhagen: Munksgaard, 1977.

25. Becerra JE, Khoury MJ, Cordero JF, Erickson JD. Diabetes mellitus during pregnancy and the risks for specific birth defects: a population based case–control study. Pediatrics 1990; 85: 1–9.

26. Martínez-Frías ML. Epidemiological analysis of outcomes of pregnancy in diabetic mothers: identification of the most characteristic and most frequent congenital anomalies. Am J Med Genet 1994; 51: 108–13.

27. Mills JL, Baker L, Goldman AS. Malformations in infants of diabetic mothers occur before the seventh gestational week. Implications for treatment. Diabetes 1979; 28: 292–3.

28. Martínez-Frías ML, Bermejo E, Rodríguez-Pinilla E et al. Epidemiological analysis of outcomes of pregnancy in gestational diabetic mothers. Am J Med Genet 1998; 78: 140–5.

29. Khoussef BG. Gestational diabetes mellitus (class A). A human teratogen? Am J Med Genet 1999; 83: 402–8.

30. Schaefer UM, Songster G, Xiang A et al. Congenital malformations in offspring of women with hyperglycemia first detected during pregnancy. Am J Obstet Gynecol 1997; 177: 1165–71.

31. Moore LL, Bradlee ML, Singer MR et al. Chromosomal anomalies among the offspring of women with gestational diabetes. Am J Epidemiol 2002; 155: 719–24.

32. Driscoll SG, Benirschke K, Curtis GW. Neonatal deaths among infants of diabetic mothers. Am J Dis Child 1960; 100: 818–34.

127. Reece EA, Pinter E, Leranth C et al. Yolk sac failure in embryopathy due to hyperglycemia: Horseradish peroxidase uptake in the assessment of yolk sac function. Obstet Gynecol 1989; 74: 755–62.

128. Smoak IW. Teratogenic effects of tolbutamide on early-somite mouse embryos in vitro. Diabetes Res Clin Pract 1992; 17: 161–7.

129. Ziegler MH, Grafton TF, Hansen DK. The effect of tolbutamide on rat embryonic development in vitro. Teratology 1993; 48: 45–51.

130. Smoak IW. Embryopathic effects of the oral hypoglycaemic agent chlorpropamide in cultured mouse embryos. Am J Obstet Gynecol 1993; 169 2 Pt 1: 409–14.

131. Denno KM, Sadler TW. Effects of the biguanide class of oral hypoglycaemic agents on mouse embryogenesis. Teratology 1994; 49: 260–6.

132. Bedaiwy MA, Miller KF, Goldberg JM et al. Effect of metformin on mouse embryo development. Fertil Steril 2001; 76: 1078–9.

133. Navarrete VN, Paniagua HE, Alger CR, Manzo PB. The significance of metabolic adjustment before a new pregnancy. Prophylaxis of congenital malformations. Am J Obstet Gynecol 1970; 107: 250–63.

134. Steel JM, Parboosingh J, Cole RA, Duncan LJP. Prepregnancy counselling—A logical prelude to the management of the pregnant diabetic woman. Diabetes Care 1980; 3: 371–3.

135. Steel JM, Johstone FD, Smith AF, Duncan LJP. Five years' experience of a "prepregnancy" clinic for insulin-dependent diabetes. BMJ 1982; 285: 353–6.

136. Fuhrmann K, Reiher H, Semmler K et al. Prevention of congenital malformations in infants of insulin-dependent diabetic mothers. Diabetes Care 1983; 6: 219–23.

137. Fuhrmann K, Reiher H Semmler K et al. The effect of intensified conventional insulin therapy before and during pregnancy on the malformation rate in offspring of diabetic mothers. Exp Clin Endocrinol 1984; 83: 173–7.

138. Goldman JA, Dicker D, Feldberg D et al. Pregnancy outcome in patients with insulin-dependent diabetes mellitus with preconceptual diabetic control: a comparative study. Am J Obstet Gynecol 1986; 155: 293–7.

139. Jensen BM, Kuhl C, Molsted-Pedersen L et al. Preconceptional treatment with insulin infusion pumps in insulin-dependent diabetic women with particular reference to prevention of congenital malformations. Acta Endocrinol Suppl (Copenh) 1986; 277: 81–5.

140. Rowe BR, Rowbotham CJ, Barnett AH. Preconception counselling, birth weight, and congenital abnormalities in established and gestational diabetic pregnancy. Diabetes Res 1987; 6: 33–5.

141. Mills JL, Knopp RH, Simpson JL et al. Lack of relation of increased malformation rates in infants of diabetic mothers to glycemic control during pregnancy. N Engl J Med 1988; 318: 671–6.

142. Steel JM, Johnstone FD, Hepburn DA, Smith AF. Can prepregnancy care of diabetic women reduce the risk of abnormal babies? BMJ 1990; 301: 1070–4.

143. Rosenn B, Miodovnik M, Combs C et al. Preconception management of insulin-dependent diabetes: improvement of pregnancy outcome. Obstet Gynecol 1991; 77: 846–9.

144. Willhoite MB, Herman WH, Bennert Jr HW et al. The impact of preconception counseling on pregnancy outcomes. Diabetes Care 1993; 16: 450–5.

145. The Diabetes Control and Complications Trial Research Group. Pregnancy outcomes in the Diabetes Control and Complications Trial. Am J Obstet Gynecol 1996; 174: 1343–53.

146. García-Patterson A, Corcoy R, Rigla M et al. Does preconceptional counselling in diabetic women improve perinatal outcome? Ann Ist Super Sanita 1997; 33: 333–6.

147. Dunne FP, Brydon P, Smith T et al. Preconception diabetes care in insulin-dependent diabetes mellitus. QJM 1999; 92: 175–6.

148. Herman WJ, Janz NK, Becker MP et al. Diabetes and pregnancy: pre-conception care, pregnancy outcomes, resource utilization and costs. J Reprod Med 1999; 44: 33–8.

149. Ray JG, O'Brien TE, Chan WS. Preconception care and the risk of congenital anomalies in the offspring of women with diabetes mellitus: a meta-analysis. QJM 2001; 94: 435–44.

150. Elixhauser A, Weschler JM, Kitzmiller J et al. Cost-benefit analysis of preconception care for women with established diabetes mellitus. Diabetes Care 1993; 16: 1146–57.

151. Cousins L. The California Diabetes and Pregnancy Program: a statewide collaborative programme for the preconception and prenatal care of diabetic women. Bailliere's Clin Obstet Gynecol 1991; 5: 443–59.

152. Damm P, Molsted-Pedersen L. Significant decrease in congenital malformations in newborn infants of an unselected population of diabetic women. Am J Obstet Gynecol 1989; 161: 1163–7.

153. St James PJ, Younger MD, Hamilton BD, Waisbren SE. Unplanned pregnancies in young women with diabetes. An analysis of psychosocial factors. Diabetes Care 1993; 16: 1572–8.

154. Kimmerle R, Zass RP, Cupisti S et al. Pregnancies in women with diabetic nephropathy: long-term outcome for mother and child. Diabetologia 1995; 38: 227–35.

155. MRC Vitamin Study Research Group. Prevention of neural tube defects: results of the MRC Vitamin Study. Lancet 1991; 338: 132–7.

156. Czeizel AE, Dudás I. Prevention of the first occurrence of neural tube defects by periconceptional vitamin supplementation. N Engl J Med 1992; 327: 1832–5.

157. Kaplan JS, Iqbal S, England BG et al. Is pregnancy in diabetic women associated with folate deficiency? Diabetes Care 1999; 22: 1017–21.

158. American Academy of Pediatrics Committee on Genetics. Folic acid for the prevention of neural tube defects. Pediatrics 1993; 92: 493–4.

159. Wills CJ, Page SR. Peri-conceptual folic acid supplementation in Type 1 diabetes. Practical Diabetes Int 2001; 18: 123–5.

160. Shaw GM, Schaffer D, Velie EM et al. Periconceptional vitamin use, dietary folate and the occurrence of neural tube defects. Epidemiology 1995; 6: 205–7.

161. Persson B. Prevention of fetal malformation with antioxidants in diabetic pregnancy. Pediatr Res 2001; 49: 742–3.

162. Kontush A, Finckh B, Karten B et al. Antioxidant and prooxidant activity of alpha-tocopherol in human plasma and low density lipoprotein. J Lipid Res 1996; 37: 1436–8.

163. Otero P, Viana M, Herrera E, Bonet B. Antioxidant and prooxidant effects of ascorbic acid, dehydroascorbic acid and flavonoids on LDL submitted to different degrees of oxidation. Free Radical Res 1997; 27: 619–26.

14

Inflammation and vaccination: cause and cure for Type 1 diabetes

Irun R Cohen, Sol Efroni

Introduction

Type 1 diabetes refers to two related, but nosologically different entities: the inflammatory process that destroys the insulin-producing β-cells and the consequences of the insulin deficiency that results from the loss of β-cells. In other words, Type 1 diabetes encompasses two different diseases: a primary immunological disease and a secondary endocrine disease. One might argue that Type 1 diabetes also includes a third disease – a vascular disease that results in the long-term complications associated with Type 1 diabetes. However, most investigators would probably attribute the late vascular complications of Type 1 diabetes to the cumulative damage to blood vessels brought about by hyperglycemia. Daily injections of insulin can never match the degree of glucose and energy homeostasis naturally managed by the β-cells. Others might put at least some of the blame on the immune disease; the immune process active in Type 1 diabetes might target blood vessels and other tissues and not only β-cells. Here, we shall focus on the primary immune disease responsible for Type 1 diabetes.

This chapter opens with four questions:

- What is an autoimmune disease?
- Is Type 1 diabetes an autoimmune disease?
- How does an autoimmune disease start?
- How can an autoimmune disease be stopped?

It then goes on to describe:

- Vaccination therapy of Type 1 diabetes with a peptide of the 60 kDa heat shock protein (HSP60).
- Test-of-concept.

The chapter closes with a diagrammatic review of its message.

What is an autoimmune disease?

Traditionally in immunology, autoimmunity and autoimmune disease were considered as one. Autoimmunity may be defined as the recognition of self-antigens by antibodies or by the antigen receptors of clones of T-cells or B-cells. Immune recognition refers to the binding of an antigen receptor or antibody to an antigen with sufficient affinity or avidity to activate or block an immune response of some kind.[1] From this point of view, autoimmune disease is a clonal property of the lymphocyte repertoire.

Any time or place where there is autoimmunity, so it was taught, there will be autoimmune disease. The immune response was linked causally to the ability of clones of T-cells or B-cells to recognize antigens by way of their antigen receptors. There could be no adoptive immune response without antigen recognition and there could be no antigen recognition without antigen receptors. Therefore, a healthy state free of autoimmune disease would require that there be no recognition of self-antigens.[2] Freedom from autoimmune disease was believed to be the equivalent of freedom from autoimmunity. Consequently, autoimmunity had to be forbidden because autoimmune disease is forbidden.[2] But things have changed. The traditional view is still logical, but it is demonstrably wrong; it is not related to the facts.

Contrary to classical teaching, the repertoires of healthy immune systems are filled with autoantibodies and clones of T-cells and B-cells, which bear receptors capable of recognizing self-antigens.[1,3,4] True, the autoantibodies produced in autoimmune disease differ from the healthy autoantibodies in amount, affinity and isotype, and the clone size of autoimmune T-cells is larger and their cytokine profiles differ in autoimmune disease. Yet, the self-antigens recognized in disease do not seem to differ markedly from those recognizable by the healthy repertoire.[1,3,4] The potential for the prevalent autoimmune diseases is built into the healthy repertoire. In fact, autoimmune T-cells and autoantibodies may have a physiological role in maintaining the body.[5] Thus, autoimmunity is compatible with health and does not necessarily cause disease. So autoimmune disease cannot be defined in terms of autoimmunity. Autoimmune disease is not a disease of the clonal repertoire. How then is it to be defined?

I would like to propose that autoimmune disease be defined in terms of inflammation – autoimmune disease is a special kind of inflammation.

Inflammation in general has been defined as a dynamic process that is initiated in the wake of tissue injury and that leads, ideally, to complete healing.[6] Inflammation is the body's response to injury of any type. The physiology of inflammation is linked to the immune system. Quite simply, the inflammatory process is orchestrated by cells and molecules of the immune system. The inflammatory cells include the adaptive lymphocytes (T and B) and the innate leukocytes (macrophages, dendritic cells, neutrophils, eosinophils, basophils, mast cells, and others). One might argue that blood vessel endothelial cells and connective tissue cells also perform primary functions in inflammation. The inflammatory molecules are of two types: antigens, which are recognized by lymphocytes, and innately recognized signal molecules such as cytokines, chemokines, complement components, antibodies, clotting factors, adhesion molecules, proteases and a host of other enzymes and extracellular matrix components. The innate inflammatory molecules would also include the receptors for the above molecules, and other molecules, such as toll-like receptors and their ligands. These immune-system molecules act to make cells move, proliferate, differentiate, activate specific genes, or die.[1] The effects of inflammation are the sum of these actions. The inflammatory response debrides and molds tissues, induces tissue regeneration, triggers angiogenesis, generates scar tissue and bone, disposes of waste and kills body cells that are old, infected, stressed, or transformed. Immune system molecules also activate phagocytes to engulf and destroy infectious agents. In short, inflammation maintains the body and protects it in response to the grind of existence. That is the function of the immune system – to maintain the body by dispensing appropriate inflammation. Now we can define autoimmune disease.

Autoimmune disease is a process of damage to tissues or cells resulting from an inflammatory response that is inappropriate in its quality, quantity or dynamics and that takes place at the wrong time and/or in the wrong place.

The term *inappropriate* is the key concept. The cells, molecules and activities that mediate autoimmune disease are the same cells, molecules and activities found in health. Health or disease emerges from the way these components are connected and flow together – by the pattern of the process.[1] Disease results from a lack of regulation of the otherwise natural inflammatory process – from a disorganized pattern.

Any aspect of the inflammatory cascade can be disorganized and hence pathogenic. The pannus that destroys joints in rheumatoid arthritis is scar tissue growing unnecessarily in the wrong place; the lesions of systemic sclerosis are due to the proliferation of connective tissue where no healing is needed; cirrhosis of the liver is caused by healing gone wrong; an excess of angiogenesis can destroy the retina, and unnecessary apoptosis or cytolysis, for example, can kill β-cells and bring on Type 1 diabetes. Inappropriate healing can cause disease as easily as inappropriate killing.

The inflammation triggered by autoimmune T-cells in the central nervous system provides an example of the quantitative balance between beneficial autoimmunity and autoimmune disease. Clones of T-cells specific for the myelin antigen myelin basic protein (MBP) can protect the spinal cord of a rat from traumatic damage when a certain amount of the T-cells is administered; yet the same clones of T-cells can cause experimental autoimmune encephalomyelitis (EAE) when a greater number of the T-cells is administered.[5] It's all a matter of degree.

Inappropriate inflammation means that the inflammation visiting the target tissue serves no physiological purpose: an infection, injury or abnormality may have triggered the inflammatory response, but the inflammation does the wrong thing chronically or recurrently, and so the tissues and cells are damaged. Autoimmune disease reflects poorly regulated inflammation. Autoimmune disease clearly is not the equivalent of autoimmunity per se.

Is Type 1 diabetes an autoimmune disease?

The answer to the above question from most experts is yes.[7] The assignment of the disease to the autoimmune category is based on the stigmata of autoimmunity that mark the disease: the local inflammation around and within the islets, the genetic susceptibility associated with MHC 'immune response' genes, the studies in experimental animals showing adoptive transfer by immune system cells, and the demonstration that general suppression of the immune system can arrest the process.[8]

Now, if Type 1 diabetes is truly an autoimmune disease, then the most efficient way to understand Type 1 diabetes and to design rational therapies is linked to the way we understand autoimmunity as a general phenomenon. Our approach to Type 1 diabetes is linked to our approach to autoimmunity.

How does an autoimmune disease start?

If autoimmune disease is a type of inflammation, than an autoimmune disease can be triggered by any stimulus that triggers inflammation. Many factors can activate the immune system to produce inflammation, but for our present purpose we can divide the inciting stimuli into two groups of molecules: those that activate the innate receptors of leukocytes and those that activate the antigen receptors of lymphocytes (or antibodies). The molecules that induce inflammation via the lymphocytes are simply called antigens. The molecules that induce inflammation via innate receptors, as mentioned above, are very diverse and include any signals that activate leukocytes. The innate response is not restricted to particular clones. In contrast to innately induced inflammation, inflammation induced by antigens is clonal; it is initiated by lymphocytes with receptors for the antigens.

Once activated, the adaptive lymphocytes and the innate leukocytes activate one another by way of cytokines, enzymes, and by the expression of antigens or by the processing and presentation of antigens by other cells to lymphocytes. So the downstream events eventually enter a final common pathway of inflammation that reflects innate receptors and their ligands. It then becomes difficult, if not impossible, to decipher the initial trigger of the inflammation by looking at the inflammation itself. The presence of a specific autoimmune reaction, for example, cannot tell us itself whether that autoimmunity triggered the inflammation, or was activated by inflammation triggered by some other factor. Indeed, it has been reported that the first cells of the immune system in the insulitis of NOD mice are macrophages, and not lymphocytes.[9] This finding is compatible with the idea that the autoimmune T-cells found activated in Type 1 diabetes in NOD mice might be secondary to islet inflammation initiated by some other factor, a virus for example.[10] It has been reported that a very low dose of the β-cell toxin streptozotocin in genetically susceptible mice can secondarily activate specific autoimmunity to insulin and to HSP60.[11] The

activated autoimmune T-cells then go on to maintain the inflammatory process and kill β-cells.[12] If an observer was ignorant of the history of the streptozotocin intoxication, that observer might diagnose a 'primary' autoimmune disease as the cause of the Type 1 diabetes in the subjects, whether mice or humans. In short, how the inflammatory cascade began makes little difference to the end stage of the disease. The distinction between health and disease depends on how the process is dynamically tuned to the evolving state of the inflamed tissue – regulation is the name of the game.

Although innate signal molecules and innate receptors are the major mediators of inflammation, the fine-tuning of the process is strongly influenced by the adaptive lymphocytes that recognize antigens. T-cells and B-cells tune inflammation in two ways: by the antigen they recognize and by the phenotype of their response to the antigen – the cytokines or antibodies and other molecules they produce. Lymphocytes are adaptive because they learn from experience and remember their lessons.[1] Memory T-cells and B-cells, on meeting their antigen a second time, respond according to the way they were imprinted by the primary response.[13] For example, Th1 and Th2/Th3 polarized T-cell populations produce different types of cytokines and chemokines (and express different types of innate receptors) and so influence the type of inflammatory process to which they are party.[1,14] Antigen recognition can direct the inflammatory cascade.

However, inflammation itself also directs antigen recognition. Macrophages and dendritic cells activated in different ways by inflammation can migrate to different compartments of the body, process and present antigens differently, and trigger different clones of lymphocytes to produce different immune-response phenotypes. For example, the bacterial CpG motif, which activates toll-like receptor 9,[15] can shift the cytokine phenotype of specific autoimmune T-cells in NOD mice and arrest Type 1 diabetes.[16] Indeed, the interplay between autoimmune and inflammatory mechanisms has been proposed in the past to be a major factor in the development of Type 1 diabetes.[17] The inflammation triggered by trauma to the central nervous system, for another example, can activate clones of T-cells that recognize myelin antigens.[18] The anti-MBP T-cells activated in this way do not normally produce EAE (they probably help the healing process),[5] but they can cause EAE upon adoptive transfer to naive animals. Myocardial infarction activates autoantibodies to cardiac myosin; but this autoimmunity also does not normally lead to autoimmune myocarditis.[19] Inflammation often activates autoimmunity, but such activation rarely leads to autoimmune disease. Inflammation and autoimmunity are turned on and off together, without disease. Disease occurs when the *on* is without the *off*.

Let us now ask specifically: how might the autoimmune disease of Type 1 diabetes become activated? In general, by any process that activates inflammation in the islets. Candidate processes are virus infection,[10] toxic insult,[12] or trauma. It is possible that over-exertion of the β-cells and cellular stress could trigger insulitis. For example, the insulin-resistance of Type 2 diabetes could force the β-cells to produce abnormally large amounts of insulin, leading to β-cell stress (up-regulation of HSP60, for example), triggering in turn inflammation and activation of autoimmunity to HSP60, insulin, and other 'target' self-antigens, leading to a positive feedback amplification of the inflammation, β-cell death and Type 1 diabetes, as a complication of Type 2 diabetes.[20] A viral infection of β-cells could activate the same cascade.

In summary, the activation of inflammation and autoimmunity is necessary for autoimmune disease, but is not *sufficient* for autoimmune disease. Particular immune response genes are also necessary, but not sufficient for autoimmune disease.[21] Inflammation and autoimmunity get turned on all the time, but they also get turned off all the time. Disease emerges when autoimmunity and inflammation fail to get turned off. The natural mechanisms that down-regulate the process fail. This does not occur very often, and that is why autoimmune diseases, including Type 1 diabetes, are not more common.

Why would the inflammatory process fail to get turned off in some people? Why do some people and not others with the same genes suffer from particular autoimmune diseases? There is no simple answer to this question. We can say that the pattern of inflammation forms a chronic or recurrent loop,[1] but at the present time, we do not really know what this means at the molecular level.

How can an autoimmune disease be stopped?

To prevent an autoimmune disease, we need to stop two factors: the cascade of innate signal molecules that constitute the inflammation, and the antigen-specific activities of the autoimmune lymphocytes (predominantly, but not only, T-cells) that spur the inflammation on. Dealing with either factor alone probably will not solve the problem. Ongoing inflammation will recruit new autoimmune clones of T-cells, and the persistence of activated T-cells will awaken dormant inflammation. How can we both arrest the innate inflammatory cascade and change the behavior of the autoimmune T-cells? One way to accomplish this twin task is to activate immune modulation[22] using a molecule that interacts both with adaptive T-cell receptors and with innate receptors. HSP60 is an instructive example.

Vaccination therapy with an HSP60 peptide

Itamar Raz and associates have recently reported the results of a trial of therapeutic vaccination of new-onset Type 1 diabetes patients using a peptide derived from human HSP60 called p277.[23] The vaccine consisted of 1 mg of peptide p277 in a vegetable oil vehicle approved for human use with 40 mg mannitol as filler – the combination is called DiaPep277.

Peptide p277 is composed of the 24 amino acids of HSP60, positions 437–460, with two cysteine residues substituted by valines. The cysteine–valine substitution is only to stabilize the peptide; the modified p277 molecule has the immunological properties of the native sequence,[24,25] and is not an altered peptide ligand.[26]

The trial was randomized, blinded, and placebo-controlled; the placebo consisted of the vehicle and filler alone, without p277. Thirty-one subjects with Type 1 diabetes (males, 16–55 years old, with residual C-peptide above 0.1 nmol/l) received DiaPep277 or placebo injections upon entry, one month later and six months later.[23] The aim was to stop β-cell destruction and to document the immunological modifications induced by the vaccination.

Arrest of the destruction of β-cells was determined by preservation of C-peptide as a measure of endogenous insulin production.[27] The amount of exogenous insulin needed for optimal control was also used as a measure of endogenous insulin production. Immunologically, the cytokines produced by T-cells stimulated with HSP60 or peptide p277 were measured using a quantitative Elispot assay.

The results showed that those persons treated with DiaPep277 maintained significantly more C-peptide and required significantly less exogenous insulin than did the placebo-treated controls. It is reasonable to conclude that the beneficial response to the peptide vaccination was caused by a cessation of the damaging autoimmune inflammation in the islets. Indeed, the DiaPep277–treated subjects manifested an enhancement of Th2 ('anti-inflammatory') cytokines (IL-10, IL-13 and IL-4) and a decrease of a Th1 ('pro-inflammatory') cytokine, IFNγ, produced by subject T-cells in response to stimulation *in vitro* with peptide p277 or with the HSP60 molecule from which peptide p277 was derived.[23] The enhancement of the Th2 cytokine phenotype was specific; the T-cell responses of the treated subjects to bacterial antigens remained in the Th1 mode. There has been no toxicity associated with DiaPep277 vaccination in this or in the other clinical trials presently underway. Without unblinding the study, a fourth injection was given at 12 months, and the subjects were evaluated at 12 months and at 18 months. The results at these additional time points showed an even more marked statistical difference in favor of the DiaPep277-treated group compared with the placebo-treated group.

A test-of-concept

The clinical trial of DiaPep277 therapeutic vaccination grew out of a merger between an immunological concept and a sequence of research findings. The immunological concept led us to the vaccination protocol; the research led us to the HSP60 peptide vaccine.

The natural existence of autoimmunity in the lymphocyte repertoire suggests that natural regulatory mechanisms must also exist to control autoimmunity. This idea is personified in the theory of the immunological homunculus.[1,3,4,28,29] The theory proposes that natural autoimmunity is focused on a particular set of dominant self-antigens. Anti-idiotypic networks[30] and antiergotypic T-cells,[31] combined with CD25+ T cells[32] and anti-inflammatory cytokine networks,[14] work to turn off safely homuncular autoimmune activation after it has been turned on. The dominant autoimmune repertoire and its regulatory mechanisms form a functional representation of the body inscribed in the immune system. We have called this picture of the body the immunological homunculus.[3]

A corollary of the immunological homunculus concept is that autoimmune disease, as discussed above, results from a failure to turn off a natural autoimmune inflammatory process. Rather than trying to suppress the autoimmune clones, the homunculus concept recommends reactivating natural regulation.[22] Vaccination is the essence of immune activation, and so we devised a protocol for therapeutic vaccination.

In contrast to the vaccination protocol, the idea of using a peptide of HSP60 as the vaccine was not driven by a clear hypothesis. We came across HSP60 by good fortune. We were acquainted with HSP60 as a possible self-antigen in autoimmunity by the discovery that Mycobacterial HSP65, a variant of HSP60, was a target of autoimmunity in the experimental disease called adjuvant arthritis.[33] Shortly after we became aware of HSP65 in adjuvant arthritis, we read reports of a yet undefined 64 kDa antigen targeted by autoantibodies in Type 1 diabetes patients.[34] Could our 65 kDa heat shock protein, discovered in arthritis, be related to the 64 kDa self-antigen in Type 1 diabetes? This question rests on curiosity and not on hypothesis. However we went ahead and tested whether NOD mice developing Type 1 diabetes might produce antibodies to HSP65. By the time we discovered that NOD mice did make such antibodies,[35] the 64 kDa antigen was identified as glutamic acid decarboxylase.[36] We were left with unexplained autoreactivity to HSP65,[37] and we were very curious.

Subsequent research showed that T-cell autoimmunity in NOD mice was directed more to mammalian HSP60; reactivity to Mycobacterial HSP65 was only cross-reactive with true autoimmunity to HSP60.[24] It is intriguing that autoimmunity to HSP60 seems to have a role in the pathogenesis of atherosclerosis.[38] Thus, HSP60 autoimmunity can target the blood vessels in addition to β-cells. Could this face of HSP60 autoimmunity contribute to the vascular complications of diabetes, the 'third' Type 1 disease mentioned at the outset?

We put aside the connection of HSP60 to adjuvanticity detected in experimental arthritis[37] and focused on HSP60 as a T-cell autoantigen in Type 1 diabetes. We used pathogenic clones of anti-HSP60 T-cells as probes to identify the p277 sequence as containing a key target epitope.[24] Based on our earlier experience that a peptide of HSP65 could vaccinate against adjuvant arthritis,[39] we tested p277 as a vaccine and found that it could induce resistance to Type 1 diabetes in NOD mice.[24] Indeed, p277 vaccination could arrest β-cell destruction even in mice already clinically diabetic.[25] Therapeutic vaccination with p277 was also found to be effective in Type 1 diabetes induced by very low-dose streptozotocin in C57BL/ksJ mice.[40] These observations paved the way for the clinical use of p277 (DiaPep277) in newly diagnosed Type 1 subjects.[23]

The mechanism of action of p277 treatment was identified as a shift in cytokine phenotype both in the spleen[41] and in the islet inflammatory infiltrate[42] in treated NOD mice. NOD mice designed transgenically to hyper-express

HSP60 in the thymus and elsewhere manifested resistance to Type 1 diabetes.[43] Thus, HSP60 vaccination could be effective even when administered genetically. HSP60 treatment could even delay rejection of a skin allograft.[44]

The discovery by other researchers that HSP60 was a ligand for an innate receptor on macrophages,[45] returned our attention to HSP60 as an adjuvant signal[37] in addition to its immune function as a T-cell epitope. Most recently, we have discovered that peptide p277 can itself activate an innate receptor on T-cells as well as on other leukocytes (in preparation).

Now, we can propose a hypothesis that might account for the effectiveness of p277 in regulating Type 1 diabetes: an HSP60 epitope such as p277 works by simultaneously interacting both with the antigen receptors of clones of autoimmune T-cells involved in islet inflammation and with innate immune receptors involved in the inflammatory cascade. This type of vaccination deals both with adaptive autoimmunity and with innate inflammation signaling. Future research will focus on the molecular basis for this dual effect of HSP60. Whether or not this hypothesis will emerge confirmed or rejected, the beneficial effect of p277 treatment in arresting β-cell destruction is an empirical matter.

Diagrammatic review

Figure 14.1 depicts the immune system as composed of two interacting segments that together orchestrate the inflammatory response:

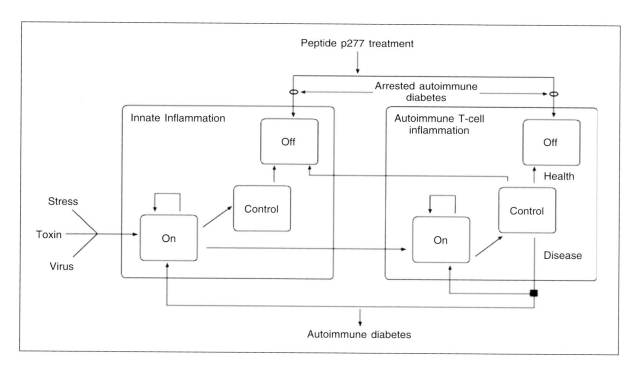

Figure 14.1
Diagrammatic review.

Innate inflammation and *Autoimmune T-cell inflammation*. Noxious stimuli of any kind, exemplified by *Virus*, *Toxin* and *Stress*, activate *Innate inflammation* into the *On* state. The *On* state is expressed by the elaboration of a variety of molecules such as cytokines, chemokines, adhesion molecules and cell-interaction signals that constitute inflammation. Inflammation often arises, like blood clotting, in an emergency that needs a quick response, and so, like blood clotting, inflammation proceeds with positive feedback: the products of inflammation generate more inflammation – a small flame can ignite a blaze. This positive feedback is depicted by the *On* arrow that loops back onto *On*. Like the clotting cascade, however, inflammation also must be regulated by *Control* mechanisms that turn the inflammation *Off*. But once turned *On*, *Innate inflammation* also activates *Autoimmune T-cell inflammation*: activated macrophages, for example, activate T-cells. Thus, the autoimmune clones in the healthy repertoire get turned *On* in response to tissue damage. *Autoimmune T-cell inflammation* also proceeds through positive feedback: activated T-cells produce cytokines that facilitate the activation of additional T-cells. The activation of autoimmune T-cells activates *Control* mechanisms that normally operate to turn *Off* both the *Autoimmune T-cell inflammation* and *Innate inflammation* once the healthy inflammatory response has healed the injury. However, it occasionally happens that individuals expressing certain immune response genes suffer a failure of healthy *Control*, and then both arms of inflammation are pushed into persistent *On*. The qualitative aspect of the abnormal *On* can include not only unneeded 'healing' but also unneeded 'destruction'; in either case, the de-regulated inflammation can cause a disease. In our example, the destruction of β-cells leads to *Autoimmune diabetes*. Administration of

Peptide p277 treatment arrests the damaging inflammation by activating the *Autoimmune T-cell inflammation* into an anti-inflammatory *Off* mode. Peptide p277 also pushes the *Innate inflammation* into an *Off* mode. The advantage of p277 treatment lies in this dual control of factors driving both the innate and the antigen-specific arms of the damaging inflammatory reaction that produced the disease.

Acknowledgements

Irun R Cohen is the incumbent of the Mauerberger Chair in Immunology and Director of the Robert Koch Minerva Center for Research in Autoimmune Disease, at the Weizmann Institute of Science, Director of the Center for the Study of Emerging Diseases, Jerusalem, and a consultant for Peptor, LTD, Rehovot, Israel.

References

1. Cohen IR. Tending Adam's Garden: Evolving the Cognitive Immune Self. London: Academic Press, 2000.
2. Burnet FM. Self and Not-Self. Cambridge: Cambridge University Press, 1969.
3. Cohen IR. The cognitive paradigm and the immunological homunculus. Immunol Today 1992; 13:490–4.
4. Cohen IR. Discrimination and dialogue in the immune system. Sem Immunol 2000; 12: 215–9; 269–71; 321–3.
5. Schwartz M, Cohen IR. Autoimmunity can benefit self-maintenance. Immunol Today 2000; 21: 265–8.
6. Florey HW. Inflammation. In: Florey HW, eds. General Pathology. London: Lloyd-Duke Ltd, 1970: 22–39.
7. Bach JF. Insulin-dependent diabetes mellitus as an autoimmune disease. Endocr Rev 1994; 15: 516–42.

8. Bougneres PF, Carel JC, Castano L et al. Factors associated with early remission of Type I diabetes in children treated with cyclosporine. N Engl J Med 1988; 318: 663–70.

9. Kolb H, Burkart V, Appels B et al. Essential contribution of macrophages to islet cell destruction in vivo and in vitro. J Autoimmun 1990; 1: 117–20.

10. Fairweather D, Rose NR. Type 1 diabetes: virus infection or autoimmune disease? Nat Immunol 2002; 3: 338–40.

11. Elias D, Prigozin H, Polak N et al. Autoimmune diabetes induced by the beta-cell toxin streptozotocin: immunity to the 60 KDa heat shock protein and to insulin. Diabetes 1994; 43: 992–8.

12. Kolb H. Mouse models of insulin dependent diabetes: low-dose streptozocin-induced diabetes and nonobese diabetic (NOD) mice. Diabetes Metab Rev 1987; 3: 751–78.

13. Friedman A, Cohen IR. T cell Ir phenotype modified by excising primary antigen deposit. Immunogenetics 1984; 19: 449–54.

14. Weiner HL. Induction and mechanism of action of transforming growth factor-beta-secreting Th3 regulatory cells. Immunol Rev 2001; 182: 207–14.

15. Hemmi H, Takeuchi O, Kawai T et al. A Toll-like receptor recognizes bacterial DNA. Nature 2000; 408: 740–5.

16. Quintana FJ, Rotem A, Carmi P et al. Vaccination with empty plasmid DNA or CpG oligonucleotide inhibits diabetes in NOD mice: Modulation of spontaneous HSP60 autoimmunity. J Immunol 2001; 165: 6148–55.

17. Kolb H, Kolb-Bachofen V, Roep BO. Autoimmune versus inflammatory Type 1 diabetes: a controversy? Immunol Today 1994; 16: 170–2.

18. Popovich PG, Stokes BT, Whitacre CC. Concept of autoimmunity following spinal cord injury: possible roles for T lymphocytes in the traumatized central nervous system. J Neurosci Res 1996; 45: 349–63.

19. Elahi AW, Vijayakumar AN, Lichstein E et al. Interplay of antibody and T cell responses in acute myocardial infarction. J Lab Clin Med 2001; 138: 112–18.

20. Schernthaner G, Hink S, Kopp HP et al. Progress in the characterization of slowly progressive autoimmune diabetes in adult patients (LADA or Type 1,5 diabetes). Exp Clin Endocrinol Diabetes 2001; 109: S94–S108.

21. Todd JA, Wicker LS Genetic protection from the inflammatory disease Type 1 diabetes in humans and animal models. Immunity 2001; 15: 387–95.

22. Cohen IR. Treatment of autoimmune disease: to activate or to deactivate? Chem Immunol 1995; 60: 150–60.

23. Raz I, Elias D, Avron A et al. Beta-cell function in new-onset Type 1 diabetes and immunomodulation with a heat-shock protein peptide (DiaPep277): a randomised, double-blind, phase II trial. Lancet 2001; 24: 1749–53.

24. Elias D, Reshef T, Birk OS et al. Vaccination against autoimmune mouse diabetes with a T-cell epitope of the human 65 kDa heat shock protein. Proc Natl Acad Sci USA 1991; 88: 3088–91.

25. Elias D, Cohen IR. Peptide therapy for diabetes in NOD mice. Lancet 1994; 343: 704–6.

26. Bielekova B, Martin R. Antigen-specific immunomodulation via altered peptide ligands. J Mol Med 2001; 79: 552–65.

27. Berger B, Stenstrom G, Sundkvist G. Random C-peptide in the classification of diabetes. Scand J Clin Lab Invest 2000; 60: 687–93.

28. Cohen IR, Young DB. Autoimmunity, microbial immunity and the immunological homunculus. Immunol Today 1991; 12: 105–10.

29. Cohen IR. The cognitive principle challenges clonal selection. Immunol Today 1992; 13: 441–4.

30. Lider O, Reshef T, Beraud E et al. Anti-idiotypic network induced by T cell vaccination against experimental autoimmune encephalomyelitis. Science 1988; 239: 181–3.

31. Lohse AW, Mor F, Karin N et al. Control of experimental autoimmune encephalomyelitis by T cells responding to activated T cells. Science 1989; 244: 820–2.

32. Sakaguchi S, Sakaguchi N, Shimizu J et al. Immunologic tolerance maintained by CD25+ CD4+ regulatory T cells: their common role in controlling autoimmunity, tumor immunity, and transplantation tolerance. Immunol Rev 2001; 182: 18–32.

33. Van Eden W, Thole JER, Van Der Zee R et al. Cloning of the mycobacterial epitope recognized by T lymphocytes in adjuvant arthritis. Nature 1988; 331: 171–3.

34. Christie MR, Pipeleers DG, Lernmark A, Baekkeskov S. Cellular and subcellular localization of an Mr 64,000 protein autoantigen in insulin-dependent diabetes. J Biol Chem 1990; 265: 376–81.

35. Elias D, Markovits D, Reshef T et al. Induction and therapy of autoimmune diabetes in the non-obese diabetic (NOD/LT) mouse by a 65-kDa heat shock protein. Proc Natl Acad Sci USA, 1990; 87: 1576–80.

36. Baekkeskov S, Aanstoot HJ, Christgau S et al. Identification of the 64K autoantigen in insulin-dependent diabetes as the GABA-synthesizing enzyme glutamic acid decarboxylase. Nature 1990; 13: 151–6.

37. Cohen IR. Autoimmunity to chaperonins in the pathogenesis of arthritis and diabetes. Annu Rev Immunol 1991; 9: 567–89.

38. Wick G, Perschinka H, Millonig G. Atherosclerosis as an autoimmune disease: an update. Trends Immunol 2001; 22: 665–9.

39. Van Eden W, Hogervorst EJ, Van Der Zee R et al. The mycobacterial 65 kD heat-shock protein and autoimmune arthritis. Rheumatol Int 1989; 9: 187–91.

40. Elias D, Cohen IR. The hsp60 peptide p277 arrests the autoimmune diabetes induced by the toxin streptozotocin. Diabetes 1996; 45: 1168–72.

41. Elias D, Meilin A, Ablamunits V et al. Hsp60 peptide therapy of NOD mouse diabetes induces a Th2 cytokine burst and down-regulates autoimmunity to various β-cell antigens. Diabetes 1997; 46: 758–64.

42. Ablamunits V, Elias D, Reshef T, Cohen IR. Islet T cells secreting IFN-gamma in NOD mouse diabetes: arrest by p277 peptide treatment. J Autoimmun 1998; 11: 73–81.

43. Birk OS, Douek DC, Elias D, et al. The role of hsp60 in autoimmune diabetes: analysis in a transgenic model. Proc Natl Acad Sci USA 1996; 93: 1032–7.

44. Birk O, Gur SL, Elias D et al. The 60 kDa heat shock protein modulates allograft rejection. Proc Nat Acad Sci USA 1999; 96: 5159–63.

45. Habich C, Baumgart K, Kolb H, Burkart V. The receptor for heat shock protein 60 on macrophages is saturable, specific, and distinct from receptors for other heat shock proteins. J Immunol 2002; 15: 168: 569–76.

15

Islet and pancreas transplantation
Reinhard G Bretzel

Introduction

Long-term studies strongly suggest that tight control of blood glucose achieved by conventional intensive insulin treatment, self-blood glucose monitoring and patient education can significantly prevent the development and retard the progression of chronic complications of Type 1 diabetes mellitus.[1,2] However, the expense for this benefit was a three-fold increase in the number of severe hypoglycemic episodes, a significant increase of the body weight, and dietary and other lifestyle restrictions affecting the quality of life.[3]

By contrast, replacement of a patient's islets of Langerhans either by pancreas transplantation or by isolated islet transplantation (Figure 15.1), is the only treatment of Type 1 diabetes mellitus to achieve an insulin-independent, constant normoglycemic state, while avoiding hypoglycemic episodes.[4,5] The expense of this benefit is the need for immunosuppressive treatment of the recipient with all its potential risks.

Results of pancreas transplantation have continued to improve, especially in the combined pancreas and kidney graft category. Results in this group are approaching those of other solid organs, but results of solitary pancreas grafting in non-uremic diabetic patients have been slow to follow and this method is still restricted to special centers. It has been demonstrated that successful pancreas transplantation exerts beneficial effects on secondary complications of diabetes and

improves quality of life. However, despite significant progress, pancreas transplantation is still associated with peri-operative mortality and significant morbidity.[6-8]

In contrast, islet cell transplantation offers an added advantage in that it can be performed as a minimally invasive procedure, in which islets are perfused percutaneously into the liver via the portal vein.[9] For the last three decades, islet cell transplantation has been proposed for the scientific community and promised to patients and their families. However, even the most convincing results in small animal studies did not translate at the same level to the clinical setting. Nonetheless, a few case reports of insulin independence achieved by intraportal islet allotransplants in Type 1 diabetic recipients do exist.[5,10-14] Recent data analysis from the International Islet Transplant Registry based at our institution showed that insulin independence after one year was achieved in only 11% of the patients.[15]

The concept of islet cell transplantation is, however, most attractive since it offers many perspectives:[16]

(1) In contrast to pancreas organ transplantation, islet cell availability could become unlimited, when strategies such as the use of xenogenic islets, engineered beta-cell lines or *in vitro* stem cell expansion and differentiation into insulin producing cells reach the stage of clinical applicability.
(2) Islet cells may be transplanted without chronic immunosuppressive treatment of

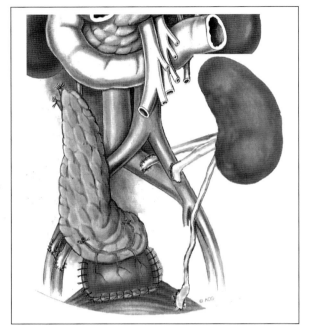

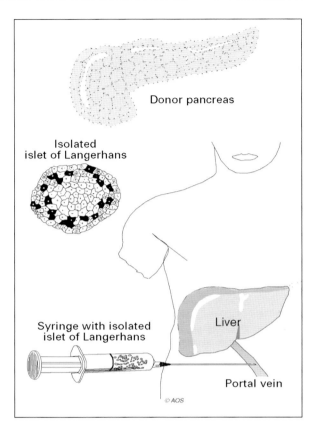

Figure 15.1
Pancreas–kidney transplantation into the pelvis with pancreatic duct drainage into the bladder (left). Islet transplantation into the portal venous system (right).

the recipient by making use of donor-specific tolerance induction strategies or immunoisolation systems. This unique set of characteristics could finally make it possible to offer islet transplants alone to adults and even adolescents and children with Type 1 diabetes, prior to the development, and with the prospect of preventing, such devastating diabetic secondary complications such as end-stage renal disease, lower limb ischemia and amputations or blindness.

This review will summarize the current status and the perspectives of both pancreatic organ and islet cell transplantations in patients with Type 1 diabetes mellitus.

Pancreas transplantation

The history of pancreas organ transplantation

The first human vascularized pancreas transplant in a patient with diabetes mellitus was performed by Kelly and co-workers at the University of Minnesota in Minneapolis, USA, in 1966.[17] The body and tail of the pancreas from a cadaveric donor (with the pancreatic duct ligated), was transplanted into the iliac fossa of a uremic diabetic woman, contralateral to a kidney graft. The patient became normoglycemic and insulin independent, but died two months after transplantation from graft rejection and sepsis. From then until 1977, a total of 57 pancreas transplants were notified to the Organ Transplant Registry, maintained by the American College of Surgeons at the National Institutes of Health.[18] During that pioneering era, only 40% of patients remained alive, and only 3% of pancreatic grafts were still functioning one year after transplantation.[19] At that time, kidney transplantation was also in its infancy and protocols for immunosuppression were only beginning to emerge.

Surgical techniques

For a long time, the major difficulty in pancreas organ transplantation was getting rid of the autoaggressive pancreatic juice. Three main duct management techniques have emerged: duct injection (DI), as advocated by Dubernard et al.;[20] intestinal drainage (ID), further developed by the Stockholm group;[21] and bladder drainage (BD), reintroduced and refined by Cook et al.,[22] Sollinger et al.[23] and Corry et al.[24] Choices also exist for the position of pancreas and the site of vascular anastomoses. The peritoneal cavity is better able to cope with enzymes released from the pancreas and is now the position of choice. The use of the iliac

vessels for vascular anastomosis, however, remains a contentious issue. Early attempts to provide portal venous drainage with anastomosis to the mesenteric circulation demonstrated high rates of venous thrombosis.[25] Nevertheless, the technique has been revisited by several groups.[26–28] These authors reported equivalent graft survival to the more conventional bladder drained technique with less incidence of reflux pancreatitis, avoidance of metabolic acidosis and a reduction in fasting hyperinsulinemia.[26] At present, enteric-drained pancreas transplant along with portal venous drainage seems to be the procedure of first choice in almost 100% of the pancreas transplants ($n = 332$) performed in 2000 in the Eurotransplant region (Belgium, The Netherlands, Luxembourg, Austria, Germany, Slovenia) as enteric-drained grafts.

Survival of patients and grafts

The evolution of pancreas organ transplantation has been documented by the International Pancreas Transplant Registry (IPTR) based at the University of Minnesota in Minneapolis, USA. As of August 2001, more than 15,000 pancreas transplants have been reported to the IPTR as shown in Figure 15.2. These include

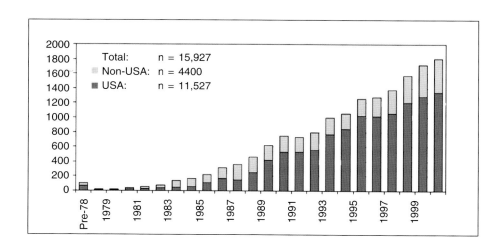

Figure 15.2
Total number of pancreas transplants performed in the USA ■ and other countries ■ between 1978 and 2000 (n = 15,927). These cases were notified by the International Pancreas Transplant Registry (IPTR), Minneapolis, USA. (Source: ref. 29).

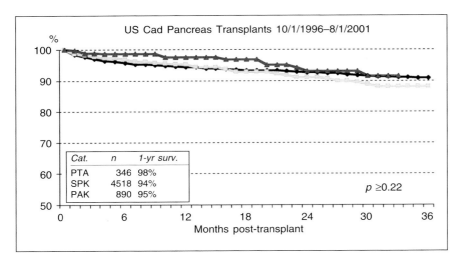

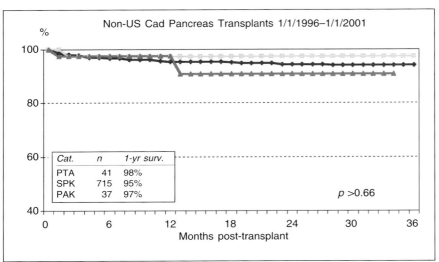

Figure 15.3
Patient survival rates at one year by recipient category for 1996–2001 US and non-US cadaveric pancreas transplants. PTA ▲; SPK ◆; PAK ■. (Source: ref. 29).

over 11,000 performed in the USA and over 4000 from outside the USA.[29] Pancreas transplant cases in 2000 reported as of August 2001, totalled 1661; 1346 US and 315 non-US. Reported cases were included in analyses where completed records were available. Data analysis provided for three main recipient categories: pancreas transplants alone (PTA); simultaneous pancreas–kidney (SPK); and pancreas after kidney (PAK).

Patient survival rates at one year for 1996–08/01/2001 US cadaveric pancreas transplants ($n = 5754$) were at least 94% in all categories (Figure 15.3): PTA 98%; SPK 94%; PAK 95%. For non-US 1996–08/01/2001 SPK cadaveric pancreas transplants ($n = 793$), the comparable results were 98%, 95% and 97% respectively (Figure 15.3).

Pancreas graft survival at one year for 1996–08/01/2001 US cadaveric pancreas transplants ($n = 5740$): SPK 84% (kidney graft survival

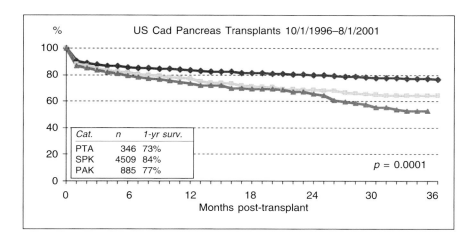

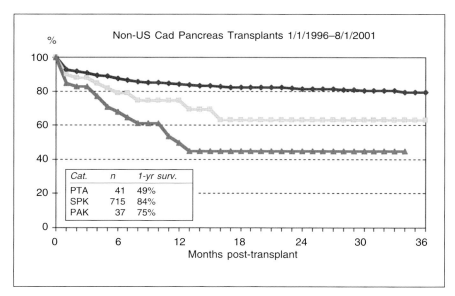

Figure 15.4
Pancreas graft survival at one year by recipient category for 1996–2001 US and non-US cadaveric pancreas transplants. PTA ▲; SPK ◆; PAK ■. (Source: ref. 29).

was 92%); PAK 77%; PTA 73%. The differences in pancreas graft survival in the three categories at one year were significant, but overall outcome for PAK and PTA has improved from previous years (Figure 15.4). For 1996–08/01/2001 non-US cadaveric pancreas transplants (n = 793), pancreas graft survival at one year was 84% (kidney graft survival was 90%); PAK 75% and PTA 49%. PTA results are significantly lower compared with the US PTA rate of 73% (Figure 15.4).

From 1987–93 the great majority of pancreas transplants were performed using bladder drainage (BD) as a duct management technique. However, since 1994 the proportion of enteric-drained (ED) US pancreas transplant cases has increased. For US cadaveric cases with a complete record for analysis (n = 3481) from 1996–2000, 55% of SPKs were reported to be using ED as the duct management method. For PAKs and PTAs, ED was 46% and

41%, respectively. The use of a Roux-en-Y loop with ED has been decreasing in cases where a duct management method was reported; since 1996 most have been done without the Roux-en-Y.

Overall, the 1996–2000 outcome for pancreas transplantation was excellent for patient, pancreas and kidney graft survival in all categories. Non-US and US pancreas transplant results were basically similar. Duct management technique had little effect on outcome for SPK; for PAK and PTA, US pancreas graft survival rates were significantly higher for BD versus ED. Immunosuppression regimens showed improved outcome for SPK cases who received anti-T-cell induction therapy and CSA/MMF for maintenance immunosuppression, while PAK and PTA pancreas graft survival rates were highest in recipients who received anti-T-cell agents for induction plus both MMF and TAC for maintenance immunosuppression. HLA matching, especially at the B locus, was important to PAK and PTA transplants, but not SPK outcomes.

Metabolic effects

Several metabolic indices can be used to measure the function of pancreas transplants. Successful grafting eliminates the need for exogenous insulin and can normalize or greatly improve glucose metabolism, as indicated by glucose tolerance tests and glycated hemoglobin concentrations.[30–32] Twenty-four hour glucose profiles have shown to be virtually normal in most patients and diurnal patterns of free fatty acids, 3-hydroxybutyrate and alanine were found to be normal, with blood lactate and glycerol slightly higher after combined renal and pancreatic grafting in comparison with kidney transplanted nondiabetic patients.[33] However, many studies have shown that glucose homeostasis after, for example, simultaneous pancreas–kidney transplantation is not entirely normal.[34–36] Pancreas transplant recipients often show fasting hyperinsulinemia, abnormal insulin and glucagon responses to a glucose challenge when compared to a control group, and a delayed return to baseline levels. Possible reasons include the denervation of the transplanted pancreas, the use of immunosuppressive drugs (particularly glucocorticoids), which can affect both beta cell function and insulin sensitivity, and the fact that in most cases, insulin is secreted by the graft into the systemic rather than the portal circulation. Debate, however, continues as to which of these factors is the most important and whether or not hyperinsulinemia is deleterious. At least the latter can be avoided by portal venous drainage techniques. A recent prospective randomized study comparing portal versus systemic venous drainage in kidney–pancreas recipients, however, did not reveal any significant difference between the two groups. Fasting and stimulated glucose or glycosylated hemoglobin were the same and no hyperinsulinemia and lipid abnormalities were evidenced in either group's long-term studies.[37]

Effect on secondary complications

With the increase in graft survival rates in pancreas transplantation, the potentially beneficial effect of successful long-term normoglycemia on secondary complications of diabetes has been studied in several centers. There is clear evidence on the prevention of recurrence of the diabetic nephropathy in the transplanted kidney.[38–40] Pancreas transplants alone can ameliorate established diabetic glomerular lesions in patients with their own kidneys.[41] It was also demonstrated that pancreas transplantation can even reverse the lesions of diabetic nephropathy, but reversal requires more than five years of normoglycemia, as demonstrated in a biopsy-proven study.[42]

Studies of the effect of pancreas transplantation on diabetic autonomic and peripheral neuropathy provide the best objective evidence of the benefits of pancreas transplantation.[43–47]

Advanced diabetic retinopathy appears to be stabilized or at least slowed down in recipients with long-term functioning pancreas grafts reassessed after several years.[48,49]

A positive effect of pancreas grafting on skin microcirculation was shown.[50] However, a disappointing feature of pancreas transplantation has been the inability to prevent progressive macroangiopathy or large vessel disease.[51]

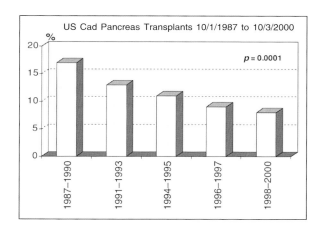

Figure 15.5
Overall technical failure rates for 1987–2000 US cadaveric pancreas transplants. (Source: ref. 29).

Safety and quality-of-life aspects

The reason for the significantly prolonged bed-stay after pancreas transplantation compared with kidney transplants alone is the frequency of complications.[52] These relate specifically to the pancreas, an organ with a low blood flow, and a great majority of its parenchymal cells associated with production of proteolytic enzymes which may induce autodigestion. The majority of the complications occur in the first few months after transplantation.

An analysis of the IPTR indicated that technical failure rates have decreased significantly over time for 1987–2000 US cadaveric pancreas transplants, from 15% for 1987–1989 to 7% for 1998–2000 (Figure 15.5). In all categories, technical failure rate has declined in each era since 1990; earlier technical failure rates for PAK and PTA groups may have been higher due to early rejections being reported as technical.

Graft thrombosis was the most common cause of technical failure for 1996–2000 US cadaveric pancreas transplant cases, ≥ 70%, whether by duct management (BD, ED) or transplant category (SPK, PAK, PTA) (Table 15.1). The incidence of any one of the remaining technical failure reasons – infection/pancreatitis, anastomotic leak, bleed – was < 3% in each transplant category. For PAK and PTA categories, the graft thrombosis and anastomotic leak rates were lower for BD versus ED. For ED in the PTA group, some early thrombosis may actually be early rejection since the diagnosis of early rejection is more difficult in the ED–PTA group. An extended overview on the surgical risk of pancreas transplantation has recently been published.[6]

The mortality rate after pancreas transplantation is about 3–5% after one year and 5–7% after three years. The most common cause of death is overwhelming sepsis, with cardiovascular causes kept to a minimum by careful screening prior to transplantation.[53] However, long-term studies clearly demonstrated the markedly improved survival rate ten years after successful simultaneous pancreas–kidney transplantation compared with kidney transplants alone.[54]

	SPK			PAK			PTA		
	BD (%)	ED (%)	p	BD (%)	ED (%)	p	BD (%)	ED (%)	p
Graft thrombosis	5.4	6.3	0.264	5.0	8.8	0.050	4.6	15.8	0.001
Infection/ pancreatitis	0.6	1.1	0.144	1.1	2.9	0.091	0.0	0.8	0.226
Anastomotic leak	0.4	0.9	0.058	0.0	0.7	0.126	0.6	0.8	0.766
Bleed	0.3	0.2	0.492	0.6	0.0	0.190	0.0	0.0	–

Notes: BD bladder drained; ED enteric drained.

Table 15.1
Reasons for technical failures for 1996–2000 US cadaveric pancreas transplants by recipient category (Source: ref. 29)

The life-long immunosuppression required by kidney-graft recipients carries significant risks in terms of increased incidence of infections and neoplasms. But these are generally outweighed by the poor quality of life and high mortality of end-stage renal failure of non-transplanted diabetic patients. Furthermore, improvement in quality of life after pancreas transplantation can be dramatic.[55,56] There is no longer the threat of hypoglycemia and the shackles of the restrictive lifestyle, and health risk from hypoglycemia has been removed. For the patient, it is perhaps the single most important benefit of pancreas transplantation and the recipients are exceptionally appreciative.

Present problems and new strategies in pancreas organ transplantation

Continuing concerns of hyperinsulinemia and exocrine complications will dictate that greater numbers of portal venous-drained pancreas transplants be performed, together with enteric drainage of the exocrine portion of the gland. For the major urinary tract complications, often seen in bladder-drained pancreas transplant recipients, enteric conversion procedures are now recommended. Recurrence of autoimmune diabetes with insulitis and the sequelae of islet function has been observed also after pancreas transplantation.[57] The number of HLA mismatches most likely influences the recurrence of autoimmune diabetes. The limited number of donor pancreas and the restrictions of using living-donor pancreas will probably lead to a plateauing of about 2000 pancreas organ transplants per year performed worldwide.

Islet transplantation
The history of islet cell transplantation

It was Rudolf Virchow (1821–1902) who first suspected an incretory capacity of the pancreatic organ in addition to its known excretory capacity. Virchow's student, Paul Langerhans, first described in his doctoral thesis (1869) clusters of cells, later named after him as islets of Langerhans. However, Paul Langerhans had no idea about the function of these cell clusters.

In April 1889, Joseph von Mering was working in Hoppe Seyler's Institute at the University of Strasbourg when Oskar Minkowski visited. Following one of their discussions on the metabolic role of the pancreatic gland, they began an investigation of the surgical removal of the pancreas from a dog. They found that diabetes mellitus develops after total pancreatectomy, providing final evidence that this disease is located in the pancreas.[58] Two years later, Oskar Minkowski gave a lecture on December 18, 1891 at the Strasbourg Society of Natural Science and Medicine which was published in the *Berliner Klinische Wochenschrift*.[59] He informed the audience that his and von Mering's series of experimental studies provided further evidence that diabetes mellitus develops after pancreatectomy and also demonstrated for the first time that pancreatectomy-induced diabetes can be prevented by autografting pancreatic fragments under the skin. Furthermore, Minkowski concluded that something seems to be delivered by the pancreatic gland which facilitates sugar consumption by the peripheral tissue. Today, of course, we all know that this 'something' is the hormone insulin, which 30 years later was extracted from pancreatic tissue and successfully injected in patients with insulin-requiring diabetes.[60]

The pioneering work by Oskar Minkowski and Joseph von Mering, in particular their experimentation with the autotransplantation of pancreatic fragments, paved the way toward clinical islet transplantations. Almost exactly two years after Minkowski's lecture, the first recorded human pancreatic fragment transplant was performed on December 20, 1893. Dr P Watson Williams and his colleague, Mr Harsant, treated a 15-year-old boy in the Bristol Royal Infirmary in Great Britain with the subcutaneous implantation of three pieces of freshly slaughtered sheep's pancreas, each 'the size of a Brazil nut'.[61] They observed that glycosuria was lowered, however, the patient died after a few days.

Current status of clinical islet transplantation

As of December 31, 2000, a total of 445 human islet cell transplantations performed between 1974 and 2000 in patients with Type 1 diabetes mellitus have been reported to the International Islet Transplant Registry (ITR) established in 1989 and maintained at our department of Giessen University, Germany. An annual updated newsletter has been published.[15] The introduction of an automated method has permitted retrieval of a sufficient number of islets even from a single human donor pancreas to allow reversal of diabetes after allotransplantation in a Type 1 diabetic patient and has made insulin independence more likely.[62]

With this method available a new era of clinical islet transplantation, either simultaneous with (SIK) or after kidney transplantation (IAK), started in the early 1990s and a total of 355 islet allotransplants in Type 1 diabetes mellitus have been performed between 1990 and December 31, 2000. There are only 10 institutions worldwide, six in the USA and Canada and four in Europe, to have performed a minimum of 10 cases (Table 15.2).

Data analysis has shown that at one year after islet transplantation the patient survival rate was 96%, the islet graft maintained function in 41% of the cases, and in 11% of the patients the ultimate goal, insulin independence, was achieved (Table 15.3). The longest insulin independence observed is now more than six years (Table 15.3).

Institution (transplantation/isolation)	Year of transplantation											Σ
	1990	1991	1992	1993	1994	1995	1996	1997	1998	1999	2000	
1. Giessen	–	–	1	5	5	12	11	17	6	4	5	66
2. Milan	4	3	2	4	4	4	1	–	5	5	10	42
3. Minneapolis	1	3	5	5	2	10	5	1	–	–	3	35
4. Miami	4	2	1	1	1	6	2	–	3	5	7	32
5. Pittsburgh	7	5	3	3	4	3	1	–	–	–	–	26
6. Edmonton	2	–	1	–	1	1	–	–	–	5	10	20
7. Geneva	–	–	–	–	–	–	4	2	4	5	4	19
8. St Louis	3	3	2	4	2	–	–	–	–	–	–	14
9. Brussels	–	–	–	–	1	3	3	3	?	?	?	10
10. Indianapolis	–	–	–	–	–	–	4	5	1	–	–	10
11. Madrid	–	–	2	1	1	2	2	–	–	–	–	8
12. Oxford	–	1	1	1	1	2	–	1	1	–	–	8
13. Stockholm/Giessen	–	–	–	–	–	–	2	2	1	2	–	7
14. Grenoble/Geneva (Gragil)	–	–	–	–	–	–	–	–	–	2	3	5
15. Odense/Milan	–	–	–	–	–	5	–	–	–	–	–	5
16. San Francisco/LA (UCLA–VA)	–	–	–	1	1	1	–	–	–	2	–	5
17. Buenos Aires	–	–	–	–	–	1	1	2	–	–	–	4
18. London (Ontario)/St Louis	2	1	1	–	–	–	–	–	–	–	–	4
19. Perugia	1	1	–	–	2	–	–	–	–	–	–	4
20. Innsbruck/Milano	–	–	–	–	–	2	1	–	–	–	–	3
21. Leicester	–	2	1	–	–	–	–	–	–	–	–	3
22. Lille	–	–	–	–	–	–	–	–	1	1	1	3
23. Los Angeles (UCLA–VA)	–	–	2	–	–	–	1	–	–	–	–	3
24. Paris	3	–	–	–	–	–	–	–	–	–	–	3
25. Lyon (Gragil)	–	–	–	–	–	–	–	–	–	–	2	2
26. Nantes	–	–	–	–	–	1	–	–	1	–	–	2
27. Strasbourg/Geneva (Gragil)	–	–	–	–	–	–	–	–	1	1	–	2
28. Berlin	–	–	–	–	–	–	–	–	–	1	–	1
29. Bethesda (NIH)	–	–	–	–	–	–	–	–	–	1	–	1
30. Charlestown	–	1	–	–	–	–	–	–	–	–	–	1
31. Chicago (NWH)	–	–	–	–	–	–	1	–	–	–	–	1
32. Chicago University	–	–	–	–	–	–	–	–	–	1	–	1
33. Harvard	–	–	–	–	–	–	–	–	–	1	–	1
34. Homburg (Saar)	–	–	–	1	–	–	–	–	–	–	–	1
35. Omaha	–	–	–	–	1	–	–	–	–	–	–	1
36. Seoul	–	–	–	–	–	–	–	–	1	–	–	1
37. Zurich	–	–	–	–	–	–	–	–	–	1	–	1
Σ	27	22	22	26	26	52	40	33	22	34	51	355

Total number of adult islet allografts from 1974–1989: 90

Note: ?, cases no longer reported to the Registry.

Σ 445

Table 15.2

Summary of adult islet allografts in Type 1 diabetic recipients according to institution and year from 1990 to December 31, 2000. (Source: ref. 15)

• Patient survival	96%
• Islet function*	41%
• Off insulin	11%
• Longest insulin independent case	[6 years]

Note: *Patients with post-Tx basal C-peptide ≥ 0.5 ng/ml

Table 15.3
Adult SIK or IAK transplantation in Type 1 diabetic patients in the era 1990–2000: results one year post-transplantation in 237 pre-Tx C-peptide negative recipients. Source: Data from ref. 15

As seen in previous ITR analyses, establishment of insulin independence was largely facilitated if:

(1) islets were isolated from pancreata with a mean preservation time ≤ 8 hours;
(2) ≥ 6000 islet equivalents (IEQ) per kg bodyweight of the recipient were transplanted;
(3) islets were implanted into the liver via the portal vein; and
(4) induction immunosuppression comprised monoclonal or polyclonal antibodies.

These four factors could predict full success (in terms of insulin independence) with a high likelihood. Factors determined not to influence insulin independence at one year included patient age and body mass index, duration of diabetes, pre-transplant HbA1c and daily insulin requirements, donor age, cold storage time of donor pancreas, and islet equivalent per kg bodyweight of the recipient.

Furthermore, the analyses may underscore the notion that intrinsic characteristics of the islet preparation (e.g. viability, apoptosis cascades triggered during islet isolation, purification and storage procedures) of the immediate post-transplant engraftment period (e.g. inflammatory

and other response of the recipient toward an intravascular islet graft, 'effective' engraftment), and factors during long-term islet survival (e.g. immune-mediated allo- and autoresponse of the recipient, susceptibility of islet grafts toward adverse diabetogenic effects of current immunosuppressive drugs, and functional exhaustion) may determine clinical success.

Undoubtedly, full (metabolic) success of islet transplantation is characterized by insulin independence. Partial success may be defined as islet endocrine function characterized by basal C-peptide secretion not accompanied by insulin independence in a specific recipient with Type 1 diabetes mellitus. Nevertheless, patients with partially successful islet transplants may benefit in the long run since basal serum C-peptide levels with a threshold of 0.5 ng/ml exerts significant biological effects[63–66] (Figure 15.6). Translated to the clinical situation, significant basal C-peptide levels after partially successful islet allotransplantation was followed by a decrease of daily insulin requirements, led to a stable metabolic control and was accompanied by less frequent or no hypoglycemic episodes.[67] Even in cases with

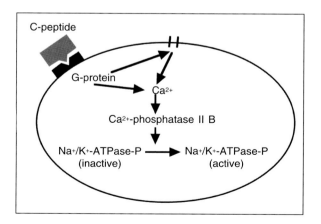

Figure 15.6
Proposed mechanism of C-peptide action. Source: adapted from refs 63 and 64.

partial success, progression of diabetic secondary complications might be halted in the long run.

Islet transplantation at Giessen University Center

The above mentioned detailed analysis of the ITR demonstrated that detectable graft function was lost in about 50% of the cases during the initial three months following transplantation (Figure 15.7). Several reasons for this early graft loss have been discussed (Figure 15.8).

Therefore, after more than ten years of experience in islet isolation from the pancreas of large mammals and humans,[68] we implemented into our clinical islet transplant protocol at Giessen University Center strategies to

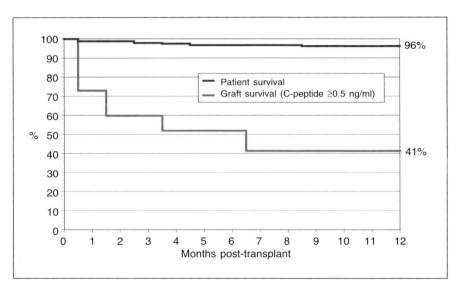

Figure 15.7
Cumulative one-year patient and graft survival in 237 pretransplant C-peptide negative Type 1 diabetic recipients, transplanted in the era 1990–1999.

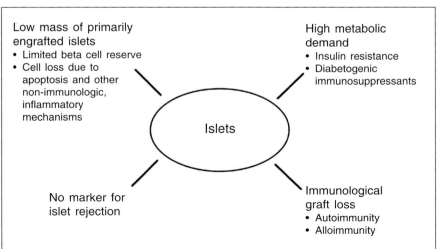

Figure 15.8
Possible reasons for early and late islet graft failure and obstacles to the success of clinical islet cell transplantation.

	Endotoxin-free reagents
• Islet preparation	Endotoxin-free reagents
• Pre-Tx	ATG/ALG
• Peri-Tx	Total Parenteral Nutrition (TPN)
• Post-Tx	Prednisolone
	CYA (300–400 ng/ml WB trough level)
	Azathioprine or MMF
	IV insulin
	Nicotinamide
	Verapamil
	Pentoxifylline
	Antioxidants

Table 15.4
The Giessen Protocol for islet allotransplantations in Type 1 diabetic subjects of the recipient categories SIK and IAK, respectively

facilitate human islet isolation, purification and storage and a refined peritransplant management, in order to promote early islet engraftment and to make insulin independence more likely (Table 15.4).[69] Islet transplantation into the liver through portal vein access was performed under local anesthesia by percutaneous transhepatic catheterization of the portal vein[9] (Figures 15.9 and 15.10).

Almost all recipients received only one islet preparation yielded from a single donor pancreas. Using this protocol, we recently

reported a markedly improved three months islet cell function rate of 100% for SIK recipients and 75% for IAK recipients, respectively.[70]

A follow-up of our first 56 consecutive cases (SIK/n = 35 and IAK/n = 21) illustrates a significantly improved one-year islet allograft survival of 86% for SIK cases and 47% for IAK cases, respectively (Table 15.5). The comparative numbers for non-Giessen SIK and IAK cases are 38% and 34%, respectively (Table 15.5).

Islet transplants alone (ITA) in non-uremic Type 1 diabetic subjects

The ultimate aim of islet cell transplantation and the most appealing aspect of this treatment concept is to achieve long-term function of the grafted tissue in non-uremic Type 1 diabetic patients early in the course of the disease, before significant microvascular, macrovascular and neurological complications are developed (Figure 15.11). We have recently performed for the first time islet transplants alone (ITA) in non-uremic patients with long-standing Type 1 diabetes mellitus and hypoglycemia-associated syndrome, suffering from hypoglycemia unawareness, defect counter-regulation and experiencing recurrent episodes of severe hypoglycemia.[67] We found that intraportal islet transplantation did not restore hypoglycemia-induced glucagon secretion, but it significantly

	SIK (n = 35)	IAK (n = 21)
• Patient survival	35/35	19/21
• Islet function	86% (38%)	47% (34%)
• Insulin independence	17% (7%)	21% (7%)
• Kidney function	97%	100%

Table 15.5
Adult SIK or IAK transplantation in Type 1 diabetic patients at Giessen University Hospital Center: one-year results. For comparison, results of non-Giessen centers (ITR data) given in brackets

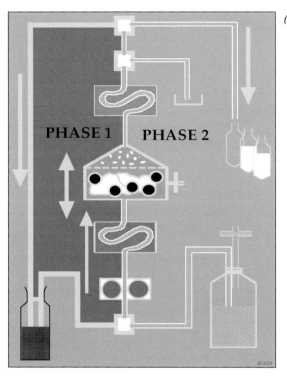

(a)

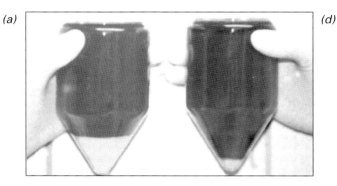

(d)

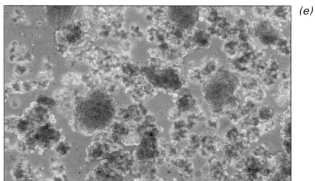

(e)

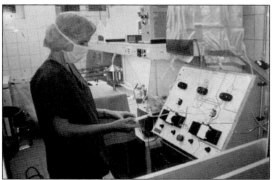

(b)

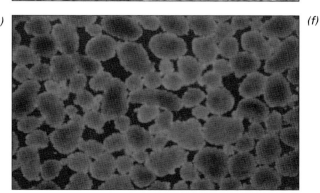

(f)

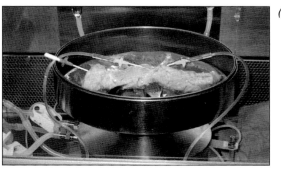

(c)

Figure 15.9
The Giessen Protocol: islet isolation and purification.
(a) Schematic drawing of enzyme digestion of the pancreas and islet isolation (modified according to Ricordi et al. (ref. 62); (b) view at the clean rooms; (c) retrieved human pancreatic organ (70–100 g) with ductal system cannulated for perfusion; (d) beta cell mass after collagenase (enzyme) digestion (left) and consecutive purification on a density gradient system (right); (e) crude preparation showing isolated islets contaminated with exocrine tissue; (f) highly purified islet preparation.

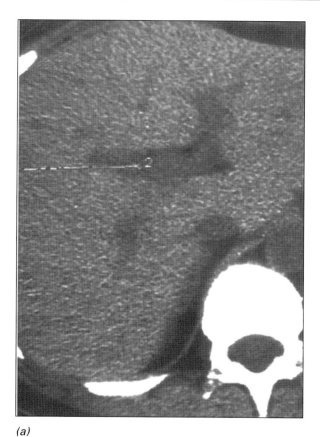

(a)

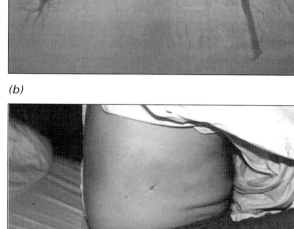

(b)

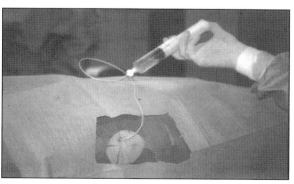

(d)

Figure 15.10
The Giessen Protocol: islet (cell) implantation by percutaneous transhepatic catheterization of the portal venous system in local anesthesia. (a) CT-guided imaging of the portal venous system; (b) fluoroscopy-guided localization of the catheter; (c) infusion of the islet (cell) suspension; (d) closure of the small cutaneous incision.

(c)

improved the responses of most counter-regulatory hormones and re-established both autonomic and neuroglucopenic hypoglycemia warning symptoms even in long-standing Type 1 diabetes (Figure 15.12). However, we were permitted by the local ethics committee to treat these recipients by a monoclonal anti-CD4 mouse antibody together with cyclosporine A

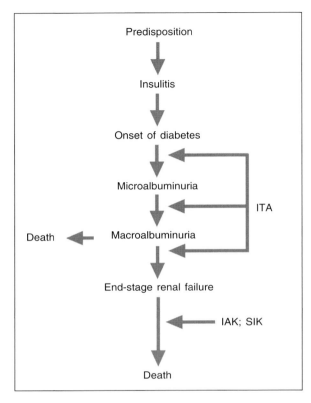

Figure 15.11
Indications and timing of islet (cell) transplantations in the natural course of Type 1 diabetes mellitus. Notes: ITA = islet transplants alone; IAK = islet after kidney transplants; SIK = simultaneous islet kidney transplants.

only for four weeks. After drug withdrawal all patients consecutively lost islet graft function over the following three months, indicating that no permanent immunotolerance state was established.

New strategies for circumventing the obstacles to the success of clinical islet cell transplantation

In Figure 15.8, the major obstacles to the success of islet transplantation in subjects with

Type 1 diabetes mellitus have been illustrated. First, the imbalance between the islet mass engrafted and the metabolic demand determines the clinical outcome. From animal experiments, it was calculated that approximately 50% of the islets transferred will not engraft and primary non-function may be the result of low functional capacity of beta cells after the isolation procedure, of local inflammatory and apoptotic mechanisms, cytokines, clotting elements of the blood and hypoxia before revascularization of the islets in the hepatic microenvironment.[71–77] A high metabolic demand imposed on the islet graft results from the insulin resistance in diabetic recipients as well as from diabetogenic and probably toxic effects of high portal vein concentrations of conventional immunosuppressive agents (cyclosporine A, tacrolimus, glucocorticoids).[78,79] Second, isolated islet grafts seem to be more prone to destruction by autoimmune recurrence and allograft rejection than whole pancreatic organ allotransplants.[80–86]

These factors of islet graft failure have been targeted in new strategies to promote islet cell transplants. Some of these promising novel strategies will be described here.

Sequential islet transplants and steroid-free immunosuppression

Recently, the Islet Transplant Center of the University of Alberta in Edmonton, Canada, reported an increased success rate of islet allotransplantations.[87] They developed a novel protocol of sequential islet allotransplants prepared from two or more pancreata performed 2–10 weeks apart in order to achieve an adequate mass of (engrafted) islets. In order to overcome the problems with conventional immunosuppressives, these patients were given a glucocorticoid-free immunosuppressive regimen, which included an interleukin-2-receptor antibody (daclizumab), sirolimus (rapamycin),

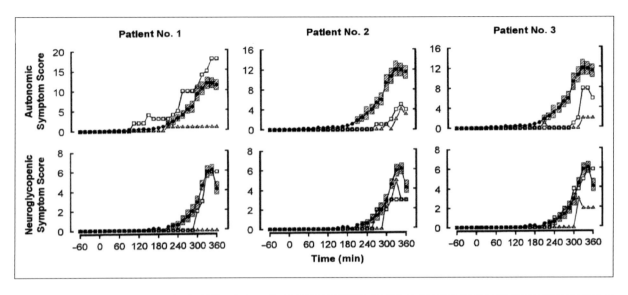

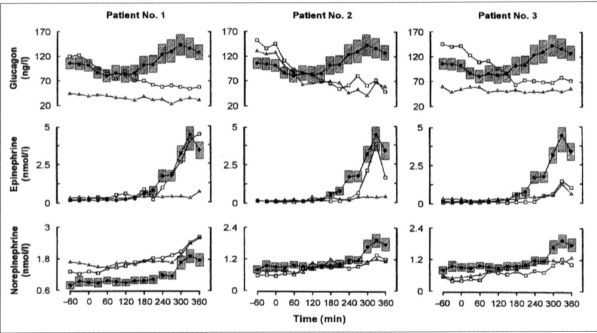

Figure 15.12
ITA in patients with long-standing Type 1 diabetes and hypoglycemia-associated syndrome. Six-hour insulin-induced hypoglycemia clamp-tests performed before (△) and after (□) islet transplantation. Upper panels: autonomic and neuroglycopenic symptom scores in response to hypoglycemia. Lower panels: response of counter-regulation hormones glucagon, epinephrine, and norepinephrine to hypoglycemia. Shaded boxes indicate test responses of age-matched healthy control subjects (n = 10). Source: adapted from ref. 67.

and low-dose tacrolimus. Seven consecutive patients with Type 1 diabetes and a history of severe hypoglycemia and metabolic instability ('Brittle-Diabetes') underwent islet transplants alone (ITA). All seven recipients quickly attained sustained insulin independence after transplantation of a mean (± SD) islet mass of 11,547 ± 1604 islet equivalents (basis: diameter of 150 µm) per kilogram of body weight.[87] HbA1c concentrations were normal. More importantly, the recipients no longer experience hypoglycemic episodes, and severe side effects were not observed in any of the recipients. Meanwhile, the authors have extended their experience with the Edmonton Protocol to a larger number of recipients with presently 100% graft survival and 75% insulin independence rates.[88]

The Immune Tolerance Network (ITN), one of the clinical research projects of the US National Institutes of Health, together with the Juvenile Diabetes Research Foundation, has now started a multicenter controlled trial to coordinate implementation of the Edmonton Protocol. Seven centers in the USA/Canada and three centers in Europe (Geneva, Giessen, Milan) have been selected to participate.

New immunosuppressive agents – immunotolerance induction – encapsulation of islets

Several strategies for prevention of autoimmune recurrence following islet transplantation have been proven in the 'preclinical' model of Type 1 diabetes, the spontaneously diabetic NOD mouse. Among the few effective strategies (possibly through the regeneration of immunoregulatory T cells) are immunotherapy with antilymphocyte serum weeks before islet transplantation, Complete Freund's Adjuvant (CFA) and Bacille-Calmette-Guerin (BCG) adjuvant immunotherapy, (FCR)-non-binding anti-CD3 antibodies, combined therapy with

IL-4 and IL-10, GAD65-based immunotherapy and combined administration of vitamin D3 analog and cyclosporine (for overview see reference 89). A combination therapy with low-dose sirolimus and tacrolimus was recently described as synergistic in preventing recurrent autoimmune diabetes in non-obese diabetic (NOD) mice.[90] The following has been suggested to overcome the problem of autoimmune diabetes recurrence: transplanting human islets rendered glutamate-decarboxylase (GAD)-less through introduction of an antisense transgene *in vitro*.[91] Indeed, it has been shown that NOD knockout mice or GAD antigene do not develop autoimmune diabetes.[92]

The next step on the way to better outcomes in clinical islet transplantation is to develop effective protocols for stemming the tide of rejection. Immunosuppressive regimens are likely to undergo significant improvements with the advent of more selective and less toxic agents, such as humanized interleukin-2-receptor antibodies which proved effective with no adverse effects on islet function and glucose metabolism in animal experiments.[93–96]

Finally, tolerance induction is central to the thesis of islet transplantation. Meanwhile, the mechanisms of islet allograft rejection are better understood. At least, three levels of cell-to-cell crosstalk, between the antigen presenting cells (APCs) and the recipient's T cells have to be taken into account (Figure 15.13). Blockage of the co-stimulatory signal (signal 2) for T cell activation, and induction of hematopoietic chimerism are the two main and most promising strategies for tolerance induction[97,98] (see also Table 15.6). Recent studies in non-human primates demonstrated that immunotolerance toward islet cells can be established by CD40–CD40 ligand (CD154) blockade.[99,100] Pre-implantation-stage stem cells surprisingly were capable of inducing long-term allogeneic graft acceptance with supplementary host conditioning.[101] However, most strategies

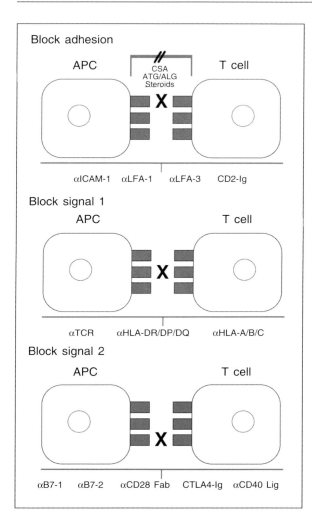

Figure 15.13
Crosstalk of donor antigen-presenting cells (APC) and recipient T cells on different levels and principles of blocking (immunosuppressive) agents.

- Induction of micro- or macrochimerism deletion of mature T cells by immunotoxin/ irradiation + donor antigen (graft or bone marrow)
- Modifying signal 1
  anti-CD4 monoclonal antibody (lck56)
- Blocking signal 2
  blocking CD28/B7 (CTLA4Ig) or
  CD40L (CD154)/CD40 (anti-CD40LmAb)
- Donor antigen (activation induced apoptosis?) donor specific blood transfusion; dendritic cells (vIL-10 etc.); soluble MHC molecules

Table 15.6
Some principles of transplant tolerance induction

Therefore, the ITN is committed to supporting clinical research focusing on the following points:

(1) novel immunotherapeutic strategies aiming at early withdrawal of immunosuppression with a suggested 40 patients as control group transplanted in the 10 centers, according to the Edmonton Protocol;
(2) therapeutic establishment of hematopoietic chimerism, with emphasis on depletion- and irradiation-free conditioning protocols.

Another approach to avoid life-long immunosuppressive treatment of the recipient would be to immunoisolate islets by means of macroencapsulation or microencapsulation, prior to transplantation.[105–108] Porcine encapsulated islets have been reported to induce normoglycemia without immunosuppression in spontaneously diabetic monkeys for more than 800 days.[109] However, successful studies in several animal models were not followed by clinical studies. So far, a single case, for which the authors claimed full success in terms of insulin independence after transplantation of

that successfully induce transplant tolerance in murine models have so far failed on translation into clinical therapies[102] and all clinical trials with a humanized anti-CD154 (CD40 ligand) antibody were completely halted due to unexpected high rates of thromboembolic complications in kidney transplant recipients.[103,104]

- Xenogenic (porcine) islets
- Differentiation and expansion of embryonic or adult stem cells
- Genetically engineered artificial beta cell lines
- Gene therapy for *in vivo* or *ex vivo/in vitro* converting patient cells to beta cells

Table 15.7
Possible beta cell sources beyond cadaveric donor tissue

microencapsulated islets in a patient with previous kidney graft, was reported in 1994.[110] However, the case was not well documented and there was no consecutive report on the follow-up of this recipient. The main problems with microencapsulation are the limited biocompatibility of the membranes, a lack of nutrients and oxygen supply of the islets, and the fact that small molecules, such as cytokines and other pro-inflammatory mediators, can still enter and exit the protective membranes and impair the function of the encapsulated islets or exert fibrotic membrane overgrowth on the outer layer. Even a combination of islet pre-treatment and islet encapsulation in barium alginate membranes did not establish long-lasting islet function in animal studies.[111]

Xenotransplants – stem cell therapy – gene therapy

Provided the problems with islet autoimmune destruction and allogeneic rejection are solved and the indication for islet allotransplants is extended to non-uremic Type 1 diabetic patients, a further problem may emerge: huge amounts of donor islet tissue are needed, but from where should the islets come? (See also Table 15.7.)

The pig is considered the primary alternative donor species for islet xenografts to humans, due to ethical considerations, breeding characteristics,

infectious disease concerns and its compatible size and physiology.[112] Porcine insulin has been widely used in humans and the pig insulin molecular structure only differs from human insulin in one amino-acid position.

A major barrier to progress in pig-to-human transplants is the presence of the terminal carbohydrate epitope, α-1,3-galactosyl (gal) on the surface of pig cells.[113] Humans (and Old World monkeys) have lost their corresponding galactosyl transferase activity in the course of evolution and therefore produce preformed natural antibodies against the epitope that are responsible for hyperacute rejection of porcine organs. Measures such as temporary removal of natural antibodies through affinity absorption, expression of complement regulators, competitive inhibition of galactosyl transferase or blocking the expression of gal epitopes, resulted in only partial reduction in epitope numbers but failed to significantly extend xenograft survival in primate recipients.[114] There is also no clear-cut advantage of isolated islet xenografts over that of a whole pancreatic organ. CD40+ T cells of the recipient seem to play a major role in xenoislet rejection, and conventional immunosuppressive agents allowed only a modest, if any, prolongation of islet xenograft survival in most pig-to-rodent models.[115–119] However, with the production of α-1,3-galactosyl transferase knockout pigs by nuclear transfer, as reported recently, there is now hope to overcome at least major problems with adult porcine islet xenograft hyperacute rejection.[120]

Another source for islet xenograft tissue might be the fetal pancreas.[121] The cultured fetal porcine pancreas bears several potential advantages:

(1) it contains a larger proportion of endocrine tissue;
(2) the exocrine tissue undergoes atrophy during culture;

(3) the fetal tissue inherits a considerable growth potential; and

(4) it might be less immunogenic.

It should be noted that cell aggregates (fetal porcine islet-like cell clusters (FPCCs)) do not trigger a hyperacute rejection when transplanted to rodents and it is likely that they are revascularized from the surrounding tissues thus containing recipient endothelial cells.[122] This would make such cultured fetal islet tissue ideal for clinical trials with xenotransplantations.

Fetal pig proislets, which can be easily produced to a large scale, further differentiate, mature and grow in culture or *in vivo* after grafting and may be stored long term in liquid nitrogene can persistently reverse diabetes after xenografting and may be more resistant to diabetogenic agents than adult islet tissue.[123–129] However, preliminary experience with fetal pig proislets in a preclinical xenograft model using cynomolgus monkeys as recipients was not very promising.[130]

The first clinical experience of fetal porcine pancreatic microfragment xenotransplantation into a conventionally immunosuppressed Type 1 diabetic patient was reported more than two decades ago.[131] During 40 days after transplantation, insulin requirements did not change, but C-peptide appeared (at very low concentrations) in the urine, suggesting at least low function of the transplanted tissue.[131] Finally, the same group transplanted a total of ten diabetic patients with porcine fetal pancreatic fragments, but again, no reduction in insulin requirement was observed in any of these patients.[132]

However, the use of pigs as a source for organs and cells to be xenografted to humans has provoked ethical and epidemiological controversies.[133] Transfer of Porcine Endogenous Retroviruses (PERV) from porcine cells

to human cells has been demonstrated *in vitro* and *in vivo* after xenotransplantation into immuno-incompetent and immunodeficient SCID mice.[134–137] However, there is until now no evidence of infection with PERV in those Swedish patients who were treated with porcine islet cell xenografts or in patients treated with living pig tissue.[138,139] Another option to prevent recipient infection might be the use of specially breeded PERV-free pigs.

Stem cell therapy, the use of either embryonic or adult progenitor cells differentiated and expanded under special conditions to fully functional, insulin-producing beta cells is a second approach to overcome the problems with limited tissue supply for clinical islet transplantation in diabetes mellitus.[140]

It is generally accepted that the pancreatic endocrine cells are of endodermal origin. The pathway from precursor cells to distinguished cell types, the genes and transcription factors involved, and the spatial and sequential temporal order meanwhile has become clear[141–145] (see also Figure 15.14). Recent reports on the *in vitro* differentiation and expansion of embryonic stem cells of murine or human origin to insulin-producing beta cells are very promising.[146–148] Transplanted into diabetic animals, these cells normalized blood glucose of the recipients.[146,147]

However, ethical concerns with the research on human embryonic material brought up the question as to whether adult ('old') cells can learn new tricks, i.e. can differentiate to insulin-producing cells. So-called Nestin-positive cells in the pancreatic duct or within the islets of Langerhans may be relevant progenitor cells.[149] By *in vitro* cultivation of ductal epithelial cells from adult mice, islets could be obtained which responded *in vitro* to glucose stimulation and reversed diabetes when transplanted into diabetic NOD mice.[150] A method to yield islets through *in vitro* cultivation of adult human pancreatic ductal cells was described recently.[151]

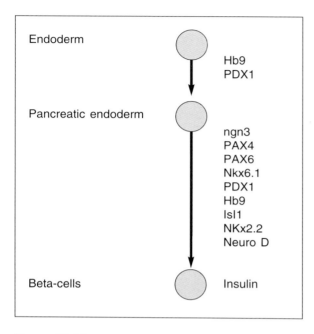

Figure 15.14
Relevant genes and transcription factors for the development of insulin-producing beta cells.

A third approach to overcome the problems with limited donor tissue supply is to make use of gene therapy for engineering pancreatic islets (for an overview see reference 152). The principal advantage of this approach is that autologous tissue and cells can be used and the problems with graft rejection and disease recurrence would probably no longer exist. For example, gut, liver or muscle cells have been successfully targeted for transfection with the insulin/pro-insulin gene.[153–156] A group in Israel recently described expression of insulin genes in the liver and amelioration of hyperglycemia in mice after viral transfection of the hepatocytes with the pancreatic and duodenal homeobox (PDX)-1 gene.[157] This is proof-of-principle for converting hepatocytes to beta cells.[158]

Conclusion

Islet cell transplantation has raised hope for a cure of diabetes for over three decades. The failure to reach this goal quickly has been an enormous disappointment to scientists, clinicians and patients. But, the field of islet transplantation has evolved and matured tremendously, it has witnessed significant progress and the results of recent human islet allotransplantations in patients with Type 1 diabetes mellitus are encouraging. At the dawn of the millennium, with the synergy of a number of important innovative tools, including stem cell expansion, immunomodulation, and gene therapy, it is my belief that we enter this new century with a solid foundation for expanding fundamental research and for translating basic knowledge into clinical applications. The challenges will still be many, but the potential benefit for patients with Type 1 diabetes will be extraordinary. Finally, it is necessary that the importance, potential, and feasibility of islet transplantation be better appreciated so that the urgent need to develop this therapy will be more accepted.[159]

Acknowledgements

We gratefully acknowledge grant support by JDRF (large individual grant), NIH-NIDDK (R01-DK56962–01 and ITN-Trial), and BMBF (FKZ07024806).

References

1. The Diabetes Control and Complications Trial Research Group. The effect of intensive treatment of diabetes on the development and progression of long-term complications in insulin-dependent diabetes mellitus. N Engl J Med 1993; 329: 977–86.

2. Wang PH, Lau J, Chalmers TC. Meta-analysis of effects of intensive blood-glucose control on late complications of type-1 diabetes. Lancet 1993; 341: 1306–9.

3. The Diabetes Control and Complications Trial Research Group. Hypoglycemia in the Diabetes Control and Complications Trial. Diabetes 1997; 46: 271–86.

4. Sutherland DE, Gores PF, Farney AC et al. Evolution of kidney, pancreas, and islet transplantation for patients with diabetes at the University of Minnesota. Am J Surg 1993; 166: 456–91.

5. Bretzel RG, Browatzki CC, Schultz A et al. Clinical islet transplantation in diabetes mellitus – report of the Islet Transplant Registry and the Giessen Center experience. Diabetes Stoffw 1993; 2: 378–90.

6. Gruessner RWG, Sutherland DER, Troppmann C et al. The surgical risk of pancreas transplantation in the cyclosporine era: an overview: J Am Coll Surg 1997; 185: 128–44.

7. Manske CL. Risks and benefits of kidney and pancreas transplantation for diabetic patients. Diabetes Care 1999; 22: B114–120.

8. Humar A, Kandaswamy R, Granger D et al. Decreased surgical risks of pancreas transplantation in the modern era. Ann Surg 2000; 231: 342–4.

9. Weimar B, Rauber K, Brendel MD et al. Percutaneous transhepatic catheterization of the portal vein: a combined CT- and fluoroscopy-guided technique. Cardiovasc Intervent Radiol 1999; 22: 342–4.

10. Scharp DW, Lacy PE, Santiago JV et al. Insulin independence after islet transplantation into Type I diabetic patient. Diabetes 1990; 39: 515–18.

11. Socci C, Falqui L, Davalli AM et al. Fresh human islet transplantation to replace pancreatic endocrine function in Type 1 diabetic patients. Report of six cases. Acta Diabetol 1991; 28: 151–7.

12. Warnock GL, Kneteman NM, Ryan EA et al. Long-term follow-up after transplantation of insulin-producing pancreatic islets into patients with Type 1 (insulin-dependent) diabetes mellitus. Diabetologia 1992; 35: 89–95.

13. Gores PF, Najarian JS, Stephanian E et al. Insulin independence in Type I diabetes after transplantation of unpurified islets from single donor with 15-deoxyspergualin. Lancet 1993; 341: 19–21.

14. Alejandro R, Lehmann R, Ricordi C et al. Long-term function (6 years) of islet allografts in Type 1 diabetes. Diabetes 1997; 46: 1983–9.

15. Brendel MD, Hering BJ, Schultz AO, Bretzel RG. International Islet Transplant Registry Newsletter 2001; No. 9: 1–20.

16. Bretzel RG. Biological alternatives to insulin therapy. Exp Clin Endocrinol Diabetes 1999; 107: S39–S43.

17. Kelly WD, Lillehei RC, Merkel FK et al. Allotransplantation of the pancreas and duodenum along with the kidney in diabetic nephropathy. Surgery 1967; 61: 827–37.

18. American College of Surgeons/National Institutes of Health. Organ Transplant Registry: first scientific report. JAMA 1971; 217: 1520–9.

19. Sutherland DER. International Human Pancreas and Islet Transplant Registry. Transplant Proc 1980; 12: 229–36.

20. Dubernard JM, Traeger J, Neyra P et al. A new method of preparation of segmental pancreatic grafts for transplantation and trials in dogs and in man. Surgery 1978; 84: 633–9.

21. Groth CG, Lungren G, Colliste H. Successful outcome on segmental human pancreatic transplantation with enteric exocrine diversion after modifications in technique. Lancet 1982; 1: 522–4.

22. Cook K, Sollinger HW, Warner T et al. Pancreaticocystostomy: an alternative method fo exocrine drainage of segmental pancreatic allografts. Transplantation 1983; 35: 634–6.

23. Sollinger HW, Stratta RJ, Kalayoglu M et al. Pancreas transplantation with pancreaticocystostomy and quadruple immunosuppression. Surgery 1987; 102: 674–9.

24. Corry RJ, Nghiem DD, Schulak JA. Surgical treatment of diabetic nephropathy with simultaneous pancreatic, duodenal and renal transplantation. Surg Gynecol Obstet 1986; 162: 547–55.

25. Mühlbacher F, Gnant MFX, Auinger M et al. Pancreatic venous drainage to the portal vein;

a new method in human pancreas transplantation. Transplant Proc 1990; 22: 636–7.

26. Gabr OA, Shokouh-Amiri MH, Hathaway DK et al. Results of pancreas transplantation with portal venous and enteric drainage. Ann Surg 1995; 221: 613–24.

27. Corry RJ, Egidi MF, Shapiro R et al. Enteric drainage of pancreas transplants revisited. Transplant Proc 1995; 27: 3048–9.

28. Newell KA, Bruce DS, Cronin DC et al. Comparison of pancreas transplantation with portal venous and enteric exocrine drainage to the standard technique utilizing bladder drainage of exocrine secretions. Transplantation 1996; 62: 1353–6.

29. Bland BJ. International Pancreas Transplant Registry Newsletter 2001; 13: 1–24.

30. Pozza G, Bosi E, Secchi A et al. Metabolic control of Type I (insulin dependent) diabetes after pancreas transplantation. BMJ 1985; 291: 510–13.

31. Morel P, Goetz FC, Moudry-Munns K et al. Long-term glucose control in patients with pancreatic transplants. Ann Intern Med 1991; 115: 694–9.

32. Katz H, Homan M, Velosa J et al. Effects of pancreas transplantation on postprandial glucose metabolism. N Engl J Med 1991; 325: 1278–83.

33. Ostman J, Bolinder J, Gunnarsson R et al. Effect of pancreas transplantation on metabolic and hormonal profiles in IDDM patients. Diabetes 1989; 38 Suppl. 1: 88–93.

34. Pfeffer F, Nauck MA, Benz S et al. Determinants of a normal (versus impaired) oral glucose tolerance after combined pancreas-kidney transplantation in IDDM patients. Diabetologia 1996; 39: 462–8.

35. Rooney DP, Robertson RP. Hepatic insulin resistance after pancreas transplantation in Type I diabetes. Diabetes 1996; 45: 134–8.

36. Hawthorne WJ, Griffin AD, Lau H et al. The effect of venous drainage on glucose homeostasis after experimental pancreas transplantation. Transplantation 1996; 62: 435–41.

37. Martin X, Petruzzo P, Dawahra M et al. Effects of portal versus systemic drainage in kidney-pancreas recipients. Transplant Int 2000; 13: 64–8.

38. Bohmann SO, Tyden G, Wilczek H. Prevention of kidney graft diabetic nephropathy by pancreas transplantation in man. Diabetes 1985; 34: 306–8.

39. Bohmann SO, Wilczek H, Tyden G et al. Recurrent diabetic nephropathy in renal allografts placed in diabetic patients and protective effect of simultaneous pancreatic transplantation. Transplant Proc 1987; 19: 2290–3.

40. Bilous RW, Mauer SM, Sutherland DER et al. The effects of pancreas transplantation on the glomerular structure of renal allografts in patients with insulin dependent diabetes. N Engl J Med 1989; 321: 80–5.

41. Fioretto P, Mauer SM, Bilous RW et al. Effects of pancreas transplantation on glomerular structure in insulin-dependent diabetic patients with their own kidneys. Lancet 1993; 342: 1193–6.

42. Fioretto P, Steffes MW, Sutherland DE et al. Reversal of lesions of diabetic nephropathy after pancreas transplantation. N Engl J Med 1998; 339: 69–75.

43. Gabr OA, El-Gebely S, Sugathan P et al. Early improvement in cardiac function occurs for pancreas-kidney but not diabetic kidney-alone transplant recipients. Transplantation 1995; 59: 1105–12.

44. Solders G, Tyden G, Tibell A et al. Improvement in nerve conduction 8 years after combined pancreatic and renal transplantation. Transplant Proc 1995; 27: 3091.

45. Laftavi MR, Chapuis F, Vial C et al. Diabetic polyneuropathy outcome after successful pancreas transplantation: 1 to 9 year follow up. Transplant Proc 1995; 27: 1406–9.

46. Navarro X, Kennedy WR, Aeppli D, Sutherland DER. Neuropathy and mortality in diabetes: influence of pancreas transplantation. Muscle Nerve 1996; 19: 1009–16.

47. Allen RD, Al-Harbi IS, Morris JG et al. Diabetic neuropathy after pancreas transplantation: determinants of recovery. Transplantation 1997; 63: 830–8.

48. Ulbig M, Kampik A, Landgraf R, Land W. The influence of combined pancreatic and renal transplantation on advanced diabetic retinopathy. Transplant Proc 1987; 19: 3554–6.

49. Scheider A, Meyer-Schwickerath E, Nasser J et al. Diabetic retinopathy and pancreas transplantation: a 3 year follow-up. Diabetologia 1991; 34: 95–9.

50. Abendroth D, Landgraf R, Illner WD, Land W. Beneficial effect of pancreatic transplantation in insulin dependent diabetes mellitus patients. Transplant Proc 1990; 22: 696–7.

51. Larsen JL, Lynch T, Al'Halawi M et al. Carotid intima-media thickness by ultrasound measurement in pancreas transplant candidates. Transplant Proc 1996; 27: 2996.

52. Douzdjian V, Abecassis MM, Corry RJ et al. Simultaneous pancreas-kidney versus kidney-alone transplants in diabetics: increased risk of early cardiac death and acute rejection following pancreas transplants. Clin Transplant 1994; 8: 246–51.

53. Lumbreras C, Fernandez I, Velosa J et al. Infectious complications following pancreatic transplantation; incidence, microbiological and clinical characteristics, and outcome. Clin Infect Dis 1995; 20: 514–20.

54. Smets YFC, Westendorp RGJ, van der Pijl JW et al. Effect of simultaneous pancreas-kidney transplantation on mortality of patients with type-1 diabetes mellitus and end-stage renal failure. Lancet 1999; 353: 1915–19.

55. Milde FK, Hart LK, Zehr PS. Pancreatic transplantation. Impact on the quality of life of diabetic renal transplant recipients. Diabetes Care 1995; 18: 93–5.

56. Adang EMM, Engel GL, van Hooff JP, Kootstra G. Comparison before and after transplantation of pancreas-kidney and pancreas-kidney with loss of pancreas – a prospective controlled quality of life study. Transplantation 1995; 62: 754–8.

57. Tyden G, Reinholt FP, Sundkvist G, Bolinder J. Recurrence of autoimmune diabetes mellitus in recipients of cadaveric pancreatic grafts. N Engl J Med 1996; 335: 860–3.

58. von Mering J, Minkowski O. Diabetes mellitus nach Pankreasexstirpation. Arch Exp Pathol Pharmakol 1890; 26: 37.

59. Minkowski O. Weitere Mittheilungen über den Diabetes mellitus nach Exstirpation des Pankreas. Berliner Klin Wochenschr 1892; 29: 90–4.

60. Banting FG, Best CH. The internal secretion of the pancreas. J Lab Clin Invest 1922; 7: 251–66.

61. Williams PW. Notes on diabetes treated with extract and by grafts of sheep's pancreas. BMJ 1894; 2: 1303.

62. Ricordi C, Lacy PE, Finke EH et al. Automated method for isolation of human pancreatic islets. Diabetes 1988; 37: 413–20.

63. Johansson BL, Borg K, Fernqvist-Forbes E et al. C-peptide improves autonomic nerve function in IDDM patients. Diabetologia 1996; 39: 687–95.

64. Wahren J, Johansson BL. New aspects of C-peptide physiology. Horm Metab Res 1998; 30: A2–A5.

65. Steiner DF, Rubenstein AH. Proinsulin C-peptide – biological activity? [comment]. Science 1997; 277: 531–2.

66. Ido Y, Vindigni A, Chang K et al. Prevention of vascular and neural dysfunction in diabetic rats by C-peptide. Science 1997; 277: 563–7.

67. Meyer C, Hering BJ, Grossmann R et al. Improved glucose counterregulation and autonomic symptoms after intraportal islet transplants alone in patients with Type I diabetes mellitus. Transplantation 1998; 66: 233–40.

68. Brandhorst D, Brandhorst H, Hering BJ et al. Islet isolation from the pancreas of large mammals and humans: 10 years of experience. Exp Clin Endocrinol Diabetes 1995; 103 Suppl. 2: 3–14.

69. Hering BJ, Bretzel RG, Hopt UT et al. New protocol toward prevention of early human islet allograft failure. Transplant Proc 1994; 26: 570–1.

70. Bretzel RG, Brandhorst D, Brandhorst H et al. Improved survival of intraportal pancreatic islet cell allografts in patients with Type 1 diabetes mellitus by refined peritransplant management. J Mol Med 1999; 77: 140–3.

71. Vargas F, Vives-Pi M, Somoza N et al. Endotoxin contamination may be responsible for the unexplained failure of human pancreatic islet transplantation. Transplantation 1998; 65: 722–7.

72. Kaufman DB, Platt JL, Rabe FL et al. Differential roles of Mac-1+ cells and CD4+ and CD8+ T lymphocytes in primary nonfunction

and classical rejection of islet allografts. J Exp Med 1990; 172: 291–302.

73. Bottino R, Fernandez LA, Ricordi C et al. Transplantation of allogeneic islets of Langerhans in the rat liver. Effects of macrophage depletion on graft survival and microenvironment activation. Diabetes 1998; 47: 316–23.

74. Menger MD, Vajkoczy P, Leiderer R et al. Influence of experimental hyperglycemia on microvascular blood perfusion of pancreatic islet isografts. J Clin Invest 1992; 90: 1361–9.

75. Berney T, Molano RD, Cattan P et al. Endotoxin-mediated delayed islet graft function is associated with increased intra-islet cytokine production and islet cell apoptosis. Transplantation 2001; 71: 125–32.

76. Bennet W, Sunberg B, Groth CG et al. Incompatibility between human blood and isolated islets of Langerhans: a finding with implications for clinical intraportal islet transplantation? Diabetes 1999; 48: 1907–14.

77. El-Ouaghlidi A, Jahr H, Pfeiffer G et al. Cytokine mRNA expression in peripheral blood cells of immunosuppressed human islet transplant recipients. J Mol Med 1999; 77: 115–7.

78. Shapiro AM, Gallant H, Hao E et al. Portal vein immunosuppressant levels and islet graft toxicity. Transplant Proc 1997; 30: 641.

79. Drachenberg CB, Klassen DK, Weir MR et al. Islet cell damage associated with tacrolimus and cyclosporine: morphological features in pancreas allograft biopsies and clinical correlation. Transplantation 1999; 68: 396–402.

80. Jaeger C, Hering BJ, Dyrberg T et al. Islet cell antibodies and GAD65 antibodies in IDDM patients undergoing kidney and islet after kidney transplantation. Transplantation 1996; 62: 424–426.

81. Jaeger C, Brendel MD, Hering BJ et al. Progressive islet graft failure occurs significantly earlier in autoantibody positive than in autoantibody negative IDDM recipients of intrahepatic islet allografts. Diabetes 1997; 46: 1907–10.

82. Jaeger C, Brendel MD, Eckhard M, Bretzel RG. Islet autoantibodies as potential markers for disease recurrence in clinical islet transplantation. Exp Clin Endocrinol Diabetes 2000; 108: 328–33.

83. Braghi S, Bonifacio E, Secchi A et al. Modulation of humoral islet autoimmunity by pancreas allotransplantation influences allograft outcome in patients with Type 1 diabetes. Diabetes 2000; 49: 218–24.

84. Tyden G, Reinholt FP, Sundkvist G, Bolinder J. Recurrence of autoimmune diabetes in recipients of cadaveric pancreatic grafts. N Engl J Med 1996; 335: 860–3.

85. Halloran PF, Homik J, Goes N et al. The 'injury response': a concept linking nonspecific injury, acute rejection, and long-term transplant outcomes. Transplant Proc 1997; 29: 79–81.

86. Roep BO, Stobbe I, Duinkerken G et al. Auto- and alloimmune reactivity to human islet allografts transplanted into type-1 diabetic patients. Diabetes 1999; 48: 484–90.

87. Shapiro AM, Lakey JR, Ryan EA et al. Islet transplantation in seven patients with Type 1 diabetes mellitus using a glucocorticoid-free immunosuppressive regimen. N Engl J Med 2000; 343: 230–8.

88. Ryan EA, Lakey JRT, Rajotte RV et al. Clinical outcomes and insulin secretion after islet transplantation with the Edmonton protocol. Diabetes 2001; 50: 710–19.

89. Hering BJ, Ricordi C. Results, research priorities, and reasons for optimism: islet transplantation for patients with Type 1 diabetes. Graft 1999; 2: 12–27.

90. Shapiro AMJ, Suarez-Pinzon WL, Power R, Rabinovitch A. Combination therapy with low dose sirolimus and tacrolimus is synergistic in preventing spontaneous and recurrent autoimmune diabetes in non-obese diabetic mice. Diabetologia 2002; 45: 224–30.

91. Boehmer H von, Sarukhan A. GAD, a single autoantigen for diabetes. [comment]. Science 1999; 384: 1135–7.

92. Yoon JW, Yoon CS, Lim HW et al. Control of autoimmune diabetes in NOD mice by GAD expression or suppression in beta cells. Science 1999; 284: 1183–7.

93. Yakimets WJ, Lakey JRT, Yatscoff RW et al. Prolongation of canine pancreatic islet allograft survival with combined rapamycin and cyclosporine therapy at low doses. Transplantation 1993; 56: 1293–8.

94. Kneteman NM, Lakey JR, Wagner T, Finegood D. The metabolic impact of

rapamycin (sirolimus) in chronic canine islet graft recipients. Transplantation 1996; 61: 1206–10.

95. Guo Z, Chong AS, Shen J et al. In vivo effects of leflunomide on normal pancreatic islet and syngeneic islet graft function. Transplantation 1997; 63: 716–21.

96. Guo Z, Chong AS, Shen J et al. Prolongation of rat islet allograft survival by the immuno-suppressive agent leflunomide. Transplantation 1997; 63: 711–16.

97. Waldmann H. Transplantation tolerance: where do we stand? Nat Med 1999; 11: 1245–8.

98. Acholonu IN, Ildstad ST. The role of bone marrow transplantation in tolerance: organ-specific and cellular grafts. Curr Opin Organ Transplant 1999; 4: 189–96.

99. Kenyon NS, Chatzipetron M, Masetti M et al. Long-term survival and function of intrahep-atic islet allografts in rhesus monkeys treated with humanized anti-CD 154. Proc Natl Acad Sci USA 1999; 96: 8132–7.

100. Kenyon NS, Fernandez LA, Lehmann R et al. Long-term survival and function of intrahep-atic islet allografts in baboons treated with humanized anti-CD 154. Diabetes 1999; 48: 1473–81.

101. Fändrich F, Lin X, Chai GX et al. Pre-implantation-stage stem cells induce long-term allogenic graft acceptance without supplementary host conditioning. Nat Med 2002; 8: 171–8.

102. Chong AS, Yin D, Boussy IA. Transplantation tolerance: of mice and men. Graft 2002; 5: 27–33.

103. Kawai T, Andrews D, Colvin RB et al. Thromboembolic complications after treat-ment with monoclonal antibody against CD40 ligand. Nat Med 2000; 6: 114.

104. Kirk AD, Harlan DM. Thromboembolic complications after treatment with mono-clonal antibody against CD40 ligand (reply). Nat Med 2000; 6: 114.

105. Zekorn T, Horcher A, Siebers U et al. Islet transplantation in immunoseparating mem-branes for treatment of insulin-dependent diabetes mellitus. Exp Clin Endocrinol Diabetes 1995; 103 Suppl. 2: 136–9.

106. Siebers U, Horcher A, Bretzel RG et al. Alginate-based microcapsules for immunopro-tected islet transplantation. In: Prokop A, Hunkeler D, Cherrington AD, eds. Bioartificial organs. Ann NY Acad Sci 1997; 831: 304–12.

107. Siebers U, Horcher A, Brandhorst H et al. Analysis of the cellular reaction towards microencapsulated xenogeneic islets after intraperitoneal transplantation. J Mol Med 1999; 77: 215–18.

108. de Vos P, Hamel AF, Tatarkiewicz K. Considerations for successful transplantation of encapsulated pancreatic islets. Diabetologia 2002; 45: 159–73.

109. Sun Y, Ma X, Zhou D et al. Normalization of diabetes in spontaneously diabetic cynomolgus monkeys by xenografts of microencapsulated porcine islets without immunosuppression. J Clin Invest 1996; 98: 1417–22.

110. Soon-Shiong P, Heintz RE, Merideth N et al. Insulin independence in a Type 1 diabetic patient after encapsulated islet transplanta-tion. Lancet 1994; 343: 950–1.

111. Zekorn TD, Horcher A, Siebers U et al. Synergistic effect of microencapsulation and immunoalteration on islet allograft survival in bioartificial pancreas. J Mol Med 1999; 77: 193–8.

112. Evans RW. In: Platt JL, ed. Xeno-transplantation. Washington: ASM Press, 2001: 29–51.

113. Good AH, Cooper DKC, Malcolm AJ et al. Identification of carbohydrate structures which bind human anti-porcine antibodies: implications for discordant xenografting in man. Transplant Proc 1992; 24: 559–62.

114. Miyagawa S, Murakami H, Takahagi Y et al. Remodeling of the major pig xenoantigen by N-acetylglucosaminyltransferase III in trans-genic pig. J Biol Chem 2001; 276: 39310–9.

115. Wennberg L, Wallgren AC, Sundberg B et al. Efficacy of immunosuppressive drugs in islet xenotransplantation: a study in the pig-to-rat model. Xenotransplantation 1995; 2: 222–9.

116. Wennberg L, Karlsson-Parra A, Sundberg B et al. Efficacy of immunosuppressive drugs in islet xenotransplantation. Transplantation 1997; 63: 1234–42.

117. Friedman T, Smith RN, Colvin RB, Iacomini J. A critical role for human CD4+ T-cells in rejection of porcine islet cell xenografts. Diabetes 1999; 48: 2340.

118. Jahr H, Brandhorst D, Brandhorst H et al. Abstossungsreaktionen bei der tierexperimentellen xenogenen Transplantation von isolierten Langerhansschen Inseln des Schweins. Zentralbl Chir 1998; 123: 823–9.

119. Lau D, Hering BJ, El-Ouaghlidi A et al. Isokinetic gradient centrifugation prolongs survival of pig islets xenografted into mice. J Mol Med 1999; 77: 175–7.

120. Lai L, Kolber-Simonds D, Kwang-Wook P et al. Production of α-1,3-galactosyltransferase knockout pigs by nuclear transfer cloning. Science 2002; 295: 1089–92.

121. Brown J, Danilovs JA, Clark WR, Mullen YS. Fetal pancreas as a donor organ. World J Surg 1984; 8: 152–7.

122. Korsgren O. Xenotransplantation of fetal porcine islet-like cell clusters in diabetes mellitus: an experimental and clinical study. Acta Univ Upsal 1991; 295: 1–40.

123. Korsgren O, Sandler S, Landström A et al. Large-scale production of fetal porcine pancreatic islet-like cell clusters. An experimental tool for studies of islet cell differentiation and xenotransplantation. Transplantation 1988; 45: 509–14.

124. Korsgren O, Jansson L, Eizirik D, Andersson A. Functional and morphological differentiation of fetal porcine islet-like cell clusters after transplantation into nude mice. Diabetologia 1991; 34: 379–86.

125. Liu X, Federlin KF, Bretzel RG et al. Persistent reversal of diabetes by transplantation of fetal pig proislets into nude mice. Diabetes 1991; 40: 858–66.

126. Liu X, Brendel MD, Hering BJ et al. Comparison of the potency of fetal pig pancreatic proislets and fragments to reverse diabetes. Transplant Proc 1992; 24: 987.

127. Liu X, Brendel MD, Brandhorst H et al. Successful cryopreservation of fetal porcine proislets. Cryobiology 1993; 30: 262–71.

128. Liu X, Brendel MD, Brandhorst D et al. Reversal of diabetes in nude mice by transplantation of cryopreserved fetal porcine proislets. Transplant Proc 1994; 26: 707–8.

129. Bretzel RG, Liu X, Hering BJ et al. Cryopreservation transplantation and susceptibility to diabetogenic agents of fetal porcine proislets. Xenotransplantation 1995; 2: 133–8.

130. Soderlund J, Wennberg L, Castanos-Velez E et al. Fetal porcine islet-like cell clusters transplanted to cynomolgus monkeys: an immunohistochemical study. Transplantation 1999; 67: 784.

131. Groth CG, Andersson A, Björken C et al. Transplantation of fetal pancreatic microfragments via the portal vein to a diabetic patients. Diabetes 1980; 29: 80–3.

132. Groth CG, Korsgren O, Tibell A et al. Transplantation of porcine fetal pancreas to diabetic patients. Lancet 1994; 344: 1402–4.

133. Bach FH, Fishman JA, Daniels N et al. Uncertainty in xenotransplantation: individual benefit versus collective risk. Nat Med 1998; 4: 141–4.

134. Patience C, Takeuchi Y, Weiss RA. Infection of human cells by an endogenous retrovirus of pigs. Nat Med 1997; 3: 275–6.

135. Martin U, Kiessig V, Blusch JH et al. Expression of pig endogenous retrovirus by primary porcine endothelial cells and infection of human cells. Lancet 1998; 352: 666–7.

136. Van der Laan LJ, Lockey C, Griffeth BC et al. Infection by porcine endogenous retroviruses after islet xenotransplantation in SCID mice. Nature 2000; 407: 90–4.

137. Deng YM, Tuch BE, Rawlinson WD. Transmission of porcine endogenous retroviruses in severe combined immunodeficient mice xenotransplanted with fetal porcine pancreatic cells. Transplantation 2000; 70: 1010–16.

138. Heneine W, Tibell A, Switzer WM et al. No evidence of infection with porcine endogenous retrovirus in recipients of porcine islet-cell xenografts. Lancet 1998; 352: 695–9.

139. Paradis K, Langford G, Long Z et al. Search for cross-species transmission of porcine endogenous retrovirus in patients treated with living pig tissue. Science 1999; 285: 1236–41.

140. Soria B, Skoudy A, Martin F. From stem cells to beta cells: new strategies in cell therapy of diabetes mellitus. Diabetologia 2001; 44: 407–15.

141. Edlund H. Transcribing the pancreas. Diabetes 1958; 47: 1817–23.

142. Stoffers DA, Zinkin NT, Stanojevic V et al. Pancreatic agenesis attributable to a single nucleotide deletion in the human IPF1 gene

coding sequence. Nat Genet 1997; 15: 106–10.

143. Apelqvist A, Li H, Sommer L et al. Notch signalling controls pancreatic cell differentiation. Nature 1999; 400: 877–81.

144. Gradwohl G, Dierich A, Le Meur M, Guillemot F. Neurogenin 3 is required for the development of the four endocrine cell lineages of the pancreas. Proc Natl Acad Sci USA 2000; 97: 1607–11.

145. Sosa-Pineda B, Chowdhury K, Torres M et al. The Pax 4 gene is essential for differentiation of insulin-producing beta cells in the mammalian pancreas. Nature 1997; 386: 399–402.

146. Soria B, Roche E, Berna G et al. Insulin-secreting cells derived from embryonic stem cells normalize glycemia in streptozotocin-induced diabetic mice. Diabetes 2000; 49: 157–62.

147. Lumelsky N, Blondel O, Laeng P et al. Differentiation of embryonic stem cells to insulin-secreting structures similar to pancreatic islets. Science 2001; 292: 1389–94.

148. Assady S, Maor G, Amit M et al. Insulin production by human embryonic stem cells. Diabetes 2001; 50: 1691–7.

149. Zulewski H, Abraham EJ, Gerlach MJ et al. Multipotential nestin-positive stem cells isolated from adult pancreatic islets differentiate ex vivo into pancreatic endocrine, exocrine, and hepatic phenotypes. Diabetes 2001; 50: 521–33.

150. Ramiya VK, Maraist M, Arfors KE et al. Reversal of insulin-dependent diabetes using islets generated in vitro from pancreatic stem cells. Nat Med 2000; 6: 278–82.

151. Bonner-Weir S, Taneja M, Weir GC et al. In vitro cultivation of human islets from expanded ductal tissue. Proc Natl Acad Sci USA 2000; 97: 7999–8004.

152. Soria B, Andreu E, Berna G et al. Engineering pancreatic islets. Eur J Physiol 2000; 440: 1–18.

153. Cheung AT, Dayanandan B, Lewis JT et al. Glucose-dependent insulin release from genetically engineered K cells. Science 2000; 290: 1959–62.

154. Lee HC, Kim SJ, Kim KS et al. Remission in models of Type 1 diabetes by gene therapy using a single-chain insulin analogue. Nature 2000; 408: 483–8.

155. Shaw JAM, Delday MI, Hart AW, Docherty K. Secretion of bioactive human insulin following plasmid-mediated gene transfer to non-neuroendocrine cell lines, primary cultures and rat skeletal muscle in vivo. J Endocrinol 2002; 172: 653–72.

156. Riu E, Mas A, Ferre T et al. Counteraction of Type 1 diabetic alterations by engineering skeletal muscle to produce insulin: insights from transgenic mice. Diabetes 2002; 51: 704–11.

157. Ferber S, Halkin A, Cohen H et al. Pancreatic and duodenal homeobox gene 1 induces expression of insulin genes in liver and ameliorates streptozotocin-induced hyperglycemia. Nat Med 2000; 6: 568–72.

158. Kahn A. Converting hepatocytes to β-cells—a new approach for diabetes? Nat Med 2000; 6: 505–6.

159. Weir GC, Bonner-Weir S. Scientific and political impediment to successful islet transplantation. Diabetes 1997; 46: 1247–56.

16

Advances in methods and procedures for beta-cell transplantation

Norma Sue Kenyon

Introduction

Biological replacement of beta-cells that have been destroyed by the autoimmune attack of Type 1 diabetes has the potential to alter the lives of millions of people. Recent advances in clinical islet cell transplantation have focused public awareness on diabetes itself and on the intensive research efforts to cure and ameliorate the disease. The heightened expectations generated by reports of reproducible insulin independence are balanced by the shortage of organ donors for islet procurement and the requirement for lifelong immunosuppression of the recipient to prevent islet rejection and recurrent autoimmunity. Along with the first published reports of 100% insulin independence in non-human primates and patients came a dramatic shift in research priorities; that is, while great emphasis was previously given to islet transplant studies in rodent models, with many centers participating, relatively few dollars were relegated to larger animal/preclinical and clinical studies and to identification of alternative sources of insulin-producing tissue. The advent of insulin independence resulted in a shifting of efforts to obtain a more equitable distribution between basic, translational and clinical islet studies and to a dramatically increased focus on identification of alternative sources of insulin-producing tissue. The goal of this chapter is not to provide a detailed historical perspective on islet cell transplantation but to give an update on recent advances that have led to heightened interest in, and funding for, the study of biological replacement strategies as a cure for Type 1 diabetes.

For many years, the success of islet cell transplantation in non-human primates and humans was limited, with minimal, short-term engraftment and sporadic insulin independence achieved in non-human primate models[1] and reports of 8–10% insulin independence at one year post-transplant in patients.[2] Inconsistencies in outcome could be attributed partly to differences in islet quality, with few laboratories worldwide capable of isolating islets suitable for transplantation. Despite the use of multiple donors in some trials, rates of insulin independence at one year post-transplant remained low. Together with the relative lack of efficacy of standard immunosuppressive drugs for prevention of islet rejection and recurrence of autoimmunity, the diabetogenicity[3] of these same drugs contributed significantly to the lack of success by effectively decreasing functional islet mass. Early islet loss, owing to infusion-mediated activation of intrahepatic macrophages and endothelial cells, and subsequent production of proinflammatory mediators that are detrimental to islet function and survival, can result in further decreases in functional islet mass post-transplant.[4,5] The challenges to successful islet transplantation, therefore, included isolation of a sufficient number of viable, functional islets, engraftment and survival of an adequate islet mass to result reproducibly in insulin independence, and effective prevention of rejection and recurrent autoimmunity, without the increased metabolic demands posed by steroids and calcineurin inhibitors.

The first reports of reproducible insulin independence in C-peptide negative non-human primates[6,7] validated the feasibility of islet allotransplantation and generated increased enthusiasm for this therapeutic strategy. The subseqeunt report of 100% insulin independence in clinical islet allotransplant trials[8] resulted in an impassioned, worldwide response by patients and scientists alike. Different anti-rejection agents were used in the preclinical and clinical studies, but importantly both therapeutic strategies avoided the use of steroids. For the non-human primate (NHP) studies, calcineurin inhibitors were also eliminated; the clinical trials incorporated low doses of the calcineurin inhibitor tacrolimus, in combination with sirolimus and anti-IL2 receptor monoclonal antibody induction therapy. In addition, a minimum of 10,000 islet equivalents (IEQ)[9] from a single donor were transplanted per kg recipient body weight in the NHP studies in order to attain reproducibly insulin independence. Patients received sequential islet preparations from different donors until insulin independence was achieved, with a mean of 11,547 +/- 1604 IEQ required.[8] As additional centers have utilized steroid-free immune suppression, the requirement for 9000–10,000 IEQ/kg to achieve insulin independence reproducibly, whether this mass is achieved with a single or multiple donors, has been verified. Both in animals and in humans, it is possible to reverse diabetes in some individuals with fewer islets.

As scientists and physicians work to identify and test agents that do not adversely affect islet function, that are highly effective for prevention of rejection and recurrent autoimmunity, and

that limit early islet loss, it should be possible to reverse diabetes consistently with fewer islets. Ideally, we would delineate strategies that result in the induction of immunological tolerance to the transplanted islets, thereby enabling patients to discontinue immunosuppression and decrease the risks associated with these drugs.

Advances in clinical islet cell transplantation

Dramatic advances have been made in clinical islet cell transplantation. A significant improvement in islet allograft survival was first obtained when recipients undergoing upper abdominal exenteration for malignancy received islet cell transplants;[10] in this series, autoimmunity was not a barrier to graft survival and six out of nine patients experienced periods of insulin independence. Results for C-peptide negative patients with Type 1 diabetes were not as encouraging,[2] although long-term stabilization of metabolic control and normalization of HbA1c has been observed for patients with functioning islet allografts.[11] In one series, refinement of peri-transplant management with agents aimed at limiting early islet loss resulted in periods of insulin independence in 33% of C-peptide negative patients with Type 1 diabetes.[12]

As mentioned previously, the first report of 100% insulin independence originated from clinical trials in which steroids were excluded and tacrolimus was used at reduced dosages, thereby decreasing the diabetogenicity of the immunosuppressive regimen. The anti-IL2 receptor-specific monoclonal antibody, daclizumab, was used as induction therapy.[8,13] In addition to the efficacious prevention of rejection and recurrent autoimmunity, transplantation of freshly isolated islets that were not exposed to xenogeneic proteins (fetal calf serum), coupled with sequential infusions to achieve an adequate functional mass to reverse diabetes, contributed to the success of the trial.[8] By initiating immunosuppression and giving the first infusion, followed by a settling-in period and a subsequent transplant when another donor becomes available, it is highly likely that a favorable intrahepatic milieu is established, in which infusion-related, nonspecific inflammatory events are limited due to ongoing immune suppression. In addition, the presence of revascularized islets in the liver may contribute to the engraftment of islets that arrive later, and the metabolic demands on the islets would be lessened due to the stabilized metabolic control that is commonly observed after the first transplant. With some variations unique to individual programs, several centers worldwide have achieved similar results. Significant efforts are being made to verify, in controlled trials, that these promising results can be duplicated at several centers by using the exact same isolation and transplant procedures.

As the field continues to advance, studies will be driven by efforts to modify immunosuppression to incorporate agents that limit early islet loss and effectively prevent rejection and recurrent autoimmunity, without causing nephrotoxicity, diabetogenicity and other adverse effects associated with generalized immunosuppression. A follow-up report on the initial seven insulin-independent patients, plus five others, highlighted the need for such strategies. Of 12 patients with elevated creatinine pre-transplant, two had significant increases in creatinine in the long term, and cholesterol increased in five patients, with three requiring lipid-lowering agents.[13] One promising observation was the lack of cytomegalovirus (CMV) infection in CMV-negative recipients of islets from CMV-positive donors.[13] Insulin independence at one year post-transplant is approximately 85%.[13] As overviewed in subsequent sections on experimental models of islet cell transplantation (ICT), several new approaches are being taken

to prevent rejection, many of which have proven successful in non-human primate models. Some of the approaches under study are: incorporation of monoclonal antibodies and chimeric molecules that block immune mediators/cells, genetic modification of the graft to enhance survival post-transplant or create an immunomodulatory microenvironment, and immunoisolation.

The success of these trials should put islet cell transplantation closer to being covered by medical insurance programs. In the USA, islet cell transplants are regulated by the Food and Drug Administration (FDA). To date, the majority of studies require that patients have had Type 1 diabetes for five years or more and been under the care of a physician for six months to a year prior to enrollment. Patients must suffer from hypoglycemia unawareness (blood glucose <54 mg/dl that goes unrecognized and requires the assistance of another individual) or have documented evidence of hospitalizations due to ketoacidosis. Poor metabolic control that results from a lack of compliance would result in the exclusion of a patient from a trial. A body mass index in the low to mid-20s and an exogenous insulin requirement of <0.7–1 unit of insulin per kg per day is essential, as it is otherwise difficult to transplant an adequate number of islets to reverse diabetes.

Organizations that have traditionally focused on establishing standards for hematopoietic cell processing and transplantation are now moving toward development of standards for all forms of cellular therapies, including islet cells; for example, the International Society for Hematotherapy and Graft Engineering has become the International Society for Cellular Therapy, and the American Association of Blood Banks is involved with the establishment of standards for islet transplantation. The emphasis on standard operating procedures, QA/QC, and careful documentation, which have long been a staple in blood banking and hematopoietic cell processing, creates a natural bridge between these different cellular therapies. In fact, many of the issues that are critical to successful islet cell transplantation are equally as crucial in hematopoietic cell transplants; for example, issues related to viable, functional cell mass to achieve engraftment and the need for increasing numbers of cells as the level of genetic disparity increases, are similar for both fields.

Advances in experimental models of islet cell transplantation

Now that reproducible insulin independence is attainable in people, we are faced with the challenge of decreasing the toxicity of immunosuppressive agents so that more people are eligible for an islet cell transplant. At the present time, a patient must have had diabetes for five or more years, be over the age of 18, and experience frequent, severe hypo- or hyperglycemia to justify being considered for a trial. In addition to prevention of rejection, transplanted islets must be protected from recurrent autoimmunity. Ideally, patients could be treated to alter their immune systems so that donor tissues would remain unperturbed and immune responses to infectious agents or neoplastic cells would remain intact, without the need for continued administration of immunosuppressive drugs, many of which are diabetogenic and nephrotoxic. As previously mentioned, the first successful demonstration of 100% clinical insulin independence was the direct result of elimination of steroids from the immunosuppressive regimen and the use of agents that targeted the immune response at sequential points in the series of events that can lead to rejection or recurrent autoimmunity. Experimental models of islet cell

transplantation are valuable in that they provide support for the use of various agents in clinical trials. Two key issues emerge in considering the design, execution and interpretation of experiments in these models. The first is concerned with the fact that results gained from rodent models, although highly informative with regard to potential mechanisms of immunity, have rarely and inconsistently translated to larger animals and humans.[14] The second is related to the fact that spontaneous models of autoimmune diabetes do not exist for NHP; therefore, islet transplant studies in NHP are limited to assessment of the impact of immune intervention protocols on islet allograft rejection. The islet transplant models are as follows:

- Non-autoimmune models of diabetes
  - Streptozotocin-induced diabetes in rodents
  - Streptozotocin-induced diabetes in dogs, non-human primates
  - Pancreatectomy-induced diabetes in dogs, non-human primates
- Autoimmune models of diabetes
  - BB rat
  - NOD mouse.

Interventions that effectively prevent a primary immune response to newly transplanted tissue may not be as efficacious against the pre-existing anti-islet response of Type 1 diabetes. Whether or not rodent data are adequate to justify a new clinical trial is still a topic of debate; ideally, data from both larger animal, preclinical and autoimmune rodent models would be available to support the use of new agents in humans with Type 1 diabetes.

Prevention of rejection and recurrent autoimmunity/tolerance induction

Identification of novel immune intervention agents continues to be an extremely active area of investigation, both academically and at the corporate level. Steroids and calcineurin inhibitors have been the mainstay of clinical transplantation for several years now, but these drugs have toxic effects on islets and kidneys. The immune response leading to islet rejection is a complex one, with many cell types involved; however, it is generally accepted that T-lymphocytes are critical effectors of rejection and autoimmunity.[15–17]

T-cells must interact with transplanted islets via unique T-cell receptors (TCR) that are specific for islet autoantigens and for mismatched donor major histocompatibility (MHC) antigens expressed on various cells within the islet. These autoantigen and donor antigen-specific receptors will be expressed on a low percentage of recipient T-cells. Generalized immunosuppressants, however, do not discriminate between T-cells, and also target cellular pathways that are not unique to leukocytes, thus contributing to generalized suppression of T-cells and to the side effects associated with immunosuppression. T-cells cannot recognize and respond to antigen without the help of antigen presenting cells (APC); antigen is presented to the T-cell in association with MHC molecules expressed on the APC surface.[16,18–20] Two major classes of MHC molecules govern immunity – class I and class II, with class I expressed on all nucleated cells of the body and class II expressed only on specialized cells, such as APC. In addition to TCR interaction with antigen/MHC, T-cells and APC communicate further via a plethora of receptor:ligand pairs, with each interaction leading to activation and/or continued progression of the immune response. The CD3 complex, associated with the TCR, is required for initiation of intracellular signaling upon engagement of the TCR with antigen/MHC.[21] Co-receptors, known as CD4 and CD8, are uniquely expressed on T-cells (i.e. the mature T-cell expresses CD4 or CD8), and are integral in the interaction

between T-cells and MHC antigens on APC, with class I and II molecules preferentially engaging CD8+ and CD4+ T-cells, respectively. The initial interaction between the TCR complex, and MHC/antigen on APC is known as signal 1; additional T-cell surface molecules are involved in signal 1, including CD45 and its isoforms. T-cells that only receive signal 1 are rendered anergic, or unresponsive. Signal 2, also known as co-stimulation, is primarily mediated via the CD28:CD80/86 and CD154:CD40 (T-cell:APC) pathways. Additional cell surface molecules must subsequently engage, causing the T-cell to proliferate and divide, followed by differentiation to effector cells capable of killing islets or producing immune mediators that augment immunity. Further complicating the islets' potential for survival in a patient with Type 1 diabetes are the facts that:

(1) donor MHC antigens expressed on islet cells can be directly recognized as antigen by recipient T-cells (direct pathway) or can be processed and presented by recipient APC to recipient T-cells (indirect pathway), thereby increasing the repertoire of T-cells capable of mediating rejection; and
(2) existing autoimmune T-cells, which have already expanded, are primed and ready to mediate islet destruction.

Inhibiting a primary immune response has proven simpler than inhibiting an existing one. Monoclonal antibodies (moabs) and chimeric molecules that interfere with T-cell:APC interactions have been used extensively in attempts to prevent rejection or induce tolerance[22] and many promising results have been obtained. Usage of such agents can still result in generalized immune suppression if all T-cells express the targeted molecule, but theoretically should not result in adverse effects on non-hematopoietic tissues.

Approaches that successfully prevent rodent islet allograft rejection in non-autoimmune strains do not always work to prevent destruction of syngeneic or allogeneic islets in autoimmune models such as the NOD mouse.[23,24] Data emerging from studies that involve interference with signal 1 are showing promise for both prevention of islet allograft rejection and recurrent autoimmunity.

- Agents that interfere with signal 1
  - non-depleting anti-CD3
  - depleting anti-CD3-immunotoxin conjugate
  - anti-CD4
  - anti-CD45RB;
- Agents that interfere with signal 2
  - CTLA4-Fc, CTLA4-Ig
  - anti-CD80, 86
  - anti-CD154;
- Other:
  - Hematopoietic chimerism.

Treatment of diabetic NOD mice with anti-CD3 induced durable remission of recent onset diabetes and prevented destruction of syngeneic islet grafts.[25,26] In NHP models, treatment of diabetic rhesus monkeys (streptozotocin induced diabetes) with peri-transplant anti-CD3 conjugated to an immunotoxin, plus 15-deoxyspergualin, resulted in operation tolerance to allogeneic islets.[27] Clinically, therapy with non-depleting anti-CD3 (hOKT3gamma1(Ala-Ala)) has been shown to be beneficial in patients with new onset Type 1 diabetes, with nine out of 12 treated patients demonstrating improved or maintained insulin production, as well as decreased hemoglobin A1c and insulin dosages, compared with the control group, in which only two out of 12 patients fared as well.[28] Taken together, the aforementioned data lends strong support to the use of anti-CD3 for clinical islet allotransplant trials in patients with Type 1

diabetes. Non-depleting anti-CD4 specific moabs have also been shown to prevent islet allograft destruction in diabetic NOD mice[29] and preliminary data from a small series of patients with Type 1 diabetes that received allogeneic islets in conjunction with anti-CD4 therapy[30] suggest that this may be another promising approach. Although not yet tested in clinical islet trials, the use of antibodies specific for the signal 1 molecule CD45RB,[31,32] has proven effective for prevention of murine islet allograft rejection.[33,34] Addition of anti-CD154 to the treatment regimen, resulting in interference with both signal 1 and 2, has proven synergistic in murine islet allograft models[35] and is required for enhancement of islet allograft survival in NOD mice.[36]

The engagement of CD154 on T-cells with CD40 on APC is the earliest co-stimulatory (signal 2) interaction. Unlike CD3 or CD28, CD154 is not constitutively expressed on the T-cell surface but is rapidly and transiently upregulated on activated T-cells. Theoretically, treatment of animals with agents that target CD154 should lead to specific interference with those cells that are activated subsequent to encountering transplanted islets.[37,38] The CD28:B7 co-stimulatory pathway[39,40] is operative subsequent to CD154:CD40 signaling. CD28 is constitutively expressed on T-cells; CTLA4, which also interacts with B7 molecules, is upregulated on activated T-cells and plays a key role in immune regulation. Interference with these signal 2 pathways has shown beneficial effects in both allograft and autoimmune diabetes models (see promising therapeutics list above).

Treatment with CTLA4-Fc allowed for long-term islet allograft survival and donor-specific tolerance in a murine model.[41] Treatment of mice with anti-CD86 (B7.2) or anti-CD86 and anti-CD80 (B7.1), but not with anti-CD80 alone, also resulted in allogeneic islet survival.[42]

Treatment with CTLA4-Ig was minimally effective in a cynomolgus monkey model of islet allotransplantation, with only two out of five monkeys demonstrating some islet function for 30 and 50 days.[43] Administration of CTLA4-Ig, in combination with sirolimus and anti-IL2 receptor induction therapy, to rhesus monkey islet allograft recipients resulted in stable islet engraftment and insulin independence during therapy.[44]

With regard to diabetes onset and progression, variable effects have been obtained in NOD mice treated with agents that alter the CD28:B7 co-stimulatory pathway.[45] Treatment with CTLA4-Ig (a CD28 antagonist) or anti-CD86 prevented onset of diabetes when NOD mice were treated at the onset of insulitis; however, if treated later in the course of disease progression, these agents had no inhibitory effect. Similar results have been observed in NOD mice treated with anti-CD154.[46] Strikingly, treatment with anti-CD80 or a combination of anti-CD80/86 accelerated disease progression. These results highlight the need to understand better alterations in immune status during the different phases of disease onset and progression. Treatments that might be efficacious in preventing diabetes onset or halting progression early in the course of disease may not be effective once a full blown immune response, replete with memory T-cells, has been generated. This particular point generates significant discussion when immune interventions aimed at prevention of islet allograft rejection in patients with Type 1 diabetes are considered.

With regard to transplants, co-administration of donor cells was required in order to achieve tolerance to islet allografts in mice treated with anti-CD154.[47] NOD mice continuously treated with anti-CD154 experienced prolonged syngeneic and allogeneic islet survival,[23] but attainment of tolerance to allogeneic islets in the NOD model required establishment of hematopoietic chimerism via sublethal irradiation and treatment with anti-CD154.[48] In the BB rat model, however, anti-CD154 prevented diabetes recurrence in syngeneic islets transplanted into animals with established autoimmunity.[49] With regard to larger animal models, anti-CD154 monotherapy with humanized antibody led to the first demonstration of 100% insulin independence in C-peptide negative baboons and rhesus monkeys with pancreatectomy-induced diabetes.[6,7] This result was most likely due to the efficacy of anti-CD154 for prevention of islet allograft rejection in the absence of diabetogenic effects. Evidence for alteration of antidonor-specific immune reactivity was obtained, although animals eventually rejected subsequent to discontinuation of therapy. Unlike the results obtained for murine islet allograft models,[50] addition of donor-specific transfusion to anti-CD154 therapy did not lead to tolerance in cynomolgus monkeys.[51]

Co-existence of donor and recipient hematopoietic cells in the recipient's body is referred to as mixed hematopoietic chimerism. This state, which can be challenging to achieve without the use of toxic pre-transplant conditioning regimens, can allow for acceptance of allografts from animals of the same strain as the original hematopoietic cell donor, without the need for immune suppression. Establishment of mixed hematopoietic chimerism prevents diabetes in NOD mice.[52,53] In non-autoimmune strain combinations[54] as well as in NOD mice,[48,55] mixed hematopoietic chimerism prevents islet allograft rejection. Islet allograft acceptance in the absence of immune suppression has been reported for a monkey that had previously been made tolerant to a renal allograft via a rigorous conditioning regimen involving irradiation, multiple immunosuppressive drugs and transient chimerism.[56] Several years later, having maintained stable renal function, the recipient was given islets from the original kidney donor and accepted them without antirejection agents.

Application of this approach to the clinical islet setting has been hindered by the requirement for rigorous conditioning of the recipient to enable donor hematopoietic cell engraftment, and as often seen, approaches that successfully enable engraftment in rodents have not translated to larger animals and man.[57] Nevertheless, this remains an area of great interest, and several of the reagents being employed to enhance islet allograft survival are also being applied to hematopoietic cell transplantation.

Overall, great progress has been made in delineation of agents that effectively prevent islet rejection in the absence of adverse effects on islet cell function. Induction of donor-specific tolerance is readily achieved in non-autoimmune murine islet allotransplant models and is more difficult in autoimmune NOD mice and NHP. Ultimately, identification of strategies that effectively target allorejection and recurrent autoimmunity in rodent models, and in addition, prevent islet allorejection in larger animal models, will have the most potential to affect positively islet allograft survival in patients.

Achieving an adequate mass of insulin-producing tissue to reverse diabetes

In addition to definition of less toxic immune intervention strategies and tolerance induction protocols, the limited supply of islets for transplantation must be overcome in order to apply more broadly biological replacement therapies as a cure for patients with Type 1 diabetes. The following factors are those affecting our ability to attain/engraft an adequate mass of functional insulin-producing tissue.

- Pancreas procurement
  - core temperature during harvest
  - donor variables
  - cold ischemia time
  - preservation methods
  - optimization of organ donation
  - non-heart beating donors
- Islet isolation and culture
  - enzyme
  - isolation media and reagents
  - inhibitors of apoptosis
  - purification
  - culture media
- Early post-transplant engraftment
  - complement-mediated damage
  - pro-inflammatory cytokines produced by activated macrophages, endothelial cells
  - other mediators that damage insulin-producing cells.

Increasing the number of available organs and refining procurement and islet isolation and culture techniques should all contribute to our ability to transplant a greater number of patients. In addition to these technical issues, delineating treatment regimens that limit early islet loss could significantly enhance our ability to reverse diabetes with the use of one-half of the islets required in current trials. Identification of alternative sources of insulin-producing cells, e.g. tissue derived from adult or embryonic stem cells, genetically engineered cell lines, or xenogeneic islets, would significantly increase the number of patients that could be transplanted.

Optimizing organ donation is an obvious area of concentration, but in addition, identifying methods to increase the number of organs that can be used for islet isolation is important. Traditionally, donors between the ages of 25 and 45, with cold ischemia times of eight hours or less, have yielded the best results with regards to functional islet yield.[58] Several additional variables, including body mass index, cause of death and prolonged hypotensive episodes requiring high vasopressors, as well as hyperglycemia in the donor prior to harvest, were found to significantly impact islet isolation outcome.[58-60] Maintaining a low pancreatic core temperature has also been shown to be beneficial with regards to islet yield.[61] As first demonstrated in dogs, a two-layer method incorporating perfluorocarbon, to increase oxygenation of harvested pancreata, and UW solution is showing promise as a means for enhanced preservation of organs, including prolonged storage times and enhancement of isolation from less than optimal donors.[62] In order to add to the available donor pool, some centers are exploring the potential of using non-heart beating donors[63,64] and preliminary results show a positive potential for this category of organ, both for renal and islet transplantation.

Although various modifications have been introduced over the years, the method of Ricordi et al.[65] has continued to be the gold standard by which islets are obtained. Although not the final answer, improved enzyme blends[66] have contributed significantly to the reproducibility of islet isolation. Islet yield remains a problem, as recently reviewed in the context of islet autotransplantation for chronic pancreatitis,[67] with an estimated recovery of 35–40% of pancreatic islets reported among the most experienced centers. Addition of agents with cytoprotective properties during the isolation procedure is one approach to improving recovery of viable islets.[68-70] Continued efforts to improve enzyme quality and all aspects of islet isolation, including digestion and purification, are ongoing in an effort to maximize recovery of functional islets.

Once islets have been obtained, culture techniques become a determining factor in islet survival and function. Optimization of media used in all steps of isolation and culture is essential[71] if functional islet survival is to be improved, and this is an area of active study. Extended culture of human islets in serum-free medium for a period of one to two months yielded islets capable of reversing diabetes in NOD–SCID mice, and in some cases, the cultured islets were more effective than short-term cultured islets from the same preparation.[72]

Strategies to limit non-specific inflammatory events, mediated by intrahepatic macrophages and endothelial cells that are activated by infusion-related events, may significantly decrease the number of islets required to attain insulin independence.[5] Attempts to address this issue have primarily been studied using marginal mass models, in which the smallest number of islets capable of reversing diabetes, usually with a prolonged engraftment period required to achieve insulin independence, is transplanted into diabetic animals, with or without an intervention aimed at limiting early islet loss.[36,73-76] The roles of complement-mediated events,[77,78] heme oxygenase-1,[36] and the graft-promoting potential of, e.g. macrophage inhibitory agents such as dexoyspergualin,[76] are being evaluated in an attempt to define and alter early events that lead to islet loss.

Finally, a critical area for biological replacement strategies in the treatment of Type 1 diabetes is the identification of alternative sources of insulin-producing tissue:

- embryonic stem cells
- adult stem cells
- engineered cell lines
- stimulation of islet neogenesis
- xenogeneic tissue.

Production of insulin-producing tissue from embryonic stem cells, with variable ability to produce insulin in response to glucose and/or reverse diabetes in murine models, has been achieved, although major strides must be made before such approaches reach clinical application,[79-82] independent of the ethical issues surrounding this area of research. The potential for islet neogenesis and derivation of insulin-producing cells from adult pancreatic stem cells has been reported[83–87] and would provide an acceptable alternative to embryonic stem cell approaches if limitations concerning the number of cells that can be generated can be overcome. In addition to stem cell-derived tissue, genetic engineering approaches to production of insulin-producing tissue have also met with limited success.[88,89] Understanding the factors that regulate beta-cell differentiation may lead to the development of strategies to incorporate administration of factors, stimulating islet neogenesis to patients with Type 1 diabetes, either at onset (in combination with tolerance induction strategies), or in recipients of marginal mass islet transplants.

Summary

To conclude, significant advances in islet cell transplantation have been achieved, with 100% insulin independence now attainable for patients with Type 1 diabetes. However, application of biological replacement strategies as a cure for the majority of these patients awaits identification of alternative sources of insulin-producing tissue and delineation of immune intervention therapies that effectively prevent rejection and recurrent autoimmunity, and ultimately, induce donor-specific tolerance.

References

1. Kenyon NS, Ricordi CR. Nonhuman primate models of islet transplantation:preclinical testing of novel immunotherapies. Diabetes Rev 1999; 7: 183–6.
2. Kenyon NS, Alejandro R, Ricordi C, Mintz DH. Islet cell transplantation. JB Lippincott Co, 2000.
3. Jindal RM, Sidner RA, Milgrom ML. Post-transplant diabetes mellitus. The role of immunosuppression. Drug Saf 1997; 16: 242–57.
4. Kaufman DB, Platt JL, Rabe FL et al. Differential roles of Mac-1+ cells, and CD4+ and CD8+ T lymphocytes in primary nonfunction and classic rejection of islet allografts. J Exp Med 1990; 172: 291–302.
5. Bottino R, Fernandez LA, Ricordi C et al. Transplantation of allogeneic islets of Langerhans in the rat liver: effects of macrophage depletion on graft survival and microenvironment activation. Diabetes 1998; 47: 316–23.
6. Kenyon NS, Chatzipetrou M, Masetti M et al. Long-term survival and function of intrahepatic islet allografts in rhesus monkeys treated with humanized anti-CD154. Proc Natl Acad Sci USA 1999; 96: 8132–7.
7. Kenyon NS, Fernandez LA, Lehmann R et al. Long-term survival and function of intrahepatic islet allografts in baboons treated with humanized anti-CD154. Diabetes 1999; 48: 1473–81.
8. Shapiro AM, Lakey JR, Ryan EA et al. Islet transplantation in seven patients with type 1 diabetes mellitus using a glucocorticoid-free immunosuppressive regimen. N Engl J Med 2000; 343: 230–8.
9. Ricordi C, Gray DW, Hering BJ et al. Islet isolation assessment in man and large animals. Acta Diabetol Lat 1990; 27: 185–95.
10. Tzakis AG, Ricordi C, Alejandro R et al. Pancreatic islet transplantation after upper abdominal exenteration and liver replacement. Lancet 1990; 336: 402–5.
11. Alejandro R, Lehmann R, Ricordi C et al. Long-term function (6 years) of islet allografts in type 1 diabetes. Diabetes 1997; 46: 1983–9.
12. Hering BJ, Eckhard M, Brandhorst H et al. Improved survival of single donor islet allografts in IDDM recipients by refined peritransplant management. Diabetes 1997; 46: 64A.
13. Ryan EA, Lakey JR, Rajotte RV et al. Clinical outcomes and insulin secretion after islet transplantation with the Edmonton protocol. Diabetes 2001; 50: 710–9.
14. Greiner DL, Rossini AA, Mordes JP. Translating data from animal models into methods for preventing human autoimmune diabetes mellitus: caveat emptor and primum non nocere. Clin Immunol 2001; 100: 134–43.

15. Gill RG, Coulombe M, Lafferty KJ. Pancreatic islet allograft immunity and tolerance: the two-signal hypothesis revisited. Immunol Rev 1996; 149: 75–96.

16. Nicolls MR, Coulombe M, Gill RG. The basis of immunogenicity of endocrine allografts. Crit Rev Immunol 2001; 21: 87–101.

17. Yoon JW, Jun HS. Cellular and molecular pathogenic mechanisms of insulin-dependent diabetes mellitus. Ann NY Acad Sci 2001; 928: 200–11.

18. Hudson AW, Ploegh HL. The cell biology of antigen presentation. Exp Cell Res 2002; 272: 1–7.

19. Chakraborty AK. How and why does the immunological synapse form? Physical chemistry meets cell biology. Sci STKE 2002; 2002: PE10.

20. Mellman I, Steinman RM. Dendritic cells: specialized and regulated antigen processing machines. Cell 2001; 106: 255–8.

21. Garcia KC. Molecular interactions between extracellular components of the T-cell receptor signaling complex. Immunol Rev 1999; 172: 73–85.

22. Kenyon N, ed. Experimental Approaches to the Prevention of Rejection. Oxford: Oxford University Press, 2002.

23. Molano RD, Berney T, Li H et al. Prolonged islet graft survival in NOD mice by blockade of the CD40-CD154 pathway of T-cell costimulation. Diabetes 2001; 50: 270–6.

24. Markees TG, Serreze DV, Phillips NE et al. NOD mice have a generalized defect in their response to transplantation tolerance induction. Diabetes 1999; 48: 967–74.

25. Chatenoud L, Primo J, Bach JF. CD3 antibody-induced dominant self tolerance in overtly diabetic NOD mice. J Immunol 1997; 158: 2947–54.

26. Chatenoud L, Thervet E, Primo J, Bach JF. Anti-CD3 antibody induces long-term remission of overt autoimmunity in nonobese diabetic mice. Proc Natl Acad Sci USA 1994; 91: 123–7.

27. Thomas JM, Contreras JL, Smyth CA et al. Successful reversal of streptozotocin-induced diabetes with stable allogeneic islet function in a preclinical model of type 1 diabetes. Diabetes 2001; 50: 1227–36.

28. Herold KC, Hagopian W, Auger JA et al. Anti-CD3 monoclonal antibody in new-onset type 1 diabetes mellitus. N Engl J Med 2002; 346: 1692–8.

29. Guo Z, Wu T, Kirchhof N et al. Immunotherapy with nondepleting anti-CD4 monoclonal antibodies but not CD28 antagonists protects islet graft in spontaneously diabetic nod mice from autoimmune destruction and allogeneic and xenogeneic graft rejection. Transplantation 2001; 71: 1656–65.

30. Meyer C, Hering BJ, Grossmann R et al. Improved glucose counterregulation and autonomic symptoms after intraportal islet transplants alone in patients with long-standing type 1 diabetes mellitus. Transplantation 1998; 66: 233–40.

31. Alexander DR. The CD45 tyrosine phosphatase: a positive and negative regulator of immune cell function. Semin Immunol 2000; 12: 349–59.

32. Luke PP, O'Brien CA, Jevnikar AM, Zhong R. Anti-CD45RB monoclonal antibody-mediated transplantation tolerance. Curr Mol Med 2001; 1: 533–43.

33. Auersvald LA, Rothstein DM, Oliveira SC et al. Indefinite islet allograft survival in mice after a short course of treatment with anti-CD45 monoclonal antibodies. Transplantation 1997; 63: 1355–8.

34. Basadonna GP, Auersvald L, Khuong CQ et al. Antibody-mediated targeting of CD45 isoforms: a novel immunotherapeutic strategy. Proc Natl Acad Sci USA 1998; 95: 382–6.

35. Rothstein DM, Livak MF, Kishimoto K et al. Targeting signal 1 through CD45RB synergizes with CD40 ligand blockade and promotes long term engraftment and tolerance in stringent transplant models. J Immunol 2001; 166: 322–9.

36. Pileggi A, Molano RD, Berney T et al. Heme oxygenase-1 induction in islet cells results in protection from apoptosis and improved in vivo function after transplantation. Diabetes 2001; 50: 1983–91.

37. Yamada, Sayegh MH. The CD154-CD40 costimulatory pathway in transplantation. Transplantation 2002; 73 (1 Suppl.): S36–9.

38. Kirk AD, Blair PJ, Tadaki DK et al. The role of CD154 in organ transplant rejection and acceptance. Philos Trans R Soc Lond B Biol Sci 2001; 356: 691–702.

39. Lenschow DJ, Walunas TL, Bluestone JA.

CD28/B7 system of T cell costimulation. Annu Rev Immunol 1996; 14: 233–58.

40. Salomon B, Bluestone JA. Complexities of CD28/B7: CTLA-4 costimulatory pathways in autoimmunity and transplantation. Annu Rev Immunol 2001; 19: 225–52.

41. Tran HM, Nickerson PW, Restifo AC et al. Distinct mechanisms for the induction and maintenance of allograft tolerance with CTLA4-Fc treatment. J Immunol 1997; 159: 2232–9.

42. Lenschow DJ, Zeng Y, Hathcock KS et al. Inhibition of transplant rejection following treatment with anti-B&-2 and anti-B7-1 antibodies. Transplantation 1995; 60: 1171–8.

43. Levisetti MG, Padrid PA, Szot GL et al. Immunosuppressive effects of human CTLA4Ig in a non-human primate model of allogeneic pancreatic islet transplantation. J Immunol 1997; 159: 5187–91.

44. Adams AB, Shirasugi N, Durham MM et al. Calcineurin inhibitor-free CD28 blockade-based protocol protects allogeneic islets in nonhuman primates. Diabetes 2002; 51: 265–70.

45. Lenschow DJ, Ho SC, Sattar H et al. Differential effects of anti-B7-1 and anti-B7-2 monoclonal antibody treatment on the development of diabetes in the nonobese diabetic mouse. J Exp Med 1995; 181: 1145–55.

46. Balasa B, Krahl T, Patstone G et al. CD40 ligand-CD40 interactions are necessary for the initiation of insulitis and diabetes in nonobese diabetic mice. J Immunol 1997; 159: 4620–7.

47. Zheng XX, Markees TG, Hancock WW et al. CTLA4 signals are required to optimally induce allograft tolerance with combined donor-specific transfusion and anti-CD154 monoclonal antibody treatment. J Immunol 1999; 162: 4983–90.

48. Seung E, Ikakoshi N, Woda BA et al. Allogeneic hematopoietic chimerism in mice treated with sublethal myeloablation and anti-CD154 antibody: absence of graft-versus-host disease, induction of skin allograft tolerance, and prevention of recurrent autoimmunity in islet-allografted NOD/Lt mice. Blood 2000; 95: 2175–82.

49. Kover KL, Geng Z, Hess DM et al. Anti-CD154 (CD40L) prevents recurrence of diabetes in islet isografts in the DR-BB rat. Diabetes 2000; 49: 1666–70.

50. Parker DC, Greiner DL, Phillips NE et al. Survival of mouse pancreatic islet allografts in recipients treated with allogeneic small lymphocytes and antibody to CD40 ligand. Proc Natl Acad Sci USA 1995; 92: 9560–4.

51. Kenyon NS, Alejandro R, Ricordi C. On the preclinical results if islets and anti-CD154. Graft 2000; 3: 230–4.

52. Li H, Kaufman CL, Boggs SS et al. Mixed allogeneic chimerism induced by a sublethal approach prevents autoimmune diabetes and reverses insulitis in nonobese diabetic (NOD) mice. J Immunol 1996; 156: 380–8.

53. Mathieu C, Casteels K, Bouillon R, Waer M. Protection against autoimmune diabetes in mixed bone marrow chimeras: mechanisms involved. J Immunol 1997; 158: 1453–7.

54. Li H, Colson YL, Ildstad ST. Mixed allogeneic chimerism achieved by lethal and nonlethal conditioning approaches induces donor-specific tolerance to simultaneous islet allografts. Transplantation 1995; 60: 523–9.

55. Li H, Kaufman CL, Ildstad ST. Allogeneic chimerism induces donor-specific tolerance to simultaneous islet allografts in nonobese diabetic mice. Surgery 1995; 118: 192–7; discussion 197–8.

56. Kawai T, Sogawa H, Koulmanda M et al. Long-term islet allograft function in the absence of chronic immunosuppression: a case report of a nonhuman primate previously made tolerant to a renal allograft from the same donor. Transplantation 2001; 72: 351–4.

57. Kenyon NS, Chatzipetrou M, Tzakis A et al. Allogeneic hematopoietic stem cell transplantation in recipients of cellular or solid organ allografts. Cancer Treat Res 1999; 101: 109–32.

58. Lakey JR, Warnock GL, Rajotte RV et al. Variables in organ donors that affect the recovery of human islets of Langerhans. Transplantation 1996; 61: 1047–53.

59. Zeng Y, Torre MA, Karrison T, Thistlethwaite JR. The correlation between donor characteristics and the success of human islet isolation. Transplantation 1994; 57: 954–8.

60. Benhamou PY, Watt PC, Mullen Y et al. Human islet isolation in 104 consecutive cases. Factors affecting isolation success. Transplantation 1994; 57: 1804–10.

61. Lakey JR, Kneteman NM, Rajotte RV et al.

Effect of core pancreas temperature during cadaveric procurement on human islet isolation and functional viability. Transplantation 2002; 73: 1106–10.

62. Tanioka Y, Sutherland DE, Kuroda Y et al. Excellence of the two-layer method (University of Wisconsin solution/perfluorochemical) in pancreas preservation before islet isolation. Surgery 1997; 122: 435–41; discussion 441–2.

63. Clayton HA, Swift SM, Turner JM et al. Non-heart-beating organ donors: a potential source of islets for transplantation? Transplantation 2000; 69: 2094–8.

64. Alvarez J, del Barrio R, Arias J et al. Non-heart-beating donors from the streets: an increasing donor pool source. Transplantation 2000; 70: 314–7.

65. Ricordi C, Lacy PE, Finke EH et al. Automated method for isolation of human pancreatic islets. Diabetes 1988; 37: 413–20.

66. Linetsky E, Bottino R, Lehmann R et al. Improved human islet isolation using a new enzyme blend, liberase. Diabetes 1997; 46: 1120–3.

67. Morrison CP, Wemyss-Holden SA, Dennison AR, Maddern GJ. Islet yield remains a problem in islet autotransplantation. Arch Surg 2002; 137: 80–3.

68. Paraskevas S, Maysinger D, Wang R et al. Cell loss in isolated human islets occurs by apoptosis. Pancreas 2000; 20: 270–6.

69. Thomas FT, Contreras JL, Bilbao G et al. Anoikis, extracellular matrix, and apoptosis factors in isolated cell transplantation. Surgery 1999; 126: 299–304.

70. Arita S, Une S, Ohtsuka S et al. Increased islet viability by addition of beraprost sodium to collagenase solution. Pancreas 2001; 23: 62–7.

71. London NJ, Swift SM, Clayton HA. Isolation, culture and functional evaluation of islets of Langerhans. Diabetes Metab 1998; 24: 200–7.

72. Gaber AO, Fraga DW, Callicutt CS et al. Improved in vivo pancreatic islet function after prolonged in vitro islet culture. Transplantation 2001; 72: 1730–6.

73. Berney T, Molano RD, Pileggi A et al. Absence of CSF-1-dependent macrophages does not improve function of transplanted islets of Langerhans. Cell Transplant 2001; 10: 633–7.

74. Berney T, Molano RD, Cattan P et al. Endotoxin-mediated delayed islet graft function

is associated with increased intra-islet cytokine production and islet cell apoptosis. Transplantation 2001: 71: 125–32.

75. Pileggi A, Ricordi C, Alessiani M, Inverardi L. Factors influencing islet of Langerhans graft function and monitoring. Clin Chim Acta 2001; 310: 3–16.

76. Kaufman DB, Gores PF, Field MJ et al. Effect of 15-deoxyspergualin on immediate function and long-term survival of transplanted islets in murine recipients of a marginal islet mass. Diabetes 1994; 43: 778–83.

77. Bennett W, Groth CG, Larsson R et al. Isolated human islets trigger an instant blood mediated inflammatory reaction: implications for intra-portal islet transportation as a treatment for patients with type 1 diabetes. Ups J Med Sci 2000; 105: 125–33.

78. Bennet W, Sundberg B, Groth CG et al. Incompatibility between human blood and isolated islets of Langerhans: a finding with implications for clinical intraportal islet transplantation? Diabetes 1999; 48: 1907–14.

79. Peshavaria M, Pang K. Manipulation of pancreatic stem cells for replacement therapy. Diabetes Technol Ther 2000; 2: 453–60.

80. Soria B, Skoudy A, Martin F. From stem cells to beta cells: new strategies in cell therapy of diabetes mellitus. Diabetologia 2001; 44: 407–15.

81. Ramiya VK, Maraist M, Arfors KE et al. Reversal of insulin-dependent diabetes using islets generated in vitro from pancreatic stem cells. Nat Med 2000; 6: 278–82.

82. Lumelsky N, Blondel O, Laeng P et al. Differentiation of embryonic stem cells to insulin-secreting structures similar to pancreatic islets. Science 2001; 292: 1389–94.

83. Bonner-Weir S, Baxter LA, Schuppin GT, Smith FE. A second pathway for regeneration of adult exocrine and endocrine pancreas. A possible recapitulation of embryonic development. Diabetes 1993; 42: 1715–20.

84. Bonner-Weir S, Taneja M, Weir GC et al. In vitro cultivation of human islets from expanded ductal tissue. Proc Natl Acad Sci USA 2000; 97: 7999–8004.

85. Wang RN, Kloppel G, Bouwens L. Duct- to islet-cell differentiation and islet growth in the pancreas of duct-ligated adult rats. Diabetologia 1995; 38: 1405–11.

86. Rosenberg L. In vivo cell transformation: neogenesis of beta cells from pancreatic ductal cells. Cell Transplant 1995; 4: 371–83.
87. Rafaeloff R, Pittenger GL, Barlow SW et al. Cloning and sequencing of the pancreatic islet neogenesis associated protein (INGAP) gene and its expression in islet neogenesis in hamsters. J Clin Invest 1997; 99: 2100–9.
88. Newgard CB. Cellular engineering and gene therapy strategies for insulin replacement in diabetes. Diabetes 1994; 43: 341–50.
89. Demeterco C, Levine F. Gene therapy for diabetes. Front Biosci 2001; 6: D175–91.

17

Postprandial hyperglycemia: present treatment and its importance in the future

Stefano Del Prato, Luca Benzi, Giuseppe Penno, Roberto Miccoli

Although multiple metabolic alterations contribute to the overall risk to develop long-term complications, hyperglycemia remains the hallmark of diabetes mellitus. Increased plasma concentration of glucose is used for diagnostic purposes and it is associated with the risk to develop both micro- and macrovascular complications. Such an association, though appreciated for a long time, has received solid support by the use of glycated hemoglobin (HbA1c), an integrated marker of overall glucose exposure over a certain period of time, in large epidemiological surveys. For example, in the Finnish population the incidence of mortality and morbidity for coronary heart disease increased in a linear manner with the worsening of glycemic control as indicated by progressive increase of HbA1c levels.[1] From such a strong relationship one could infer that reduction of HbA1c by intervention should be associated with a reduction in the number of cardiovascular events.

Glycated hemoglobin really represents an integrated measure of glucose exposure during the day with both interprandial and postprandial glucose levels contributing to its absolute level. Thus, it is not surprising that correlations have been reported between HbA1c and fasting,[2,3] preprandial,[4] and postprandial[5] plasma glucose concentrations. More recently, however, emphasis has been placed on the possible independent association of fasting and postprandial glucose concentration with overall and cardiovascular mortality. In their meta-analysis, Coutinho et al.[6] have analyzed a total of 20 studies including 95,783 non-diabetic subjects and 3707 cardiovascular events during a mean follow-up period of 12.4 years. According to that analysis, both fasting and 2-h post-OGTT plasma glucose levels appeared to be independently associated with an increased risk for cardiovascular events. The distinction between an independent role of fasting versus post-challenge plasma glucose levels has become a hot issue following the recent Report of the Expert Committee on the diagnosis and classification of diabetes mellitus from the American Diabetes Association.[7] While suggesting that fasting plasma glucose measurements are as important as the oral glucose tolerance test (OGTT), a new category at risk to develop diabetes was identified: impaired fasting glucose (IFG; ≥ 6.1, <7 mmol/l or ≥ 110, <126 mg/dl). Nonetheless, it soon became apparent that IFG and impaired glucose tolerance (IGT; 2-h OGTT plasma levels ≥ 7.8, <11.1 mmol/l or ≥ 140, <200 mg/dl) did not identify the same population with a limited overlap of the two groups of individuals.[8] This observation has triggered extensive epidemiological research in the attempt to define whether IFG and IGT patients also differed in terms of cardiovascular risk. In the Funagata Diabetes Study,[9] 2534 subjects over 40 years of age entered a 7-year follow-up for estimation of the survival rate, upon identifi-

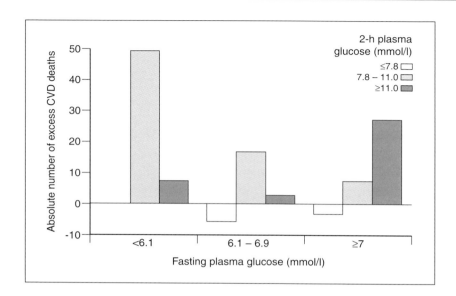

Figure 17.1

Estimated number of excess cardiovascular deaths as a function of fasting and 2-h glucose categories in the DECODE database. Source: adapted from ref. 11.

cation of subjects with normal (NFG), IFG, IGT, and overt diabetes. After the seven years of observation, the cumulative survival rates from cardiovascular disease (CVD) related to IGT and diabetes were 0.962 and 0.954, respectively, both significantly lower than that of NGT (0.988). The Cox's proportional hazard model analysis showed that the hazard ratio of IGT to NGT on death from CVD was 2.219 (95% CI 1.076–4.577). However, the cumulative survival rate of IFG from CVD was 0.977, not significantly lower than that of NFG (0.985). The Cox's hazard ratio of IFG to NFG on death from CVD was 1.136 (0.345–3.734), which was not significant either. Thus, at least in this Japanese population, IGT was a risk factor for CVD, but IFG was not. DECODE (Diabetes Epidemiology: Collaborative analysis Of Diagnostic criteria in Europe) includes OGTT data from more than 25,000 subjects collected all over Europe that have been used to analyze the respective association of fasting and 2-h OGTT plasma glucose levels with overall[10] and cardiovascular mortality.[11] The DECODE study indicated that an increased mortality risk was associated with 2-h post-load plasma glucose levels to a much greater extent than with FPG (fasting plasma glucose).[10] The latter, after adjustment for the 2-h glucose value, lost any association with all-cause mortality. After adjusting for possible confounders, the excess death for CVD was not affected by progressive increase in fasting plasma glucose levels when subjects with normal glucose tolerance were considered (Figure 17.1). The greatest excess mortality occurred in subjects with normal fasting plasma glucose concentration (FPG <6.1 mmol/l) but impaired glucose tolerance.[11] These results are in complete agreement with findings from many other epidemiological studies (see ref. 12 for review) and support the concept that excessive glucose excursion after the ingestion of an oral glucose load is associated with an independent risk for CVD that is significantly greater than the one associated with FPG. Based on these results it has been suggested that individuals with isolated post-challenge hyperglycemia should be identified and that post-meal glucose concentration should be a target for therapy in the attempt to reduce the cardiovascular risk of these subjects.

Post-challenge or post-meal hyperglycemia?

The bulk of data linking glucose excursions and cardiovascular diseases is derived from epidemiological studies employing OGTT. The assumption that similar glucose excursions may also occur after the ingestion of a mixed meal is, therefore, an extrapolation. In the study by Wolever et al.,[13] however, the relationship between 2-h plasma glucose after an OGTT and following a standard mixed meal was calculated in 36 subjects. The two values were shown to be highly correlated ($r = 0.97$; $p < 0.0001$) suggesting that people with excessive glucose excursion after an OGTT also tend to have a greater glucose excursion during daily life. Bonora et al.[4] have assessed daily glucose profile in 856 Type 2 diabetic patients on different treatments (diet, sulfonylureas, metformin, or the combination of the two). Average fasting plasma glucose was 8.8 ± 1.9 mmol/l and increased to 10.2 ± 3.0 mmol/l 2-h after breakfast. Before lunch, plasma glucose averaged 8.1 ± 2.8 mmol/l while 2 h later it was 10.0 ± 3.2 mmol/l. These figures indicate that even in treated Type 2 diabetic patients the increase in plasma glucose after meals is quite consistent. Of interest was the fact that high postprandial glucose levels could often be found even in patients with apparently satisfactory metabolic control (HbA1c <7.0%). This finding is in full agreement with the recent analysis performed on the diabetic population of the NHANES III, showing that 39% of patients with HbA1c <7.0% had a 2-h OGTT plasma glucose level higher than 11.1 mmol/l, a percentage increasing to 99% in subjects with HbA1c 7.0–7.9%.[14] In diabetic patients also, post-meal glucose

seems to be a better predictor of CVD. In the Diabetes Intervention Study,[15] no association could be found between FPG at entry and myocardial infarction or mortality, while a significant association was apparent when 1-h post-meal glucose levels were considered. These data clearly indicate that the majority of Type 2 diabetic patients, even many with low HbA1c levels, have higher-than-recommended post-meal glucose levels and that the degree of post-meal hyperglycemia is related to the overall cardiovascular risk. Nonetheless, the possibility remains that post-meal hyperglycemia is a marker for a risk rather than a cardiovascular risk itself. In a survey of 107 individuals with normal glucose tolerance, Yudkin and Coppack[16] found that 2-h post-load hyperglycemia but not fasting plasma glucose was directly correlated with adiposity, adipose tissue distribution, lipid profile, C-reactive protein, and cellular fibronectin. It was concluded from this finding that 2-h hyperglycemia may reflect alteration typical of the Metabolic Syndrome and that these should be the true target for therapy. Though this highlights the value of a simple determination such as post-meal glucose concentration for identification of subjects at risk for cardiovascular disease (CVD), a possible cause–effect relationship between this parameter and cardiovascular outcome remains to be established.

Post-meal glucose: a marker or a target for therapy?

In order to establish post-meal hyperglycemia as CVD risk factor at least three criteria must be met:

1. evidence for an independent relationship,
2. a plausible causal mechanism, and
3. risk reversibility by intervention.

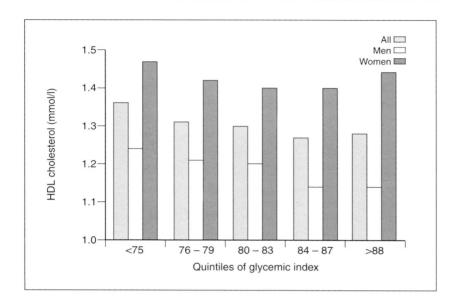

Figure 17.2
Mean serum levels of HDL cholesterol according to quintiles of glycemic index in the 13,907 participants in the Third National Health and Nutrition Examination Survey (1988–1994). Data are adjusted for age, race or ethnicity, smoking status, BMI, alcohol intake, physical activity, energy fraction from protein and carbohydrates, and total energy intake. Source: adapted from ref. 18.

Evidence for an independent relationship

Studies have looked at the intima-media thickness (IMT) as a proxy for activation of the atherosclerotic process. In a large cohort of diabetic patients, the relationships of overall glycemic control (HbA1c) and 2-h post-load hyperglycemia with IMT were determined. While IMT increased for each tertile of HbA1c, within each tertile the higher the 2-h plasma glucose the higher was the IMT value.[17] Similar results have been reported for Japanese patients.[18] In this study, however, other post-load parameters (C-reactive protein, total cholesterol, and triglycerides) appeared to be directly related with IMT. These results seem to be in keeping with those of Yudkin and Coppack,[16] suggesting that multiple metabolic alterations associated in the Metabolic Syndrome may play the role. However, on a multiple regression analysis only post-load glucose and post-load triglyceride remained independently associated with IMT, supporting a role for post-meal hyperglycemia in building

up the CVD risk of Type 2 diabetic patients. The possibility also exists that the excessive post-meal glucose excursion may contribute to generating a poor lipid profile. A recent analysis was performed among the NHANES III population to assess the impact of ingestion of foods with different glycemic index on the concentration of the HDL cholesterol.[19] A detailed analysis of the diet record of 13,907 individuals was carried out and the population divided into quintiles of glycemic index. Upon adjustment for age, race or ethnicity, smoking status, BMI, alcohol intake, physical activity, energy fraction from protein, and carbohydrates, and total energy intake, HDL cholesterol decreased as a function of increasing glycemic index. This was apparent in the population as a whole, though the effect was more pronounced in men than in women (Figure 17.2). Since high glycemic index is associated with larger glucose excursion after food ingestion, one might argue that excessive glucose swings may favor a less favorable lipid profile, increasing the CVD risk of these subjects.

Mechanisms through which post-meal hyperglycemia may contribute to the atherosclerotic process

Different metabolic pathways are activated by hyperglycemia that may contribute to development of long-term micro- and macroangiopathic complications. They include activation of the polyol pathway, the hexosamine pathway, the protein kinase C (PKC), and the formation of advanced glycation end products (AGE), as recently reviewed by Brownlee.[20] At least two of these pathways can be activated by rapid glucose excursions.

In normal subjects, 2-h elevation of plasma glucose by a hyperglycemic clamp results in a sustained activation of several PKC isoforms and of PKC-β2 in particular.[21] Post-meal glucose excursions are directly correlated with post-meal levels of highly reactive molecules (2-deoxyglucosone, methylglyoxal)[22] that represent a potent trigger for dicarbonyl stress and subsequent oxidative stress and AGE formation.[23] When Type 2 diabetic patients with similar overall glycemic control (HbA1c 8.2 ± 1.2 versus 8.2 ± 1.7%) but different glucose variability based on the standard deviation of plasma glucose levels (±92 versus ±49 mg/dl) were compared, a much greater serum concentration of D-fructosone, D-deoxyglucose, and D-lactate was observed in patients with less stable plasma glucose control, suggesting a greater degree of carbonyl stress.[24] Of note is the fact that carbonyl stress can be generated by not only excess glucose excursion but also increased levels of lipids and amino acids, suggesting a more complex post-meal metabolic condition. The negative effects of acute hyperglycemia are likely the result of labile non-enzymatic glycation[25] and production of free-radicals[26] with ensuing oxidative stress.[27] AGEs affect protein function and gene expression. AGEs, PKC, and oxidative stress are potent stimuli for the production of reactive oxygen species (ROS), all common culprits in vascular pathology. PKC activation interferes with cell signaling, stimulates the conversion of smooth muscle and endothelial cells to a proliferative phenotype in peripheral conduit vasculatures, and causes release of vasoconstrictor substances.[28] In keeping with these effects are the data by Risso et al.[29] Incubation of human umbilical vein endothelial cells (HUVEC) in the presence of 20 mM glucose led to increased DNA fragmentation, a marker for apoptosis. An even greater fragmentation was documented when glucose was presented to the cells in a cycling manner, simulating glucose fluctuation. These alterations can explain the impairment in metacholine-induced vasodilatation that acute elevation of plasma glucose concentration can also cause in normal individuals.[29] Acute hyperglycemia causes endothelial dysfunction,[30,31] possibly through a reduction of nitric oxide availability.[32] The implication of PKC activation by acute glucose increase in the impairment of endothelium-dependent vasodilatation has been recently demonstrated by prevention of this effect by PKC-β inhibitor LY333531.[33]

Mealtime glucose excursions exert marked effects on the coagulation process by shortening the half-life of fibrinogen[34] and increasing the circulating levels of fibrinopeptide A,[35] thrombin,[36] prothrombin fragments,[37] and factor VII.[38] Hence, the acute changes in plasma glucose concentrations may result in a thrombophilic condition as platelet adhesion is also enhanced by hyperglycemia.[39] The atherogenic process may be facilitated by the increase in adhesion proteins triggered by hyperglycemic peaks.[40] A significant increase in P-selectin serum levels has been reported in Type 2 diabetic patients with high coefficient of

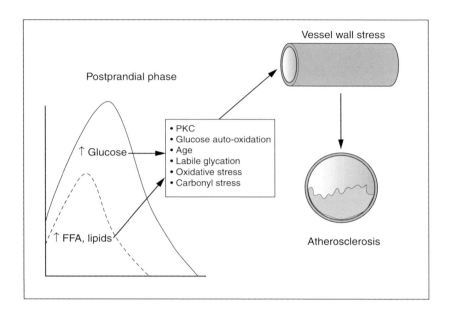

Figure 17.3
Mechanisms triggered by metabolic alterations occurring in the postprandial phase leading to vessel wall stress and atherosclerosis.

variation (CV), of fasting plasma glucose >25% as compared with low plasma glucose variability (CV <10%).[41]

In summary, the post-meal phase appears to be a complex metabolic condition where acute increase not only in plasma glucose, but also in lipids and, possibly, amino acids, can trigger an array of cellular and molecular mechanisms which may lead to vessel wall stress and, in the long term, atherosclerosis (Figure 17.3).

Intervention studies

Large intervention trials assessing the impact of glycemic control on cardiovascular disease in Type 2 diabetes are limited. The largest available study still remains the UKPDS where maintenance of an average HbA1c level of 7% over the 10-year follow-up was associated with a 12% reduction in any diabetes-related event, 25% reduction in microangiopathic complications, and 16% reduction of myocardial infarction; although only the first two reached statistical significance.[42] However, the UKPDS

may not have reached the necessary glycemic control required to exert a manifest effect on cardiovascular complications. Following the first year follow-up, glycemic control progressively deteriorated suggesting that a delay rather than a prevention of events was to be expected. In the UKPDS, the target for treatment was fasting plasma glucose concentration, and only at the end of the study was HbA1c used to assess the relationship between glycemic control and complications. This approach assumes fasting plasma glucose is the main determinant of HbA1c. Figure 17.4 presents the percentage changes in fasting plasma glucose and HbA1c following the initial improvement in the intensive treatment and clearly demonstrates that the two curves progressively separate. This suggests that fasting plasma glucose is not the only parameter affecting HbA1c, and we propose that the gap between the two lines can be explained by unmet post-meal glucose control. Moreover, HbA1c does not necessarily account for glucose fluctuations, and mealtime glycemic excursions. Avignon et al. evaluated the

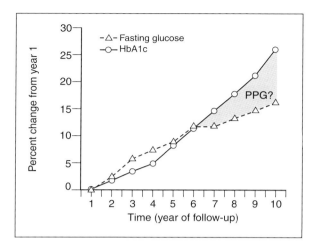

Figure 17.4
Dissociation between changes in fasting plasma glucose and HbA1c following the first year of follow-up in the United Kingdom Prospective Diabetes Study. PPG: postprandial glucose. Source: recalculated from ref. 41.

relationship between HbA1c and plasma glucose in patients with Type 2 diabetes, measured at four time points during the day.[5] A correlation between plasma glucose and HbA1c could be seen at each time point. However, after multiple regression analysis, HbA1c was found to be significantly predicted by plasma glucose levels measured only at post-lunch (2-h) and extended post-lunch (5-h) time points. A recent analysis performed in the Hoorn Study[43] has indicated that the strongest age- and sex-adjusted relative risk (RR) for both all-cause and cardiovascular mortality was associated with the 2-h post-load plasma glucose levels. After additional adjustment for hypertension, body mass index, triglycerides, LDL cholesterol, and cigarette smoking, the correlation remained statistically significant. Interestingly, when newly diagnosed diabetic patients were excluded from the analysis, the age- and sex-adjusted RR for mortality had an even higher

correlation with 2-h plasma glucose (statistically significant) and with HbA1c. The Kumamoto Study[44] differs from the UKPDS in term of size, and ethnic population. The two studies were also very different because of the treatment strategies (intensive treatment with bedtime insulin or oral hypoglycemic agents versus conventional treatment, mainly diet, in the UKPDS; multiple versus conventional insulin injection regimens in the Kumamoto Study), and also in terms of therapeutic goals. While fasting plasma glucose concentration was the only therapeutic goal in the UKPDS, in the Japanese study goals were set in terms of fasting, post-meal plasma glucose, and mean amplitude glucose excursion (MAGE). The recently reported 8-year follow-up of the latter study has confirmed the maintenance of good metabolic control in intensively treated patients (HbA1c, 7.0 versus 9.2%), and very interestingly, a smaller number of cardiovascular events, though no statistical significance could be ascertained due to the still limited number of events.[45] Though suggestive, this cannot be taken as proof that improvement in postprandial glucose may per se be associated with better outcomes in terms of long-term diabetic complications. Nonetheless, it clearly demonstrates that a more comprehensive approach, aiming at controlling both fasting and post-meal glucose concentrations, may be more effective in ensuring long-term reduction of HbA1c. More direct evidence for an independent effect of post-meal glucose excursion is provided by the study of de Veciana et al.[46] Tackling post-meal glucose concentration during diabetic pregnancy was associated with lower occurrence of neonatal hypoglycemia, cesarean section, and fewer babies for larger gestational age.

In summary, little attention has been paid to post-meal glucose control until recently. This was due to a poor understanding of its role and mechanisms in the development of diabetic complications. Moreover, the lack of therapeutic agents capable of substantially affecting postprandial metabolic abnormalities have led to concentrate most of the efforts in controlling plasma glucose levels. Finally, accurate monitoring of postprandial glucose excursion may be cumbersome and strictly dependent upon patients' compliance.

Monitoring glucose excursion

A possible role for glucose excursion in generating overall risk for long-term complications in diabetes has been recognized for a long time. Integrated expressions of daily glucose profile were attempted in the 1960s with the calculation of MAGE[47] and the M-value of Schlichtkrull et al.[48] Unfortunately, both measures require several capillary blood glucose readings per day, making them unusable over a long period of time. In our own experience, the average number of blood glucose readings in young insulin-treated diabetic patients is 1.7/day.[49] The absolute number of readings was inversely related to HbA1c (r = 0.45; p <0.05), suggesting that more readings are obtained when the need develops for recovering

from looser control. Continuous interstitial glucose reading has been proven to highlight otherwise unrecognized large glucose swings,[50] but the application of the subcutaneous dyalitic membrane still remains limited in time. Ideally, one would like to base judgment of postprandial glucose excursion on a parameter with the same feature of HbA1c, that is reliability and a sufficient retrospective parameter. Rapid glucose excursion may cause labile protein glycation. We have tested the relationship between labile glycated hemoglobin (labile GH) and parameters of glucose oscillation of the previous day and found a correlation between labile GH and standard deviation (r = 0.51; p = 0.006) and coefficient of variation (r = 0.47; p = 0.04) of mean daily plasma glucose (Figure 17.5). However, the time span covered by labile GH is likely to be limited as the highest correlation coefficient was found with pre-bedtime glucose level, i.e. the last blood glucose determination. 1,5-anhydro-D-glucitol (AG) has been proposed as a better marker for glucose instability than HbA1c.[51] AG is a polyol present in human plasma. It is derived largely from ingestion and its main route of elimination is urinary excretion. Therefore, under the condition of hyperglycemia a competition between glucose and AG for

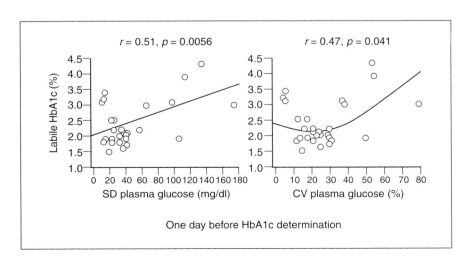

Figure 17.5
Correlation between labile glycated Hb and parameters of glucose instability: SD (standard deviation) and CV (coefficient of variation) of the mean plasma glucose levels during the day before determination of labile glycated Hb. (Personal data).

tubular reabsorption occurs. Therefore, high glucose increases AG excretion and leads to a net AG depletion. Based on kinetics models it has been proposed that AG monitoring should be able to indicate the presence of past glucosuric hyperglycemic excursions during a period of days to weeks.[52] In a group of 101 Type 2 diabetic patients (Karrei K, Temelkova-Kurktschiev TS, Del Prato S, personal communication), AG and HbA1c were significantly correlated ($r = -0.49$; $p < 0.001$), but only the former was related to glucose excursions ($r = -0.25$; $p = 0.012$). Moreover, in a multivariate analysis carried out in 20 diabetic patients, AG correlation with the M-value of Schlichtkrull was maintained ($r = 0.50$; $p < 0.0005$), while both correlations between HbA1c and labile GH were lost. Other parameters may turn out to represent a useful marker to be used in combination with HbA1c in determining the glycemic control. Glucose excursions were, indeed, highly correlated with both methylglyoxal and 3-deoxyglucosone in a recent study where fast-acting insulin analogs were employed in order to reduce post-meal hyperglycemia.[22] Thus, the development of an integrated measure of glucose instability may simplify the monitoring of postprandial hyperglycemia, offering further opportunities to describe the risk profile for diabetic complications. Such a measure would also be extremely valuable in assessing the impact of specific treatment for post-meal hyperglycemia.

Present and future treatment of postprandial hyperglycemia

If a primary goal of diabetes therapy is control of post-meal glucose excursion, the regulation of glucose absorption from the gut and entry into the circulation is an important mechanism to consider. The goal of dietary modifications is reduction of post-meal glucose peaks. The value of using an adequate amount of fibers has recently been confirmed in a study comparing a 6-week standard ADA diet and fiber-supplemented diet.[53]

Alpha-glucosidase inhibitors, such as acarbose, delay intestinal glucose absorption and reduce mealtime glucose excursion without affecting pancreatic β-cell secretion.[54] Although these agents may be useful in the early stages of the disease when hyperglycemia is mainly limited to the absorptive state, their use in the more severe diabetic condition may not be sufficient. The UKPDS has recently indicated that the average reduction in HbA1c seen in patients who tolerated the drug was 0.3%.[55] Amylin and its analog, pramlintide, slow down gastric emptying, and the latter has been suggested to suppress plasma glucagon concentration after ingestion of a mixed meal.[56] In a larger study of patients with Type 2 diabetes, administration of pramlintide before each meal was associated with a 0.5% reduction in HbA1c.[57]

Taken together, the above considerations point out the need for agents capable of intervening on more basic defects responsible for post-meal hyperglycemia. An excessive rise in plasma glucose concentration may recognize several mechanisms, but loss of rapid insulin release after ingestion of a meal is associated with impaired suppression of endogenous glucose production.[58] Since the appreciation of the primary role of such a mechanism, restoration of early insulin release was seen as a rational therapeutic goal as indicated by an active pharmaceutical armamentarium (Table 17.1).

Sulfonylureas

Over the past two decades, sulfonylureas have been used to enhance insulin secretion in patients with Type 2 diabetes. Data suggest

	Route of administration	Hypoglycemic potency	Early insulin	Late insulin	Glucagon suppression	Side effects
Insulin lispro	subcutaneous	++++	++	+	direct	hypoglycemia
Insulin aspart	subcutaneous	++++	++	+	direct	hypoglycemia
GLP-1	subcutaneous, i.m.	+++	+++	++	direct	G.I.
Repaglinide	oral	+++	+++	++	indirect	(hypoglycemia)
Nateglinide	oral	+++	++++	+	indirect	(hypoglycemia)
Metiglinide	oral	(+++)	(+++)	(+)	indirect	(hypoglycemia)

Note: Brackets indicate unconformed data

Table 17.1
Drugs affecting early phase insulin secretion

that some second-generation sulfonylureas may exert a stimulatory effect on first-phase insulin secretion. Hosker et al.[59] reported that first-phase insulin secretion in response to different degrees of hyperglycemia was enhanced, though not normalized, by administration of gliclazide. In our experience,[60] the acute administration of gliclazide in newly diagnosed patients prior to receiving a constant infusion of glucose was associated with an improvement in glucose tolerance, expressed as the incremental plasma glucose area above baseline compared with placebo (352 ± 42 versus 461 ± 52 mmol/240 min). However, no significant differences were observed in the insulin secretion rate, which only became apparent after two months of treatment. These data suggest that the amelioration of first- and second-phase insulin secretion that occurs with sulfonylureas may be partly mediated by relief of glucose toxicity.

The presumed clinical advantages of sulfonylureas are not fully supported by other experimental results. Endogenous glucose production (EGP) and peripheral glucose disposal in response to different plasma insulin concentrations were assessed before and after treatment with either tolazamide or insulin in patients with Type 2 diabetes.[61] Although a certain degree of improvement in EGP and glucose utilization was observed with both treatments, the use of tolazamide did not provide significant advantages over insulin treatment. This sulfonylurea is unlikely to exert a preferential stimulation of first-phase insulin secretion.

Glinides

More recently, meglitinide, a non-sulfonylurea benzoic acid derivative, has been shown to elicit an acute insulin release.[62] This compound and its analogs increase insulin secretion in a glucose-dependent manner by reducing membrane conductance in pancreatic β-cells.[63] These features suggest that meglitinide analogs may be the agents of choice for acute stimulation of insulin secretion in response to a meal.

Repaglinide
Repaglinide was the first analog of meglitinide to be made available. It stimulates insulin secretion upon closure of the K^+_{ATP} channels on the β-cell. Plasma insulin peaks at 1–2 h and returns to baseline after 6 h. The short

duration of the drug is associated with much lower frequency of hypoglycemia as compared to sulfonylureas.[64,65] In an early comparative study with glibenclamide, repaglinide exhibited a greater effect on post-meal plasma glucose concentration,[66] although a more recent study reported no significant differences after a one-year treatment.[67] In a one-year comparison study with glipizide, repaglinide led to a lower HbA1c and fasting plasma glucose levels. Similar results have been confirmed in 5985 Type 2 diabetic patients switched to flexible-dose rather than a fixed-dose regimen of pre-meal administration of repaglinide.[68]

Mitiglinide

Mitiglinide is a more recent meglitinide analog on phase II evaluation in Europe and phase III in Japan. Preliminary studies have shown that pre-meal administration of the compound can effectively reduce post-meal glucose excursion.[69]

Nateglinide

Nateglinide, a D-phenylalanine derivative,[70] is characterized by a rapid and short-lasting stimulatory effect on insulin secretion.[71] Though the mechanism of action is also related to closure of K^+_{ATP} channels, the drug binding is quickly reversed, leading to restoration of early phase insulin secretion.[72] When administered to non-diabetic volunteers, nateglinide produced a more rapid and short-lived stimulation of insulin secretion than repaglinide, resulting in lower meal-related glucose excursions.[73] Similar results have been observed in Type 2 diabetic patients.[74,75] In these studies postprandial glucose was much lower, as compared to both placebo[74] and glibenclamide.[75] As for repaglinide, the available data suggest a much lower risk of hypoglycemia compared with traditional sulfonylureas.

Glucagon-like peptide-1

Oral glucose elicits a larger insulin response than intravenous glucose. Plasma glucose concentrations after i.v. glucose tend to remain at higher levels than when following the ingestion of the same amount of glucose, and plasma insulin concentrations are greater after oral than i.v. glucose administration.[76] This observation has been explained by the operativity of the so-called entero-insular axis.[77] Several hormonal factors (incretins) have been shown to play a potentiating effect on β-cells after ingestion of a carbohydrate meal.[77] Glucagon-like peptide-1 (GLP-1), the most potent incretin, is an insulinotropic intestinal hormone released in response to an enteral nutrient challenge.[78] Nathan et al.[79] clearly demonstrated the potentiating effect of GLP-1 on insulin secretion in Type 2 patients. A 30-min infusion of GLP-1 was associated with a prompt and sustained increase in mealtime insulin secretion. The increased insulin concentration dropped to basal levels after interruption of GLP-1 infusion and remained lower than in control individuals. As expected, the initial rise was followed by a second phase of plasma insulin increase, which was primarily supported by prevalent hyperglycemia. The initial increase in plasma insulin concentrations abolished the early rise in plasma glucose levels that followed the ingestion of a mixed meal. After the interruption of GLP-1 infusion, plasma glucose concentrations remained lower compared with control individuals, suggesting that early modulation of the post-meal glucose concentration may result in an overall improvement in glucose tolerance in the face of lower circulating insulin levels. GLP-1 has been shown to enhance insulin action and to suppress plasma glucagon concentration.[80] Nauck et al.[81] showed that plasma elevations of exogenous, infused GLP-1 are associated with a constant decline in plasma glucose levels, a possible consequence of the effects on insulin secretion and the concomitant suppression of plasma glucagon levels. Evidence supporting the clinical use of GLP-1, however, is lacking because of its rapid proteolytic degradation.[82] Peptidase-resistant analogs are being currently tested[83] along with exendin, a peptide with 53% homology to GLP-1 and a prolonged glucose-lowering action.[84]

Reconstructing early post-meal insulin rise: fast-acting insulin analogs

Sulfonylureas, glinides, GLP-1 all act by stimulating the β-cells. Therefore, their effect is a function of spare mass and function of insulin-secreting pancreatic β-cells. The possibility then arises that no significant rapid insulin secretion can be elicited to support the option for insulin treatment. The importance of the timing of insulin administration in glucose control following a meal has been appreciated for many years in the treatment of Type 1 diabetes. It has been demonstrated that adjustments in the timing as well as in the amount of insulin administered before the meal are necessary in the management of the disease. In a study by Bruce et al.,[85] patients with Type 2 diabetes received an identical dose of insulin in three distinct regimens at mealtimes. Insulin was given i.v. over 30 min at the beginning of a meal, in a profile that simulated a normal insulin response; in the profile but delayed by 30 min; or as a constant infusion over the entire duration of the study. A significant improvement in post-meal glucose tolerance was demonstrated only with early administration of insulin, in keeping with the proposed regulatory role of the acute insulin peak on EGP. The use of fast-acting

insulin analogs may produce similar benefits,[86] due to a much quicker rise of insulin concentration. In type 2 diabetic patients, s.c. injection of no more than 3 U of lispro insulin analog 5 min before a 50 g oral glucose load, was associated with a more rapid rise in plasma insulin concentration and lower post-load glucose excursion compared with the administration of an equivalent amount of regular insulin.[87] The earlier rise in plasma insulin concentration after the glucose load was associated with a faster and short-lived suppression of EGP. Similar results have been obtained with aspart insulin, the other available fast-acting insulin analogs.[88] A significant reduction of post-meal glucose excursion has been maintained over a six-month treatment with lispro insulin analog.[89] The advantage of reconstructing a more physiologic insulin profile is highlighted by the results of combination therapy, a procedure more frequently employed in patients with failure to oral agents. In general, adding a second anti-hyperglycemic agent to the current treatment, lowers HbA1c. However, when fast-acting insulin analogs are used to focus on postprandial blood glucose, a greater impact on overall metabolic control is attained.[90,91]

In summary, several therapeutic tools are or will be available to tackle post-meal hyperglycemia. These tools are designed to restore a more physiologic plasma insulin profile after meal ingestion, that is to ensure a rapid rise of plasma insulin level to mimic first-phase insulin secretion and ensure prompt suppression of endogenous glucose production. This effect is likely to be potentiated by concomitant use of insulin sensitizers, as insulin resistance is a common feature in Type 2 diabetes. Moreover, the latter may contribute to the control of not only hyperglycemia but also the more complex metabolic perturbation that accompanies the postprandial phase.

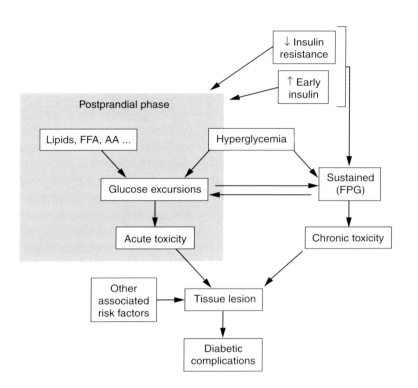

Figure 17.6
Synopsis of comprehensive approach to Type 2 diabetes for reduction of the risk of diabetic complications. This includes control of sustained and acute (postprandial) metabolic alterations by correction of the dual pathogenic defect: insulin resistance and loss of first-phase insulin secretion. Care must be taken in controlling other associated risk factors.

Future importance

Hyperglycemia is the hallmark of diabetes and a main cause for long-term complications. The deleterious effect of hyperglycemia is likely to be exerted both in a chronic and sustained way as well as through rapid fluctuation of plasma glucose levels. Glucose variability is largely attributed to post-meal glucose excursion and it may differentiate among diabetic patients with comparable HbA1c, thus contributing to different glucose susceptibility to complications. Epidemiological evidence supports a relationship of post-load (and post-meal) plasma glucose and CV mortality and morbidity, while *in vitro* studies clearly demonstrate that isolated glucose excursion can trigger molecular mechanisms involved in the pathogenesis of

diabetic complications. Finally, data from intervention studies are still limited though compatible with a causal relationship between postprandial glucose and diabetic complications. However, it is very likely that not only glucose but also the excursion of other metabolic parameters can contribute to overall risk of long-term complications. For instance, both postprandial glucose and postprandial triglycerides are independently associated with IMT. In view of this complex picture, a complex and comprehensive approach must be envisaged as depicted in Figure 17.6. Strict glycemic control will require more focus on postprandial hyperglycemia. To this purpose, restoration of the early phase insulin release appears to be a rational approach. This can be accomplished by quick-acting secretagogues (glinides, GLP-1) as far as β-cell mass and function are retained, while fast-acting insulin analogs may be required if reconstruction of more physiologic insulin profiles are needed. Concomitant use of insulin sensitizers may be of value because they may contribute to the control of fasting and inter-prandial glucose levels. Moreover, insulin sensitizers may be important in tackling the complex postprandial phase which includes not only glucose, but also lipid and amino acid excursions.[92]

The complexity of the metabolic alteration in Type 2 diabetes must be fully recognized. Though hyperglycemia is a simple diagnostic criterion and it plays a main role in the pathogenesis of diabetic micro- and macrovascular complications, other factors (dyslipidemia, arterial hypertension, obesity, impaired coagulation and fibrinolysis, endothelial dysfunction, inflammatory responses, and many others) do contribute to the overall risk in diabetic individuals. Therefore, specific skill and continuous surveillance must be put to work to reduce the burden of diabetic complications.

References

1. Laakso M. Hyperglycemia and cardiovascular disease in type 2 diabetes. Diabetes 1999; 48: 937–4.
2. Ito C, Maeda R, Ishida S et al. Correlation among fasting plasma glucose, two-hour plasma glucose levels in OGTT and HbA1c. Diabetes Res Clin Pract 2000; 50: 225–30.
3. American Diabetes Association. Postprandial blood glucose. Diabetes Care 2001; 24: 775 8.
4. Bonora E, Calcaterra F, Lombardi S et al. Plasma glucose levels thorughout the day and HbA1c interrelationships in Type 2 diabetes. Implications for treatment and monitoring of metabolic control. Diabetes Care 2001; 24: 2023–9.
5. Avignon A, Radauceanu A, Monnier L. Nonfasting plasma glucose is a better marker of diabetic control than fasting plasma glucose in type 2 diabetes. Diabetes Care 1997; 20: 1822–6.
6. Coutinho M, Gerstein HC, Wang Y, Yusuf S. The relationship between glucose and incident cardiovascular events. A metaregression analysis of published data from 20 studies of 95,783 individuals followed for 12.4 years. Diabetes Care 1999; 22: 233–40.
7. The Expert Committee on the diagnosis and classification of diabetes mellitus. Report of the Expert Committee on the diagnosis and classification of diabetes mellitus. Diabetes Care 1997; 20: 1183–97.
8. Vaccaro O, Ruffa G, Imperatore G et al. Risk of diabetes in the new diagnostic category of impaired fasting glucose: a prospective analysis. Diabetes Care 1999; 22: 1490–3.
9. Tominaga M, Eguchi H, Manaka H et al. Impaired glucose tolerance is a risk factor for cardiovascular disease, but not impaired fasting glucose. The Funagata Diabetes Study. Diabetes Care 1999; 22: 920–4.
10. DECODE Study Group. Glucose tolerance and mortality: comparison of WHO and American Diabetes Association diagnostic criteria. Lancet 1999; 354: 617–21.
11. DECODE Study Group. Glucose tolerance and cardiovascular mortality. Comparison of fasting and 2-hour diagnostic criteria. Arch Intern Med 2001; 161: 397–404.
12. Bonora E, Muggeo M. Postprandial blood glucose as a risk factor for cardiovascular disease in Type II diabetes: the epidemiological evidence. Diabetologia 2001; 44: 2107–14.
13. Wolever TMS, Chiasson J-L, Csima A et al. Variation of postprandial glucose, palatability, and symptoms associated with a standardized mixed test meal versus 75g oral glucose. Diabetes Care 1998; 21: 336–40.
14. Erlinger TP, Brancati FL. Postchallenge hyperglycemia in a national sample of U.S. adults with Type 2 diabetes. Diabetes Care 2001; 24: 1734–8.
15. Hanefeld M, Fischer S, Julius U et al. Risk factors for myocardial infarction and death in newly detected NIDDM: the Diabetes Intervention Study, 11-year follow-up. Diabetologia 1996; 39: 1577–83.
16. Yudkin JS, Coppack S. Insulin resistance and

impaired glucose tolerance. Lancet 1994; 344: 1294–5.

17. Temelkova-Kurktschiev TS, Koehler C, Henkel E et al. Postchallenge plasma glucose and glycemic spikes are more strongly associated with atherosclerosis than fasting glucose or HbA1c level. Diabetes Care 2000; 23: 1830–4.

18. Teno S, Uto Y, Nagashima H et al. Association of postprandial hypertriglyceridemia and carotid intima-media thickness in patients with type 2 diabetes. Diabetes Care 2000; 23: 1401–6.

19. Ford ES, Liu S. Glycemic index and serum high-density lipoprotein cholesterol concentration among us adults. Arch Intern Med 2001; 161: 572–6.

20. Brownlee M. Biochemistry and molecular cell biology of diabetic complications. Nature 2001; 414: 813–20.

21. Assert R, Scherk G, Bumbure A. et al. Regulation of protein kinase C by short term hyperglycaemia in human platelets in vivo and in vitro. Diabetologia 2001; 44: 188–95.

22. Beisswenger PJ, Howell SK, O'Dell RM et al. α-Dicarbonyls increase in the postprandial period and reflect the degree of hyperglycemia. Diabetes Care 2001; 24: 726–32.

23. Baynes JW, Thorpe SR. Role of oxidative stress in diabetic complications: a new perspective on an old paradigm. Diabetes 1999; 48: 1–9.

24. Beisswenger PJ, Szwergold BS, Yeo KT. Glycated proteins in diabetes. Clin Lab Med 2001; 21: 53–78.

25. Ceriello A, Quatraro A, Giugliano D. New insights on non-enzymatic glycosylation may lead to therapeutic approaches for the prevention of diabetic complications. Diabet Med 1992; 9: 297–9.

26. Lipinski B. Pathophysiology of oxidative stress in diabetes mellitus. J Diabetes Complications 2001; 15: 203–10.

27. Giugliano D, Ceriello A, Paolisso G. Oxidative stress and diabetic vascular complications. Diabetes Care 1996; 19: 257–67.

28. Gutterman DD. Vascular dysfunction in hyperglycemia: is protein kinase C the culprit? Circ Res 2002; 90: 5–7.

29. Risso A, Mercuri F, Quagliaro L et al. Intermittent high glucose enhances apoptosis in human umbilical vein endothelial cells in culture. Am J Physiol Endocrinol Metab 2001; 281: E924–30.

30. Williams SB, Goldfine AB, Timimi FK et al. Acute hyperglycemia attenuates endothelium-dependent vasodilation in humans in vivo. Circulation 1998; 97: 1695–1701.

31. Akbari CM, Saouaf R, Barnhill DF et al. Endothelium-dependent vasodilatation is impaired in both microcirculation and macro-circulation during acute hyperglycemia. J Vasc Surg 1998; 28: 687–94.

32. Du XL, Edelstein D, Dimmeler S et al. Hyperglycemia inhibits endothelial nitric oxide synthase activity by posttranslational modification at the Akt site. J Clin Invest 2001; 108: 1341–8.

33. Beckman JA, Goldfine AB, Gordon MB et al. Inhibition of protein kinase Cbeta prevents impaired endothelium-dependent vasodilation caused by hyperglycemia in humans. Circ Res 2002; 90: 107–11.

34. Jones RL, Peterson CM. Reduced fibrinogen survival in diabetes mellitus. A reversible phenomenon. J Clin Invest 1979; 63: 485–93.

35. Ceriello A, Giugliano D, Quatraro A et al. Hyperglycemia may determine fibrinopeptide A plasma level increase in humans. Metabolism 1989; 38: 1162–3.

36. Ceriello A, Taboga C, Tonutti L et al. Post-meal coagulation activation in diabetes mellitus: the effect of acarbose. Diabetologia 1996; 39: 469–73.

37. Ceriello A, Giacomello R, Stel G et al. Hyperglycemia-induced thrombin formation in diabetes. The possible role of oxidative stress. Diabetes 1995; 44: 924–8.

38. Ceriello A, Giugliano D, Quatraro A et al. Blood glucose may condition factor VII levels in diabetic and normal subjects. Diabetologia 1988; 31: 889–91.

39. Pirags V, Assert R, Haupt K et al. Activation of human platelet protein kinase C-beta 2 in vivo in response to acute hyperglycemia. Exp Clin Endocrinol Diabetes 1996; 104: 431–40.

40. Ceriello A, Falleti E, Motz E et al. Hyperglycemia-induced circulating ICAM-1 increase in diabetes mellitus: the possible role of oxidative stress. Horm Metab Res 1998; 30: 146–9.

41. Brun E, Zoppini G, Zamboni C et al. Glucose

instability is associated with a high level of circulating p-selectin. Diabetes Care 2001; 24: 1685.

42. UK Prospective Diabetes Study (UKPDS) Group. Intensive blood-glucose control with sulphonylureas or insulin compared with conventional treatment and risk of complications in patients with type 2 diabetes (UKPDS 33). Lancet 1998; 352: 837–53.

43. de Vegt F, Dekker JM, Ruhé HG et al. Hyperglycaemia is associated with all-cause and cardiovascular mortality in the Hoorn population: the Hoorn study [abstract]. Diabetologia 1999; 42: 926–31.

44. Ohkubo Y, Kishikawa H, Araki E et al. Intensive insulin therapy prevents the progression of diabetic microvascular complications in Japanese patients with non-insulin-dependent diabetes mellitus: a randomized prospective 6-year study. Diabetes Res Clin Pract 1995; 28: 103–17.

45. Shichiri M, Kishikawa H, Ohkubo Y, Wake N. Long-term results of the Kumamoto Study on optimal diabetes control in type 2 diabetic patients. Diabetes Care 2000; 23 Suppl 2: B21–9.

46. de Veciana M, Major CA, Morgan MA et al. Postprandial versus preprandial blood glucose monitoring in women with gestational diabetes mellitus requiring insulin therapy. N Engl J Med 1995; 333: 1237–41.

47. Service FJ, O'Brien PC, Rizza RA. Measurements of glucose control. Diabetes Care 1987; 10: 225–37.

48. Schlichtkrull J, Munch O, Jersild M. The M-value, an index of blood sugar control in diabetics. Acta Med Scand 1965; 177: 95–102.

49. Bruttomesso D, Barberio S, Fongher C et al. Retrospective analysis of daily glucose profile in type 1 diabetic patients with continuous subcutaneous insulin infusion (CSII). Diabetes Res Clin Pract 1992; 16: 197–202.

50. Maran A, Crepaldi C, Tiengo A et al. Continuous subcutaneous glucose monitoring in diabetic patients: a multicenter analysis. Diabetes Care 2002; 25: 347–52.

51. Yamanouchi T, Ogata N, Tagaya T et al. Clinical usefulness of serum 1,5–anhydroglucitol in monitoring glycaemic control. Lancet 1996; 347: 1514–18.

52. Stickle D, Turk J. A kinetic mass balance model for 1,5–anhydroglucitol: applications to monitoring of glycemic control. Am J Physiol 1997; 273: E821–30.

53. Chandalia M, Garg A, Lutjohann D et al. Beneficial effects of high dietary fiber intake in patients with type 2 diabetes mellitus. N Engl J Med 2000; 342: 1392–8.

54. Bischoff H. Pharmacology of alpha-glucosidase inhibition. Eur J Clin Invest 1994; 24 Suppl 3: 3–10.

55. Holman RR, Cull CA, Turner RC. A randomized double-blind trial of acarbose in type 2 diabetes shows improved glycemic control over 3 years (U.K. Prospective Diabetes Study 44). Diabetes Care 1999; 22: 960–4.

56. Nyholm B, Orskov L, Hove KY et al. The amylin analog pramlintide improves glycemic control and reduces postprandial glucagon concentrations in patients with type 1 diabetes mellitus. Metabolism 1999; 48: 935–41.

57. Thompson RG, Pearson L, Schoenfeld SL, Kolterman OG. Pramlintide, a synthetic analog of human amylin, improves the metabolic profile of patients with type 2 diabetes using insulin. The Pramlintide in Type 2 Diabetes Group. Diabetes Care 1998; 21: 987–93.

58. Del Prato S, Tiengo A. The importance of first-phase insulin secretion: implications for the therapy of type 2 diabetes mellitus. Diabetes Metab Res Rev 2001; 17: 164–74.

59. Hosker JP, Rudenski AS, Burnett MA et al. Similar reduction of first- and second-phase B-cell responses at three different glucose levels in type II diabetes and the effect of gliclazide therapy. Metabolism 1989; 38: 767–72,.

60. Riccio A, Lisato G, Vigili de Kreutzenberg S et al. Gliclazide potentiates suppression of hepatic glucose production in non-insulin-dependent diabetic patients. Metabolism 1996; 45: 1196–1202.

61. Firth RG, Bell PM, Rizza RA. Effects of tolazamide and exogenous insulin on insulin action in patients with non-insulin-dependent diabetes mellitus. N Engl J Med 1986; 314: 1280–6.

62. Malaisse WJ. Stimulation of insulin release by non-sulfonylurea hypoglycemic agents: the meglitinide family. Horm Metab Res 1995; 27: 263–6.

63. Bakkali-Nadi A, Malaisse-Lagae F, Malaisse

WJ. Insulinotropic action of meglitinide analogs: concentration-response relationship and nutrient dependency. Diabetes Res 1994; 27: 81–7.

64. Moses R. A review of clinical experience with the prandial glucose regulator, repaglinide, in the treatment of type 2 diabetes. Expert Opin Pharmacother 2000; 1: 1455–67.

65. Landgraf R, Frank M, Bauer C, Dieken ML. Prandial glucose regulation with repaglinide: its clinical and lifestyle impact in a large cohort of patients with Type 2 diabetes. Int J Obes Relat Metab Disord 2000; 24 Suppl 3: S38–44.

66. Wolffenbuttel BH, Nijst L, Sels JP et al. Effects of a new oral hypoglycaemic agent, repaglinide, on metabolic control in sulphonylurea-treated patients with NIDDM. Eur J Clin Pharmacol 199; 345: 113–16.

67. Wolffenbuttel BHR, Landgraf R, on behalf of the Dutch and German Repaglinide Study Group. A 1-year multicenter randomized double-blind comparison of repaglinide and glyburide for the treatment of type 2 diabetes. Diabetes Care 1999; 22: 463–7.

68. Madsbad S, Kilhovd B, Lager I et al. Comparison between repaglinide and glipizide in Type 2 diabetes mellitus: a 1-year multicentre study. Diabet Med 2001; 18: 395–401.

69. Yamada N, Shigeta Y, Kaneko T. Hypoglycemic effects and safety of a novel rapid-acting insulinotropic agent, KAD-1299, for NIDDM. Diabetes 1996; 45 Suppl. 2: 74.

70. Hu S, Wang S, Fanelli B et al. Pancreatic beta-cell K(ATP) channel activity and membrane-binding studies with nateglinide: a comparison with sulfonylureas and repaglinide. J Pharmacol Exp Ther 2000; 293: 444–52.

71. Dunn CJ, Faulds D. Nateglinide. Drugs 2000; 60: 607–15.

72. Whitelaw DC, Clark PM, Smith JM, Nattrass M. Effects of the new oral hypoglycaemic agent nateglinide on insulin secretion in Type 2 diabetes mellitus. Diabet Med 2000; 17: 225–9.

73. Kalbag JB, Walter YH, Nedelman JR, McLeod JF. Mealtime glucose regulation with nateglinide in healthy volunteers: comparison with repaglinide and placebo. Diabetes Care 2001; 24: 73–7.

74. Hanefeld M, Bouter KP, Dickinson S, Guitard C. Rapid and short-acting mealtime insulin

secretion with nateglinide controls both prandial and mean glycemia. Diabetes Care 2000; 23: 202–7.

75. Hollander PA, Schwartz SL, Gatlin MR et al. Importance of early insulin secretion: comparison of nateglinide and glyburide in previously diet-treated patients with type 2 diabetes. Diabetes Care 2001; 24: 983–8.

76. DeFronzo RA, Ferrannini E, Hendler R et al. Influence of hyperinsulinemia, hyperglycemia, and the route of glucose administration on splanchnic glucose exchange. Proc Natl Acad Sci USA 1978; 75: 5173–7.

77. Creutzfeldt W. The entero-insular axis in Type 2 diabetes - incretins as therapeutic agents. Exp Clin Endocrinol Diabetes 2001; 109 Suppl. 2: 288–303.

78. Nauck MA. Is glucagon-like peptide 1 an incretin hormone? Diabetologia 1999; 42: 373–9.

79. Nathan DM, Schreiber E, Fogel H et al. Insulinotropic action of glucagonlike peptide-I-(7–37) in diabetic and nondiabetic subjects. Diabetes Care 1992; 15: 270–6.

80. Juhl CB, Hollingdal M, Sturis J et al. Bedtime administration of NN2211, a long-acting GLP-1 derivative, substantially reduces fasting and postprandial glycemia in type 2 diabetes. Diabetes 2002; 51: 424–9.

81. Nauck MA, Kleine N, Orskov C et al. Normalization of fasting hyperglycaemia by exogenous glucagon-like peptide 1 (7–36 amide) in type 2 (non-insulin-dependent) diabetic patients. Diabetologia 1993; 36: 741–4.

82. Holst JJ, Deacon CF. Inhibition of the activity of dipeptidyl-peptidase IV as a treatment for type 2 diabetes. Diabetes 1998; 47: 1663–70.

83. Siegel EG, Scharf G, Gallwitz B et al. Comparison of the effect of native glucagon-like peptide 1 and dipeptidyl peptidase IV-resistant analogues on insulin release from rat pancreatic islets. Eur J Clin Invest 1999; 29: 610–4.

84. Egan JM, Clocquet AR, Elahi D. The insulinotropic effect of acute exendin-4 administered to humans: comparison of nondiabetic state to type 2 diabetes. J Clin Endocrinol Metab 2002; 87: 1282–90.

85. Bruce DG, Chisholm DJ, Storlien LH, Kraegen EW. Physiological importance of deficiency in

early prandial insulin secretion in non-insulin-dependent diabetes. Diabetes 1988; 37: 736–44.

86. Bolli GB, Di Marchi RD, Park GD et al. Insulin analogues and their potential in the management of diabetes mellitus. Diabetologia 1999; 42: 1151–67.

87. Bruttomesso D, Pianta A, Mari A et al. Restoration of early rise in plasma insulin levels improves the glucose tolerance of type 2 diabetic patients. Diabetes 1999; 48: 99–105,.

88. Rosenfalck AM, Thorsby P, Kjems L et al. Improved postprandial glycaemic control with insulin Aspart in type 2 diabetic patients treated with insulin. Acta Diabetol 2000; 37: 41–6.

89. Anderson JHJ, Brunelle RL, Keohane P et al. Mealtime treatment with insulin analog improves postprandial hyperglycemia and hypoglycemia in patients with non-insulin-dependent diabetes mellitus. Arch Intern Med 1997; 157: 1249–55.

90. Bastyr EJ III, Stuart CA, Brodows RG et al. Therapy focused on lowering postprandial glucose, not fasting glucose, may be superior for lowering HbA1c. IOEZ Study Group. Diabetes Care 2000; 23: 1236–41.

91. Bastyr EJ III, Johnson ME, Trautmann ME et al. Insulin lispro in the treatment of patients with type 2 diabetes mellitus after oral agent failure. Clin Ther 1999; 21: 1703–14.

92. Heine RJ, Balkau B, Ceriello A et al. What does post-prandial hyperglycaemia mean? Diabet Med 2002; in press.

18

Blood glucose control: relation to cardiovascular morbidity and mortality*

Robert J Heine, Jacqueline M Dekker

Introduction

The elevated risk of CVD in patients with Type 2 diabetes is of the same magnitude as the increased risk observed in persons with a history of CVD.[1] The risk is two- and four-fold for men and women, respectively, compared with persons without diabetes.[2–4] Less than half of this excess risk can be attributed to the higher prevalence of classic risk factors, for example dyslipidemia (high triglycerides (TG), low HDL cholesterol) and hypertension.[5,6]

The elevated risk of CVD disease, associated with high glucose levels, extends into the non-diabetic range. Many large-scale epidemiological studies have shown a relationship between glucose levels 2 hours after the 75 g oral glucose tolerance test (2hPG) and the occurrence of CVD in the general population.[7–18] A meta-analysis including more than 95,000 people from 22 studies confirmed the association between the 2hPG and incident cardiovascular events.[19] Even persons with non-diabetic fasting glucose levels but with elevated 2hPG, had about a two-fold risk of CVD.[20–22]

In some population studies the fasting glucose level was also associated with CVD.[16,23]

In addition, a few studies of persons with manifest diabetes have also shown an association of 2hPG, and mean glucose during the day with CVD.[24,25]

First we briefly review the possible mechanisms explaining the observed relationships between meal related metabolic changes and CVD. Then we address the question of whether postprandial hyperglycemia is an independent risk factor, i.e. causally related to CVD, or a marker for elevated CVD risk. If postprandial hyperglycemia is a risk factor, when can we consider the enhanced meal related glucose excursions as a treatment target in persons with Type 2 diabetes? If it is just a risk marker, other factors need to be identified which can explain the epidemiological observations. Finally, the therapeutic consequences, if any, will be discussed.

How are plasma glucose and TG levels associated with CVD risk?

Plasma glucose as predictor of CVD

There is a substantial discrepancy in the classification of individuals based on the fasting glucose, as proposed by the American Diabetes Association in 1997, or based on both fasting

*This paper has been adapted with permission from Heine RJ, Dekker JM. Beyond postprandial hyperglycaemia: metabolic factors associated with cardiovascular disease. Diabetologia 2002; 45: 461–75. © Springer-Verlag.

Study	n	Age (years)	Follow-up (years)	End point	Reference category FPG/2hPG (mmol/l)	RR DM WHO-85	RR DM ADA-97	RR IGT	RR IFG
DECODE study[17]	25,364	>30	10	mortality	<6.1/<7.8	2.0*	1.6	1.6	1.2
Hoorn study[26]**	2468	50–75	9	mortality	<6.1 /<7.8 <6.1	1.7	1.6	1.3	1.5
Mauritius, Fiji and Nauru[20]	9179	>20	5–12	mortality	<7.0/<11.1	male 2.7* female 2.0*	male 1.6 female 1.2	–	–
				CVD-mort		male 2.3* female 2.6*	male 1.3 female 1.4		
Funagata Diabetes study[14]	2534	>40	7	mortality	<7.8/<7.8 <6.1	1.2	1.7	1.3	1.2
				CVD-mort	<7.8/<7.8 <6.1	2.3	2.5	2.2	1.1
Cardiovascular Health study[18]	4515	>65	8	CVD	<7.8/<7.8 <6.1	1.7	1.5	1.2	1.4
Strong Heart study[27]	6483	45–74	5	CHD	<6.1/<7.8 <6.1/<7.8	1.7 2.7	1.7 2.7	1.2 0.7	1.5 0.7

Notes: FPG, fasting plasma glucose; 2hPG, 2-hour postload glucose; DM, diabetes; IGT, impaired glucose tolerance; IFG, impaired fasting glucose; RR, relative risk; mort, mortality; CVD, cardiovascular disease; CHD, coronary heart disease
*IPH, isolated postload hyperglycaemia (FPG <7.0 mmol/l, 2hPG ≥11.1 mmol/l)
** The Hoorn study is participating in the DECODE study

Table 18.1
Published risks of mortality and cardiovascular disease in glucose intolerance categories according to the WHO-85 and ADA-97 diagnostic criteria

and postload (2hPG) levels, as advocated by the WHO. This raises the question of whether the risk for mortality and for macrovascular complications is more closely associated with fasting or with postload hyperglycemia. Several prospective studies have now addressed this question.[14,17,18,20,26–28] Summarizing the results of these studies (Table 18.1), according to either set of diagnostic criteria diabetes was associated with an increased risk for mortality and cardiovascular complications. In the Hoorn study and in the DECODE study, the subjects fulfilling either set of criteria had similar mortality risks of 2.2 and 2.3, respectively, relative to subjects with normal glucose levels.[26,28] Furthermore, in the DECODE study mortality significantly increased in all categories of fasting plasma glucose with increasing 2hPG levels, which was not seen for increasing levels of fasting plasma glucose in categories of 2hPG.[17] In the Cardiovascular Health study and the Strong Heart study the degree of risk for incident CVD was similar for subjects diagnosed with diabetes by the WHO-85 or ADA-97 criteria.[18,27] However, in the Cardiovascular Health study more subjects with incident CVD were classified as having abnormal glucose levels by the WHO-85 criteria than by the fasting ADA-97 criteria.[18] In the Funagata Diabetes study in Japan only impaired glucose tolerance (IGT), and not impaired fasting glucose (IFG), was a statistically significant predictor for death from CVD.[14] Taken together, these and other studies, show that 2hPG is a good predictor for mortality, which has been attributed to the association between postload glucose levels and insulin resistance.[16,17,20,26,29,30] Both the elevated fasting glucose and 2hPG identify subjects at risk for mortality and cardiovascular complications, but 2hPG seems to have a greater ability to detect subjects at risk for these complications. Clearly, the 75 g oral glucose

tolerance test provides additional prognostic information for mortality and macrovascular disease.

The association between 2hPG and the actual presence of atherosclerosis was studied in 582 subjects with various degrees of glucose (in)tolerance, ranging from normal glucose tolerance to diabetes.[31] A surrogate marker of atherosclerosis, the carotid intima-media thickness (IMT) was determined by an ultrasound technique. The 2hPG was found to be the most important glycemic determinant of IMT, more so than HbA1c or fasting plasma glucose. An increase of the 2hPG was associated with an increase of the IMT within each tertile of HbA1c. In contrast, fasting plasma glucose was not associated with a rise of IMT in the HbA1c tertiles. The other independent determinants of IMT were: age, male gender, proinsulin, albuminuria, total and HDL cholesterol. This study confirms the findings of the DECODE study, showing an association between the 2hPG and atherosclerotic vascular disease. Later we will discuss the potential factors explaining this association.

Also in persons with manifest Type 2 diabetes a few studies have demonstrated 2hPG to be an independent predictor of myocardial infarction. In the Diabetes Intervention study, 1139 newly diagnosed patients were followed for 11 years. The independent predictors identified for death were blood pressure, smoking, male sex, age, TG and postprandial glucose.[24] Another study from the same group went on to study whether isolated post-challenge hyperglycemia constituted a risk factor for atherosclerosis as reflected by IMT. For this they studied 119 asymptomatic diabetic subjects with either isolated fasting (IFH), post-challenge (IPH) or combined hyperglycemia (FH/PH).[32] The IMT increased with the deterioration of glucose tolerance; the lowest IMT value was found in those with normal glucose tolerance, intermediate values in subjects with IFH and IPH and the highest values in persons with combined hyperglycemia. In multiple regression analysis the most important determinants were 2hPG, in addition to age, gender, total and HDL cholesterol and blood pressure. The fasting plasma glucose level did not contribute to the IMT measure in any class of 2hPG. Not surprisingly, the authors strongly favor the oral glucose tolerance test for the assessment of the cardiovascular risk in persons at risk of diabetes.

An important and often overlooked group consists of mostly elderly persons with isolated post-challenge hyperglycemia. These persons are characterized by a normal fasting glucose level and a diabetic 2hPG. At least three studies have shown that these subjects suffer about a two-fold risk of mortality from cardiovascular and other causes.[20,21]

From the above it is evident that the 2hPG is a much stronger determinant of either mortality (population based studies) or IMT (studies in specific groups) than the other glycemic indices, as for example fasting plasma glucose levels and HbA1c.

Postprandial plasma TG levels as predictors of CVD

The known inverse relationship between HDL cholesterol and triglyceride (TG) makes it very difficult to determine whether TG is an independent risk factor for atherosclerotic vascular disease.[33] It therefore required a meta-analysis including data of 57,000 persons from 17 studies to demonstrate that the TG level is an independent risk factor for CVD, also when adjusted for HDL cholesterol.[34] A 1 mmol/l increase was associated with a relative risk of 1.3 for men and 1.8 for women.

In diabetes, postprandial dyslipidemia is a frequent feature, even in patients with appar-

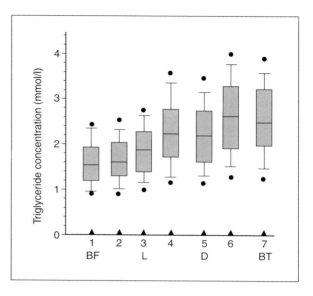

Figure 18.1

Box and whisker plots (median, box, (25–75th percentiles), whiskers (10–90th precentiles) and dots (5–95th percentiles) of the home measured triglyceride concentrations in patients with Type 2 diabetes, selected on the basis of normal fasting triglyceride concentrations (<2.2 mmol/l). Measurements were made before and two hours after the main meals and at bedtime. Since the triglyceride concentrations show a gradual rise over the day, the fasting concentrations severely underestimate the triglyceride exposure in persons with Type 2 diabetes. Numbers 1–7 indicate the time points of the measurements: fasting, post-breakfast (BF), before and after lunch (L), before and after dinner (D), and at bedtime (BT), respectively.

ently normal fasting TG values. This was clearly shown in 81 persons with Type 2 diabetes with fasting TG levels <2.2 mmol/l (Figure 18.1). The daytime TG profiles were assessed with an ambulatory measurement device.[35] The average 24 h TG concentrations were 2.2 +/– 0.65 mmol/l with mean fasting levels of 1.3 +/– 0.51 mmol/l. Following breakfast, the TG levels gradually rose to reach peak levels between dinner and bedtime. This illustrates the long duration of the so-called postprandial state, which probably can be explained by the insulin resistant state. The major contributing factors to the elevated TG-rich lipoproteins in the diabetic state are increased VLDL production and competition of chylomicron and VLDL particles for the removal mechanisms, as for example lipoprotein lipase and hepatic receptors.[36] A meal related increase of chylomicron levels will saturate the catabolic pathways resulting in a longer residence time of TG-rich remnant particles. These alterations in the kinetics will promote the cholesterol ester transfer protein (CETP)-mediated transfer of cholesteryl esters and TG between the TG-enriched lipoproteins and LDL and HDL. This exchange will ultimately result in small dense LDL and HDL, and low HDL cholesterol concentrations, all of which are now known to be independent predictors of CVD. Postprandial hypertriglyceridemia and the associated atherogenic alterations of the lipoproteins are now considered to be part of the insulin resistance syndrome,[37,38] but the evidence for a direct atherogenic effect of remnant particles is accumulating.[39–41]

This issue was addressed by applying new assays for measuring remnant particles in the Framingham Heart study. Remnant Like Particles (RLP) – cholesterol (C) and RLP-TG were measured in samples of 1567 women of whom 83 had CVD.[42] Indeed, fasting RLP-C was significantly associated with prevalent CVD, also after adjustment for other risk factors. Also several clinical studies have suggested that high postprandial TG-rich lipoproteins are related to the presence of coronary heart and/or carotid artery disease in non-diabetic subjects.[43–45] Moreover, an association could be demonstrated between postprandial chylomicron remnants and the

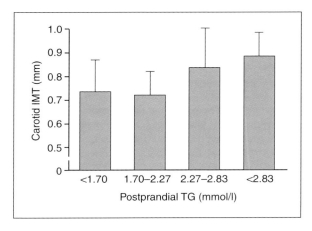

Figure 18.2
Association between carotid intima-media thickness (IMT), measured with ultrasonography and triglyceride levels in the fasting state fTG, and four hours following a meal (pTG) in 42 Type 2 diabetic patients with normal fasting triglyceride levels (<1.7 mmol/l) Source: reproduced with permission from Diabetes Care 2000; 23: 1401–6.[48] © 2000 American Diabetes Association.

progression of angiographically determined coronary heart disease.[46] More recently Mero et al. compared the postprandial apolipoprotein B48 and B100 response in 43 Type 2 diabetic subjects with that in healthy controls to differentiate between intestinal (B48) and liver-derived TG-rich lipoproteins (B100), in relation to the presence of coronary heart disease, as estimated by quantitative coronary angiography.[47] Patients with mild and severe coronary heart disease had similar postprandial responses of B48- and B100-containing lipoprotein particles. In both groups the responses were greater than in the healthy control group. Of great interest was the finding of a correlation between maximal stenosis in the coronary angiogram (%) and postprandial levels of apolipoprotein B100 of IDL. The latter finding suggests that in particular the smaller remnant particle is atherogenic.

In patients with Type 2 diabetes, Teno et al. investigated the association between postprandial TG levels and the carotid (IMT) by ultrasonography.[48] (Figure 18.2). In 61 non-obese Type 2 diabetic patients in Japan, plasma glucose and serum lipid levels were measured before and four hours after a standardized meal. In univariate analysis fasting total cholesterol, LDL cholesterol and TG levels were associated with IMT. The postprandial variables, which were associated with IMT included plasma levels of glucose, TG, cholesterol, and C-peptide. In multivariate analysis only fasting, LDL cholesterol, and postprandial levels of TG and glucose were significantly and independently associated with carotid IMT. Postprandial TG had the strongest association with carotid IMT.[48] Interestingly, an association was also found between postprandial TG levels and carotid IMT in patients with normal fasting TG levels.

These associations between postprandial lipid metabolism and atherosclerosis support the concept that atherosclerosis is a postprandial phenomenon.

Are the associations of 2hPG and TG levels with CVD explained by insulin resistance?

Insulin resistance has been shown to be associated with different cardiovascular risk factors. These include hypertension and dyslipidemia (notably high TG levels and low HDL cholesterol concentrations), a high waist circumference and waist to hip circumference ratio.[49,50,51] This clustering of risk factors for CVD, commonly referred to as the insulin resistance syndrome or IRS, has repeatedly been demonstrated, using different methods and in various ethnic groups.[52,53] However, collectively these only explain a part of the excess risk of CVD associated with abnormal glucose tolerance.

The San Antonio Heart study demonstrated, during a seven-year follow-up of 1734 non-diabetic subjects that persons who converted to diabetes were more likely to harbor CVD risk factors than those who did not.[54] Of great interest was the finding that only those who were insulin resistant, as reflected by the HOMA-IR (homeostatic model assessment for insulin resistance), showed an adverse CVD risk profile in the pre-diabetic state. In contrast, those with a predominant decrease in insulin secretion (delta insulin 0–30 min/delta glucose 0–30 min, following a 75 g glucose load) with similar 2hPG values had a more favorable profile. These findings confirm the well-known fact that the Type 2 diabetic population is heterogeneous with respect to insulin resistance and β-cell dysfunction. Moreover, the presence of atherogenic risk factors, i.e. high waist circumference, low HDL cholesterol, high TG, and elevated blood pressure are more closely related to the presence of insulin resistance than to the presence of an insulin secretory defect (Figure 18.3).

In the newly diagnosed persons with diabetes in the United Kingdom Prospective Diabetes Study (UKPDS) the major predictor of coronary heart disease was LDL cholesterol; other independent predictors apart from age and gender were low HDL cholesterol, high HbA1c and systolic blood pressure, and smoking.[55] In the UKPDS no information is available on glucose excursions. LDL cholesterol has previously been shown to be a risk factor for coronary artery disease in non-diabetic and diabetic subjects,[56] but has not always been identified as such in diabetic cohorts.[57] LDL cholesterol has now more convincingly been recognized as a risk factor in Type 2 diabetes because of the post hoc analyses of the secondary prevention trials using cholesterol

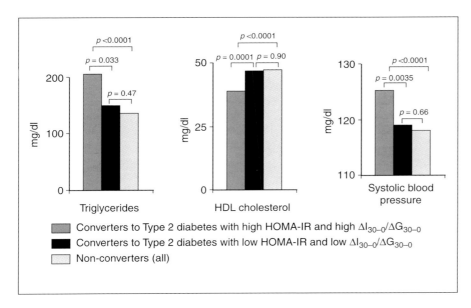

Figure 18.3
Cardiovascular risk factors by insulin resistance (HOMA-IR), insulin secretion (delta insulin/delta glucose 0–30 minutes $\Delta I_{30-0}/\Delta G_{30-0}$) and conversion status. The persons converting to diabetes with a high HOMA-IR, indicating insulin resistance, show a worse cardiovascular risk profile than those who converted with a relatively normal insulin sensitivity (low HOMA-IR) (Reproduced with permission from Haffner SM et al.[54]

lowering drugs (HMGCoA reductase inhibitors) as for example in the 4S and CARE study, showing that LDL lowering effectively reduces recurrence of coronary heart disease events.[58,59] To some extent it is remarkable that LDL cholesterol has emerged as an independent risk factor in Type 2 diabetes. Most cross-sectional studies have not, or have only to a very modest extent, demonstrated an elevated total and/or LDL cholesterol in persons with abnormal glucose tolerance.[60,61] In summary, the observed association between postload excursions of glucose with CVD is at least partly explained by the presence of insulin resistance and related cardiovascular disease risk factors.

Biochemical and physiological responses to meal

Different mechanisms can potentially contribute to the observed associations of meal related metabolic changes and CVD. These include oxidative stress, glycation, depressed NO availability, and prolongation of the QTc interval. These mechanisms are strongly interrelated, but will be discussed separately for reasons of clarity (Figure 18.4).

Oxidative stress

Diabetes is associated with an enhanced production of reactive oxygen species and an impaired antioxidant defence.[62,63] Hyperglycemia is known to stimulate the production of reactive oxygen species through several pathways. These include non-enzymatic glycation, auto-oxidation of glucose and stimulation of the polyol pathway. It has been suggested that the antioxidant status in the postprandial state is diminished and the susceptibility of LDL to oxidation is enhanced,[64] especially in patients with diabetes.[65] In particular, the total radical trapping antioxidant parameter, which is a global measure of plasma antioxidant capacity, decreased considerably during the

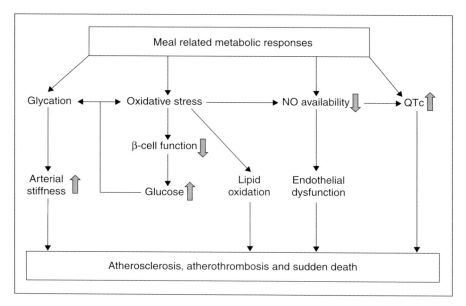

Figure 18.4
Meal related metabolic changes contributing to glycation, oxidative stress, depressed nitric oxide (NO) availability, and prolongation of the QTc interval. These interrelated abnormalities may in turn lead to arterial stiffness, lipid oxidation, endothelial dysfuncion, and manifestations of cardiovascular disease, respectively.

meal. These changes were attributed to the concomitant hyperglycemia. However, also FFA and TG responses can contribute to oxidative stress.[66]

We recently suggested that intracellular accumulation of long chain fatty acyl CoA in obesity is the starting point of enhanced oxidative stress and adenosine release.[66,67] One of the adverse consequences of obesity, and in particular central fat distribution, is increased cytosolic TG storage in tissues like muscle, liver and pancreatic β-cells. Elevated levels of intracellular long chain acyl CoA esters inhibit the mitochondrial adenine nucleotide translocator, resulting in an intramitochondrial rise of the ATP/ADP ratio. Intramitochondrial ADP deficiency stimulates oxygen free-radical production.[68] Tissues, which are likely to be susceptible to oxidative stress, are those that have a high-energy demand and/or a poor free-radical scavenging capacity. These include the pancreatic β-cells. Thus according to our hypothesis intracellular TG accumulation

induced oxidative stress contributes to the gradual decline in β-cell function.

A second phenomenon related to intracellular long chain acyl CoA accumulation induced impairment of oxidative phosphorylation is a chronic systemic increase of adenosine.[67] Chronic elevation of adenosine release is known to stimulate, amongst others, the sympathetic nervous system and to induce renal vasoconstriction. The enhanced production of adenosine may therefore also contribute to the hemodynamic alterations involved in insulin resistance syndrome.

Thus, obesity and meal related perturbation in different substrates via several routes stimulate the production of reactive oxygen species and in turn accelerate atherogenesis.[64,66]

Glycation

Meal related glucose excursions may potentially contribute to the glycation of apolipoproteins and transfer proteins enhancing the clearance of LDL via the scavenger pathway and the exchange of cholesteryl ester for TG via CETP, rendering LDL more atherogenic.[69,70] Also, the glycation process involving small dense LDL may enhance the susceptibility to oxidative stress, further contributing to the atherogenicity of these particles.[71] However, the clinical relevance of these changes remains to be established.

Accumulation of advanced glycation end products (AGE) is known to adversely affect several tissues and to be involved in the development of the well-known microvascular complications of diabetes.[72] The formation of AGE is also accompanied by production of reactive oxygen species. AGE may affect large vessel function in several ways, for example by inducing abnormalities in extracellular matrix function, affecting the structure (enhance stiffness) and function of large vessels. This has been shown in animals, where AGE decreased the elasticity and vasodilatory response to nitric oxide.[73] Also, the administration of drugs, which break the AGE cross-links in diabetic rats, reversed the diabetes induced increase of large artery stiffness.[74]

Even in non-diabetic subjects, fasting glucose and HbA1c have been found to be associated with the carotid intima media thickness (IMT).[31,75,76] In persons with impaired glucose tolerance, characterized by moderately elevated postprandial glucose only, the major determinants of the changes in carotid artery diameter and in distensibility (stiffness) occurring over a follow-up period of three years were, apart from blood pressure, fasting blood glucose and HbA1c, and insulin levels.[76] The suggestion was made that, especially in women, insulin resistance, as reflected by high insulin levels, may contribute to arterial stiffening. Insulin has been suggested to stimulate collagen synthesis and smooth muscle cell proliferation.[29] Thus, here again, the observed vascular changes cannot solely be attributed to the small elevations of glucose values. It is very likely that other mechanisms, and insulin resistance in particular, are involved.

Depressed NO availability

In patients with diabetes, a diminished vasodilatory response, measured with ultrasound techniques, has been documented.[77] This is suggestive of depressed nitric oxide (NO) availability. In both Type 1 and Type 2 diabetes, chronic hyperglycemia has been shown to impair endothelial function.[78,79]

A measure of endothelial function is the post-ischemic flow-mediated endothelium dependent vasodilatation.[80,81] The vascular response to different meals has been studied using this technique in persons with and without diabetes. In healthy volunteers, a fatty meal has been shown to induce vasodilatation and to increase forearm blood flow.[82] These changes could be related to the insulin and TG responses. Possibly these hemodynamic responses may be attributed to the vasodilatory effect of insulin.[83] In vitro studies have shown that both hyperglycemia and insulinopenia can suppress NO production in human coronary endothelial cells, whereas high insulin levels stimulate NO production.[84] Also obesity, insulin resistance and dyslipidemia without manifest hyperglycemia have been associated with endothelial dysfunction.[80,82,85–90] In vivo and in vitro studies have shown that remnant lipoproteins affect endothelial function, as reflected by lowered NO production and activity.[86,91–93] These observations have been confirmed in a study of 20 healthy volunteers submitted to a fat load of 50 g/m² body surface whipped cream. The consumption resulted in a rise of TG levels from 1.0 to 1.8 mmol/l at four hours. The flow-mediated dilatation (FMD) of the brachial artery decreased from 10.6%

before the meal to 5.8% at four hours following the fat load.[88] These authors extended the observation by demonstrating that the attenuation of FMD can be abolished by folic acid pre-treatment, which, albeit speculatively, may be attributed to an increase of NO production. These findings are in apparant contrast to the earlier mentioned results from studies in healthy volunteers showing a vasodilatory response following a high fat meal.[82] This may be explained by differences in meal composition resulting in different insulin-induced NO-mediated vascular responses.

A study of 34 healthy men assessed the association between LDL particle size and endothelial function.[90] LDL size was found to be the only significant determinant of endothelium-dependent vasodilatation, strongly suggesting that small and dense LDL cholesterol may, partly, mediate the adverse effects of insulin resistance associated dyslipidemia on vascular function.[76,91,94] These studies uniformly show that endothelial dysfunction can be related to abnormal lipid metabolism, both in the fasting state (relationship with small dense LDL) and postprandially, following a fatty meal.

Perticone et al. addressed the question to what extent insulin resistance associated factors are related to endothelial function.[95] The main determinants in this study of 76 healthy subjects, as determined by forearm blood flow changes during intra-arterial acetylcholine infusions, were BMI, waist to hip ratio, fasting insulin and insulin resistance (HOMA-IR model). Fasting plasma levels of cholesterol and TG were not related to the forearm blood flow changes. The investigators also showed that vitamin C and indomethacin administration restored the attenuated forearm blood flow response in the obese. The results of this study suggest that insulin resistance in the obese is responsible for the demonstrated endothelial dysfunction and that oxidative stress, due to quenching and deactivating NO, is one of the contributing factors.

Prolongation of the QTc interval

In non-diabetic and diabetic subjects a prolonged heart rate adjusted QT interval (QTc) has been shown to be predictive of sudden death and to correlate with measures of CVD.[96-97] These studies have also demonstrated a prolonged QTc associated with hyperinsulinemia and hyperglycemia.[98,99] In persons with diabetes, the prevalence of QTc prolongation is high (about 35%), and has been found to be associated with autonomic neuropathy.[100]

Acute hyperglycemia of about 15 mmol/l, induced by an intravenous glucose load in healthy individuals, increased the QTc, and several sympathetic tone dependent hemodynamic parameters.[101] In control experiments, the rise of insulin was prevented by an octreotide infusion. Nevertheless, the QTc prolongation, the blood pressure rise, and the elevation of plasma concentrations of epinephrine and norepinephrine were very similar. These data strongly suggest that hyperglycemia alone can enhance the risk of sudden death in vulnerable persons by enhancing the sympathetic tone and by prolongation of the QTc interval. One of the suggested mechanisms that may explain these effects of acute hyperglycemia is depressed NO formation resulting in increased intracellular calcium content.[102] In support of this hypothesis these authors found, in another set of experiments, that in patients with newly diagnosed diabetes the adverse hemodynamic effects of acute hyperglycemia, i.e. blood pressure rise and baroreflex responses, can be reversed by L-arginine infusion, a precursor of nitric oxide. Moreover, the adverse effects of acute hyperglycemia could also here be prevented by glutathione, an antioxidant, enhancing NO availability.[103] Insulin may also, as suggested by Gastaldelli et al., have a direct effect on QTc. Insulin lowers potassium levels, which in turn causes hyperpolarization of the cell membrane.[104]

From the above, it is clear that glucose and especially the factors associated with insulin resistance may, via several biochemical pathways, affect endothelial dysfunction and promote the development of CVD (Figure 18.4). The proportional contributions of the different, but interrelated factors that lead to the severely elevated risk of CVD in diabetic patients, have to be determined.

The importance of lowering glucose and the possible contribution of lowering meal related glucose excursions

What do we know about the blood glucose lowering interventions that have been applied to lower CVD risk and CVD risk factors? The UKPDS has taught us that maintaining good glycemic control lowers the incidence rate of microvascular complications in Type 2 diabetes.[105] This was independent of the allocated treatments; no difference was observed between the blood glucose lowering agents sulfonylurea and insulin. Perhaps due to the gradual deterioration of glycemic control and the small contrast in HbA1c value between the intensive and conventional treatment groups (0.9%) only a modest difference (16%) in the occurrence of myocardial infarctions was seen. Nevertheless it is now well established that long-term complications of diabetes can be reduced in proportion to the achieved decrease in HbA1c. Patients targeting for normalization of the postprandial glucose levels may obtain a lower HbA1c. Only one study in women with

gestational diabetes demonstrated that women who adjusted insulin therapy in accordance with postprandial levels, rather than preprandial, achieved a lower HbA1c and better pregnancy outcome.[106] In Type 2 diabetes patients, no benefits have been reported so far of postprandial glucose monitoring. In contrast, metformin is in fact the only blood glucose lowering drug that has been shown in the UKPDS to lower diabetes related end points and all cause mortality and stroke in overweight Type 2 diabetic patients.[107] Even among patients allocated to intensive blood glucose lowering, metformin showed a greater effect than chlorpropamide, glibenclamide, or insulin for all cause mortality, stroke and the so-called combined (diabetes related) end points. As the glucose lowering potency of metformin is not greater than that of other blood glucose lowering agents, and certainly not in terms of meal related glucose excursions, it is of great interest to understand the mechanisms, which may explain the observed benefits. Studies over the years have shown metformin to lower the meal related TG-rich lipoproteins and TG excursions,[108] and to decrease the methylglyoxal levels in Type 2 diabetic patients.[109] This latter finding is of particular interest since methylglyoxal levels are elevated in diabetic patients and may contribute to the development of complications as a precursor of advanced glycation end products (AGE). Methylglyoxal and glyoxal are dicarbonyl compounds, known to be very reactive glycating agents and involved in the formation of AGE products.

In vitro and animal studies have shown that metformin is able to react strongly with dicarbonyl compounds and may thus decrease AGE formation.[110] The question then remains can we lower the risk more considerably and consistently by lowering the meal-related glucose excursions and, if yes, how should this be done? The drugs which have been specifically targeted on restoring the meal-related glucose excursions are the α-glucosidase inhibitors, the short acting insulin analogs, inhaled insulin, pramlintide, and the meglitinides (repaglinide and nateglinide).[111–113] These drugs have all proved to be effective in reducing the meal related glucose excursions. The metiglinides, for example, have been shown to lower the postprandial glucose values in Type 2 diabetes by improving the insulin response to a meal. This resulted in a modest 0.5–0.6% decline in HbA1c.[114] This observation is an important proof of concept. However, the long-term benefit remains to be established.

Few studies have addressed the efficacy of blood glucose lowering drugs on meal related lipoprotein level excursions. A Japanese study in persons with Type 2 diabetes found a modest lowering of postprandial TG and insulin levels with acarbose treatment.[115] To our knowledge, the postprandial lipid response has not been studied with the other mentioned drugs, apart from metformin. In contrast, the meal related glucose and insulin responses have been studied extensively. Does this in itself justify the propagation of these drugs in the treatment arsenal of Type 2 diabetes?[116–118] Before jumping to any kind of clinical recommendation it is pivotal to learn more about these specific drugs, particularly because of their intended use in the treatment of a high risk population, i.e. the Type 2 diabetic patient. Lowering a risk indicator may not provide the benefit that one would hope for or one would wrongly predict from epidemiological studies (Figure 18.5). More evidence, which can only be obtained from randomized clinical trials, is certainly required. We also need to accept that the various compounds targeted at the correction of postprandial hyperglycemia act in different ways and thus it is likely that they will

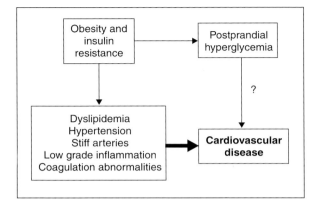

Figure 18.5
Obesity and insulin resistance contribute to both postprandial hyperglycemia and, as depicted in Figure 18.4, a cluster of CVD risk factors. Lowering the postprandial hyperglycemia only, without influencing the established risk factors, will not provide the benefit one would predict from the epidemiological association between 2hPG and mortality.

affect the discussed established risk factors, and outcomes, differently. For example, insulin secretion enhancers will probably affect the postprandial lipid responses and vascular function differently from compounds, which affect the gastric emptying or glucose absorption rate. The required evidence does not necessarily include mortality or morbidity data from long-term intervention trials, but it at least needs to include the effect on potential mechanisms, for example lipoproteins and coagulation factors, and intermediate end points, for example endothelial function parameters (FMD) and/or IMT measurements.

Therefore, we have to conclude that postprandial hyperglycemia per se cannot, at least as yet, be considered to be a treatment target in itself. We have to await the evidence from convincing long-term studies showing amelioration of clinically relevant end points. This conclusion should in no way distract from the therapeutic aim to achieve target HbA1c values in patients with Type 2 diabetes.

Acknowledgements

The Dutch Diabetes Research Foundation and Roche Diagnostics, Mannheim, Germany supported a few studies mentioned in the manuscript. We thank Dr F de Vegt and M Diamant for their contributions and critical comments on earlier drafts of this review.

References

1. Haffner SM, Lehto S, Ronnemaa T et al. Mortality from coronary heart disease in subjects with Type 2 diabetes and in non-diabetic subjects with and without prior myocardial infarction. N Engl J Med 1998; 339: 229–34.
2. Kannel WB, McGee DL. Diabetes and CVD. The Framingham study. JAMA 1979; 241: 2035–8.
3. Stamler J, Vaccaro O, Neaton JD, Wentworth D. Diabetes, other risk factors, and 12-yr cardiovascular mortality for men screened in the Multiple Risk Factor Intervention Trial. Diabetes Care 1993; 16: 434–44.
4. Lee WL, Cheung AM, Cape D, Zinman B. Impact of diabetes on coronary artery disease in women and men: a meta-analysis of prospective studies. Diabetes Care 2000; 23: 962–8.
5. Laakso M, Lehto S. Epidemiology of risk factors for cardiovascular disease in diabetes and impaired glucose tolerance. Atherosclerosis 1998; 137 Suppl. S65–S73.
6. Lehto S, Ronnemaa T, Pyorala K, Laakso M. Cardiovascular risk factors clustering with endogenous hyperinsulinaemia predict death from coronary heart disease in patients with Type II diabetes. Diabetologia 2000; 43: 148–55.
7. Stamler R, Stamler J, Lindberg HA et al. Asymptomatic hyperglycemia and coronary heart disease in middle-aged men in two employed populations in Chicago. J Chronic Dis 1979; 32: 805–15.
8. Yano K, Kagan A, McGee D, Rhoads GG. Glucose intolerance and nine-year mortality in Japanese men in Hawaii. Am J Med 1982; 72: 71–80.
9. Fuller JH, Shipley MJ, Rose G. Coronary-heart-disease risk and impaired glucose tolerance. The Whitehall Study. Lancet 1982; 1: 1373–6.
10. Donahue RP, Abbott RD, Reed DM, Yano K. Postchallenge glucose concentration and coronary heart disease in men of Japanese ancestry. Honolulu Heart Program. Diabetes 1987; 36: 689–92.
11. Lowe LP, Liu K, Greenland P. Diabetes, asymptomatic hyperglycemia, and 22-year mortality in black and white men. The Chicago Heart Association Detection Project in Industry Study. Diabetes Care 1997; 20: 163–9.
12. Balkau B, Shipley M, Jarrett RJ et al. High blood glucose concentration is a risk factor for mortality in middle-aged nondiabetic men. 20-year follow-up in the Whitehall Study, the Paris Prospective Study, and the Helsinki Policemen Study. Diabetes Care 1998; 21: 360–7.
13. Rodriguez BL, Lau N, Burchfiel CM et al. Glucose intolerance and 23-year risk of coronary heart disease and total mortality: the Honolulu Heart Program. Diabetes Care 1999; 22: 1262–5.
14. Tominaga M, Eguchi H, Manaka H et al. Impaired glucose tolerance is a risk factor for cardiovascular disease, but not impaired fasting glucose. The Funagata Diabetes Study. Diabetes Care 1998; 22: 920–4.
15. Balkau B, Bertrais S, Ducimetiere P, Eschwege E. Is there a glycemic threshold for mortality risk? Diabetes Care 1999; 22: 696–9.
16. de Vegt F, Dekker JM, Ruhe HG et al. Hyperglycaemia is associated with all-cause and cardiovascular mortality in the Hoorn population: the Hoorn Study. Diabetologia 1999; 42: 926–31.
17. The DECODE study group. Glucose tolerance

and mortality: comparison of WHO and American Diabetes Association diagnostic criteria. European Diabetes Epidemiology Group. Diabetes Epidemiology: Collaborative analysis Of Diagnostic criteria in Europe. Lancet 1999; 354: 617–21.

18. Barzilay JI, Spiekerman CF, Wahl PW. Cardiovascular disease in older adults with glucose disorders: comparison of American Diabetes Association criteria for diabetes mellitus with WHO criteria. Lancet 1999; 354: 622–5.

19. Coutinho M, Gerstein HC, Wang Y, Yusuf S. The relationship between glucose and incident cardiovascular events. A metaregression analysis of published data from 20 studies of 95,783 individuals followed for 12.4 years. Diabetes Care 1999; 22: 233–40.

20. Shaw JE, Hodge AM, de Courten M et al. Isolated post-challenge hyperglycaemia confirmed as a risk factor for mortality. Diabetologia 1999; 42: 1050–4.

21. Barrett-Connor E, Ferrara A. Isolated postchallenge hyperglycemia and the risk of fatal cardiovascular disease in older women and men. The Rancho Bernardo Study. Diabetes Care 1998; 21: 1236–9.

22. Balkau B, Jouven X, Ducimetiere P, Eschwege E. Diabetes as a risk factor for sudden death. Lancet 1999; 354: 1968–9.

23. Folsom AR, Szklo M, Stevens J et al. A prospective study of coronary heart disease in relation to fasting insulin, glucose, and diabetes. The Atherosclerosis Risk in Communities (ARIC) Study. Diabetes Care 1997; 20: 935–42.

24. Hanefeld M, Fischer S, Julius U et al. Risk factors for myocardial infarction and death in newly detected NIDDM: the Diabetes Intervention Study, 11-year follow-up. Diabetologia 1996; 39: 1577–83.

25. Bonora E, Muggeo M. Postprandial blood glucose as a risk factor for cardiovascular disease in Type II diabetes: the epidemiological evidence. Diabetologia 2001; 44: 2107–14.

26. de Vegt F, Dekker JM, Stehouwer CD et al. Similar 9-year mortality risks and reproducibility for the World Health Organization and American Diabetes Association glucose tolerance categories: the Hoorn Study. Diabetes Care 2000; 23: 40–4.

27. Hu D, Zhang Y, Yeh F et al. Comparison of ADA and WHO diagnostic criteria for predicting CHD risk: the Strong Heart Study. Diabetes 2000; 49 Suppl. 1: A186.

28. Balkau B. New diagnostic criteria for diabetes and mortality in older adults. DECODE Study Group. European Diabetes Epidemiology Group. Lancet 19989 353: 68–9.

29. DeFronzo RA, Ferrannini E. Insulin resistance. A multifaceted syndrome responsible for NIDDM, obesity, hypertension, dyslipidemia, and atherosclerotic cardiovascular disease. Diabetes Care 1991; 14: 173–94.

30. Haffner SM. The insulin resistance syndrome revisited. Diabetes Care 1996; 19: 275–7.

31. Temelkova-Kurktschiev T, Koehler C, Schaper F et al. Relationship between fasting plasma glucose, atherosclerosis risk factors and carotid intima media thickness in non-diabetic individuals. Diabetologia 1998; 41: 706–12.

32. Hanefeld M, Koehler C, Henkel E et al. Post-challenge hyperglycaemia relates more strongly than fasting hyperglycaemia with carotid intima-media thickness: the RIAD Study. Diabet Med 2000; 17: 835–40.

33. Taskinen MR, Lahdenpera S, Syvanne M. New insights into lipid metabolism in non-insulin-dependent diabetes mellitus. Ann Med 1996; 28: 335–40.

34. Hokanson JE, Austin MA. Plasma TG level is a risk factor for cardiovascular disease independent of high-density lipoprotein cholesterol level: a meta-analysis of population-based prospective studies. J Cardiovasc Risk 1996; 3: 213–19.

35. Luley C, Ronquist G, Reuter W et al. Point-of-care testing of triglycerides: evaluation of the Accutrend triglycerides system. Clin Chem 2000; 46: 287–91.

36. Mero N, Syvanne M, Taskinen MR. Postprandial lipid metabolism in diabetes. Atherosclerosis 1998; 141 Suppl. 1: S53–S55.

37. Miller GJ. Postprandial lipaemia and haemostatic factors. Atherosclerosis 1998; 141 Suppl 1: S47–S51.

38. Lemieux I, Pascot A, Couillard C et al. Hypertriglyceridemic waist: a marker of the atherogenic metabolic triad (hyperinsulinemia; hyperapolipoprotein B; small, dense LDL) in men? Circulation 2000; 102: 179–84.

39. Karpe F, de Faire U, Mercuri M et al. Magnitude of alimentary lipemia is related to intima-media thickness of the common carotid artery in middle-aged men. Atherosclerosis 1998; 141: 307–14.

40. Ryu JE, Howard G, Craven TE et al. Postprandial triglyceridemia and carotid atherosclerosis in middle-aged subjects. Stroke 1992; 23: 823–8.

41. Axelsen M, Smith U, Eriksson JW et al. Postprandial hypertriglyceridemia and insulin resistance in normoglycemic first-degree relatives of patients with Type 2 diabetes. Ann Intern Med 1999; 131: 27–31.

42. McNamara JR, Shah PK, Nakajima K et al. Remnant-like particle (RLP) cholesterol is an independent cardiovascular disease risk factor in women: results from the Framingham Heart Study. Atherosclerosis 2001; 154: 229–36.

43. Patsch JR, Miesenbock G, Hopferwieser T et al. Relation of triglyceride metabolism and coronary artery disease. Studies in the postprandial state. Arterioscler Thromb Vasc Biol 1992; 12: 1336–45.

44. Groot PH, van Stiphout WA, Krauss XH et al. Postprandial lipoprotein metabolism in normolipidemic men with and without coronary artery disease. Arterioscler Thromb Vasc Biol 1991; 11: 653–62.

45. Weintraub MS, Grosskopf I, Rassin T et al. Clearance of chylomicron remnants in normolipidaemic patients with coronary artery disease: case–control study over three years. BMJ 1996; 312: 936–9.

46. Karpe F, Steiner G, Uffelman K et al. Postprandial lipoproteins and progression of coronary atherosclerosis. Atherosclerosis 1994; 106: 83–97.

47. Mero N, Malmstrom R, Steiner G et al. Postprandial metabolism of apolipoprotein B-48- and B-100-containing particles in Type 2 diabetes mellitus: relations to angiographically verified severity of coronary artery disease. Atherosclerosis 2000; 150: 167–77.

48. Teno S, Uto Y, Nagashima H et al. Association of postprandial hypertriglyceridemia and carotid intima-media thickness in patients with Type 2 diabetes. Diabetes Care 2000; 23: 1401–6.

49. Reaven GM. Banting lecture 1988. Role of insulin resistance in human disease. Diabetes 1988; 37: 1595–607.

50. Haffner SM, Valdez RA, Hazuda HP et al. Prospective analysis of the insulin-resistance syndrome (syndrome X). Diabetes 1992; 41: 715–22.

51. Ferrannini E, Haffner SM, Mitchell BD, Stern MP. Hyperinsulinaemia: the key feature of a cardiovascular and metabolic syndrome. Diabetologia 1991; 34: 416–22.

52. Haffner SM, Stern MP, Hazuda HP et al. Cardiovascular risk factors in confirmed prediabetic individuals. Does the clock for coronary heart disease start ticking before the onset of clinical diabetes? JAMA 1990; 263: 2893–8.

53. Stern MP. Do non-insulin-dependent diabetes mellitus and cardiovascular disease share common antecedents? Ann Intern Med 1996; 124: 110–6.

54. Haffner SM, Mykkanen L, Festa A et al. Insulin-resistant prediabetic subjects have more atherogenic risk factors than insulin-sensitive prediabetic subjects: implications for preventing coronary heart disease during the prediabetic state. Circulation 2000; 101: 975–80.

55. Turner RC, Millns H, Neil HA et al. Risk factors for coronary artery disease in non-insulin dependent diabetes mellitus: United Kingdom Prospective Diabetes Study (UKPDS: 23). BMJ 1998; 316: 823–8.

56. Fontbonne A, Eschwege E, Cambien F et al. Hypertriglyceridaemia as a risk factor of coronary heart disease mortality in subjects with impaired glucose tolerance or diabetes. Results from the 11-year follow-up of the Paris Prospective Study. Diabetologia 1989; 32: 300–4.

57. Kuusisto J, Mykkanen L, Pyorala K, Laakso M. NIDDM and its metabolic control predict coronary heart disease in elderly subjects. Diabetes 1994; 43: 960–7.

58. Pyorala K, Pedersen TR, Kjekshus J et al. Cholesterol lowering with simvastatin improves prognosis of diabetic patients with coronary heart disease. A subgroup analysis of the Scandinavian Simvastatin Survival Study (4S). Diabetes Care 1997; 20: 614–20.

59. Sacks FM, Pfeffer MA, Moye LA et al. The

effect of pravastatin on coronary events after myocardial infarction in patients with average cholesterol levels. Cholesterol and Recurrent Events Trial investigators. N Engl J Med 1996; 335: 1001–9.

60. Barrett-Connor E, Grundy SM, Holdbrook MJ. Plasma lipids and diabetes mellitus in an adult community. Am J Epidemiol 1992; 115: 657–63.

61. Haffner SM. Management of dyslipidemia in adults with diabetes. Diabetes Care 1998; 21: 160–78.

62. Betteridge DJ. What is oxidative stress? Metabolism 2000; 49: 3–8.

63. West IC. Radicals and oxidative stress in diabetes. Diabet Med 2000; 17: 171–80.

64. Ceriello A, Bortolotti N, Motz E et al. Meal-induced oxidative stress and low-density lipoprotein oxidation in diabetes: the possible role of hyperglycemia. Metabolism 1999; 48: 1503–8.

65. Ceriello A, Bortolotti N, Motz E et al. Meal-generated oxidative stress in Type 2 diabetic patients. Diabetes Care 1998; 21: 1529–33.

66. Bakker SJ, IJzerman RG, Teerlink T et al. Cytosolic triglycerides and oxidative stress in central obesity: the missing link between excessive atherosclerosis, endothelial dysfunction, and beta-cell failure? Atherosclerosis 2000; 148: 17–21.

67. Bakker SJ, Gans ROB, Ter Maaten JC et al. The potential role of adenosine in the pathphysiology of the insulin resistance syndrome. Atherosclerosis 2001; 155: 283–90.

68. Brand MD, Murphy MP. Control of electron flux through the respiratory chain in mitochondria and cells. Biol Rev 1987; 62: 141–93.

69. Witztum JL, Mahoney EM, Branks MJ et al. Non-enzymatic glycosylation of low density lipoprotein alters its biological activity Diabetes 1982; 31: 283–91.

70. Bakker SJ, Dekker JM, Heine RJ. Association between HbA1c and HDL-cholesterol independent of fasting triglycerides in a Caucasian population: evidence for enhanced cholesterol ester transfer induced by in vivo glycation. Diabetologia 1998; 41: 1249–50.

71. Bowie A, Owens D, Collins P et al. Glycosylated low density lipoprotein is more sensitive to oxidation: implications for the diabteic patient? Atherosclerosis 1993; 102: 63–7.

72. Brownlee M. Negative consequences of glycation. Metabolism 2000; 49: 9–13.

73. Huijberts MS, Wolffenbuttel BH, Boudier HA et al. Aminoguanidine treatment increases elasticity and decreases fluid filtration of large arteries from diabetic rats. J Clin Invest 1993; 92: 1407–11.

74. Wolffenbuttel BH, Boulanger CM, Crijns FR et al. Breakers of advanced glycation end products restore large artery properties in experimental diabetes. Proc Natl Acad Sci USA 1998; 95: 4630–4.

75. Vitelli LL, Shahar E, Heiss G et al. Glycosylated hemoglobin level and carotid intimal-medial thickening in nondiabetic individuals. The Atherosclerosis Risk in Communities Study. Diabetes Care 1997; 20: 1454–8.

76. van Dijk RA, Nijpels G, Twisk JW et al. Change in common carotid artery diameter, distensibility and compliance in subjects with a recent history of impaired glucose tolerance: a 3-year follow-up study. J Hypertens 2000; 18: 293–300.

77. Loscalzo J. Nitric oxide and vascular disease. N Engl J Med 1995; 333: 251–3.

78. Makimattila S, Virkamaki A, Groop PH et al. Chronic hyperglycemia impairs endothelial function and insulin sensitivity via different mechanisms in insulin-dependent diabetes mellitus. Circulation 1996; 94: 1276–82.

79. De Vriese AS, Verbeuren TJ, Van de Voorde J et al. Endothelial dysfunction in diabetes. Br J Pharmacol 2000; 130: 963–74.

80. Celermajer DS, Sorensen KE, Gooch VM. Non-invasive detection of endothelial dysfunction in children and adults at risk of atherosclerosis. Lancet 1992; 340: 1111–15.

81. Kawano H, Motoyama T, Hirashima O et al. Hyperglycemia rapidly suppresses flow-mediated endothelium-dependent vasodilation of brachial artery. J Am Coll Cardiol 1999; 34: 146–54.

82. Raitakari OT, Lai N, Griffiths K et al. Enhanced peripheral vasodilation in humans after a fatty meal. J Am Coll Cardiol 200; 36: 417–22.

83. Scherrer U, Randin D, Vollenweider P et al. Nitric oxide release accounts for insulin's vascular effects in humans. J Clin Invest 1994; 94: 2511–15.

84. Ding Y, Vaziri ND, Coulson R et al. Effects of simulated hyperglycemia, insulin, and glucagon on endothelial nitric oxide synthase expression. Am J Physiol Endocrinol Metab 2000; 279: E11–E17.

85. Steinberg HO, Chaker H, Leaming R et al. Obesity/insulin resistance is associated with endothelial dysfunction. Implications for the syndrome of insulin resistance. J Clin Invest 1996; 97: 2601–10.

86. Kugiyama K, Doi H, Motoyama T et al. Association of remnant lipoprotein levels with impairment of endothelium-dependent vasomotor function in human coronary arteries. Circulation 1998; 97: 2519–26.

87. Verhaar MC, Wever RM, Kastelein JJ. 5-methyltetrahydrofolate, the active form of folic acid, restores endothelial function in familial hypercholesterolemia. Circulation 1998; 97: 237–41.

88. Wilmink HW, Stroes ES, Erkelens WD et al. Influence of folic acid on postprandial endothelial dysfunction. Arterioscler Thromb Vasc Biol 2000; 20: 185–8.

89. Lewis TV, Dart AM, Chin-Dusting JP. Endothelium-dependent relaxation by acetylcholine is impaired in hypertriglyceridemic humans with normal levels of plasma LDL cholesterol. J Am Coll Cardiol 1999; 33: 805–12.

90. Vakkilainen J, Makimattila S, Seppala-Lindroos A et al. Endothelial dysfunction in men with small LDL particles. Circulation 2000; 102: 716–21.

91. Grieve DJ, Avella MA, Elliott J, Botham KM. The influence of chylomicron remnants on endothelial cell function in the isolated perfused rat aorta. Atherosclerosis 1998; 139: 273–81.

92. Plotnick GD, Corretti MC, Vogel RA. Effect of antioxidant vitamins on the transient impairment of endothelium-dependent brachial artery vasoactivity following a single high-fat meal. JAMA 1997; 278: 1682–6.

93. Vogel RA, Corretti MC, Plotnick GD. Effect of a single high-fat meal on endothelial function in healthy subjects. Am J Cardiol 1997; 79: 350–4.

94. Steinberg HO, Tarshoby M, Monestel R et al. Elevated circulating free fatty acid levels impair endothelium-dependent vasodilation. J Clin Invest 1997; 100: 1230–9.

95. Perticone F, Ceravolo R, Candigliota M et al. Obesity and body fat distribution induce endothelial dysfunction by oxidative stress: protective effect of vitamin C. Diabetes 2001; 50: 159–65.

96. Dekker JM, Schouten EG, Klootwijk P et al. Association between QT interval and coronary heart disease in middle-aged and elderly men. The Zutphen Study. Circulation 1994; 90: 779–85.

97. Festa A, D'Agostino RJ, Rautaharju P et al. Is QT interval a marker of subclinical atherosclerosis in nondiabetic subjects? The Insulin Resistance Atherosclerosis Study (IRAS). Stroke 1999; 30: 1566–71.

98. Dekker JM, Feskens EJ, Schouten EG et al. QTc duration is associated with levels of insulin and glucose intolerance. The Zutphen Elderly Study. Diabetes 1996; 45: 376–80.

99. Watanabe T, Ashikaga T, Nishizaki M et al. Association of insulin with QTc dispersion. Lancet 1997; 350: 1821–2.

100. Borra M, Gea VMB. Prevalence of Qtc prolongation in Type 2 diabetes: an Italian population based cohort. Diabetologia 2001; 42: A295.

101. Marfella R, Nappo F, De Angelis L et al. The effect of acute hyperglycaemia on QTc duration in healthy man. Diabetologia 2000; 43: 571–5.

102. Giugliano D, Marfella R, Coppola L et al. Vascular effects of acute hyperglycemia in humans are reversed by L-arginine. Evidence for reduced availability of nitric oxide during hyperglycemia. Circulation 1997; 95: 1783–90.

103. Marfella R, Nappo F, De Angelis L et al. Hemodynamic effects of acute hyperglycemia in Type 2 diabetic patients. Diabetes Care 2000; 23: 658–63.

104. Gastaldelli A, Emdin M, Conforti F et al. Insulin prolongs the QTc interval in humans. Am J Physiol Regul Integr Comp Physiol 2000; 279: R2022–R2025.

105. Prospective Diabetes Study (UKPDS) Group. Intensive blood-glucose control with sulphonylureas or insulin compared with conventional treatment and risk of complications in patients with Type 2 diabetes (UKPDS 33). Lancet 1998; 352: 837–53.

106. De Veciana M, Major CA, Morgan MA et al. Postprandial versus preprandial blood glucose monitoring in women with gestational diabetesmellitus requiring insuln therapy. N Engl J Med 1995; 333: 1237–41.

107. Prospective Diabetes Study (UKPDS) Group. Effect of intensive blood-glucose control with metformin on complications in overweight patients with Type 2 diabetes (UKPDS 34). Lancet 1998; 352: 854–65.

108. Jeppesen J, Zhou MY, Chen YD, Reaven GM. Effect of metformin on postprandial lipemia in patients with fairly to poorly controlled NIDDM. Diabetes Care 1999; 17: 1093–9.

109. Ruggiero-Lopez D, Lecomte M, Moinet G et al. Reaction of metformin with dicarbonyl compounds. Possible implication in the inhibition of advanced glycation end product formation. Biochem Pharmacol 1999; 58: 1765–73.

110. Jyothirmayi GN, Soni BJ, Masurekar M et al. Effects of Metformin on collagen glycation and diastolic dysfunction in diabetic myocardium. J Cardiovasc Pharmacol Ther 1998; 3: 319–26.

111. Kalbag JB, Walter YH, Nedelman JR, McLeod JE. Mealtime glucose regulation with nateglinide in healthy volunteers. Diabetes Care 2001; 24: 73–7.

112. Heinemann L, Klappoth W, Rave K et al. Intra-individual variability of the metabolic effect of inhaled insulin together with an absorption enhancer. Diabetes Care 2000; 23: 1343–7.

113. Thompson RG, Pearson L, Schoenfeld SL, Kolterman OG. Pramlintide, a synthetic analog of human amylin, improves the metabolic profile of patients with Type 2 diabetes using insulin. The Pramlintide in Type 2 Diabetes Group. Diabetes Care 1998; 21: 987–93.

114. Horton ES, Clinkingbeard C, Gatlin M et al. Nateglinide alone and in combination with metformin improves glycemic control by reducing mealtime glucose levels in Type 2 diabetes. Diabetes Care 2000; 23: 1660–5.

115. Kado S, Murakami T, Aoki A et al. Effect of acarbose on postprandial lipid metabolism in Type 2 diabetes mellitus. Diabetes Res Clin Pract 1998; 41: 49–55.

116. Breuer HWM. The postprandial blood glucose level. A new target for optimizing treatment of diabetes mellitus. Eur Heart J 2001; 2 Suppl. D: D36–38.

117. Bruttomesso D, Pianta A, Mari A et al. Restoration of early rise in plasma insulin levels improves the glucose tolerance of Type 2 diabetic patients. Diabetes 1999; 48: 99–105.

118. Hanefeld M, Temelkova-Kurktschiev T. The postprandial state and the risk of atherosclerosis. Diabet Med 1997; 14 Suppl 3: S6–11.

19

Obesity-induced diabetes mellitus: a nutritional disease with lifestyle treatments

Gal Dubnov, Dorit Adler, Keren Hershkop, Elliot M Berry

Introduction

Around the year 1550 BC, the first description of diabetes and its treatment was written in Egypt. As described in the Ebers Papyrus, found in 1862, the treatment consisted of drinking the water mixture of bone, grain, grit, wheat, green lead and earth. This was, indeed, an impressive 'nutritional' treatment for diabetes. Until the identification and utilization of insulin for diabetics, nutritional therapy was the only option. As recognized in the American Diabetes Association position statement: Nutrition Recommendations and Principles for People with Diabetes Mellitus,[1] nutritional therapy is still an essential component of successful diabetes management. It is only after the patient has tried significant lifestyle changes that drug control of diabetes should be initiated. Even after the addition of drug therapy, lifestyle changes should still be encouraged, especially as weight loss and prevention of weight gain can lower the need for these and other medications. Since the risk of cardiovascular mortality in diabetics is similar to that of subjects with established coronary disease,[2] every effort should be made to reduce the number of all modifiable risk factors.

This chapter will discuss the cause of most Type 2 diabetes cases today – obesity – as well as the role of nutrition, physical activity and lifestyle modification in its treatment.

Obesity: prevalence, causes and complications

Obesity is a global epidemic

Obesity is the most common nutritional disorder in the modern world and its prevalence is growing rapidly. The WHO has declared that obesity is an epidemic on a global scale,[3] posing one of the greatest long-term threats to human health and well-being. In 1998, the American Heart Association called for action from clinicians, researchers and the public to combat obesity as an emerging major risk factor for cardiovascular disease.[4] Obesity is commonly defined using the Body Mass Index (BMI = weight in kg divided by square of height in meters). Overweight is when the BMI is >25 kg/m^2 and obesity when the BMI is >30 kg/m^2. Data from the third NHANES showed that in the beginning of the 1990s, almost 60% of men and 51% of women were overweight and obese, which is close to 100 million Americans.[5] The prevalence of obesity in the USA grew by 56% in the decade that followed, increasing by 5.6% on average every year – from 17.9% in 1998, to 18.9% in 1999.[6] In Israel, about 50% of women and 60% of men are overweight or obese. In European countries these percentages vary; up to 43% of women (Naples, Italy) and 57% of men (Latina, Italy) are overweight, and up to 37% of women and 20% of men are obese (Latina, Italy).[7] The lowest values among these study centers were in France and Geneva, suggesting a north–south gradient in obesity prevalence across Europe. A conservative summary is that about a half of the Western world's population is overweight or obese and the number is growing.

The causes of obesity

The major causes of the obesity epidemic are 'bad' genes, and a 'too-good' environment. The genetic part accounts for between 40 and 70% of the risk of becoming obese, and 250 chromosome loci found on all but the Y-chromosomes may contribute to an obese phenotype.[8] Genes may influence appetite regulation, food selection, energy metabolism, physical activity (PA) tolerance and more. Still, an annual increase of over 5% in obesity prevalence cannot be blamed on genetic effects, as these could not possibly change over this short time period.

The environmental basis for the growing number of obese individuals is of great importance.[9] The abundance of large food chains offering 'supersize deals' or 'all you can eat', in the competition for the consumers' patronage, obviously play a role in the increased food intake. On the other side of the energy balance equation – that of expenditure – the use of transport, escalators and lifts greatly decrease the amount of energy spent throughout the day. An example of the environmental effects on obesity were seen in a study by Luke et al., in which the authors compared black adults from Nigeria and the USA – two totally different environments, but with a similar genetic background.[10] The amount of body fat in black US women was twice that in the Nigerians, and the prevalence of obesity among these women was 50%, compared with only 5% in the Nigerians. These striking differences were attributed to environmental influences.

Environmental effects are getting to our children as well. Children are also gaining weight at an increasing rate, and sadly, an obese child has an excellent chance of becoming an obese adult. A follow-up of children into their young adulthood showed that BMI at the age of 13 correlated well with that at the age of 22 and with insulin resistance, as determined by a euglycemic insulin clamp.[11] The prevalence of obesity and its accompanying insulin resistance in children has grown significantly in the last decades, resulting in a need for major actions in the field of public health.[12] Primary prevention is the best form of prevention, so lowering the prevalence of obesity should begin at childhood, where lifestyle may still be more easily modified.

Obesity-related illnesses

It has been said that the obese 'dig their graves with their teeth'. About 280,000 annual deaths in the USA are attributed to being overweight and obese.[13] Eighty percent of these occurred in people with a BMI >30 kg/m², emphasizing the importance of this cut-off point. A large prospective study of over 1 million US adults related mortality to high BMI.[14] The safest BMI in this study proved to be between 22.0 to 23.4 kg/m² for women, and 23.5–24.9 kg/m² for men. A BMI of 25 kg/m² or more in women, and 26.5 kg/m² or more in men, carried statistically significant elevated mortality risks. In British men, however, the safest BMI was shown to be 30 kg/m² for all-cause mortality in a cohort of 7700 men.[15] For protection against cardiovascular disease, diabetes and death from any cause, the required BMI was 20–23.9 kg/m². Among the causes for obesity-related mortality, cardiovascular disease is a leading one.[14,16]

There is a significant disease burden associated with obesity, but also with being 'only' overweight:[17,18] diabetes, hypertension, hypercholesterolemia, gallbladder disease and osteoarthritis are the more common. For the overweight and obese, the occurrence of these conditions, varying by sex and degree of obesity, was 5–20% for diabetes, 34–64% for hypertension, 35–45% for hypercholesterolemia, 3–23% for gallbladder disease, and 4.5–17% for osteoarthritis. Of extreme importance is the relationship between obesity and malignancies in hormone-dependent tissues. Among the tumors more prevalent among the obese are those of the breast, uterus, prostate, colon, esophagus and gastric cardia, kidney and lung.[19–26] In a large Swedish cohort, additional obesity-related tumors were those of the small intestine, gallbladder, pancreas, bladder, larynx, brain, connective tissue and lymphoma.[27]

The epidemiological link between overweight and development of Type 2 diabetes is solid: two-thirds of Type 2 diabetics have a BMI >27, and almost half have a BMI >30.[18] The article by the National Task Force on the Prevention and Treatment of Obesity, listed diabetes first among obesity-related diseases, followed by coronary artery disease (CAD). The growing prevalence of Type 2 diabetes parallels the spread of obesity: the prevalence of diabetes rose from 4.9% in 1990, to 6.5% in 1998.[28] This growth, of 33%, can be attributed almost solely to the obesity epidemic. The relative risk of developing diabetes, based on the NHANES III, was 3.72 for overweight men and 3.82 for overweight women under the age of 55.[17] Given the large number of people in this 'weight category' in the modern world, the public health issues regarding prevention and treatment of overweight, obesity and diabetes are clear.

In the Nurses' Health Study, even a weight gain of a few kilograms increased two-fold the risk of Type 2 diabetes.[29] Gaining >8 kg increased the risk almost three-fold, and women who gained >20 kg had a relative risk of over 12 for developing Type 2 diabetes. This was true even for women who were not overweight and were within the recommended values of BMI (<25 kg/m^2). In men also, higher BMI or weight gain correlated significantly with the risk for developing diabetes.[30] The more weight gained, the higher the risk of diabetes. In the extreme, men whose BMI was >24 kg/m^2 at young adulthood and gained >11 kg, increased their risk for diabetes over 20-fold. If baseline BMI was 22–23 kg/m^2, that risk increased nine-fold.

A possible mechanism by which abdominal fat contributes to insulin resistance has been reviewed by Bergman:[31] the greater influx of free fatty acids from abdominal fat into the liver could act as a regulator of insulin levels, decreasing its breakdown and allowing for higher systemic levels. Eventually, insulin resistance develops. A pathway through which obesity causes insulin resistance has recently been discovered in mice, in the form of an adipose tissue-derived hormone named resistin – an important link between the adipocyte and diabetes.[32,33]

In summary, obesity is a major public health threat due to its numerous associated illnesses. An important relationship between obesity and diabetes exists, so preventing and treating diabetes should commence with treating obesity.

Management of obesity

Most doctors and patients would agree that the medical management of obesity is a failure. The modern epidemic of obesity necessarily implies that there is an environmental rather than a metabolic cause promoting prolonged positive energy balance. Treatment should therefore move more into the realm of behavioral psychology,[34] using paradigms taken from treatment of addictive behaviors in order to promote a healthier lifestyle.[35] Doctors still have an important role in encouraging exercise and eating habits,[36] rather than prescribing potentially dangerous 'magic bullets'. In this light, the recent attempts advocating long-term drug treatment for obesity (and when should you stop?) makes poor sense both medically and economically.[37] It is counterproductive and uneducational, deceiving patients into thinking that they have a drug-treatable disease – so that they need not make any effort to change the poor lifestyle that is at the root of obesity. Yet, most trials added drug therapy to lifestyle changes. The behavioral approach to obesity is as successful as that of drugs,[34] has minimal side effects but is obviously less attractive for research support from industry. However, it is surely the direction in which professionals must go in order to try to lessen the tremendous health burden of obesity.[38]

Several options are available for weight reduction: lifestyle modifications, medications or surgery. 'Magic diets' and special food additives are not an option, as most have not been properly proved as beneficial over the long term. This issue will be covered in greater detail below. Additionally, as anyone can lose weight, the hard part is weight maintenance. Therefore, good programs are those presenting long-term weight loss. Guidelines of the International Association for the Study of Obesity only assess treatments with a minimum of one-year follow-up. The relationship between weight loss and improved insulin sensitivity allows us to combat insulin resistance by losing some extra fat. Even a modest weight loss (5–10%) is beneficial, and reduces the major cardiovascular risk factors.[39] In diabetics, weight loss of this magnitude also

reduced levels of insulin, fasting plasma glucose and HbA1c, indicating a better glycemic control over one year of follow-up.[40] Paralleling improvements were also seen in the lipid profile, making modest weight loss an important yet achievable goal. Therefore, one does not have to return to teenage weight, but always aim to shed off a little fat or 'convert' adipose tissue to muscle.

Available therapeutic options for the obese diabetic

The medications currently approved for weight loss act to reduce energy intake, either by reducing appetite or inhibiting fat absorption.[41] Drugs are modestly effective in reducing weight, by an average addition of 2–10 kg to a weight-loss program. The additional weight loss achieved by adding the lipase inhibitor Orlistat, to a low-energy diet had also improved glucose levels across two years of follow-up.[42] Sibutramine, a centrally acting appetite suppressor, could also improve weight loss and concomitant glucose control in diabetics.[43] Currently, antiobesity drugs are not recommended for routine use, and if initiated should be combined with the lifestyle changes described below.[41] Medications are usually prescribed to those with BMI >27 kg/m[2], or with over >30% body fat for women. Patients with lower BMI, but with obesity-related conditions could also receive pharmacological treatment. It is doubtful whether drug treatment should be used for long-term management, as in the above mentioned studies, although the drug industry would like obesity to be considered in the same way as diabetes or hypertension – a disease which only a pill can fix. It is our view that medications should be likened to crutches for a person with a broken leg – temporary help until he/she can manage on their own, and probably for not more than three months. This gives an encouraging 'push', after which the person has to continue the improved lifestyle for weight reduction and maintenance.

Gastric surgery is an efficient method for weight reduction,[44,45] currently reserved for patients with a BMI of >40 kg/m², who clearly understand the need for strict follow-up. Patients with a BMI >35 kg/m² may also be candidates for surgery if they have life-threatening co-morbid conditions or a severe impairment in everyday living. Surgery has also been shown to allow 83% of diabetics to be taken off medications after the procedure.[45] Patients with impaired glucose tolerance had a 30-fold reduction in the risk of progression to diabetes after undergoing surgery, but at eight years follow-up, this reduction narrowed to only five-fold. Though effective, weight loss through surgery may not provide the additional benefits of lifestyle modification, such as proper food selection and engagement in PA. A study comparing weight loss through these two different methods showed that the surgical patients had higher amounts of fat in their food, and lower levels of PA,[46] suggesting that a healthy lifestyle may not have been fully implemented. This can reduce the chances of weight maintenance after surgery in the long term, and could eventually result in returning to the initial weight having gone through a potentially dangerous operation 'for nothing'.

The advantages of lifestyle modification are that it is simple, has no side effects, is potentially long term, and puts weight reduction under the control of the patient. The American Heart Association has set recommendations for prevention of heart disease, elaborating on limiting fat content, advocating engagement in PA and avoiding weight gain and smoking.[47] The nutritional plan for weight loss, which is rich in grains, fruits and vegetables, has additional effects such as decreased incidence of CAD,[47,48] stroke[49] and cancer.[50] The combined lifestyle

measures can offer great protection from coronary events, adding to the effects of weight loss. In the Nurses' Health Study, those who kept a healthy diet, abstained from smoking and exercised regularly, had a reduction of 57% in coronary events compared to those who did not, for the same body mass.[51] Adding the recommended BMI (<25 kg/m²) to the equation further lowered this risk. Among British men, PA, BMI and smoking are modifiable risk factors that greatly influenced the appearance of diabetes and major cardiovascular events.[52] In this study, a 50-year-old British man who had never smoked, was physically active and whose BMI was <24 kg/m², had a 90% chance of reaching the age of 65 without diabetes, stroke or myocardial infarction. A person of the same age but smoking, physically inactive and obese, has less than half that chance of remaining disease free. That the environment brings about most of obesity and diabetes cases was also shown in another follow-up from the Nurses' Health Study: it was calculated that 91% of diabetes cases were attributable to environmental, hence modifiable, causes.[53] Among the protective factors was maintenance of a BMI <25 kg/m², eating a 'healthy' diet, exercising regularly, abstaining from smoking and drinking alcohol moderately.

With all weight reduction methods, compliance to method-specific rules is crucial for the maintenance of the new weight. Overeating after surgery, cessation of drug use or of PA, will eventually lead to a return to the initial weight. Lifestyle modification is essential in maintaining the newly reduced weight, regardless of the method used for the initial weight reduction.

Lifestyle modification – a necessity for the obese diabetic

The safest and most rewarding method of reducing excess weight is through a combination of three arms: proper diet, proper behavioral changes, and adequate PA. A report on the trends of CAD and lifestyle changes among nurses reveals that the incidence of CAD has dropped by 30% between 1980 and 1994.[54] The authors attribute two-thirds of this decline to a healthier lifestyle: better food selection, cessation of smoking, and use of post-menopausal hormone replacement therapy. However, the study reveals an increasing preva-lence of obesity with age, which has attenuated this decline. This was not a specific program, only a report of the habits of this group, which seems to also be affected by the increasing prevalence of obesity in the population. For the glucose intolerant, lifestyle changes can also prevent the onset of diabetes through weight loss.[55] In this cohort of overweight and obese subjects, those who were given weight reduc-tion guidance through diet and PA had reduced their overall risk of developing diabetes by 63% for men and 54% for women.

Some general strategies exist which may help patients comply with their treatment.[56,57] The treatment setting should promote the patient to take an active role in her/his treatment, both in the doctor's office and in program groups. Patient education should include brief explana-tions of regulation of body weight, causes and complications of obesity, and the rate of expected weight loss (about 0.5 kg/week). Guidelines for proper diet and/or referral to a dietitian, along with exercise prescription and/or referral to exercise groups, may also be included, as diabet-ics have special needs in these fields. Certain aspects of behavior should also be modified, as it has a major role in the maintenance of the newly reduced body weight.[58] When observing the behavioral patterns of reduced weight maintainers, factors such as regular PA, spouse and social support, feeling in control of eating and avoiding eating during emotional stress seem to play important roles.[59,60]

Importance of physical activity

PA is recommended for diabetics, both because of its importance in weight loss management and due to its acute and chronic effects on glucose controls.[61,62] Absence of PA and low fitness have been shown to raise mortality risk among healthy[63] and diabetic men;[64] in fact, the obese and fit had a lower risk of death than lean yet unfit men.[63] Increasing levels of PA paralleled with decreasing occurrence of diabetes in British men.[52] Surprisingly, there was no accompanying dose-dependent manner of CAD risk reduction, but still, the active had a lower chance of the disease. The exercisers also had a decreased chance of smoking, or being overweight, heavy drinkers or known CAD patients at baseline. By the end of the 17-year follow-up, the physically active had lower insulin levels and diastolic blood pressure, a better lipid profile and lower chances of CAD diagnosis. In diabetic women also, increased PA offered additional protection against cardiovascular events.[65] Additional evidence from the Nurses' Health Study suggests that in both obese and non-obese, regular PA reduces the risk for developing Type 2 diabetes through the years.[66] Even non-vigorous PA, such as bowling, gardening and household work has been shown to reduce insulin resistance.[67] PA has been shown to reduce hyperinsulinemia and improve insulin peripheral activity in 65-year-old subjects,[68] which shows that even at this age, chronic diseases can be fought through a better lifestyle. As central obesity is a major contributor to insulin resistance, reduction of the former is of utmost impor-tance. Even without weight loss, PA reduced abdominal fat in men.[69] When combined with weight loss, PA reduced insulin resistance in addition. A recent meta-analysis showed that exercise reduced HbA1c levels by an amount that is expected to reduce diabetic complications, without a mean effect on body weight.[70] This further supports the notion that PA has benefits of its own, acting in addition to weight loss. Taken together, the data support that PA should be encouraged in all, due to evidence of reduced mortality, CAD risk and diabetes progression in the physically active.

PA also has a major part in weight reduction programs. In a meta-analysis assessing weight loss programs, the role of exercise was shown to be more important in the long-term rather than in the short-term.[71] When comparing diet only with diet plus exercise programs, on average both yielded the same weight loss at the end of the program – about 11 kg in 15 weeks. Both also showed similar reductions in fat and total body mass. Exercise only resulted in loss of about 3 kg, so compared with the alternatives, it was not an effective way to lose weight. This lack of weight loss could be explained in part by concomitant increases in appetite or in fat-free mass. Another meta-analysis revealed that, in women using a diet-only weight loss program, 24% of the reduction in weight resulted from loss of fat-free mass; while in those on diet plus PA, only 11% of weight reduced was attributed to this tissue.[72] For that reason, adding PA to the diet regimen is recommended, so that more fat can be shed off while conserving the energy-utilizing muscle tissue, thus attenuating the inevitable decrease in basal metabolic expenditure following weight loss. This is a crucial point in the long-term management. Indeed, when observing subjects who maintained their weight loss, it appears that most had integrated PA into their lifestyle (reviewed in ref. 73). This seems to be independent of the method by which weight had been lost. Among various strategies used by reduced-weight maintainers, PA is a major contributor.[58–60] In women, 90% of weight maintainers used PA as an aid, compared with only 34% of weight regainers.[59]

An additional benefit of PA is the enhancement of mood,[74] which is important in improving body image and adherence to the new lifestyle.

We summarize this section by emphasizing that PA is an integral part of any successful weight-loss program. PA should accompany any nutritional therapy, in order to increase the metabolic effects and to prevent loss of fat-free mass.

Nutritional treatment of diabetes mellitus Type 2

The nutritional plan and support for the obese diabetic have three roles. Firstly, given this trail of obesity–diabetes–cardiovascular disease–mortality, one should adhere to the well-established nutritional recommendations of the AHA/ADA.[1,47] This reduces the overall risk for cardiovascular disease consequences, including reduction of blood pressure and blood cholesterol – both accompanying diabetes in the growth of the atherosclerotic plaques. Second, as most Type 2 diabetics are obese, a reduced calorie diet combined with PA for weight loss yields concomitant reductions in insulin resistance and plasma glucose. Finally, there are specific food components, which have an impact on plasma glucose levels, and can therefore be included in the diet.

Reducing CAD risk

On the general nutritional aspect of CAD prevention, specific guidelines have been made public by the American Heart Association.[47] These call for weight management, limiting fat content to <30% of total daily energy intake, and, for diabetics, limiting saturated fat to <7% of energy, and that of cholesterol to <200 mg/day. Additionally, consumption of at least two fish servings per week is advocated, along with an increased intake of fruit and vegetables. Salt and alcohol should also be limited, to a maximum of 6 g of salt per day (equivalent to no added salt at the table), and one alcoholic drink per day for women, two for men. Naturally, cessation of smoking is a given, and it should be strongly discouraged among diabetics in order to reduce oxidative damage to lipoproteins.[75] These recommendations come to prevent further spiraling into the atherosclerotic process and its complications by reducing major risk factors: diabetes, hyperlipidemia, hypertension, overweight, smoking and physical inactivity.

Weight loss

Dieting only is an effective way to lose weight, but not to maintain weight loss.[71] The parallel reduction of muscle mass might lower the metabolic rate and reduce energy expenditure, resulting in lower energy needs. PA can help to restore this energy-utilizing tissue. Reduced-calorie nutrition for weight loss should be part of a slow process that can be maintained in the long term. The rate of weight reduction should approximate 0.5 kg/week, by a combination of a reduced energy diet and PA. As loss of 1 kg of body weight represents a net energy deficit of approximately 7000 kcal, this target may be achieved by about 500 kcal less per day, resulting in a total of −3500 kcal/week. It could be that reducing food intake by 500 kcal/day is much easier than increasing the expense of the same magnitude (for example, one hour of basketball playing), but a combination of increased activity and decreased intake is the optimal method. It is probably advisable for subjects on a diet for longer than a couple of months, to take a regular multivitamin supplement with extra calcium for women. Compliance to the nutritional program can be boosted by allowing at least one free day per week when three 'normal' meals may be consumed without any feelings of 'guilt'.

Specific food components

Even though the nutritional management of the obese diabetic patient requires a reduced calorie diet, the amounts of all major nutrients in the diet should be carefully monitored. The reason is that endless combinations of protein, fat and carbohydrate can be made when constructing a diet – but what is their optimal ratio? Throughout the last century, fat content has been minimized and substituted by carbohydrates (Table 19.1). Even though the nutritional therapy for each patient is individualized, some properties of various nutrients are common for all and can be described. The diet program set by a dietician can emphasize consuming foods with a good nutritional value for the diabetic.

Year	Distribution of calories (%) Carbohydrate	Protein	Fat
1914	10 g/day	(Allen Starvation Treatment)	
1921	20	10	70
1950	40	20	40
1971	45	20	35
1986	<60	12–20	<30
1994	50–60 *	10–20	<30 **

Notes: * based on nutritional assessment and treatment goals; ** additionally, saturated fat <7%, cholesterol <200 mg/day.

Table 19.1

Historical perspective of nutritional recommendations for diabetics. Throughout the last century, there has been a shift from low carbohydrate to high carbohydrate recommendations for diabetics

Protein

ADA recommendations for diabetics do not differ from the recommendations to the general public, of up to 20% protein in the diet.[1] The 'Protein Power' diet recommends even higher amounts of protein. However, care should be taken to ensure that kidney function is normal. With the onset of nephropathy detectable even by microproteinuria, protein amounts should be decreased in order to reduce glomerular filtration. There is no sound base for advising high protein diets at this time, as no scientific evidence has yet been provided for favorable metabolic effects or long-term weight loss and maintenance.[76] A high protein diet will restrict the spectrum of foods allowed, and may result in nutrient deficiency. Poor compliance is another possible result, again due to the limited variety of foods.

Fat content and specific fatty acids

Throughout the last century, the recommended percentage of fat in the diet decreased from 70% to the current <30%.[1] Yet, the importance of lowering dietary fat is still a matter of debate.[77] The problem is that commonly, lowering fat content in the diet results in a rise in carbohydrate content, and not in the anticipated replacement by fruit and vegetable consumption. As a result, triglyceride and small, dense-LDL levels increase while HDL levels decrease, resulting in a more atherogenic lipid profile. If patients are losing weight, then the amount of fat is probably far more important than the type of fat.

There are those who claim obesity should be treated with low amounts of carbohydrate and high levels of fat and protein but most of these dietary regimens have not been scientifically proven, for example, Protein Power or the Atkins Diet. The latter is high in protein and fat but low in carbohydrate, is marketed based on Dr Atkins' '30 years of experience', and

lacks long-term follow-up studies.[78] Looking at 2681 subjects who were successful at weight loss, only 25 consumed a diet low in carbohydrates, as advised by these low carbohydrate diets.[79] In general, low carbohydrate diets contribute to weight loss merely through overall energy restriction (about 500 kcal/day), through a transient diuretic effect, and by suppression of appetite due to high protein content or circulating ketones.[80] These diets may even prove harmful due to many reasons: ketones creating mental impairments, high fat intake causing LDL elevations and arrhythmias, micronutrient deficiencies, kidney stones, osteoporosis and possible renal failure. The elimination of dietary fruit, vegetables and grains from the diet is inconceivable, as these have proved so important in reducing cardiovascular morbidity and mortality.[81,82] A study observing 10,000 subjects has shown that overall diet quality was higher among those consuming a high carbohydrate diet, with an overall lower energy intake.[83] The lowest energy intake was seen among subjects consuming a vegetarian-type diet. Subjects on low-carbohydrate diets consumed twice the amount of saturated fat than those on high carbohydrate diets. Regarding body mass, vegetarians were the leanest, while subjects on low carbohydrate diets had the highest BMI. This comes to show that in general, low carbohydrate diets are not associated with other feasible dietary patterns.

Fatty acids are grouped by their degree of desaturation. It seems that a diet rich in polyunsaturated fatty acids reduces the risk for developing diabetes in healthy women, while saturated and monounsaturated fat in the diet had no effect on this risk.[84] There is emerging evidence for the importance of specific fatty acids on glucose levels. The insulin-releasing effect of fatty acids increases with chain length and decreases with degree of unsaturation.[85]

Additionally, saturated fat elevates insulin resistance, and combined with its hypercholesterolemic effect, this gives a sound basis for limiting its intake, especially among diabetics and those at risk for CAD. Fatty acids have additional effects on the other CAD risk factors,[85,86] so the fat content and type in the diet should be carefully monitored. n-3 Polyunsaturated fatty acids were shown to contribute to but also protect against vascular damage in diabetes, depending on additional fatty acids present.[86] They may be beneficial for the obese diabetic by lowering triglyceride levels and blood pressure, and have been shown to cause less weight gain in mice when compared with mice that consumed an n-6 rich diet. Supplementation with fish oil, a source of n-3 fatty acids, has been shown to decrease triglyceride levels but without an apparent effect on other plasma lipids in Type 2 diabetics.[86] Hence, they may prove useful in the hypertriglyceridemic diabetic. High n-6 diets, which were believed to be beneficial in CAD prevention, may promote LDL oxidation and accelerate its associated atherosclerosis. Additionally, n-6 fatty acids can progressively lead to insulin resistance.[87] Therefore, a diet with a high n-3 to n-6 fatty acids ratio seems advisable.[86,87]

Monounsaturated fat (MUFA), such as in olive oil, is now believed to be the most important fatty acid in dietary prevention of atherosclerosis.[86,88] It works by both lowering cholesterol levels and reducing LDL oxidation, perhaps through its antioxidant properties. Diets rich in MUFA also reduce triglyceride and VLDL levels while increasing HDL levels, when compared with high carbohydrate diets. In a group of 48 volunteers, both high MUFA and high carbohydrate diets reduced the total cholesterol levels. However, the high carbohydrate diet caused a decrease in HDL levels and an increase in TG levels, while the high MUFA diet increased HDL levels.[89] Additionally, these diets also reduced fasting and postprandial glucose levels, and were generally accompanied by a reduction in insulin, but not glipizide, requirements. Therefore, high MUFA diets show a favorable effect on the lipid profile and glucose levels, making these fatty acids an important constituent of dietary fat. However, since the general population cannot eat a daily spoonful of pure MUFA, one should be aware of certain issues. First, increasing the amount of MUFA in the diet might be associated with an increase in consumption of the unwanted trans fatty acids. Hence, it is important for the dietitian to encourage the consumption of MUFA from the *cis* configuration. Second, increasing the amount of fat in the diet might result in weight gain, by increasing energy intake. Therefore, increasing fat intake should accompany a reduction in carbohydrates or proteins.

In summary of the fat issue, saturated fat sources (mostly animal red meat, liver and high fat milk products) should be avoided, while the proportional intake of vegetable, olive and fish oils should be increased. New nutritional recommendations from the AHA call for two or more servings of fish per week, aiming for increased n-3 fat consumption.[47] The resulting effects of proper fat selection can be lowering of plasma LDL, triglycerides, and risk for developing CAD. Still, the underlying problem remains the excess weight. In order to lose weight, we still advise a low fat diet, with its fat sources carefully selected.

Carbohydrates and fiber

The glycemic index, which is not addressed in nutritional recommendations for diabetics, can also have an impact on diabetes incidence and control. This index is the ratio of the area under the curve (AUC) of plasma glucose levels after feeding, relative to eating an equi-carbohydrate portion of white bread (which is considered to have a glycemic index of 100%). The faster glucose is absorbed from the GI tract, the higher the index. Simple carbohydrates are absorbed more rapidly and therefore produce a higher glycemic response. Consuming a diet with a high dietary glycemic index was found to be associated with a higher risk for development of Type 2 diabetes in large cohorts of men[90] and women.[91] A low amount of fiber in the diet also had this unwanted effect. Combining a diet containing a high glycemic index with low fiber further increased this risk to be twice that found in the other extreme (low glycemic index with high fiber). It has also been shown that consumption of foods with a lower glycemic index was associated with a higher HDL level.[92] This effect was true after regarding other factors that influence HDL levels and after correction for total carbohydrate intake.

A crossover study, in which 13 diabetics consumed a diet with increased fiber, reinforced the recommendation for increased amounts of fiber in the diabetic patient's nutrition.[93] In comparison with a control diet containing 24 g of fiber, when subjects consumed 50 g of fiber, glucose and insulin levels dropped by 10 and 12%, respectively. Additionally, triglyceride, total- and VLDL cholesterol levels were lower at the time of high fiber consumption. The difference between LDL and HDL cholesterol levels did not reach statistical significance.

In summary of the carbohydrate issue, the total amount of carbohydrates recommended is still a subject of controversy. Nowadays, there is a tendency to reduce their total amount in order to receive a close to normal glycemic response and a better lipid profile. The actual amount of carbohydrates should be decided on an individualized basis according to the weight, blood glucose levels, lipid profile and, ultimately, compliance of the diabetic person. Carbohydrate consumption throughout the day should be regulated according to the medications taken, and according to the blood glucose levels. There should be a tendency toward a meal plan with a lower glycemic index. Among factors that influence the glycemic index of foods, processing is one. Generally, the less the grains are processed- the lower the glycemic index. Hence, it is better to choose food from natural sources as a carbohydrate source, and to use whole grains and seeds with their high fiber content and low glycemic index.

Specific micronutrients

There are many micronutrients shown to be of value for the diabetic, whether by influencing glucose levels and insulin resistance, reducing neuropathy and retinopathy, or other mechanisms; some common ones being chromium, magnesium, vitamins B, C and E, lipoic acid, and herbs such as *Atriplex hallimus*, bitter melon, soybeans, garlic and fenugreek. Although study results are still inconclusive, some evidence exists as to the potential for using these inexpensive and relatively safe methods for diabetes control. For example: 500 µg of chromium have been shown to improve HbA1c levels; garlic extracts improved diabetic condition in rats to the same extent as insulin; lipoic acid improved peripheral and autonomic neuropathy.[94] Additional studies on this matter will surely emerge, as tight diabetes control requires all the methods we can recruit.

Conclusion

The current epidemic of obesity and diabetes is a direct consequence of prolonged positive energy balance. Some medical conditions brought about by obesity and reversed by

	Obesity	Weight loss	Physical activity/ fitness
Mortality			
Overall	⇑	⇓	⇓
Cardiovascular	⇑	⇓	⇓
CAD events	⇑	⇓	⇓
Type 2 diabetes	⇑	⇓	⇓
Insulin resistance	⇑	⇓	⇓
Glucose control	⇓	⇑	⇑
HTN risk	⇑	⇓	⇓
Dyslipidemia	⇑	⇓	⇓
Stroke risk	⇑	⇓	⇓
Gallbladder disease	⇑	⇓	⇓
Cancer	⇑	⇓	⇓
Breast	⇑	⇓	⇓
Colon	⇑	⇓	⇓
Lung	⇑	⇓	⇓
Osteoarthritis*	⇑	⇓	⇓

Notes: CAD coronary artery disease; HTN hypertension. * in a carefully planned program

Table 19.2
Several common conditions influenced by gain or loss of body weight and physical activity/ physical fitness

weight loss or PA are presented in Table 19.2. In theory, the disease and its complications may be reversed, and medications reduced, by appropriate lifestyle changes in PA and nutrition. In this context, reducing the amounts consumed are of far more importance than the effects of specific nutrients – whether fatty acids or carbohydrates. The problem is that successful weight loss is beyond the capabilities of the vast majority of patients and thus, the conclusion must follow that the medical management of obesity is by and large a failure. Until behavioral and other techniques, as well as pharmacological modalities are improved, the diabetes care-giver has to use a combination of diet, exercise, drugs and insulin to achieve optimal glycemic control. Lifestyle changes require a new paradigm in the doctor–patient relationship where the doctor becomes more of an advisor/coach, and the patient must be more active and take more responsibility for his or her health and adherence to treatment. Contract relationships and shared decision making are appropriate and the nursing staff and dietitians are the most suitable case managers for these objectives. Such treatment needs to involve the skills practised by behavioral and psychological professionals in the management of smoking addiction or substance abuse. These topics must become part of the medical school and health sciences curriculum, while primary care facilities should widen the range of care-givers to include these professions to complement the efforts of the general practitioners. Group treatment is probably the most cost-effective treatment approach.

Thus, the public health challenge for the coming decades is how to motivate people to live more healthy lives. This makes both medical and economic sense, for the diseases of lifestyle are eminently preventable.

Note: The American Diabetes Association issued new nutrition guidelines for diabetes (Evidence-based nutrition principles and recommendations for the treatment and prevention of diabetes and related complications, Diabetes Care 25; 202–12, 2002 and Supplement 1). Over 50 statements were made and they were ranked according to the supporting evidence. Of the statements, 16 had the highest A rating from well-conducted studies, 17 received a B, 3 a C and 15 received an E representing recommendations based on expert opinion only. Thus, one-third of the recommendations are not necessarily based on strong evidence and therefore the area of diet and diabetes still requires more research.

References

1. American Diabetes Association. Nutrition recommendations and principles for people with diabetes mellitus (position statement). Diabetes Care 2000; 24: S44–S47.
2. Haffner SM, Lehto S, Ronnemma T et al. Mortality from coronary heart disease in subjects with Type 2 diabetes and in nondiabetic patients with and without prior myocardial infarction. N Engl J Med 1998; 339: 229–34.
3. World Health Organization. Obesity: preventing and managing the global epidemic. Report of a WHO consultation on obesity. Geneva: World Health Organization, 1998.
4. Eckel RE, Krauss RM. American Heart Association call to action: obesity as a major risk factor for coronary heart disease. Circulation 1998; 97: 2099–100.
5. Kuczmarski RJ, Carroll MD, Flegal KM et al. Varying body mass index cutoff points to describe overweight prevalence among US adults: NHANES III (1988–1994). Obes Res 1997; 5: 542–8.
6. Mokdad AH, Serdula MK, Dietz WH et al. The continuing epidemic of obesity in the United States. JAMA 2000; 284: 1650–1.
7. Beer-Borst S, Morabia A, Hercberg S et al. Obesity and other health determinants across Europe: The EURALIM project. J Epidemiol Community Health 2000; 54: 424–30.
8. Perusse L, Chagnon YC, Weisnagel SJ et al. The human obesity gene map: The 2000 update. Obes Res 2001; 9: 135–69.
9. Hill JO, Peters JC. Environmental contributions to the obesity epidemic. Science 1998; 280: 1371–4.
10. Luke A, Rotimi CN, Adeyemo AA et al. Comparability of resting energy expenditure in Nigerians and US blacks. Obes Res 2000; 8: 351–9.
11. Steinberger J, Moran A, Hong C et al. Adiposity in childhood predicts obesity and insulin resistance in young adulthood. J Pediatr 2001; 138: 469–73.
12. Ludwig DS, Ebbeling CB. Type 2 diabetes mellitus in children. JAMA 2001; 286: 1427–30.
13. Allison DB, Fontaine KR, Manson JE et al. Annual deaths attributable to obesity in the United States. JAMA 1999; 282: 1530–8.
14. Calle EE, Thun MJ, Petrelli JM et al. Body mass index and mortality in a prospective cohort of US adults. N Engl J Med 1999; 341: 1097–105.
15. Shaper AG, Wannamethee SG, Walker M. Body weight: implications for the prevention of coronary heart disease, stroke and diabetes mellitus in a cohort study of middle aged men. BMJ 1997; 314: 1311–14.
16. Willett WC, Manson JE, Stampfer MJ et al. Weight, weight change and coronary heart disease in women. Risk within the 'normal' weight range. JAMA 1995; 273: 461–5.
17. Must A, Spadano J, Coakley EH et al. The disease burden associated with overweight and obesity. JAMA 1999; 282: 1523–9.
18. National Task Force on the Prevention and Treatment of Obesity. Overweight, obesity and health risk. Ann Intern Med 2000; 160: 898–904.
19. Van den Brandt PA, Spiegelman D, Yaun SS et al. Pooled analysis of prospective cohort studies on height, weight, and breast cancer risk. Am J Epidemiol 2000; 152: 514–27.
20. Austin H, Austin JM, Partridge EE et al. Endometrial cancer, obesity, and body fat distribution. Cancer Res 1991; 51: 568–72.
21. Terry P, Baron JA, Weiderpass E et al. Lifestyle and endometrial cancer risk: a cohort study from the Swedish twin registry. Int J Cancer 1999; 82: 38–42.
22. Giovannucci E, Colditz GA, Stampfer MJ et al. Physical activity, obesity, and risk of colorectal adenoma in women. Cancer Causes Control 1996; 7: 253–63.
23. Giovannucci E, Ascherio A, Rimm EB et al. Physical activity, obesity and risk for colon cancer and adenoma in men. Ann Intern Med 1995; 122: 327–34.
24. Lagergren J, Bergstrom R, Nyren O. Association between body mass and adenocarcinoma of the esophagus and gastric cardia. Ann Intern Med 1999; 130: 883–90.
25. Vogelzang NJ, Stadler WM. Kidney cancer. Lancet 1998; 352: 1691–6.
26. Raucher GH, Mayne ST, Janerich DT. Relation between body mass index and lung cancer risk in men and women never and former smokers. Am J Epidemiol 2000; 152: 506–13.
27. Wolk A, Gridley G, Svensson M et al. A prospective study of obesity and cancer risk. Cancer Causes Control 2001; 12: 13–21.

28. Mokdad AH, Ford ES, Bowman BA et al. Diabetes trends in the US: 1990–1998. Diabetes Care 2000; 23: 1278–83.

29. Colditz GA, Willett WC, Rotnitzky A et al. Weight gain as a risk factor for clinical diabetes mellitus in women. Ann Intern Med 1995; 122: 481–6.

30. Chan JM. Obesity, fat distribution, and weight gain as risk factors for clinical diabetes in men. Diabetes Care 1994; 17: 961–9.

31. Bergman RN. Non-esterified fatty acids and the liver: why is insulin secreted into the portal vein? Diabetologia 2000; 43: 946–52.

32. Steppan CM, Bailey ST, Bhat S et al. The hormone resistin links obesity to diabetes. Nature 2001; 409: 307–12.

33. Shuldiner AR, Yang R, Gong DW. Resistin, obesity and insulin resistance – the emerging role of the adipocyte as an endocrine organ. N Engl J Med 2001; 345: 1345–6.

34. Wing RR, Goldstein MG, Acton KJ et al. Behavioral science research in diabetes: lifestyle changes related to obesity, eating behavior, and physical activity. Diabetes Care 2001; 24: 117–123.

35. Prochaska JO, DiClemente CC, Norcross GC. In search of how people change. Am Psychol 1992; 47: 1102–14.

36. Rollnick S, Heather N, Bell A. Negotiating behavior change in medical settings: the development of brief motivational interviewing. J Mental Health 1992; 1: 25–37.

37. Berry EM. Drug therapy for management of obesity. Lancet 2001; 357: 1287.

38. Thompson D, Edelsberg J, Colditz GA et al. Lifetime health and economic consequences of obesity. Arch Intern Med 1999; 159: 2177–83.

39. Mertens IL, Van Gaal LF. Overweight, obesity and blood pressure: the effects of modest weight reduction. Obes Res 2000; 8: 270–8.

40. Wing RR, Koeske R, Epstein LH et al. Long term effects of modest weight loss in Type 2 diabetic patients. Arch Intern Med 1987; 147: 1749–53.

41. National Task Force on the Prevention and Treatment of Obesity. Long term pharmacotherapy in the management of obesity. JAMA 1996; 1907–15.

42. Heymsfield SB, Segal KR, Hauptman J et al. Effects of weight loss with Orlistat on glucose tolerance and progression to Type 2 diabetes in obese adults. Arch Intern Med 2000; 160: 1321–6.

43. Fujioka K, Seaton TB, Rowe E et al. Weight loss with sibutramine improves glycemic control and other metabolic parameters in obese patients with Type 2 diabetes mellitus. Diabetes Obes Metabol 2000; 2: 175–87.

44. Gastrointestinal surgery for severe obesity. NIH Consensus Statement 1991; 9: 1–20.

45. Pinkney JH, Sjostrom CD, Gale EAM. Should surgeons treat diabetes in severely obese people? Lancet 2001; 357: 1357–59.

46. Klem ML, Wing RR, Chang CC et al. A case–control study of successful maintenance of a substantial weight loss: individuals who lost weight through surgery versus those who lost weight through non-surgical means. Int J Obes Relat Metab Disord 2000; 24: 573–9.

47. Krauss RM, Eckel RH, Howard B et al. AHA dietary guidelines. Circulation 2000; 102: 2296–311.

48. Liu S, Manson JE, Lee IM et al. Fruit and vegetable intake and risk of cardiovascular disease: the Women's Health Study. Am J Clin Nutr 2000; 4: 922–8.

49. Liu S, Manson JE, Stampfer MJ et al. Whole grain consumption and risk of ischemic stroke in women. JAMA 2000; 284: 1534–40.

50. Glade MJ. Food, nutrition and the prevention of cancer: a global perspective. Nutrition 1999; 15: 523–6.

51. Stampfer MJ, Hu FB, Manson JE et al. Primary prevention of coronary heart disease in women through diet and lifestyle. N Engl J Med 2000; 343: 16–22.

52. Wannamethee SG, Shaper AG, Walker MA, Ebrahim S. Lifestyle and 15 year survival free of heart attack, stroke and diabetes in middle aged British men. Arch Intern Med 1998; 158: 2433–40.

53. Hu FB, Manson JE, Stampfer MJ et al. Diet, lifestyle, and the risk of Type 2 diabetes mellitus in women. N Engl J Med 2001; 345: 790–7.

54. Hu FB, Stampfer MJ, Manson JE et al. Trends in the incidence of coronary heart disease and changes in diet and lifestyle in women. N Engl J Med 2000; 343: 530–7.

55. Tuomilehto J, Lindstrom J, Erikkson JG et al. Prevention of Type 2 diabetes mellitus by changes

in lifestyle among subjects with impaired glucose tolerance. N Engl J Med 2001; 344: 1343–50.

56. Berry EM. Strategies to improve patient compliance in the management of obesity. In: Oomura Y, et al, eds. Progress in Obesity Research. London: John Libbey & Co Ltd, 1990.

57. Brownell KD, Fairburn CG, eds. Eating Disorders and Obesity. New York: The Guildford Press, 1995.

58. McGuire MT, Wing RR, Klem ML et al. Behavioral strategies of individuals who have maintained long-term weight losses. Obes Res 1999; 7: 334–41.

59. Kayman S, Brovold W, Stern JS. Maintenance and relapse after weight loss in women: behavioral aspects. Am J Clin Nutr 1990; 52: 800–7.

60. Lavery MA, Loewy JW. Identifying predictive variables for long-term weight change after participation in a weight loss program. J Am Diet Assoc 1993; 93: 1017–24.

61. American College of Sports Medicine Position Stand. Exercise and Type 2 diabetes. Med Sci Sports Exer 2001; 32: 1345–60.

62. American Diabetes Association. Diabetes mellitus and exercise (position statement). Diabetes Care 2000; 24: S51–S55. See also www.diabetes.org, Clinical Practice Recommendations, accessed Sept 2001.

63. Lee CD, Blair SN, Jackson AS. Cardiorespiratory fitness, body composition, and all-cause and cardiovascular disease mortality in men. Am J Clin Nutr 1999; 69: 373–80.

64. Wei M, Gibbons LW, Kampert JB et al. Low cardiorespiratory fitness and physical inactivity as predictors of mortality in men with Type 2 diabetes. Ann Intern Med 2000; 132: 605–11.

65. Hu FB, Stampfer MJ, Solomon C et al. Physical activity and risk for cardiovascular events in diabetic women. Ann Intern Med 2001; 134: 96–105.

66. Manson JE, Rimm EB, Stampfer MJ et al. Physical activity and incidence of non-insulin dependant diabetes mellitus in women. Lancet 1991; 338: 774–8.

67. Mayer-Davis EJ, D'Agostino R, Karter AJ et al. Intensity and amount of physical activity in relation to insulin sensitivity. JAMA 1998; 279: 669–74.

68. Kirwan JP, Kohrt WM, Wojta DM et al. Endurance exercise training reduces glucose-stimulated insulin levels in 60 to 70 year old men and women. J Gerontol 1993; 48: M84–90.

69. Ross R, Dagnone D, Jones PJH et al. reduction in obesity and related comorbid conditions after diet-induced weight loss or exercise-induced weight loss in men. Ann Intern Med 2000; 133: 92–103.

70. Boule NG, Haddad E, Kenny GP et al. Effects of exercise on glycemic control and body mass in Type 2 diabetes. JAMA 2001; 286: 1218–27.

71. Miller WC, Koceja DM, Hamilton EJ. A meta-analysis of the past 25 years of weight loss research using diet, exercise or diet plus exercise intervention. Int J Obes Relat Metab Disord 1997; 21: 941–7.

72. Ballor DL, Poehlman ET. Exercise training enhances fat-free mass preservation during diet-induced weight loss: a meta-analytical finding. Int J Obes Relat Metabol Disord 1994; 18: 35–40.

73. Votruba SB, Horvitz MA, Schoeller DA. The role of exercise in the treatment of obesity. Nutrition 2000; 16: 179–88.

74. Dubnov G, Berry EM. Physical activity and mood: the endocrine connection. In: Warren MP, Constantini NW, eds. Sports Endocrinology. Totowa, New Jersey: Humana Press, 2000: 421–31.

75. American Diabetes Association. Smoking and diabetes (position statement). Diabetes Care 2000; 24: S64–S65. See also www.diabetes.org, Clinical Practice Recommendations, accessed Sept 2001.

76. St Jeor ST, Howard BV, Prewitt TE et al. Dietary protein and weight reduction. Circulation 2001; 104: 1869–74.

77. Taubes G. The soft science of dietary fat. Science 2001; 291: 2536–45.

78. Well-known diet gurus square off at ACC 2001. ACC Scientific Session News 2001; 19: 5.

79. Wyatt HR, Seagle HM, Grunwald GK et al. Long term weight loss and very low carbohydrate diets in the National Weight Control Registry. Obes Res 2000; 8 Suppl 1: 87S.

80. Denke MA. Metabolic effects of high–protein, low-carbohydrate diets. Am J Cardiol 2001; 88: 59–61.

81. deLorgeril M, Salen P, Martin JL et al. Mediterranean diet, traditional risk factors and the rate of cardiovascular complications after

myocardial infarction. Final report of the Lyon Diet Heart Study. Circulation 1999; 99: 779–85.

82. Singh RB, Dubnov G, Niaz MA et al. The effect of an Indo-Mediterranean diet on the progression of coronary artery disease in high risk patients: the Indo-Mediterranean Diet Heart Study. Lancet 2002; in press.

83. Kennedy ET, Bowman SA, Spence JT et al. Popular diets: correlation to health, nutrition and obesity. J Am Diet Assoc 2001; 101: 411–20.

84. Salmeron J, Hu FB, Manson JE et al. Dietary fat intake and risk of Type 2 diabetes in women. Am J Clin Nutr 2001; 73: 1019–26.

85. Kris-Etherton P, Daniels SR, Eckel RH et al. Summary of the scientific conference on dietary fatty acids and cardiovascular health. Circulation 2000; 103: 1034–9.

86. Berry EM. Dietary fatty acids in the management of diabetes mellitus. Am J Clin Nutr 1997; 66 Supp): 991S–7S.

87. Berry EM. Are diets high in omega-6 polyunsaturated fatty acids unhealthy? Eur Heart J Supplements 2001; 3: D37–41.

88. Garg, A. High monounsaturated fat diets for patients with diabetes mellitus: a meta-analysis. Am J Clin Nutr 1998; 67 Suppl: 577S-82S.

89. Mensink RP, Katan MB. Effect of monounsaturated fatty acids versus complex carbohydrates on high-density lipoproteins in healthy men and women. Lancet 1987; 1: 122–5.

90. Salmeron J, Ascherio A, Rimm EB et al. Dietary fiber, glycemic load, and risk of NIDDM in men. Diabetes Care 1997; 20: 545–50.

91. Salmeron J, Manson JE, Stampfer MJ et al. Dietary fiber, glycemic load, and risk of non-insulin dependent diabetes mellitus in women. JAMA 1997; 277: 472–7.

92. Ford ES, Liu S. Glycemic index and serum high-density lipoprotein cholesterol concentration among US adults. Arch Intern Med 2001; 161: 572–6.

93. Chandalia M, Garg A, Lutjohann D et al. Beneficial effects of high dietary fiber intake in patients with Type 2 diabetes mellitus. N Engl J Med 2000; 342: 1392–8.

94. Morelli V, Zoorob, RJ. Alternative therapies: Part 1. Depression, diabetes, obesity. Am Fam Phys 2000; 62: 1051–60.

20

Insulin analogues and the treatment of diabetes

Alice YY Cheng, Bernard Zinman

Introduction

The discovery of insulin in 1921 by Banting, Best, Collip and MacLeod at the University of Toronto is felt to be one of the greatest achievements of modern medicine. Collip purified the substance isolated from dog pancreas sufficiently for human administration and Leonard Thompson was the first patient with diabetes to receive insulin on 11 January 1922 at the Toronto General Hospital.[1] The substance was further purified and soon became commercially available and revolutionized the treatment of diabetes. Members of the original team received the Nobel Prize in Medicine for their achievement.

The insulin available at that time was short-acting and three or four injections were required to ensure adequate insulin concentrations. The need for a longer-acting insulin led to the discovery by Hagedorn in 1936 that the addition of fish protamine would delay the absorption of insulin from subcutaneous sites.[2] Shortly thereafter, Scott and Fisher found that the addition of zinc to protamine insulin further extended its action.[3] In 1946, neutral protamine Hagedorn (NPH) was introduced and remains in use today as an intermediate-acting insulin.[4]

The next major advance in insulin therapy was the use of recombinant DNA technology to commercially produce human insulin in the 1980s.[5] Prior to that, only bovine or porcine insulins were available which resulted in significant allergic reactions and antibody formation

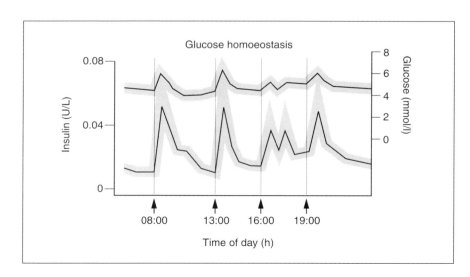

Figure 20.1
Plasma glucose and insulin levels in healthy individuals. Source: reprinted with permission from Elsevier Science from Owens et al. Lancet 2001; 358: 739–46.[7]

in certain patients. The widespread use of human insulins has generally made animal insulins obsolete.

Despite these advances in insulin formulation, production and purity, the goal of achieving physiologic insulin replacement remained elusive (Figure 20.1).[6] The available insulins when administered subcutaneously were unable to adequately mimic the physiologic characteristics of insulin secretion from the pancreas in response to meal and the overnight fasting state. Therefore, in the 1990s, insulin analogues were introduced.[8] They were biologically engineered to have certain pharmacodynamic and pharmacokinetic properties to behave better as bolus (premeal) or basal insulins.[7] The principal rapid-acting insulin analogues available today include insulin lispro (B28 Lys, B29 Pro) and insulin aspart (B28 Asp). The principal long-acting insulin analogues include glargine (A21 Gly, B31 Arg, B32 Arg) and insulin detemir (NN-304). These

insulin analogues and their use will be discussed in detail in this chapter.

Human insulin

Before discussing insulin analogues, it is important to review the structure and function of human insulin. Endogenous insulin is synthesized in the beta cells of the islets of Langerhans in the pancreas. Preproinsulin is converted to proinsulin, an 86-amino acid polypeptide including A- and B-chains of the insulin molecule plus a connecting segment known as C-peptide. The proinsulin molecule is cleaved and the result is a 51-amino acid insulin molecule and a 31-amino acid C-peptide. The insulin molecule consists of a 21-amino acid A-chain and a 30-amino acid B-chain joined by two disulfide bonds and a third disulfide bridge within the A-chain (Figure 20.2).[6] Human insulin molecules aggregate in solution and

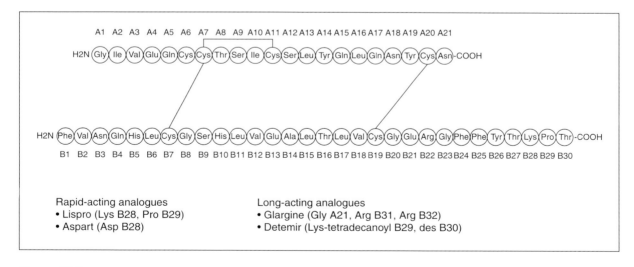

Figure 20.2

The amino acid sequence and structure of human insulin. The A-chain and B-chain are joined by two disulfide bonds and a third disulfide bridge is present within the A-chain.

Insulin	Onset of action	Peak of action	Duration of action
Mealtime insulins			
Lispro	10–15 minutes	1–1.5 hours	3–5 hours
Aspart[a]	10–15 minutes	1–2 hours	3–5 hours
Regular	15–60 minutes	2–4 hours	5–8 hours
Basal insulins			
NPH	2.5–3 hours	5–7 hours	13–16 hours
Lente	2.5–3 hours	7–12 hours	Up to 18 hours
Ultralente	3–4 hours	8–10 hours	Up to 20 hours
Detemir[b]	2–3 hours	No peak	Up to 24 hours
Glargine[c]	2–3 hours	No peak	Up to 30 hours

Source: Adapted from Heinemann et al.[9]
Notes: [a]Data from Mudaliar et al.[53]; [b]Data from Heinemann et al.[84]; [c]Data from Heinemann et al.[70]

Table 20.1
Approximate pharmacokinetic properties of human insulin and insulin analogues following subcutaneous injection

form dimers and hexamers, which delay the absorption from the subcutaneous space. The more stable the hexamer, the slower the absorption. Therefore, regular human insulin has an onset of action of 15–60 minutes with a peak at 2–4 hours and lasts for 5–8 hours. NPH, lente and ultralente are modified insulins and have an onset of action of 2.5–4 hours, peak at 5–10 hours and last up to 20 hours (Table 20.1).[9,10]

Rapid-acting insulin analogues

Insulin lispro (B28 Lys, B29 Pro)

Lispro was the first insulin analogue to become commercially available. It was approved for clinical use in the USA and Europe in 1996.[11]

Structure
The natural sequence of proline at position 28 of the B-chain (B28) and lysine at B29 is reversed in insulin lispro (see Figure 20.2). This amino acid switch causes a conformational change that reduces insulin self-association. Therefore, the dimer association factor is reduced by a factor of 300 compared to regular insulin.[12] Despite the conformational change in the insulin molecule, the affinity of lispro for the insulin receptor is similar to that of regular insulin. The affinity of lispro to the IGF-1 receptor is 1.5 times that of regular insulin but still only 10% that of IGF-1 and as a consequence, cell growth is stimulated to the same extent as regular insulin.[13]

Time-action profile
The reduced affinity for insulin lispro to self-associate accounts for its rapid absorption, onset of action, peak action and shorter duration of action. In euglycaemic clamp studies in healthy subjects, subcutaneous administration of equivalent doses of lispro produced nearly twice the peak serum insulin concentration in half the time with a faster decrease to basal levels compared to regular insulin. The glucose infusion rate (GIR) required to maintain euglycaemia followed a

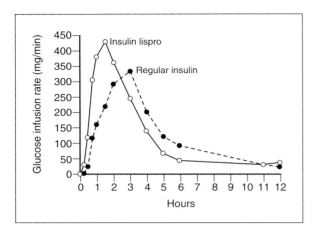

Figure 20.3
Glucose infusion rate to maintain euglycaemia after subcutaneous injection of insulin lispro in normal subjects. Source: reprinted with permission from Holleman et al. N Engl J Med 1997; 337: 176–83.[11] © 1997 Massachusetts Medical Society. All rights reserved.

similar pattern, although the total amount of glucose infused was similar in the lispro and regular insulin groups suggesting that the hypoglycaemic potencies are equivalent (Figure 20.3). The onset of action of lispro is approximately 10–15 minutes with a peak at 1–1.5 hours and duration of action of approximately 3–5 hours.[14] The time to peak action appears to be much less dependent on insulin dose unlike regular insulin with less interpatient variability.[15,16]

Clinical use
A number of studies have looked at the use of lispro in both Type 1 and Type 2 diabetes. Since its approval for clinical use in 1996, its popularity has grown substantially. Its short onset of action, quick peak and short duration of action makes it ideal for mealtimes. It fact, it is felt to be the bolus (mealtime) insulin of choice in multiple daily injection regimens. Studies have shown decreased incidence of

postprandial and nocturnal hypoglycaemia and improved postprandial plasma glucose levels in patients with Type 1 and Type 2 diabetes.[17–28] A recent meta-analysis with 2,576 patients with Type 1 diabetes showed a 30% relative risk reduction of severe hypoglycaemic episodes, defined as coma or requiring glucagon or intravenous glucose, in the lispro-treated group compared to regular insulin.[17] Since lispro acts so quickly, it should be administered at the time of the meal, unlike regular insulin which should be administered 30 minutes before the meal. This allows for much more flexibility of mealtimes and daily activities. This may partially account for the significant improvements in quality of life with lispro noted in both adults and adolescents.[20,23,29] However, controversy remains over the impact of lispro on overall glycaemic control in multiple daily injection (MDI) regimens compared to regular insulin. Some studies have shown no improvements in HbA1c but confirmed the decreased incidence of hypoglycaemia and improved quality of life.[22–25,27,28] Others have shown a significant decrease in HbA1c with use of lispro as compared to regular insulin in MDI.[18–21,30] One of the possible explanations for this discrepancy may be the different basal insulin replacement utilized in the various MDI regimens. Since lispro is such a short-acting insulin, insufficient basal replacement may cause periods of hyperglycaemia, counteracting the benefits of the postprandial glycaemic control.[30] Studies that have shown reductions in HbA1c also noted increased frequency of basal insulin use up to three times per day.[18,19,30] Either NPH or ultralente can be used as the basal insulin with lispro in an MDI regimen, although one study suggested a trend towards reduced HbA1c in patients receiving two injections of NPH per day compared to twice-daily ultralente.[31] Lispro can be mixed with NPH as long as the mixture is given shortly after it is drawn up.[32] Two recent studies have looked at the impact of lispro on glycaemic control and incidence of hypoglycaemia in a clinic setting. Chatterjee et al. demonstrated a significant reduction in HbA1c from 9.11 +/– 0.15% to 8.56 +/– 0.19% and significant reduction in incidence of hypoglycaemia after six months of therapy with lispro in 221 patients with Type 1 and Type 2 diabetes being treated in a clinic in the UK.[20] Chase et al. followed a cohort of patients presenting to a diabetes centre in the USA and noted a significant reduction in HbA1c after the release of the Diabetes Control and Complications Trial report in 1993, accompanied by a significant increase in hypoglycaemia and a further reduction in HbA1c after the introduction of lispro in 1996 without an increase in hypoglycaemia.[21] Neither of these studies were randomized controlled trials but they do provide evidence that the benefits seen in the clinical trials can be translated into real life clinic situations.

Continuous subcutaneous insulin infusion (CSII) with an external pump is currently our best tool to try to mimic physiologic insulin replacement. A number of investigators from Canada, France, Germany, Sweden and the USA have shown that lispro is superior to regular insulin in CSII, both in terms of overall glycaemic control and number of hypoglycaemic events.[33–38] Thus, lispro is the insulin of choice for CSII. When there is an interruption in insulin delivery by the pump, patients receiving lispro have a more rapid metabolic deterioration but they also have a more rapid recovery compared to regular human insulin.[39]

Safety

Pregnancy was an exclusion criteria in most of the lispro studies, so there is little clinical trial data regarding the use of lispro in pregnancy.[8,11,40] Jovanovic et al. compared the use of lispro to regular human insulin in 42 women with gestational diabetes. Anti-insulin antibody levels were similar in both groups. Lispro was not detected in the cord blood. Mean fasting and postprandial glucose concentrations and HbA1c levels were similar but the lispro group experienced fewer hypoglycaemic episodes. No fetal or neonatal abnormalities were noted in either group. The authors of the study concluded that lispro was safe to use in gestational diabetes.[41] However, the use of lispro in pregnant patients with Type 1 diabetes has come under question because of a recent report implicating lispro in the development of proliferative retinopathy during pregnancy in three of ten women with initial normal ophthalmologic examinations.[42] Other reports have shown no increase in development of proliferative retinopathy. Bhattacharyya et al. reported no progression in 15 women with Type 1 diabetes and Buchbinder et al. reported no progression in 12 women treated with lispro and progression in 6 of 42 women treated with regular insulin.[43,44] Unfortunately, the sample sizes in all of the reports are small and therefore it is difficult to draw any firm conclusions from them. Importantly, lispro has now been approved for use in pregnancy and is commonly employed in this context.

Lispro has also been studied in patients with end-stage renal disease. It has a similar time-action profile in patients on haemodialysis and also causes less hypoglycaemia.[45] It can safely be administered intraperitoneally for patients on peritoneal dialysis.

Overall, lispro has been found to be safe in patients with diabetes with few adverse effects or allergic reactions.[40] In fact, there have been several case reports of lispro being used to treat patients with severe insulin allergy.[46–49] It has been proposed that lispro may be less antigenic and have beneficial effects in immunogenic complications.[47] It has also been suggested that

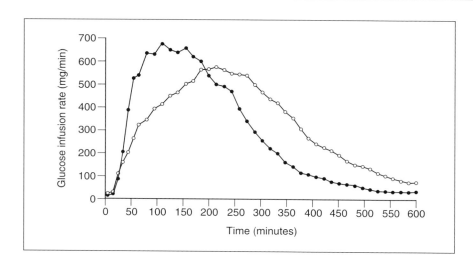

Figure 20.4
Glucose infusion rate to maintain euglycaemia after subcutaneous injection of aspart (●) and regular insulin (○). Source: reprinted with permission from Mudaliar et al. Diabetes Care 1999; 22: 1501–6.[53] © 1999 American Diabetes Association.

the faster absorption may lead to less immunogenicity.[48,49] There have also been case reports of severe insulin resistance, presumably on the basis of antibodies being effectively treated with frequent injections of lispro.[50,51]

Insulin aspart (B28 Asp)

Structure
Insulin aspart is another rapid-acting insulin analogue. The proline in position 28 of the B-chain is replaced by aspartic acid. This amino acid change reduces the tendency of the insulin molecule to self-associate into hexamers. The negative charge of aspartic acid creates a repulsion between it and other negatively charged amino acids and discourages self-association.[7,8] The affinity of aspart to the insulin receptor is similar to that of human insulin.[7,8] Its affinity to the IGF-1 receptor is also similar to that of human insulin which is considerably less than that of IGF-1 itself.[52]

Time-action profile
In euglycaemic clamp studies in healthy subjects, serum insulin levels peaked nearly twice as fast and more than twice as high with subcutaneous administration of aspart compared to regular human insulin. The maximal glucose infusion rate (GIR) was also greater and occurred at an earlier time. However, the duration of action was shorter than that of regular insulin (Figure 20.4).[53–56] The onset of action was within 10–15 minutes with a peak at 1–2 hours and a duration of action between 3 and 5 hours.[53] This time-action profile is very similar to that of lispro. Aspart injected into the abdomen appears to be absorbed more quickly than deltoid or thigh injections.[53] This time-action profile has also been confirmed in children and adolescents with Type 1 diabetes.[56]

Clinical use
The time-action profile of insulin aspart also makes it an ideal insulin to be used premeal as a bolus insulin. A number of clinical studies have shown improved postprandial glycaemic control and less hypoglycaemia with the use of aspart in MDI regimens in Type 1 diabetes.[57–61] In Type 2 diabetes, similar improvements in postprandial glycaemic control have been found.[62,63] As with lispro, aspart should be administered at the time of the meal, not 30

minutes premeal as with regular human insulin. This provides much more mealtime flexibility and partially accounts for the significant improvement in quality of life demonstrated in patients with Type 1 diabetes receiving aspart.[64] Despite the improvements in postprandial glycaemic control and reduction in frequency of hypoglycaemia, the effect of aspart in MDI on overall glycaemic control remains controversial. As with lispro, the overall glycaemic control may be more reflective of the appropriate use of basal insulin with the meal analogue. In the studies showing improvement in HbA1c, multiple injections and higher doses of basal insulin were required.[59-61] As with lispro, insulin aspart can be mixed with NPH in the syringe as long the mixture is administered promptly.[65]

Its use in CSII has also been studied. A recent single-centre randomized open-label study of insulin aspart compared to regular insulin in CSII for seven weeks demonstrated fewer hypoglycaemic events per person but no significant difference in glycaemic control in the aspart group.[66] A direct head-to-head comparison between insulin aspart and insulin lispro in CSII has not been reported.

Safety

At this time, there is insufficient data on the use of insulin aspart in pregnancy. In non-pregnant patients with diabetes, there is no evidence of increased allergic reactions or adverse effects with insulin aspart.[7]

Other rapid-acting insulin analogues

B10 Asp

B10 Asp was an analogue created by the substitution of aspartate for histidine at position 10 of the B-chain. Like other rapid-acting analogues, B10 Asp had a fast peak of action with a shorter duration of action. However, its biological action was different. Its affinity for the IGF-1 receptor was greater than that of insulin and it was 62% more potent than insulin at stimulating the incorporation of tritiated thymidine into cultured cells, a marker of DNA synthesis.[52] This raised concerns that B10 Asp might stimulate cell division and neoplasia. This was confirmed in a study showing increased incidence of benign and malignant mammary tumours in female rats that had received B10 Asp for one year.[67] Owing to this finding, B10 Asp is no longer being studied.

Long-acting insulin analogues

The goal of achieving near-physiologic replacement of insulin requires both bolus (mealtime) insulins and basal insulins. The traditional human basal insulins are NPH, lente and ultralente. Their absorption from the subcutaneous space is delayed by the addition of protamine or zinc which produces a more stable compound in the neutral pH of the subcutaneous space.[8,9] Although the duration of action is longer, each of the longer-acting human insulins has a peak 5–8 hours after injection which may contribute to hypoglycaemia. In addition, NPH and lente insulin are suspensions in solution and need to be adequately resuspended for proper dosing.[9] Therefore, the ideal basal insulin would have no peak, provide a stable insulin level for a long duration of time and have low intrasubject coefficient of variation. At this time, glargine (HOE 901) is the only long-acting insulin analogue which has some of these properties and is commercially available. Other long-acting insulin analogues are being developed.

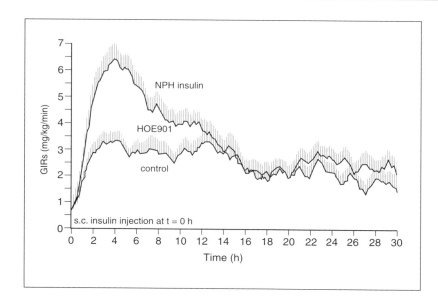

Figure 20.5
Glucose infusion rate to maintain euglycaemia after subcutaneous injection of glargine (HOE 901) and NPH insulin. Source: reprinted with permission from Heinemann et al. Diabetes Care 2000; 23: 644–9.[70] © 2000 American Diabetes Association.

Insulin glargine

Insulin glargine (A21 Gly, B31 Arg, B32 Arg) is the first long-acting insulin analogue to become commercially available. It was approved for clinical use in patients with Type 1 and Type 2 diabetes by the United States Food and Drug Administration and the European Agency for the Evaluation of Medicinal Products in 2000.[68]

Structure

Insulin glargine results from two modifications of human insulin. The first is the addition of two positively charged arginine molecules to the NH_2-terminal of the B-chain. This modification shifts the isoelectric point of glargine from a pH of 5.4 to 6.7 making the molecule more soluble at acidic pH and less soluble at physiologic pH of subcutaneous tissue.[69] The second modification is the replacement of acid-sensitive asparagine at position 21 of the A-chain by charge-neutral glycine. This change improves the stability of the analogue. Insulin

glargine is formulated at an acidic pH and is supplied as a clear colourless solution. Once injected into the neutral pH of the subcutaneous space, it forms microprecipitates, thereby delaying its absorption and prolonging its action. The addition of low amounts of zinc further prolongs its action.[69]

In vitro, insulin glargine has about 60% the affinity of human insulin for the insulin receptor. However, its *in vivo* potency is equivalent to human insulin because the plasma concentrations are twice that of human insulin.[68] It also has up to a six-fold greater affinity for the IGF-1 receptor than human insulin. However, insulin glargine given to rats and mice for up to two years did not exhibit any carcinogenic effects.[68]

Time-action profile

Euglycaemic clamp studies in healthy volunteers using insulin glargine did not show the pronounced peak in metabolic activity seen with NPH insulin.[70–72] After an initial rise in serum insulin levels and glucose insulin rate over 2–3 hours, they remained stable for up to 30 hours with no significant peak (Figure 20.5). These findings were confirmed in patients with Type 1 and Type 2 diabetes.[73,74] There was also less intersubject variability with glargine compared to NPH or lente and no difference in absorption characteristics between injection sites.[72,73] The pharmacokinetics of glargine in an MDI regimen was compared to insulin administered by CSII and a similar peakless concentration/action profile was seen.[73]

Clinical use

The peakless, prolonged time-action profile of glargine is compatible with the requirements of a basal insulin. A number of studies have compared the use of glargine and NPH as basal insulin in MDI regimens using either lispro or regular human insulin as the bolus insulin in patients with Type 1 diabetes.[75–78] They demonstrated lower fasting plasma glucose levels and less nocturnal hypoglycaemia. Some of the studies also demonstrated lower HbA1c levels.[76] All of the studies used only one injection of glargine at bedtime compared to one or two injections per day of NPH. In Type 2 diabetes, glargine at bedtime has been compared to NPH at bedtime in combination with oral hypoglycaemic agents. The glargine group experienced less nocturnal hypoglycaemia and better post-dinner plasma glucose control.[79,80] However, no significant difference was detected in overall glycaemic control. The utility of insulin glargine in MDI regimens for Type 1 diabetes is well established.[8] The role of glargine in Type 2 diabetes remains to be defined.

Safety

The safety of insulin glargine in pregnancy has not been established and pregnancy is currently not a labelled indication for its use. As mentioned earlier, insulin glargine has a significantly higher affinity for the IGF-1 receptor.[68] This raised the concern of possible mitogenic effects of glargine. This was not shown in rats and mice receiving glargine for two years.[68] However, Kurtzhals et al. recently reported increased mitogenicity of insulin glargine compared with human insulin in a malignant human osteosarcoma cell-line.[81] The clinical relevance of this observation is unknown and long-term data are needed to answer this question.

A recent case report demonstrated the benefits of insulin glargine in a man with Type 1 diabetes who had generalized allergy to animal and human insulins.[82] The use of glargine appeared to suppress the allergy to regular human insulin. The authors hypothesized that the patient's allergic epitopes contained both human insulin A-chain and animal insulin (B30 Ala), both of which are modified in insulin glargine.[82]

Insulin detemir (NN-304)

Structure

Alternative means of prolonging insulin action have been studied. The presence of albumin in the subcutaneous and intravascular comparments makes binding of insulin to albumin an attractive option to prolong action.[83] Albumin has many binding sites for non-esterified fatty acids so the addition of a fatty acid to the insulin molecule is an effective means of coupling insulin with albumin.[83] Specifically, a 14-carbon aliphatic fatty acid is acylated to the amino acid at position 29 of the B-chain and the amino acid at position 30 is removed.[84] The resulting molecule, named detemir, is combined with zinc and phenol and exists as a hexamer in the subcutaneous space.[85] Its hypoglycaemic action is prolonged by the association of the fatty acid residue to the fatty acid binding sites

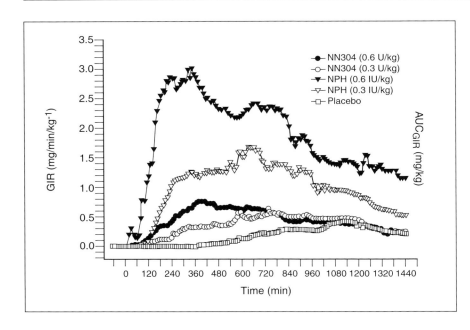

Figure 20.6
Glucose infusion rate to maintain euglycaemia after subcutaneous injection of insulin detemir (NN 304) and NPH insulin. Source: reprinted with permission from Brunner et al. Exp Clin Endocrinol Diabetes 2000; 108: 100–5.[86]

of albumin in blood and peripheral tissues. More than 98% of detemir is bound to albumin and only the free analogue binds to the insulin receptor with a binding affinity 46% that of human insulin.[84] It is formulated as a soluble preparation and does not require mixing prior to administration.

Time-action profile

In euglycaemic clamp studies of detemir in healthy volunteers, the insulin effect was delayed and prolonged and there was a less pronounced peak effect compared to NPH insulin (Figure 20.6). However, larger doses of detemir were needed for the same hypoglycaemic effect.[84,86]

Clinical use

Insulin detemir has been studied in a multicentre open-label randomized crossover trial involving 59 patients with Type 1 diabetes. Once-daily detemir was compared to NPH given once or twice daily in MDI regimens.

Mean dose requirements of insulin detemir were 2.35 times higher than NPH. With the higher doses of detemir, the two groups had similar glycaemic control but the detemir group had less intrasubject variability in fasting plasma glucose. There appeared to be less hypoglycaemia with insulin detemir but this was only demonstrated in the last week of therapy.[85] More clinical trial data on the use of detemir are required to understand fully its role in the management of diabetes.

Pre-mixed insulin analogues

Human insulins are available in pre-mixed formulations that are often preferred by elderly patients or those with difficulty mixing insulins. Pre-mixed insulins are commonly used in the treatment of Type 2 diabetes in a twice-daily fashion but are not recommended in Type 1 diabetes because they do not provide enough flexibility for adjustment and do not adequately

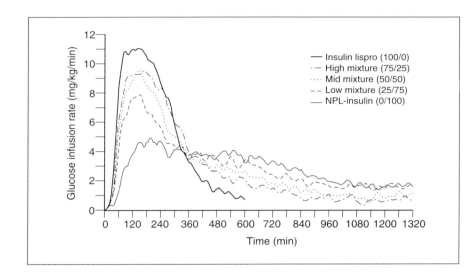

Figure 20.7
Glucose infusion rate to maintain euglycaemia after subcutaneous injection of pre-mixed insulin analogues, lispro and NPL insulin. Source: reprinted with permission from Heise et al. Diabetes Care 1998; 21: 800–3.[88] © 1998 American Diabetes Association.

mimic physiologic insulin replacement. The currently available pre-mixed human insulins are a mixture of regular human insulin and NPH insulin in ratios ranging from 50/50 to 10/90.[9] Although lispro can be mixed with NPH in the syringe and then administered immediately, they can not be pre-mixed in solution. There would be a slow exchange of the free lispro molecule and the NPH-bound human insulin molecule which would result in unpredictable ratios of free insulin lispro and free regular human insulin in the bottle.[7] In response to this, NPL (neutral protamine lispro) was developed. It replaces the human insulin molecule in NPH with lispro thereby allowing for lispro to be pre-mixed with a longer-acting insulin. NPL has been shown to have a similar time-action profile to NPH.[87] Three separate pre-mixed formulations of insulin lispro and NPL have been developed. Low mixture (Mix25) contains 25% lispro and 75% NPL. Mid mixture (Mix50) contains 50% lispro and 50% NPL. High mixture contains 75% lispro

and 25% NPL. Each formulation has a unique time-action profile which shows a rapid insulin effect with various peaks followed by the lesser more stable prolonged effect of the NPL (Figure 20.7).[88,89]

Clinical use

In patients with Type 2 diabetes, improved postprandial glycaemic control after a test meal was seen with Mix25 (25% lispro/75% NPL) compared to human insulin 30/70 (30% regular/70% NPH).[90,91] In a six-month, open-label-randomized study of 89 patients with Type 2 diabetes, Mix25 or human insulin 30/70 was given before breakfast and dinner. Treatment with Mix25 resulted in better postprandial glycaemic control after breakfast and dinner but no difference in HbA1c.[92] Other studies have also shown less nocturnal hypoglycaemia because lispro does not have the prolonged action of regular insulin which contributes to nocturnal hypoglycaemia.[93] Pre-mixed insulin analogues are commercially available and are being used with increasing frequency in patients with Type 2 diabetes.

Conclusion

Over the past 80 years, very significant advances in insulin technology have provided more effective tools to mimic the physiologic replacement of insulin. The advent of rapid-acting insulin analogues, lispro and aspart, have allowed for improved bolus replacement of insulin at mealtimes. The longer-acting insulin analogues, glargine and detemir, behave more like the ideal basal insulin with a peakless effect. Although these designer insulins have better properties than the human insulins, they are not perfect. Research continues into insulins with superior biologic and pharmacokinetic activities. In addition, alternative routes of insulin delivery are actively being investigated. Despite all of our technological advances, it is important to remember that patient education and support are critical to the success of any insulin regimen. Only with the continued cooperation of patients, health care teams and research will we be able to achieve near-normal glycaemic control and prevent the long-term complications of diabetes.

References

1. Bliss M. The Discovery of Insulin. Chicago: McClelland & Stewart, 1996.
2. Hagedorn HC, Jensen BN, Krarup NB, et al. Protamine insulinate. JAMA 1936; 106: 177–80.
3. Scott D, Fisher A. Studies on insulin with protamine. J Pharmacol Exp Ther 1936; 58: 78–92.
4. Krayenbuhl C, Rosenberg T. Crystalline protamine insulin. Rep Steno Mem Hosp 1946; 1: 60–73.
5. Riggs AD. Bacterial production of human insulin. Diabetes Care, 1984; 4: 64–8.
6. Zinman B. The physiologic replacement of insulin – an elusive goal. N Engl J Med 1989; 321: 363–70.
7. Owens DR, Zinman B, Bolli GB. Insulins today and beyond. Lancet 2001; 358: 739–46.
8. Lee WL, Zinman B. From insulin to insulin analogs: progress in the treatment of Type 1 diabetes. Diabetes Rev 1998; 6: 73–88.
9. Heinemann L, Richter B. Clinical pharmacology of human insulin. Diabetes Care 1993; 16(S3): 90–101.
10. Burge MR, Schade DS. Insulins. Endocrinol Metab Clin North Am 1997; 26: 57597.
11. Holleman F, Hoekstra JBL. Insulin lispro. N Engl J Med 1997; 337: 176–83.
12. Brems DN, Alter LA, Beckage MJ et al. Altering the association properties of insulin by amino acid replacement. Protein Eng 1992; 5: 527–32.
13. Slieker LJ, Sundell K. Modifications in the 29–20 position of the insulin B-chain alter binding to the IGF-1 receptor with minimal effect on insulin receptor binding. Diabetes 1991; 40(S1): 168A (Abstract).
14. Howey DC, Bowsher RR, Brunelle RF, Woodworth JR. [Lys(B28), Pro(B29)]-human insulin: a rapidly absorbed analogue of human insulin. Diabetes 1994; 43: 396–402.
15. Woodworth J, Howey D, Bowsher R et al. [Lys(B28), Pro(B29)]-human insulin (K): dose-ranging vs. Humulin R (H). Diabetes 1993; 42(S1): 54A (Abstract).
16. Antsiferov M, Woodworth JR, Mayorov A et al. Within patient variability in postprandial glucose excursion with lispro insulin analog compared with regular insulin. Diabetologia 1995; 38(S1): A190 (Abstract).
17. Brunelle RL, Llewelyn J, Anderson JH et al. Meta-analysis of the effect of insulin lispro on severe hypoglycaemia in patients with Type 1 diabetes. Diabetes Care 1998; 21: 1726–31.
18. Ebelin P, Jansson PA, Smith U et al. Strategies toward improved control during insulin lispro therapy in IDDM. Diabetes Care 1997; 20: 1287–9.
19. Heller SR, Amiel SA, Mansell P. Effect of the fast-acting insulin analog lispro on the risk of nocturnal hypoglycaemia during intensified insulin therapy. Diabetes Care 1999; 22: 1607–11.

20. Chatterjee S, Gallen IW, Sandler L. 2-year prospective audit of the effect of the introduction of insulin lispro in patients with specific clinical indications. Diabetes Care 1999; 22: 1226–7.

21. Chase HP, Lockspeiser T, Peery B et al. The impact of the diabetes control and complications trial and Humalog insulin on glycohemoglobin levels and severe hypoglycaemia in Type 1 diabetes. Diabetes Care 2001; 24: 430–4.

22. Lalli CM, Del Sindaco P, Torlone E et al. Contribution of postprandial versus interprandial blood glucose to HbA1c in Type 1 diabetes on physiologic intensive therapy with lispro insulin at mealtime. Diabetes Care 1999; 22: 795–800.

23. Colombel A, Murat A, Krempf M et al. Improvement of blood glucose control in Type 1 diabetic patients treated with lispro and multiple NPH injections. Diabet Med 1999; 16: 319–24.

24. Holleman F, Schmitt H, Rottiers R et al. Reduced frequency of severe hypoglycaemia and coma in well-controlled IDDM patients treated with insulin lispro. Diabetes Care 1997; 20: 1827–33.

25. Anderson JH, Brunelle RL, Koivisto VA et al. Reduction of postprandial hyperglycemia and frequency of hypolycemia in IDDM patients on insulin-analog treatment. Diabetes 1997; 46: 265–70.

26. Mohn A, Matyka KA, Harris DA et al. Lispro or regular insulin for multiple injection therapy in adolescence. Diabetes Care 1999; 22: 27–32.

27. Anderson JH, Brunelle RL, Keohane P et al. Mealtime treatment with insulin analog improves postprandial hyperglycemia and hypoglycaemia in patients with non-insulin-dependent diabetes mellitus. Arch Intern Med 1997; 157: 1249–55.

28. Bastyr EJ, Johnson ME, Trautmann ME et al. Insulin lispro in the treatment of patients with Type 2 diabetes mellitus after oral agent failure. Clin Ther 1999; 21: 1703–14.

29. Grey M, Boland EA, Tamborlane WV. Use of lispro insulin and quality of life in adolescents on intensive therapy. Diabetes Educator 1999; 25: 934–41.

30. Lalli C, Ciofetta M, Del Sindaco P et al. Long-term intensive treatment of Type 1 diabetes with the short-acting insulin analog lispro in variable combination with NPH insulin at mealtime. Diabetes Care 1999; 22: 468–77.

31. Zinman B, Ross S, Campos RV, Strack T. Effectiveness of human ultralente versus NPH insulin in providing basal insulin replacement for an insulin lispro multiple daily injection regimen. Diabetes Care 1999; 22: 603–8.

32. Joseph SE, Korzon-Burakowska A, Woodworth JR et al. The action profile of lispro is not blunted by mixing in the syringe with NPH insulin. Diabetes Care 1998; 21: 2098–102.

33. Zinman B, Tildesley H, Chiasson JL et al. Insulin lispro in CSII – results of a double-blind crossover study. Diabetes 1997; 46: 440–3.

34. Melki V, Renard E, Lassmann-Vague V et al. Improvement of HbA1c and blood glucose stability in IDDM patients treated with lispro insulin analog in external pumps. Diabetes Care 1998; 21: 977–82.

35. Renner R, Pfutzner A, Trautmann M et al. Use of insulin lispro in continuous subcutaneous insulin infusion treatment. Diabetes Care 1999; 22: 784–8.

36. Johansson UB, Adamson UC, Lins PE, Wredling RA. Improved blood glucose variability, HbA1c insuman Insfusat and less insulin requirement in IDDM patients using insulin lispro in CSII. The Swedish multicenter lispro insulin study. Diabetes Metab 2000; 26: 192–6.

37. Hanaire-Broutin H, Melki V, Bessieres-Lacombe S, Tauber JP. Comparison of continuous subcutaneous insulin infusion and multiple daily injection regimens using insulin lispro in Type 1 diabetic patients on intensified treatment. Diabetes Care 2000; 23: 1232–5.

38. Garg SK, Anderson JH, Gerard LA et al. Impact of insulin lispro on HbA1c values in insulin pump users. Diab Obes Metab 2000; 2: 307–11.

39. Guerci B, Meyer L, Salle A et al. Comparison of metabolic deterioration between insulin analog and regular insulin after a 5-hour interruption of a continuous subcutaneous insulin infusion in Type 1 diabetic patients. J Clin Endocrinol Metab 1999; 84: 2673–8.

40. Glazer NB, Zalani S, Anderson JH, Bastyr EJ. Safety of insulin lispro: pooled data from clinical trials. Amer J Health-Sys Pharm 1999; 56: 542–7.

41. Jovanovic L, Ilic S, Pettitt DJ et al. Metabolic and immunologic effects of insulin lispro in gestational diabetes. Diabetes Care 1999; 22: 1422–7.

42. Kitzmiller J, Main E, Ward B et al. Insulin lispro and the development of proliferative diabetic retinopathy during pregnancy. Diabetes Care 1999; 22: 874–6.

43. Bhattacharyya A, Vice PA. Insulin lispro, pregnancy and retinopathy. Diabetes Care 1999; 22: 2101–2.

44. Buchbinder A, Miodovnik M, McElvy S et al. Is insulin lispro associated with the development or progression of diabetic retinopathy during pregnancy? Am J Obstet Gynecol 2000; 183: 1162–5.

45. Aisenpreis U, Pfutzner A, Giehl M et al. Pharmacokinetics and pharmacodynamics of insulin lispro compared with regular insulin in haemodialysis patients with diabetes mellitus. Nephrol Dial Transplant 1999; 14(S4): 5–6.

46. Darmon P, Curtillet C, Boullu S et al. Insulin analog lispro decreases insulin resistance and improves glycemic control in an obese patient with insulin-requiring Type 2 diabetes. Diabetes Care 1998; 21: 1575.

47. Abraham MR, Al-Sharafi B, Saavedra GA, Khardori R. Lispro in the treatment of insulin allergy. Diabetes Care 1999; 22: 1916–17.

48. Lluch-Bernal M, Fernandez M, Herrera-Pombo JL, Sastre J. Insulin lispro, an alternative in insulin hypersensitivity. Allergy 1999; 54: 186–7.

49. Panczel P, Hosszufalusi N, Horvath MM, Horvath A. Advantage of insulin lispro in suspected insulin allergy. Allergy 2000; 55: 418–19.

50. Raine CH, Krzyston MJ, Amr M, Hydrick L. Improvement in severe insulin resistance with frequent injections of lispro insulin. J Nat Med Assoc 1999; 91: 410–13.

51. Hirsch IB, D'Alessio D, Eng L et al. Severe insulin resistance in a patient with Type 1 diabetes and stiff-man syndrome treated with insulin lispro. Diabetes Res Clin Pract 1998; 41: 197–202.

52. Bornfeldt KE, Gidlof RA, Wasteson A et al. Binding and biological effects of insulin, insulin analogues and insulin-like growth factors in rat aortic smooth muscle cells: comparison of maximal growth promoting activities. Diabetologia 1991; 34: 307–13.

53. Mudaliar SR, Lindberg FA, Joyce M et al. Insulin aspart (B28 Asp-Insulin): a fast-acting analog of human insulin. Diabetes Care 1999; 22: 1501–6.

54. Home PD, Barriocanal L, Lindholm A. Comparative pharmacokinetics and pharmacodynamics of the novel rapid-acting insulin analogue, insulin aspart, in healthy volunteers. Eur J Clin Pharmacol 1999; 55: 199–203.

55. Kaku K, Matsuda M, Urae A, Irie S. Pharmacokinetics and pharmacodynamics of insulin aspart, a rapid-acting analog of human insulin, in healthy Japanese volunteers. Diabetes Res Clin Pract 2000; 49: 119–26.

56. Mortensen H, Olsen B, Lindholm A. Pharmacokinetics of a rapid-acting human insulin analogue, insulin aspart, in children and adolescents with Type 1 diabetes. Diabetes 1999; 48(S1): A358 (Abstract).

57. Lindholm A, McEwen J, Riis AP. Improved postprandial glycemic control with insulin aspart. Diabetes Care 1999; 22: 801–5.

58. Raskin P, Guthrie RA, Leiter L et al. Use of insulin aspart, a fast-acting insulin analog, as the mealtime insulin in the management of patients with Type 1 diabetes. Diabetes Care 200; 23: 583–8.

59. Home PD, Lindholm A, Riis A. Insulin aspart vs. human insulin in the management of long-term blood glucose control in Type 1 diabetes mellitus: a randomized controlled trial. Diabet Med 2000; 17: 762–70.

60. Brunner G, Hirschberger S, Sendlhofer G et al. Post-prandial administration of the insulin analogue insulin aspart in patients with Type 1 diabetes mellitus. Diabet Med 2000; 17: 371–5.

61. Home PD, Lindholm A, Riis AP. Improved long-term blood glucose control with insulin aspart versus human insulin in people with Type 1 diabetes. Diabetes 1999; 48(S1): A358 (Abstract).

62. Rosenfalck AM, Thorsby P, Kjems L et al. Improved postprandial glycaemic control with insulin Aspart in Type 2 diabetic patients treated with insulin. Acta Diabetologica 2000; 37: 41–6.

63. Raskin P, McGill J, Kilo C, Boss AH. Human insulin analog (insulin aspart, Iasp) is compar-

able to human insulin (HI) in Type 2 diabetes. Diabetes 1999; 48(S1): A355 (Abstract).

64. Uwe B, Ebrahim S, Hirschberger S et al. Effect of the rapid acting insulin analogue insulin aspart on quality-of-life and treatment satisfaction in Type 1 diabetic patients. Diabetes 1999; 48(S1): A112 (Abstract).

65. Halberg IB, Jacobsen LV, Dahl UL. A study on self-mixing insulin aspart with NPH insulin in the syringe before injection. Diabetes 1999; 48(S1): A104 (Abstract).

66. Bode BW, Strange P. Efficacy, safety, and pump compatibility of insulin aspart used in continuous subcutaneous insulin infusion therapy in patients with Type 1 diabetes. Diabetes Care 2001; 24: 69–72.

67. Jorgensen LN, Dideriksen LH, Drejer K. Carcinogenic effect of the human insulin analogue B10 Asp in female rats. Diabetologia 1992; 35(S1): A3 (Abstract).

68. Bolli GB, Owens DR. Insulin glargine. Lancet 2000; 356: 443–4.

69. Buse J. Insulin glargine (HOE901). Diabetes Care 2000; 23: 576–8.

70. Heinemann L, Linkeschova R, Rave K et al. Time-action profile of the long-acting insulin analog insulin glargine (HOE 901) in comparison with those of NPH insulin and placebo. Diabetes Care 2000; 23: 644–9.

71. Coates PA, Mukherjee S, Srodzinski KA et al. Pharmacokinetics of a long-acting human insulin analogue (HOE901) in healthy subjects. Diabetes 1995; 44(S1): 130A (Abstract).

72. Owens DR, Coates PA, Luzio SD et al. Pharmacokinetics of ^{125}I-labeled insulin glargine (HOE901) in healthy men. Diabetes Care 2000; 23: 813–19.

73. Lepore M, Pampanelli S, Fanelli C et al. Pharmacokinetics and pharmacodynamics of subcutaneous injection of long-acting human insulin analog glargine, NPH insulin, and ultralente human insulin and continuous subcutaneous infusion of insulin lispro. Diabetes 2000; 49: 2142–8.

74. Luzio SD, Owens D, Evans M et al. Comparison of the sc absorption of HOE 901 and NPH human insulin in Type 2 diabetic subjects. Diabetes 1999; 48(S1): A111 (Abstract).

75. Ratner RE, Hirsch IB, Neifing JL et al. Less hypoglycaemia with insulin glargine in intensive insulin therapy for Type 1 diabetes. Diabetes Care 2000; 23: 639–43.

76. Pieber TR, Eugene-Jolchine I, Derobert E. Efficacy and safety of HOE 901 versus NPH insulin in patients with Type 1 diabetes. Diabetes Care 2000; 23: 157–62.

77. Raskin P, Klaff L, Bergenstal R et al. A 16-week comparison of the novel insulin analog insulin glargine (HOE 901) and NPH human insulin used with insulin lispro in patients with Type 1 diabetes. Diabetes Care 2000; 23: 1666–71.

78. Rosenstock J, Park G, Zimmerman J. Basal insulin glargine (HOE 901) versus NPH insulin in patients with Type 1 diabetes on multiple daily insulin regimens. Diabetes Care 2000; 23: 1137–42.

79. Yki-Jarvinen H, Dressler A, Ziemen M. Less nocturnal hypoglycaemia and better post-dinner glucose control with bedtime insulin glargine compared with bedtime NPH insulin during insulin combination therapy in Type 2 diabetes. Diabetes Care 2000; 23: 1130–6.

80. Raskin P, Park G, Zimmerman J. The effect of HOE 901 on glycemic control in Type 2 diabetes. Diabetes 1998; 47(S1): A103 (Abstract).

81. Kurtzhals P, Schaffer L, Sorensen A. Correlation of receptor binding and metabolic and mitogenic potencies of insulin analogs designed for clinical use. Diabetes 2000; 49: 999–1005.

82. Moriyama H, Nagata M, Fujihira K et al. Treatment with human analog (Gly A21, Arg B31, Arg B32) insulin glargine (HOE 901) resolves a generalized allergy to human insulin in Type 1 diabetes. Diabetes Care 2001; 24: 411.

83. Rosskamp RH, Park G. Long-acting insulin analogs. Diabetes Care 1999; 22(S2): B109–13.

84. Heinemann L, Sinha K, Weyer C et al. Time-action profile of the soluble, fatty acid acylated, long-acting insulin analogue NN304. Diabet Med 1999; 16: 332–8.

85. Hermansen K, Madsbad S, Perrild H et al. Comparison of the soluble basal insulin analog insulin detemir with NPH insulin. Diabetes Care 2001; 24: 296–301.

86. Brunner GA, Sendhofer G, Wutte A et al. Pharmacokinetic and pharmacodynamic properties of

long-acting insulin analogue NN304 in comparison to NPH insulin in humans. Exp Clin Endocrinol Diabetes 2000; 108: 100–5.

87. Defelippis MR, Bakaysa DL, Youngman KM et al. Preparation and characterization of neutral protamine lispro (NPL) suspension. Diabetes 1996; 45(S2): 74A (Abstract).

88. Heise T, Weyer C, Serwas A et al. Time-action profiles of novel premixed preparations of insulin lispro and NPL insulin. Diabetes Care 1998; 21: 800–3.

89. Rave K, Heinemann L, Puhl L et al. Pre-mixed formulations of insulin lispro. Diabetes Care 1999; 22: 865–6.

90. Malone JK, Woodworth JR, Arora V et al. Improved postprandial glycemic control with humalog Mix75/25 after a standard test meal in patients with Type 2 diabetes mellitus. Clin Ther 2000; 22: 222–30.

91. Koivisto VA, Tuominen JA, Ebeling P. Lispro Mix25 insulin as premeal therapy in Type 2 diabetic patients. Diabetes Care 1999; 22: 459–62.

92. Roach P, Yue L, Arora V. Improved postprandial glycemic control during treatment with humalog Mix25, a novel protamine-based insulin lispro formulation. Diabetes Care 1999; 22; 1258–61.

93. Roach P, Trautmann M, Arora V et al. Improved postprandial blood glucose control and reduced nocturnal hypoglycaemia during treatment with two novel insulin lispro-protamine formulations, insulin lispro Mix 25 and insulin lispro Mix50. Clin Ther 1999; 21: 523–33.

21

PPAR-γ modulators: their role in diabetes care

Philip D Home

Finding new drugs for use in Type 2 diabetes

Historical perspective

Our understanding of the pathogenesis of a disease should, by the normal logic of human thinking, give rise to the ideas which enable the development of new therapeutic options for its management. At the simple level, in the first half of the twentieth century, understanding of diabetes had gone little beyond appreciation of the role of hyperglycaemia, and the understanding that this was related to defects in insulin secretion. Nevertheless, the observations that led to the development of the biguanides and sulphonylureas were serendipitous in part, both deriving from unexpected observations of hypoglycaemic effects of related compounds.

While in the last quarter of the twentieth century there have been extensive advances in the understanding of what is now termed (somewhat vaguely) Type 2 diabetes, and in particular in the understanding of the development of insulin insensitivity (though not its mechanism), and the phenomenon of compensatory insulin hypersecretion and its subsequent relative failure,[1] these advances too have been remarkably unhelpful in the development of new pharmaceutical compounds suitable for the management of hyperglycaemia. Indeed while it can be argued that the α-glucosidase inhibitors are better understood in the context

of the impairment of meal-time insulin responses in people with Type 2 diabetes, their development was predicated only on the suggestion that the blunting of the post-meal hyperglycaemic excursion would be beneficial to overall glucose homeostasis.[2]

Until the 1990s this drug development problem was reflected in clinical practice where the mainstay of therapy (at least in Europe) was still the sulphonylureas and metformin, drug classes with no less than a 40-year track record, and little improvement in efficacy over that time. It is perhaps a paradox of modern clinical science that the mechanism of action of metformin can still be a matter for debate, and indeed is widely misunderstood by perhaps most of the clinicians who prescribe it. Accordingly acarbose (and subsequently the related compound miglitol), was the only really new introduction into the therapeutic glucose-lowering armoury, a situation paralleled by insulin therapy, largely unchanged from the 1950s until the arrival of the insulin analogues.

PPAR-γ agonists

It would be good for medical science to write that this was not the case for the PPAR-γ agonists, and that our understanding of the role of fatty acid metabolism in the pathogenesis of insulin insensitivity led to the discovery of a fatty acid binding protein, and that advanced chemical design mimicking the natural ligand led to a new series of drugs that proved to ameliorate the insulin resistance of Type 2 diabetes, and thus lower blood glucose. This however was not to be the case, for the glucose-lowering properties of the first thiazolidinedione were only noted in a search for a new lipid-lowering agent with properties related to the fibrates. Fibrates themselves were the product of classical drug-screening programmes in the early 1960s.[3]

Instead, pharmacology again provided a lead into physiology, as the real power of modern chemistry allowed a complete understanding of the molecular nature of the structure and binding site of the PPAR receptor family, although giving *en route* an unmanageable name (peroxisome proliferator-activated receptors (PPAR)) whose origins are not relevant. Coupled to modern computing and imaging power, this is now allowing the rational design of new PPAR-γ agonists, with chemical structures distinct from the thiazolidinediones.

Accordingly the terminology 'thiazolidinediones' (or more crudely 'glitazones' or 'TZDs') is now superseded, and while the origins of the term 'PPAR-γ agonists' are irrelevant to their actions, this is the preferred term for this group of drugs, and is used here. However, the two drugs approved for therapeutic use at the time of writing (rosiglitazone and pioglitazone) can be seen by their names to be thiazolidinediones, and that term and derivatives of the term are correctly applied to them.

Insulin insensitivity, PPAR-γ agonists and Type 2 diabetes

Pathogenesis of Type 2 diabetes

It is tempting, and indeed quite usual, to discuss the pathogenesis of Type 2 diabetes in terms of insulin insensitivity (often referred to as 'insulin resistance', as if the tissues defended themselves against an attack by insulin), and defective insulin secretion. The naïve view that one or other party was the dominant player has sunk with the development of more quantitative understandings of the processes involved,[1] although in the nature of the heterogeneity of Type 2 diabetes there is still a dominant role for the insulin secretion defect in some people with genetic defects affecting islet B-cell metabolism, with slow onset autoimmune islet damage in adulthood, and in the thin elderly patient. DeFronzo has neatly encapsulated the relationships between insulin insensitivity, defective insulin secretion and hyperglycaemia in the simple model by comparing the results of glucose clamps and glucose challenge in different groups of individuals from normal glucose homeostasis through to diabetes with absolute insulin deficiency.[1]

Concern with the simple approach might begin with the recognition that the glucose clamp, as normally performed, uses an insulin infusion rate which gives plasma levels at or above the maximum concentrations generally found postprandially, and that the principal physiological property measured is glucose uptake into skeletal muscle. As people with diabetes are hyperglycaemic in the fasting state, and as insulin-stimulated glucose disposal is of little importance in this physiological condition, it is clear that we must also entertain the role of basal control of hepatic glucose production by insulin, and/or hepatic autoregulation of glucose homeostasis. Indeed these may have a role in exacerbating hyperglycaemia in the fed state. Furthermore it is now clear that glucose toxicity arising from some degree of hyperglycaemia can further impair insulin insensitivity, defective insulin secretion, hepatic autoregulation, and glucose-induced glucose disposal (i.e. decreasing the mass action effect of hyperglycaemia in promoting receptor-mediated glucose uptake into the tissues).[4] These effects are quite substantial, and explain for example the effect of rapid-acting meal-related drugs like repaglinide on fasting blood glucose concentrations, or liver/gut acting drugs like metformin on peripheral insulin sensitivity.

Evidence that the thiazolidinediones improve insulin sensitivity is derived in particular from animal studies and human glucose clamp studies, which directly assess the effect of medium-term treatment with these drugs on the response of skeletal muscle to insulin.[5–8] Given the above, however, it is not surprising to find not only that insulin sensitivity improves on HOMA (metabolic modelling) analysis of fasting insulin and glucose concentrations, but also islet B-cell function after six months.[9,10] Such effects are sustained in the longer term.[11]

Evidence of efficacy in people with diabetes

Efficacy of drugs or other therapeutic interventions in people with Type 2 diabetes should be judged against the abnormalities of the metabolic syndrome, and in particular amelioration of hyperglycaemia, raised blood pressure and dyslipidaemia. More widely, effects on urinary albumin excretion, body fat distribution, coagulability, and even endothelial cell dysfunction are of interest. More recently there has been some interest in more general measures of inflammation.

Ultimately however, efficacy is judged against amelioration of increased mortality and morbidity. In conventional Type 2 diabetes this overwhelmingly means cardiovascular disease, whether that means coronary artery disease, cerebrovascular disease, limb arterial disease, or renovascular disease.[12] At present the required long-term studies are not available, although they are in progress. Meanwhile the increasingly early onset of Type 2 diabetes in some populations means that microvascular disease is likely to become more important as an outcome.

Glucose-lowering efficacy

Efficacy studies for pioglitazone and rosiglitazone (and troglitazone) in people with typical Type 2 diabetes have been reported for monotherapy, for combination with sulphonylureas, for combination with metformin, and for combination with insulin.[13–26] The patients entered into these studies generally have a mean age of 60 years and mean body mass index (BMI) of 30.0–32.0 kg/m². Notably, in these studies, glycated haemoglobin (HbA$_{1c}$), the primary outcome measure, was very high at baseline, in all therapy groups.

Study duration for the pivotal clinical trials was often 16–24 weeks. This is of some importance, as a number of the studies have demonstrated that, as a class, these drugs can take six weeks to have their full effect, while glycated haemoglobin can of course take 2–3 months to come into steady state. Sixteen weeks is then on the edge of the minimum time needed to demonstrate full effect. Furthermore some studies involved manipulating or allowing (usually stopping) other glucose therapies before or during a short run-in period, something that would invalidate the baseline HbA$_{1c}$ measurement used in the baseline-adjusted statistical analysis.

Nevertheless, it is clear that these drugs (pioglitazone and rosiglitazone) reduce HbA$_{1c}$ by a mean of 0.6–1.2% in placebo-controlled trials, with the larger effects possibly in combination with insulin therapy and sulphonylureas.[18–26] This is despite some reduction in insulin dosage in insulin treated patients, of the order of 9 U/day. These observations, suggesting more synergy with pharmaceutical preparations that increase plasma insulin concentrations, are consistent with the proposal principal effects of PPAR-γ agonists in improving insulin insensitivity. Many other studies still remain unpublished. However they have been reviewed for the UK National Centre for Excellence (NICE) in connection with reimbursement recommendations,[27,28] and where available at the time, by the licensing authorities.

An issue of interest here is whether these drugs are effective in all people with Type 2 diabetes, or, if their cost is a significant issue, whether they are similarly effective in all such patients. This is almost certainly not the case. Examination of the error bars on the HbA_{1c} curves in the published papers shows them to be very wide, particularly if it is remembered that these are often standard errors which should be quite small in studies involving hundreds of subjects (the standard deviation is divided by the square root of the subject number – for example by 20 for a 400-patient treatment arm). At least two effects may account for this. First there is a systematic relationship with BMI, such that patients with a BMI of <25.0 kg/m² show only a comparably minor effect, while those with a BMI of >30.0 kg/m² a much larger effect. It would seem likely, however, that BMI is crudely identifying people here with insulin insensitivity as part of the metabolic syndrome, so care needs to be taken not to exclude thinner people in some ethnic groups with abdominal adiposity from the potential benefits of these drugs. Secondly, and this seems to be confirmed by clinical experience, a minority of patients respond dramatically to these drugs, with falls of HbA_{1c} of 2.5% or more. It seems possible on first principles that these people are genetically different (perhaps in the PPAR-γ receptor,

the genes it controls, or the effect of some secondary mediator such as fatty acids on metabolism) from others, though no clinically applicable evidence is available on this point as yet.

An important clinical issue is whether the glucose-lowering effects are persistent. None of the controlled studies published to date are of longer duration than 26 weeks, so we have to rely on observational data for what happens over longer periods. From the Glaxo SmithKline data on rosiglitazone, at least in combination with metformin, it appears that the efficacy continues unchanged, at least out to two years.[11,29] Data from experience with troglitazone also suggested persistent efficacy out to longer periods.

Lipid-lowering efficacy

The lipid-'lowering' profiles of rosiglitazone and pioglitazone (and of other PPAR-γ agonists in development) do differ,[30–33] partly at least on account of their different PPAR-γ specificities. However all drugs have been associated with falls in plasma non-esterified fatty acid (NEFA) levels,[34] and this effect might be quite tightly related to the improvements in insulin sensitivity. With the plasma triglyceride concentrations also fall, and indeed more potent agents show improvements in triglycerides of the same order as found with the better fibrate drugs. In people in diabetes triglyceride concentrations tend to be tightly related (inversely) to HDL cholesterol concentrations, and indeed all the PPAR-γ agonists raise HDL cholesterol levels by amounts which are small but nevertheless clinically useful. Again we can expect greater changes in HDL cholesterol from the newer drugs in the development pipeline.

Rosiglitazone has been fairly consistently associated with changes in LDL cholesterol concentrations, namely a rise in calculated LDL cholesterol (as with troglitazone), but also with a change in the proportion of small, dense lipoprotein particles and thus average LDL density,[35] such that imputed atherogenicity might not be expected to have worsened. Ultimately only the long-term clinical trials can provide complete assurance here.

Blood pressure

The effect of PPAR-γ agonists is inconsistent, but where statistically significant effects are described they are in the direction of blood pressure lowering.[36] The likely explanation for this is that blood pressure measurement is of high variability, such that, except in studies explicitly designed for the purpose, power to detect small real changes is not present. The consistency of the findings leaves little doubt that these drugs do alter blood pressure in a beneficial direction, and this might be related to the fluid shifts discussed below. In one study with farglitazar (a drug not being further developed), useful dose-dependent reductions of blood pressure were found using ambulatory monitoring,[37] and it seems likely that other newer agents will demonstrate similar effects.

Fat distribution

As discussed above, weight gain tends to occur in hyperglycaemic people after starting on PPAR-γ agonists, and this is largely accounted for by a combination of fluid retention and amelioration of glycosuria. If calories previously lost as urinary glucose are retained they can only be stored as body fat (providing the patient is not previously in a grossly catabolic state due to insulin deficiency), though some calories will be lost in the inefficiency of the process of fatty acid synthesis/lipogenesis in the liver and adipose tissue. As abdominal fat is associated with cardiovascular disease, it is reassuring that there is evidence that the fat gain is largely in subcutaneous tissue.[38] In general this is also likely to mean it is more cosmetically acceptable.

Albumin excretion rate

There is evidence from both animal and human diabetes studies that PPAR-γ agonists, including those currently available clinically, can reduce albumin excretion rate (AER).[39–41] Indeed the rat study suggested some protection against nephropathy, a conclusion that cannot be reached simply by observation of AER in people with Type 2 diabetes as this measure should be regarded as non-specific in this condition. The reductions in albumin excretion rate seen with more potent PPAR-γ agonists (not available clinically) can be as great as that found with ACE-inhibitors or A2R-blockers.

Anti-inflammatory and other effects

A variety of other anti-inflammatory and putatively anti-thrombotic/anti-atherogenic effects have been reported in animal and human studies.[42–46] The clinical relevance of these is unclear, although those associated with endothelial cell dysfunction would fit into a pattern of general amelioration of features of the metabolic syndrome including the lipid, AER and fat distribution effects discussed above. It may then be the case that, prior to the results of the outcome studies to be reported in five or more years time, calculations of effectiveness of these drugs may be conservative if only the major glucose and lipid changes are factored into predictions of gains in mortality and morbidity. The effect of this would be to deny availability of drugs to some people for whom they would otherwise be judged cost-effective.

Clinical concern	Clinical action
Hepatotoxicity of troglitazone; no problems with other drugs	Check liver function tests at time of starting PPAR-γ agonists (to reduce clinical anxiety if LFTs found to be elevated later). No regular LFT monitoring
Fluid retention	Avoid if advanced cardiac failure; warn patients on starting; withdraw if clinically or cosmetically significant; caution/strong indication needed for insulin combination therapy
Dilutional anaemia	Anaemia occurring in patients on these drugs suggests another cause which may need investigation
Weight gain	Expect to be in line with reduction in glycosuria plus some fluid retention; not otherwise clinically significant
Pregnancy	Avoid if possibility of pregnancy; warn that it must be stopped immediately if any suspicion of pregnancy may have occurred on therapy; use with great caution in polycystic ovary syndrome due to possibility of ovulation being restored
Drug interactions	Be aware of possibilities of interactions with other P450 metabolized drugs, particularly with pioglitazone, but nevertheless no problems described

Table 21.1
Clinical concerns and safety in the use of PPAR-γ agonists

Concerns in the clinical use of PPAR-γ agonists (Table 21.1)

Liver toxicity

Following the introduction of the first of the PPAR-γ agonists into the US market, a combination of marketing, expectation, and frustration with current drugs led to about 1 million people with diabetes being exposed to the drugs in the first year. Amongst this population, 17 fatal events were identified as resulting from hepatic necrosis (liver toxicity).[47] This suggested a potential fatality rate of ~1 person in 60,000 exposed, although the possibility of considerable under-ascertainment cannot be ignored. Troglitazone remained on the market even after this problem was uncovered, not least because any effective glucose-lowering drug would be expected to save about 20 (5–200) times as many cardiovascular deaths, and there was no class alternative to troglitazone at the time. When pioglitazone and rosiglitazone became available, and once their hepatic toxicity was established as negligible, troglitazone was withdrawn.

On review of troglitazone data, it seems evident that major rises in alanine aminotransferase (ALT) in the pre-licensing trials were about three times as common as those of placebo,[29] a finding missed because of conventions of analyzing data using lower ALT cut-offs. This observation was helpful in providing reassurance over the potential liver safety of pioglitazone and rosiglitazone, neither of which provided any suggestion of unusual ALT rises detected, even after extensive data trawling. US exposure to these drugs has now covered over 4 million people, and there is no suggestion of severe drug-induced liver toxicity, though inevitably in such large populations some events of hepatocellular injury will be recorded by chance alone.[48–50]

As a result of the troglitazone experience, licensing authorities imposed a recommendation of rigorous monitoring of liver function tests on the manufacturers' product specifications, a recommendation now seen as not only clinically unnecessary but also highly cost-ineffective when judged by conventional health economic criteria. Nevertheless, clinical sensitivities remain, and given the high prevalence of abnormalities of liver function tests in people with Type 2 diabetes it is probably worth checking these as baseline estimates when starting a PPAR-γ agonist, so that the drug can be discounted as the problem from any abnormality noted later.

Drug interactions

Both rosiglitazone and pioglitazone are metabolized in the liver by components of the cytochrome P450 system. In theory this gives rise to the possibility of drug metabolism interactions, particularly with pioglitazone, which shares a part of the P450 system that is used by a variety of other drugs.[51] These include some for which changes in metabolism have significant effects on efficacy or safety, such as the statins and some hormones used in oral contraceptives, problems reported for troglitazone.[52–54] In practice, no clinically significant effects have been reported.[55] Both drugs are 99% bound to plasma proteins when in the circulation. No clinical problems appear to arise from this.

Pregnancy

In common with nearly all new drugs, the two thiazolidinediones have not been evaluated for efficacy and safety in pregnant women. Animal studies suggest fetal toxicity for both these agents. Given that the PPAR-γ receptor modulates gene function in some fundamental if ill understood parts of metabolism, and given the widespread expression of this and other PPAR receptors (the drugs are not entirely specific), such toxicity is perhaps not unexpected. These drugs should not be used in any woman who might become pregnant.

A problem here might arise in polycystic ovarian syndrome if these drugs are used (as metformin is) to improve insulin sensitivity in women presumed by experience to be anovulatory, but who respond to therapy and then begin to ovulate again.[56] The appropriate approach would appear to be to use non-hormonal contraceptive methods while taking these drugs, or to stop them as soon as carefully monitored ovulation/fertilization occurs. Neither drug is recommended in women who are breast feeding.

Fluid retention and cardiac failure

Some degree of fluid retention appears to be a class effect of PPAR-γ, and thus is found with every drug. There appears to be no particular advantage in extent of the problem with any drug, although some newer more potent PPAR-γ agonists have had to be abandoned because of the problem, suggesting that it is directly related to the mode of action of these drugs. The mechanism of this effect remains unclear, despite extensive review of all data by groups with expert knowledge of cardiovascular and endocrine dysfunction. The pattern of fluid accumulation, usually modest (ankle swelling) is similar to that seen with calcium channel blockers, and has thus been put down to changes in capillary permeability, but this has taken understanding no further forward.

On average, fluid retention is quite minor, and indeed in the majority of people undetectable, but probably accounts for the higher weight gain seen with the PPAR-γ agonists than with other glucose-lowering therapies. This suggests an average retention of about 1 l of fluid, but in some people it is unaccountably much higher. Interestingly in these people, reminiscent of insulin oedema and the similar state occasionally seen with chlorpropamide, the fluid retention is seemingly benign, and irreversible.

An important issue is whether such fluid retention can exacerbate cardiac failure, particularly in a group of people (with Type 2 diabetes) in whom ischaemic heart disease is particularly associated with left ventricular failure. Because clinical trial data are of poor quality in this area (some investigators tend to casually record congestive cardiac failure in people with simple ankle swelling[57]), the true incidence of cardiac failure is difficult to establish from only the large populations of patients studied, but may be up to 2% in six-month studies.[58] In people using insulin therapy, an incidence of rather more than double may be occurring, and it is this that has led to a contraindication to combination therapy with insulin being specified at the insistence of some licensing authorities.

Furthermore the pivotal clinical trials excluded people with advanced cardiac failure (New York Heart Association >stage 2). In these circumstances it is suggested that the drugs should not be used in people with evidence of advanced cardiac failure (patients requiring more than simple diuretic/ACE-I/β-adrenergic blocker therapy), and that use in people on insulin therapy should be restricted to those in whom the blood glucose control

remains problematic on very high insulin dosage, who cannot tolerate metformin and have strong characteristics of the metabolic syndrome.

The fluid retention results in a dilutional hypohaemoglobinaemia, typically of ~10 g/l, which in patients with a low blood haemoglobin concentration prior to therapy may result in reclassification as anaemia. Erythrocyte body mass, however, remains unchanged, although quite how the erythropoietic system achieves this, despite a fall in blood haemoglobin concentration, is unclear. Blood white cell concentrations can also fall slightly.

Early studies with thiazolidinediones in animals prevented the exploitation of the first experimental substances in man because of evidence of cardiac changes in rodents. Such changes are not seen in man with the presently licensed drugs, or others in the development pipeline, based on clinical observations (including electrocardiograms) in the clinical trials, or special echocardiographic studies performed in smaller numbers of patients since.

Clinical use of PPAR-γ agonists (Table 21.2)

Only rosiglitazone and pioglitazone are currently licensed and marketed globally. The use of these drugs is in part likely to be determined by reimbursement restrictions imposed by healthcare funders, and these vary from country to country. Logically these should depend on the relative cost-effectiveness of the drugs compared with alternative therapies (see above), but in practice, cost impact on the healthcare funder and licensing limitations also have an impact. Unfortunately the licensing process rarely manages to keep up with new data as it becomes available, and in Europe at least it is subject to covert political interference

Situation	Comment
Pre-diabetes, IFG and IGT	Long-term efficacy/safety ratio not established. Unlicensed. Likely to be poorly cost-effective
Monotherapy when lifestyle measures are inadequate	Major competitor is metformin, which is highly effective and much less expensive in many markets; possible role where metformin cannot be taken if the premium over the sulphonylureas can be tolerated
Combination therapy with one other glucose-lowering agent	Attractive in combination with metformin; also with sulphonylurea where metformin cannot be taken; expensive compared with combination of generic metformin + sulphonylurea
Triple combination therapy	No trials available, but highly likely to be safe and useful in this role; usually cheaper than transfer to insulin
Combination with insulin	Effective but concerns over safety often make this an off-licence prescription; useful if extreme metabolic resistance to exogenous insulin therapy; expensive

Notes: IFG = impaired fasting glycaemia; IGT = impaired glucose tolerance

Table 21.2
Clinical situations in which the use of PPAR-γ agonists might be considered

disguised as regulatory caution. For the purposes of this chapter, all possible indications will be considered, but riders added where cost-effectiveness, licensing or reimbursement issues have an impact on drug use.

Pre-diabetes

Insulin insensitivity is not just a phenomenon of diabetes, and states of hyperglycaemia short of diabetes (defined as impaired fasting hyperglycaemia and impaired glucose tolerance) carry some of the same features of the metabolic syndrome as found in Type 2 diabetes in most people in those non-diabetic categories. Furthermore there is evidence, inevitably only rather short-term, that troglitazone can prevent deterioration to diabetes in

women with previous gestational diabetes,[59] a finding that is likely to apply to all PPAR-γ agonists. That metformin has been shown to have similar effects would appear to confirm that some glucose-lowering drugs can be used in this way.

Unfortunately there is very little evidence to base sensible evaluation of the efficacy/safety ratio of these drugs when used in non-diabetic hyperglycaemic states. An alternative approach might be more intensive lifestyle advice coupled with careful monitoring of arterial risk factors including hyperglycaemia, and their management when they became overt. Inevitably cost-effectiveness is very difficult to estimate when effectiveness itself is uncertain, so that without outcome (morbidity/mortality data) for this indication it is difficult to make confident recommendations to treat at present. The indication is unlicensed.

Diabetes not controlled by lifestyle measures alone

Lifestyle measures at diagnosis are very effective in reducing hyperglycaemia, as demonstrated by the UKPDS, where the gain in HbA_{1c} was greater (around double) of that subsequently achieved by any therapeutic agent, and greater than the deterioration which subsequently occurred due the natural history of the condition over the next 15 years.

Nevertheless most people with diabetes will fail to meet preventative targets for arterial disease (an HbA_{1c} of <6.5%[60]) on lifestyle measures alone, or will deteriorate to levels of hyperglycaemia above such an intervention level within months. Because of its success in the UKPDS, metformin is now usually the drug of choice (if not contraindicated by renal function). Given the lack of outcome data for the PPAR-γ agonists, and given the extent of the advantage shown for metformin over sulphonylureas, insulin and epidemiological predictions, it is then difficult, despite all their beneficial effects on aspects of the metabolic syndrome, to recommend the new drugs rather than metformin except in the circumstance where the latter is contraindicated or intolerance is found after a careful trial.

Against the sulphonylureas (in people who cannot take metformin) the situation is more complex. Intolerance or contraindications to these drugs is rare (with the exception of hypoglycaemia, a special circumstance in itself), but while their efficacy can be regarded as proven even in reducing the risk of myocardial infarction, the small extent of the gain (mean risk reduction 16%[61]) makes it possible that drugs like the PPAR-γ agonists, which might be expected to have an outcome profile more similar to metformin, could be clinically advantageous. In these circumstances one approach is to recognize the heterogeneity of Type 2 diabetes and prefer PPAR-γ agonists in people with overt evidence of the metabolic syndrome, but sulphonylureas in those with more dominant insulin deficiency. Only the outcome studies will resolve these issues, but it is also possible that PPAR-γ agonists will before then be shown to preserve islet B-cell function in people with Type 2 diabetes, a finding which would underline their advantage.

Confirming these views is the relative cost of these therapies. Allowing that monitoring costs will be equal (monitoring of liver function is no longer indicated, see above), relative cost-effectiveness is largely determined by drug acquisition costs. Outside the USA, metformin is a generic drug, available very cheaply, and no new PPAR-γ agonist is able to match metformin given the lack of evidence of significantly greater efficacy at the present time.

The question of incremental cost-effectiveness versus the sulphonylureas is more difficult. Generic sulphonylureas, with no efficacy or safety disadvantage over newer agents, are cheap and widely available. As a minimum PPAR-γ agonists are as effective as the sulphonylureas, and at best two to three times better. At the minimum, PPAR-γ agonists cannot be as cost-effective as the sulphonylureas. At around double the effectiveness, PPAR-γ agonists even at ten times the price of sulfonylureas would probably be cost-effective at an incremental cost-effectiveness ratio of US$30,000 per QALY (quality of life adjusted life year), but the complexity of Type 2 diabetes outcomes prevents formal calculation of this at present. As a result, conservative healthcare funders currently refuse to pay for these drugs in patients in whom generic sulphonylureas can be used instead.

In a few markets, insulin is both cheap and easily available. In these circumstances the same arguments over cost-effectiveness as for the sulphonylureas apply to choice of glucose-lowering agent, insulin being cheaper in these markets (but see below) than the PPAR-γ agonists. However a small reduction in health quality of life (strictly health utility) due to insulin therapy itself needs to be factored into the equation.

Combination therapy with glucose-lowering drugs

As noted above, these drugs work well in combination with both metformin and sulphonylureas, and may have some synergy with the latter.[11,18–24] Accordingly, in patients no longer adequately controlled on lifestyle measures plus one of these drugs (usually metformin if it can be taken), the addition of a PPAR-γ agonist is a logical option. This is the only licensed indication in Europe. Where the choice is addition of a PPAR-γ agonist or a sulphonylurea/metformin, then exactly the same arguments over effectiveness/cost-effectiveness as given above apply.

One issue of importance in the use of these drugs is to take more care to introduce them as a trial of therapy. This follows quite simply from the high cost of the drugs (are they worth paying for as regards the individual person under consideration?), but also reflects experience of fairly high levels of failure of efficacy (the corollary of the very high efficacy found in a few patients (see above)), and equally high levels of individual intolerance for miscellaneous reasons.

There seems to be no logical reason why PPAR-γ agonists should not be used in combination therapy with α-glucosidase inhibitors.

Triple combination therapy

As noted above PPAR-γ agonists are effective in combination with sulphonylureas and with metformin.[11,18–24] In these circumstances they would of course be expected to be effective and safe in triple combination therapy with sulphonylureas + metformin. Curiously this is not the view of some licensing bodies, and as a result this obvious indication is not licensed in Europe, although this has not prevented it becoming the dominant usage in some countries.

In this circumstance, the cost-effectiveness argument relates to the alternative of acarbose (or miglitol) or insulin therapy. As the most commonly used insulin regimen in people with Type 2 diabetes is injection twice daily of NPH insulin or a biphasic pre-mix in a proprietary formulation, and as insulin injection carries additional costs in the way of increased self-monitoring, educational input from diabetes nurse specialists (diabetes educators), and hypoglycaemia, insulin therapy has been judged to be more costly than PPAR-γ agonists in the circumstance in which they might be considered alternatives (people whose HbA_{1c} has deteriorated to 7.5–8.5% on lifestyle measures plus other oral glucose-lowering drugs). Furthermore the evidence from UKPDS is that insulin is not particularly effective in this population (no more than sulphonylureas, worse than metformin),[61] so that its effectiveness compared with PPAR-γ agonists is at best equal and at worst inferior.

Combination with insulin therapy

This is not a licensed indication for PPAR-γ agonists in Europe, nor for rosiglitazone in the USA. Caution is advised with pioglitazone and insulin in combination, though it seems doubtful there is any real difference here between the two thiazolidinediones. The reasons for these cautions relate to fluid retention and cardiac failure and are discussed above. Licensing considerations have not, however, prevented the widespread use of this combination in North America and in Europe, in particular in obese patients requiring large amounts of

Advance	Comment
Better data on triple combination therapy with sulphonylureas and metformin	The major indication in people with limited but adequate resources
Clarification of safety and efficacy in combination with insulin	A major need in people who cannot take metformin or in whom insulin + metformin is ineffective; expensive
Clarification of relative efficacy in glucose lowering compared with conventional drugs	Will help calculations of relative cost-effectiveness
Better understanding of lipid effects	May allay concerns over crude changes in LDL cholesterol concentrations
Further studies on cardiac function in the medium term	Should allay fears of direct cardiotoxicity from these drugs
Better economic models of Type 2 diabetes	Should allow more precise evaluation of relative incremental cost-effectiveness against current drugs of lesser efficacy
Cardiovascular and microvascular outcome studies	Should determine relative efficacy in terms of true outcomes against conventional drugs, allowing more precise evaluation of relative cost-effectiveness

Table 21.3
Future prospects for PPAR-γ agonists

insulin but failing to achieve anything like adequate blood glucose control.

Anecdotal reports of remarkable efficacy in some patients in this circumstance have been confirmed by positive reports of small series of clinical experience, where HbA$_{1c}$ has fallen by a greater degree than expected from combination studies with oral agents, with some dramatic improvements, and despite large reductions in insulin dosage.[62] Cautious use of this combination in patients in whom it is not contraindicated seems appropriate.

PPAR-γ agonists and the future

Considerable uncertainty clearly still underlies details of the efficacy, relative efficacy, safety, and cost-effectiveness of these drugs, and is reflected in the large number of studies being reported in 2002 in major international meetings. Some of the areas of uncertainty being tackled along with associated comments are given in Table 21.3. While these should be answered progressively over the next five years, it is already obvious that people with diabetes have an enormous amount to gain from the appropriate use of these drugs, albeit at considerable expense to healthcare funders. This however looks acceptable by conventional criteria of incremental cost-effectiveness. Several newer PPAR-γ agonists can be expected to reach the market in the near future, but it seems unlikely that these will dissociate the problems relating to fluid balance from glucose-lowering efficacy, effectively putting a limit on gains in clinical usefulness. More promising in this regard are drugs providing ideal combinations of lipid-lowering and glucose-lowering efficacy, which could then usefully displace the fibrates (though not statins) from lengthy diabetes prescription lists, while at the same time provide cardiovascular protection through effects on diverse aspects of the metabolic syndrome.

Acknowledgements

Philip D Home, on behalf of the University of Newcastle upon Tyne, has been a consultant to, and/or received research support from, and/or lectured in association with the companies that now constitute GlaxoSmithKline, with GlaxoSmithKline, and with Takeda. He is Chairman of the Steering Committee of the rosiglitazone outcomes study, RECORD.

References

1. DeFronzo RA, Bonadonna RC, Ferrannini E. Pathogenesis of NIDDM. In: Alberti KGMM, Zimmet P, DeFronzo RA, eds. International Textbook of Diabetes Mellitus, 2nd Ed. Chichester: Wiley, 1997: 635–712.
2. Bailey C. New drugs for the treatment of diabetes mellitus. In: Alberti KGMM, Zimmet P, DeFronzo RA, eds. International Textbook of Diabetes Mellitus, 2nd Ed. Chichester: Wiley, 1997: 865–81.
3. Thorp JM, Waring WS. Modification and distribution of lipids by ethyl chlorophenoxy-isobutyrate. Nature Lond 1962; 194: 948–9.
4. Yki-Järvinen H. Glucose toxicity. Endocrinol Rev 1992; 13: 415–31.
5. Young PW, Cawthorne MA, Coyle PJ et al. Repeat treatment of obese mice with BRL 49653, a new and potent insulin sensitizer, enhances insulin action in white adipocytes. Diabetes 1995; 44: 1087–92.
6. Carey DJ, Cowin GJ, Galloway GJ et al. Rosiglitazone increases insulin sensitivity and reduces factors associated with insulin resistance in type 2 diabetes. Diabetes Res Clin Pract 2000; 50 Suppl. 1: P311.
7. Sironi AM, Vichi S, Gastaldelli A et al. Effects of troglitazone on insulin action and cardiovascular risk factors in patients with non-insulin-dependent diabetes. Pharmacol Ther 1997; 62: 194–202.
8. Miyazaki V, Mahankali A, Matsuda M et al. Improved glycemic control and enhanced insulin sensitivity in type 2 diabetic subjects treated with pioglitazone. Diabetes Care 2001; 24: 710–9.
9. Matthews DR, Bakst A, Weston WM et al. Rosiglitazone decreases insulin resistance and improves beta-cell function in patients with type 2 diabetes. Diabetologia 1999; 42 Suppl. 1: A228.
10. Rosenstock J. Improved insulin sensitivity and beta cell responsivity suggested by HOMA analysis of pioglitazone therapy. Diabetologia 2000; 43 Suppl. 1: A192.
11. Jones NP, Mather R, Owen S et al. Long term efficacy of rosiglitazone as monotherapy or in combination with metformin. Diabetologia 2000; 43 Suppl. 1: A192.
12. Stamler J, Vaccaro 0, Neaton JD et al. Diabetes, other risk factors, and 12-yr cardiovascular mortality for men screened in the Multiple Risk Factor Intervention Trial. Diabetes Care 1993; 16: 434–44.
13. Patel J, Anderson RJ, Rappaport EB. Rosiglitazone monotherapy improves glycaemic control in patients with type 2 diabetes: a twelve-week, randomized, placebo-controlled study. Diabetes Obes Metab 1999; 1: 165–72.
14. Aronoff S, Rosenblatt S, Braithwaite S et al. Pioglitazone hydrochloride monotherapy improves glycemic control in the treatment of patients with type 2 diabetes. Diabetes Care 2000; 23: 1605–11.
15. Raskin P, Rappaport EB, Cole ST et al. Rosiglitazone short-term monotherapy lowers fasting and post-prandial glucose in patients with type II diabetes. Diabetologia 2000; 43: 278–84.
16. Lebovitz HE, Dole JF, Patwardhan R et al. Rosiglitazone monotherapy is effective in patients with type 2 diabetes. J Clin Endocrinol Metab 2001; 86: 280–8.

17. Phillips LS, Grunberger G, Miller E et al. Once- and twice-daily dosing with rosiglitazone improves glycaemic control in patients with type 2 diabetes. Diabetes Care 2001; 24: 308–15.

18. Kreider M, Miller E, Patel J. Rosiglitazone is safe and well tolerated as monotherapy or combination therapy in patients with type-2 diabetes mellitus. Diabetes 1999; 48: A117.

19. Fonseca V, Rosenstock J, Patwardhan R, Salzman A. Effect of metformin and rosiglitazone combination therapy in patients with type 2 diabetes. A randomized controlled trial. JAMA 2000; 283: 1695–702.

20. Wolffenbuttel BHR, Gomis R, Squatrito S et al. Addition of low-dose rosiglitazone to sulphonylurea therapy improves glycaemic control in type 2 diabetic patients. Diabet Med 2000; 17: 40–7.

21 Einhorn D, Rendell M, Rosenzweig J et al. Pioglitazone hydrochloride in combination with metformin in the treatment of patients with type 2 diabetes mellitus: a randomized placebo-controlled study. Clin Ther 2000; 22: 1395–409.

22. Hanefeld M, Goke B. Combining pioglitazone with a sulphonylurea or metformin in the management of type 2 diabetes. Exp Clin Endocrinol Diabet 2000; 108 Suppl. 2: S256–S266.

23. Kipnes MS, Krosnick A, Rendell MS et al. Pioglitazone hydrochloride in combination with sulfonylurea therapy improves glycaemic control in patients with Type 2 diabetes mellitus: a randomised, placebo-controlled study. Am J Med 2001; 111: 10–17.

24. Schneider R, Egan J, Houser V. Combination therapy with pioglitazone and sulphonylurea in patients with type 2 diabetes. Diabetes 1999; 48 Suppl. 1: A458.

25. Raskin P, Rendell M, Riddle MC et al. A randomised trial of rosiglitazone therapy in patients with inadequately controlled insulin treated type 2 diabetes. Diabetes Care 2001; 24: 1226–32.

26. Schwartz S, Raskin P, Fonseca V, Graveline JF. Effect of troglitazone in insulin treated patients with type 2 diabetes. N Engl J Med 1998; 338: 861–6.

27. National Institute for Clinical Excellence. Guidance on the use of rosiglitazone for Type 2 diabetes mellitus. Technology Appraisal Guidance No. 9. London: NICE, 2000. (www.nice.org.uk)

28. National Institute for Clinical Excellence. Guidance on the use of pioglitazone for Type 2 diabetes mellitus. Technology Appraisal Guidance No. 21. London: NICE, 2001. (www.nice.org.uk)

29. Home PD. Thiazolidinediones: increasing insulin sensitivity. In: Amiel S, ed. Horizons in Medicine, 13. London: Royal College of Physicians, 2002: 185–94.

30. Ovalle F, Bell DSH. Differing effects of thiazolidinediones on LDL sub-fractions. Diabetes 2001; 50 Suppl. 2: A453.

31. Khan, MA, St. Peter JV, Xue JL. A prospective, randomized comparison of the metabolic effects of pioglitazone or rosiglitazone in patients with Type 2 diabetes who were previously treated with troglitazone. Diabetes Care 2002; 25: 708–11.

32. Parulkar AA, Pendergrass ML, Grand-Ayala R et al. Nonhypoglycemic effects of thiazolidinediones. Ann Intern Med 2001; 134: 61–71.

33. Mathisen A, Egan J, Schneider R, Pioglitazone 010 Study Group. The effect of combination therapy with pioglitazone and sulfonylurea on the lipid profile in patients with type 2 diabetes. Diabetes 1999; 48 Suppl. 1: A106.

34. Boden G. Free fatty acids, insulin resistance and type 2 diabetes mellitus. Proc Assoc Am Phys 1999; 111: 241–8.

35. Brunzell J, Cohen B, Kreider M et al. Rosiglitazone favorably affects LDL-C and HDL-C heterogeneity in type 2 diabetes. Diabetes 2001; 50: A141.

36. Bakris GL, Dole JF, Porter LE et al. Rosiglitazone improves blood pressure in patients with type 2 diabetes. Diabetes 2000; 49 Suppl. 1: A96.

37. Home PD, Piatidis G, Koelendorf K et al. Antihypertensive effect of farglitazar, a tyrosine-based non-thiazolidinedione PPARγ agonist, in patients with Type 2 diabetes and hypertension. Diabetes 2001; 20: A117.

38. Carey DG, Galloway G, Dodrell D et al. Rosiglitazone reduces hepatic fat and increases subcutaneous but not intra-abdominal fat depots. Diabetologia 2000; 43 Suppl. 1: A68.

39. Buckingham RE, Al-Barazanji KA, Toseland CD. Peroxisome proliferator-activated receptor-g agonist, rosiglitazone protects against nephropathy and pancreatic islet abnormalities in Zucker fatty rats. Diabetes 1998; 47: 1326–3134.

40. Bakris GL, Weston WM, Rappaport EB et al. Rosiglitazone produces long-term reductions in urinary albumin excretion in type 2 diabetes. Diabetologia 1999; 42 Suppl. 1: A230.

41. Freed MI, Weston WM, Viberti G. Rosiglitazone reduces urinary albumin excretion in type 2 diabetes. Diabetologia 1999; 42 Suppl. 1: A230.

42. Freed M, Fuell D, Menci L et al. Effects of combination therapy with rosiglitazone and glibenclamide on PAI-1 antigen, PAI-1 activity, and tPA in patients with type 2 diabetes. Diabetologia 2000; 43 Suppl. 1: A267.

43. Kruszynska YT, Yu JG, Olefsky JM, Sobel BE. Effects of troglitazone on blood concentrations of plasminogen activator inhibitor 1 in patients with type 2 diabetes and in lean and obese normal subjects. Diabetes 2000; 49: 633–9.

44. Greenberg A, Haffner S, Weston W et al. Rosiglitazone reduces C-reactive protein, a marker of systemic inflammation, in type 2 diabetic patients. Diabetologia 2001; 44 Suppl. 1: A222.

45. Fuell DL, Freed MI, Greenberg AS et al. The effects of treatment with rosiglitazone on C-reactive protein and interleukin-6 in patients with type 2 diabetes. Diabetes 2001; 50 Suppl. 2: A435.

46. Murphy GJ, Holder JC. PPAR-γ agonists: therapeutic role in diabetes, inflammation and cancer. Trends Pharmacol Sci 2000; 21: 469–74.

47. Watkins PB, Whitcomb RW. Hepatic dysfunction associated with troglitazone. N Engl J Med 1998; 338: 916–17.

48. Forman LM, Simmons DA, Diamond RH. Hepatic failure in a patient taking rosiglitazone. Ann Intern Med 2000; 132: 118–21.

49. Al-Salmon J, Arjomand H, Kemp DG, Mittal M. Hepatocellular injury in a patient receiving rosiglitazone: a case report. Ann Intern Med 2000; 132: 121–4.

50. Scheen AJ. Thiazolidinediones and liver toxicity. Diabetes Metab 2001 27: 305–13.

51. Yamazaki H, Suzuki M, Tane K et al. In vitro inhibitory effects of troglitazone and its metabolites on drug oxidation activities of human cytochrome P450 enzymes: comparison with pioglitazone and rosiglitazone. Xenobiotica 2000; 30: 61–70.

52. Loi CM, Stem R, Koup JR et al. Effect of troglitazone on the pharmacokinetics of an oral contraceptive agent. Clin Pharmacol 1999; 39: 410–17.

53. DiTusa L, Luzier AB. Potential interaction between troglitazone and atorvastatin. Clin Pharmacol Ther 2000; 25: 279–82.

54. Lin JC, Ito MK. A drug interaction between troglitazone and simvastatin. Diabetes Care 1999; 22: 2104–6.

55. Kortboyer JM, Eckland DJA. Pioglitazone has low potential for drug interactions. Diabetologia 1999; 42 Suppl. 1: A228.

56 Ehrmann DA, Schneider DJ, Sobel BE et al. Troglitazone improves defects in insulin action, insulin secretion, ovarian steroidogenesis, and fibrinolysis in women with polycystic ovary syndrome. J Clin Endocrinol Metab 1997; 82: 2108–16.

57. Caruana L, Petrie MC, Davie AP, McMurray JJ. Do patients with suspected heart failure and preserved left ventricular systolic function suffer from 'diastolic heart failure' or from misdiagnosis? A prospective descriptive study. BMJ 2000; 321: 215–18.

58. SmithKline Beecham. Rosiglitazone: A Clinician's Resource File. Welwyn Garden City: SmithKline Beecham, 1999.

59. Buchanan TA, Xiang AH, Peters RK et al. Response of pancreatic beta-cells to improved insulin sensitivity in women at high risk for type 2 diabetes. Diabetes 2000; 49: 782–8.

60. European Diabetes Policy Group 1999. A desktop guide to type 2 diabetes mellitus. Diabet Med 1999; 16: 716–30.

61. UK Prospective Diabetes Study (UKPDS) Group. Intensive blood-glucose control with sulphonylureas or insulin compared with conventional treatment and risk of complications in patients with type 2 diabetes (UKPDS 33). Lancet 1998; 352: 837–53.

62. Buch HN, Baskar V, Barton DM et al. Combination of insulin and thiazolidinedione therapy in massively obese patients with Type 2 diabetes. Diabet Med 2002; 19: 572–4.

22

Recognition, treatment and prevention of hypoglycaemia unawareness in Type 1 diabetes mellitus

Carmine G Fanelli, Francesca Porcellati, Simone Pampanelli, Geremia B Bolli

Introduction

Hypoglycaemia unawareness is the reduced ability, or failure, to recognize hypoglycaemia at the physiological plasma glucose concentration at which warning symptoms normally occur (~55 mg/dl, ~3 mmol/l). Patients unaware of hypoglycaemia either do not realize that plasma glucose is decreasing and causing neuroglycopenia, or ultimately feel the symptoms, but at lower than normal plasma glucose (high thresholds).

The problem of hypoglycaemia unawareness in Type 1 diabetes mellitus is important for several reasons. First, hypoglycaemia unaware Type 1 diabetic patients cannot correct impending hypoglycaemia (by eating food), and therefore cannot prevent neuroglycopenia (and unconsciousness). Thus, hypoglycaemia unawareness is a risky condition for severe hypoglycaemia. Second, hypoglycaemia unawareness is a frequent condition in Type 1 diabetes. A few years ago it was estimated that at least one-fourth of Type 1 diabetic patients suffer from hypoglycaemic unawareness.[1] It is likely that at the present time, e.g. the post-DCCT (Diabetes Control and Complications Trial) era,[2] this figure is increasing with the greater popularity of intensive therapy.[2–4] Third, over the last few years major progress in its pathogenesis and treatment have been

made. A special therapeutic approach to Type 1 diabetes can now be designed to successfully achieve reduction of the percentage of glycosylated haemoblobin A1c (HbA1c) with low risk of hypoglycaemia and hypoglycaemia unawareness. In this chapter, these points will be discussed. Special emphasis will be given to the treatment and prevention of hypoglycaemia unawareness in Type 1 diabetes.

The importance of glucose for brain metabolism

Tissues such as muscle and liver may easily switch from oxidation of glucose to other non-glucose fuels, i.e. non-esterified free fatty acids (NEFA), ketones and lactate. In contrast, from a practical point of view, the brain can utilize only glucose as a source of energy. In fact, although in theory the brain can oxidize ketones[5,6] and lactate,[6,7] this occurs in humans only under experimental hypoglycaemia conditions where supraphysiological concentrations of these substrates are produced in plasma by means of exogenous infusion. During insulin-induced hypoglycaemia closely mimicking the spontaneous condition of insulin-treated Type 1 diabetes, plasma ketone concentration decreases, and lactate concentration does not increase substantially.[8] Thus, these substrates cannot compensate the condition of neuro-glycopenia which follows hypoglycaemia. In addition, the rebound increase in plasma ketones during prolonged hypoglycaemia is not followed by blunting of the brain responses to hypoglycaemia such as release of counter-regulatory hormones, generation of specific symptoms, and cognitive dysfunction.[8] This suggests that the greater availability of ketones in response to hypoglycaemia[8] does not help the brain when it is already neuroglycopenic. In keeping with this line, a recent study inves-tigating the utilization of substrates by the brain using arterio-venous differences for substrates,[9] there was no evidence for a substantial utilization of substrates such as lactate, pyruvate and amino acids during hypoglycaemia. Therefore, it was concluded that glucose, which accounted for most of oxidative metabolism during hypoglycaemia, is the absolute substrate used by the brain under this condition. Because the brain cannot operate gluconeogenesis, or store considerable amounts of glucose in the form of glycogen, it is clear that the brain is strictly dependent on continuous glucose delivery from the circula-tion for its metabolism and function.

Physiology of responses to hypoglycaemia in humans

Because maintenance of plasma glucose concentration above a given threshold is crucial for brain function (and survival of the whole body), it is no surprise that multiple mecha-nisms cooperate to prevent hypoglycaemia in mammals, especially under adverse conditions, such as prolonged fasting, failure of vital organs (kidney, heart, liver), or after adminis-tration of glucose-lowering drugs. These homoeostatic mechanisms include: first, release of counterregulatory hormones (reviewed in ref. 10) and, second, generation of specific symptoms. The latter includes the autonomic (anxiety, palpitations, hunger, sweating, irritability, tremor), and neuroglycopenic (dizzi-ness, tingling, blurred vision, difficulty in thinking, faintness) symptoms.

An important concept is that the brain responses to hypoglycaemia are hierarchic.[11] During progressive decrements in plasma glucose, the release of counterregulatory hormones begins before the symptoms of hypoglycaemia are generated.[11] Several studies have concordantly indicated that all counter-regulatory hormones (glucagon, adrenaline, cortisol, growth hormone) are released at a (arterial) plasma glucose threshold of approxi-mately 65 mg/dl (~3.5 mmol/l); that symptoms (both autonomic and neuroglycopenic) appear only when plasma glucose decreases at approx-imately 55 mg/dl (~3.0 mmol/l); and that cognitive function deteriorates when plasma glucose decreases below 50 mg/dl (~2.7 mmol/l).[11–13]

Definition of hypoglycaemia

In classic textbooks, hypoglycaemia is usually defined as plasma glucose concentration below 50 mg/dl (~2.7 nmol/l).[14,15] However, normally the release of counterregulatory hormones in response to hypoglycaemia is already evident for modest decrements in plasma glucose below normal, post-absorptive values by ~20 mg/dl (~1 mmol/l), i.e. at a plasma glucose concentration of 65 mg/dl (~3.5 mmol/l). Thus, a modern, physiological definition of hypoglycaemia is any decrease in plasma glucose concentration below 65 mg/dl (~3.5 mmol/l). This concept is important not only in physiology, but also to define safe glycaemic targets for intensive therapy of Type 1 diabetes.[4,16]

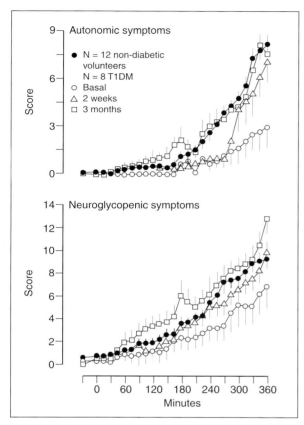

Figure 22.2

Autonomic and neuroglycopenic symptoms scores in response to the experimental hypoglycaemia of Figure 22.1, before, and two weeks and three months after meticulous prevention of hypoglycaemia in a group of Type 1 diabetic patients. Source: Reprinted with permission from © 1993 American Diabetes Association. Diabetes 1993; 42: 1683–9.[30].

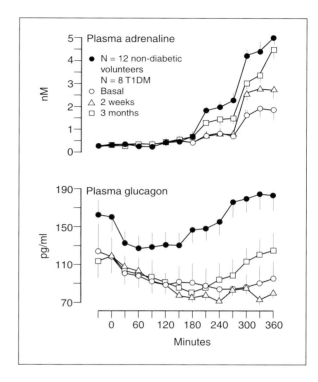

Figure 22.3

Plasma adrenaline and glucagon responses to the experimental hypoglycaemia of Figure 22.1, before, and two weeks and three months after meticulous prevention of hypoglycaemia in a group of Type 1 diabetic patients. Source: Reprinted with permission from © 1993 American Diabetes Association. Diabetes 1993; 42: 1683–9.[30].

in whom two episodes of mild and brief insulin-induced hypoglycaemia (~50 mg/dl, ~2.7 mmol/l for ~90 min, one episode in the morning, the other in the afternoon),[33] or a single episode of nocturnal hypoglycaemia,[22,25] blunt the hormonal and symptom responses to hypoglycaemia induced on the following day. Similar observations have been made in Type 1 diabetic patients.[34,35] This pattern of responses mimicks

closely the spontaneous responses of Type 1 diabetic patients unaware of hypoglycaemia.[18,30]

Taken together, these observations indicate that frequent hypoglycaemia in Type 1 diabetes, caused either by inappropriate treatment and/or impaired counterregulation, rapidly induces loss of symptoms and blunts the release of counterregulatory hormones in response to hypoglycaemia. The good news for patients and the important information for diabetologists, is that prevention of hypoglycaemia largely, if not fully, reverses unawareness of, and improves counterregulation to, hypoglycaemia.

Hypoglycaemia unawareness and impaired glucose counterregulation

Type 1 diabetic patients, unaware of hypoglycaemia, suffer from greater impairment of the glucose counterregulatory system, primarily because of more suppressed release of adrenaline.[10,17] Meticulous prevention of hypoglycaemia, which recovers symptoms, improves the responses of glucagon, although only slightly, at least in short-term Type 1 diabetes.[30] Prevention of hypoglycaemia also normalizes, or at least improves, responses of adrenaline to hypoglycaemia.[18,30,31] However, the effect of prevention of hypoglycaemia on responses of adrenaline is stronger in short-term compared with long-term diabetes,[31] and in diabetes without, rather than with, clinically overt autonomic neuropathy.[36] Taken together, these observations indicate that prevention of hypoglycaemia reverses most of the suppressed adrenaline responses reported to occur in diabetes.[10,17] The fact that some responses of adrenaline to hypoglycaemia are apparently irreversibly lost despite meticulous prevention of hypoglycaemia in diabetes, and especially in diabetes of long duration in the absence of autonomic neuropathy[30,36] cannot easily be explained at the present time. However, these data[30,36] indicate that loss of adrenaline responses to hypoglycaemia are not necessarily the result of autonomic neuropathy, although autonomic neuropathy importantly contributes to this.[36] In addition, these data indicate that it

is long-term diabetes in particular that requires a careful approach with insulin treatment to prevent hypoglycaemia.

Mechanisms of hypoglycaemia unawareness

The mechanisms of hypoglycaemia unawareness are not fully established. To date, there is evidence that rates of glucose transport from the blood to the brain may be affected by prevailing antecedent glucose concentration. In fact, in rats, chronic hypoglycaemia increases,[37] whereas chronic hyperglycaemia[38] decreases, glucose transport to the brain. In particular, chronic hypoglycaemia appears to increase the expression of glucose transporters localized in the microvessels of the blood–brain barrier (GLUT1, 55-kDa form)[37,39,40] as well as the neuron-specific glucose transporters (GLUT3).[41] In humans, prolonged hypoglycaemia (56 h of intermittent hypoglycaemia) prevents the expected decrease in brain glucose uptake, measured by the arteriovenous difference technique, during a subsequent episode of hypoglycaemia.[42] In diabetic patients with low values of glycosylated haemoglobin (HbA1c) due to antecedent, frequent hypoglycaemia, brain glucose uptake does not decrease during hypoglycaemia as it does in diabetic patients with elevated HbA1c (less frequent hypoglycaemia) and non-diabetic subjects.[43] Taken together, these observations support the view that brain glucose transport is influenced by antecedent prevailing plasma glucose concentration. Hypoglycaemia accelerates delivery of glucose to the brain. Thus, during subsequent hypoglycaemia, the brain is not, or at least is less, neuroglycopenic than normal, and does not need to generate the counterregulatory responses and the autonomic symptoms to defend and alert the subject about hypoglycaemia. However, these findings are at variance with recent data in healthy subjects and patients with Type 1 diabetes demonstrating that blood-to-brain glucose transport and cerebral glucose metabolism, as measured by a positron emission tomography (PET) technique after intravenous injection of [1–[11]C]glucose using a validated model that includes a fourth-rate constant to account for regional egress of ^{11}C metabolites, are not affected by either antecedent hypoglycaemia[44] or chronic hyperglycaemia.[45] However, since the study by Segel et al.[44] was carried out in non-diabetics, it does not rule out a putative increase in blood-to-brain glucose transport in diabetes associated with hypoglycaemia unawareness. In addition, because the [1–[11]C] glucose PET technique does not allow the quantitation of regional changes in blood-to-brain glucose transport, increments in regional blood-to-brain glucose transport cannot be excluded. Indeed, regional changes in [18F]-fluorodeoxyglucose uptake have been reported in Type 1 diabetic men with hypoglycaemia unawareness.[46]

An additional mechanism of hypoglycaemia unawareness has been provided by Davis et al.[47] who found that the responses of cortisol to antecedent hypoglycaemia blunts the autonomic hormone responses to subsequent hypoglycaemia. Similarly, preventing the increase in plasma cortisol during hypoglycaemia preserves counterregulatory and symptomatic responses to subsequent hypoglycaemia.[48] Recently, McGregor et al. found reduced autonomic neuroendocrine and autonomic symptom responses to hypoglycaemia after antecedent increase of cortisol levels by infusion of adrenocorticotropic hormone (ACTH) in healthy subjects.[49] In contrast, in rats, intracerebroventricular infusion of corticosterone failed to reduce the neuroendocrine response to subsequent hypoglycaemia, whereas antecedent hypoglycaemia blunted those responses most likely by decreasing activation of paraventricular nucleus (PVN) of the hypothalamus.[50]

Conceivably, the mechanism of cortisol-mediated hypoglycaemia unawareness is not necessarily alternative, but possibly complementary to that of accelerated brain glucose transport. The mechanisms by which antecedent response of cortisol affects responses to subsequent hypoglycaemia are not clear. *In vitro* studies have shown that glucocorticoids inhibit deoxyglucose uptake into cultures containing both neurons and glia.[51] In contrast, dexamethasone increased GLUT1 expression in vessels of brain tumours (gliomas).[52] In addition, chronic treatment with dexamethasone *in vivo* increases blood-to-brain glucose transport in the setting of hyperinsulinaemia and hyperglycaemia.[53] Therefore, currently the evidence does not allow any conclusion to be drawn about a possible influence of an increase in plasma cortisol during hypoglycaemia on changes of blood-to-brain glucose transport rates to subsequent hypoglycaemia. It is likely that the effect of antecedent-increased cortisol on the neuroendocrine and autonomic responses to subsequent hypoglycaemia is independent of changes in blood-to-brain glucose transport. It is possible to speculate that increased levels of cortisol during antecedent hypoglycaemia could blunt those responses by down-regulating hypothalamic glucocorticoid stress receptors (type II receptors)[54] to subsequent hypoglycaemia. Epinephrine and epinephrine-mediated responses to subsequent hypoglycaemia would also be reduced since the conversion of noradrenaline to adrenaline requires the glucocorticoid-mediated induction of phenylethanolamine-N-methyltransferase (PMNT). Finally, since glucocorticoid receptors are ubiquitous in the brain,[54] some aspects of cognitive adaptation to antecedent hypoglycaemia might be directly linked to lower cortisol release following antecedent hypoglycaemia.

In fact, it is well known that increased cortisol levels impair cognitive function, most commonly memory.[55] The hippocampus, which plays a critical role in the process of acquisition and recall of new information (declarative memory) may be affected by a mechanism involving neuronal calcium regulation.[56]

Interestingly, over the last decade, several studies have shown that alpha-adrenergic sensitivity, as measured by cardiac chronotropic responses to intravenous injections of the non-selective alpha-adrenergic agonist isoproterenol, is reduced in Type 1 diabetics[57] and that antecedent hypoglycaemia itself reduces alpha-adrenergic sensitivity in Type 1 diabetics but not in healthy subjects.[58] This would suggest that antecedent hypoglycaemia could alter to some extent the responses mediated by alpha-adrenergic sensitivity to subsequent hypoglycaemia, thus favouring generation of hypoglycaemia unawareness. Indeed, avoidance of hypoglycaemia restores hypoglycaemia unawareness by increasing alpha-adrenergic sensitivity in Type 1 diabetes mellitus.[59]

Taken together, the above observations indicate that the pathophysiology of hypoglycaemia unawareness is not yet well understood. Most likely, multiple mechanisms cooperate for the generation of this syndrome. At present, the relative role of individual mechanisms and their potential interactions in the development of the clinical phenomenon of hypoglycaemia unawareness in diabetes mellitus, remain to be established.

The vicious circle of 'recurrent hypoglycaemia unawareness'

Intensive insulin therapy[2-4] aims at (near-) normoglycaemia. Because subcutaneous insulin replacement is so imperfect,[16] mild hypoglycaemia is inevitably induced from time to time. In turn, if hypoglycaemia is frequent (e.g. one episode per day), unawareness of hypoglycaemia is induced.

Prevention of hypoglycaemia is an important part of modern intensive diabetes therapy.[4] In theory, if one were able to prevent hypoglycaemia from the clinical onset of diabetes, hypoglycaemia unawareness should never appear. In fact, meticulous prevention of hypoglycaemia in diabetic patients previously suffering from recurrent hypoglycaemia, fully reverses the syndrome of hypoglycaemia unawareness and impaired release of adrenaline in short-term diabetes.[30] In addition, if intensive therapy is conducted in a way that prevents the decrease in HbA1c below 6.0%, i.e. frequency of hypoglycaemia is minimized, secretion of adrenaline and generation of symptoms in response to hypoglycaemia appear to be appropriate.[4]

How to prevent hypoglycaemia in intensive therapy of Type 1 diabetes mellitus

The following steps are of primary importance in the prevention of recurrent hypoglycaemia while aiming at the goal of long-term near-normoglycaemia.

Physiological models of insulin replacement

It is easier to prevent hypoglycaemia if insulin is delivered to mimic the physiology of endogenous insulin secretion of normal non-diabetic subjects (Figure 22.4).[60] At present, there are three models of physiological insulin

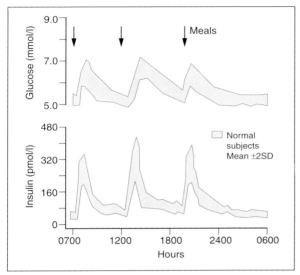

Figure 22.4
Glucose homoeostasis in normal non-diabetic subjects. Source: Reprinted with permission from © 1999 American Diabetes Association. Diabetes Care 1999; 22: 795–800.[60]

replacement in T1DM (Figure 22.5). These models have in common use of a short-acting insulin analogue at each meal, in doses related to carbohydrate content. The number of daily injections of short-acting analogue is related to the number of meals per day, including snacks. The three models differ regarding substitution of basal insulin. Therefore, lispro (or aspart) at mealtime can be combined with basal insulin replaced under the form of either (i) CSII, or (ii) multiple daily injections of NPH, or (iii) glargine once a day.

(i)   *Continuous s.c. insulin infusion.* It is much easier to maintain long-term near-normo-glycaemia in T1DM if basal insulin is replaced by mimicking the physiology of insulin secretion of normal, non-diabetic subjects in the post-absorptive state. This

Figure 22.5
Physiological models of insulin replacement in Type 1 diabetes mellitus.

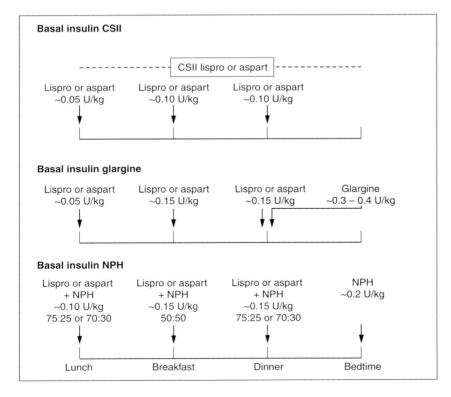

can be best achieved with CSII. As stated earlier, CSII should be presented to T1DM as the gold standard of insulin replacement, particularly as the gold standard of basal insulin substitution, especially when short-acting insulin analogues are used at mealtimes.

(ii) *Multiple daily insulin injections with NPH as basal insulin.* This model is extensively being used[61] and has recently been reviewed.[62] Short-acting insulin analogues should be preferred to human regular insulin at mealtime, primarily because of better lifestyle, and also for better postprandial blood glucose control with lower risk for hypoglycaemia. However, use of short-acting insulin analogues requires optimization of basal insulin at the same time.[61,62] T1DM patients who refuse or cannot have access to CSII should use the model of multiple daily injections of NPH. This approach successfully reproduces what CSII does during the daily hours, but is less than optimal as compared to CSII at night. The risk for nocturnal hypoglycaemia and

fasting hyperglycaemia are somehow direct consequences of the pharmacokinetic and pharmacodynamic properties of NPH insulin. Specific measures to limit the risk for nocturnal hypoglycaemia with bedtime NPH injection include:

• NPH doses no greater than 0.20–0.25 U/kg;
• NPH injection at bedtime, not at dinner time[63] (Figure 22.6);
• injection in the internal part of thigh, not abdomen;
• administration of snack with slowly-absorbed carbohydrate (i.e. 20–40 g of bread) if blood glucose is <120 mg/dl (in this case the night NPH dose should not be reduced);
• if excessive fasting hyperglycaemia persists despite blood glucose at bedtime <150 mg/dl and NPH dose up to 0.25 U/kg, 2–3 units of insulin lispro (or aspart) should be injected at 03:00 h, rather than increasing the bedtime NPH.

(iii) *Multiple daily insulin injections with glargine as basal insulin.* In this model

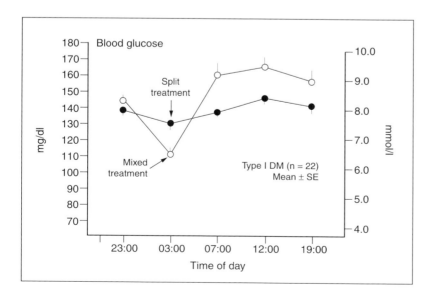

Figure 22.6
Daily blood glucose (from home blood glucose monitoring) with either the evening split treatment (human regular insulin administered at dinner and NPH (Neutral Protamine Hagedorn) insulin administered at bedtime) or mixed insulin administration (a mixture of human regular and NPH insulin administered before dinner). Source: modified with permission from Annals of Internal Medicine 2002; 136: 104–14.[63]

lispro (or aspart) at each meal is combined with s.c. injection of the long-acting insulin analogue glargine once daily. Based on data of pharmacokinetic/pharmacodynamic studies, it is expected that s.c. injection of glargine insulin mimics the effects of CSII at a single rate (Figure 5.4).[64] Lower frequency of nocturnal hypoglycaemia and lower fasting blood glucose should occur as compared to night-time administration of NPH.[65] Recently, it has been shown that glargine reduces the percentage of HbA1c.[66] In addtion, it has been shown that the more convenient dinner-time injection of glargine reproduces closely the effects of bedtime injection.[67]

Blood glucose monitoring

T1DM patients should check regularly their blood glucose concentration prior to each insulin injection. This is necessary to establish the dose of basal insulin, and also the dose of short-acting insulin analogue to be given with the next meal (in addition to carbohydrate content of the meal and insulin sensitivity). Because the short-acting insulin analogues improve the 2-h post-meal blood glucose to a greater extent than human regular insulin, patients should check also the 2-h after-meal blood glucose to titrate the meal dose of lispro (or aspart).

Blood glucose targets

The above discussed models of physiological insulin replacement should be used for both intensive and non-intensive therapy. The terms 'intensive' and 'non-intensive' refer to the long-term glycaemic goals, not to the model of insulin replacement.

Intensive therapy

Treatment of T1DM is intensive when long-term blood glucose is near-normal (Table 22.1). The blood glucose targets should be 'realistic', i.e. not strictly at normoglycaemia, but at moderate hyperglycaemia. Because our current treatment of T1DM is so imperfect, we should make prevention of hypoglycaemia, not absolute normoglycaemia our primary goal, while aiming at long-term good glycaemic control. The DCCT has shown that with HbA1c <7.0%, i.e. a slightly greater than normal value, the risk for onset and/or progression of complications appears to be largely, if not fully prevented. Thus, there seems to be a 'window' of values of HbA1c just above the upper limit of the non-diabetic range where patients are, at once, protected against onset/progression of complications[2,68] by one side, and against the risk for severe hypoglycaemia[4] by the other. Until new, safer means of therapy are available, there is no reason to decrease the percentage of HbA1c to the normal range where the risk for hypoglycaemia is greater.[69]

Non-intensive therapy

Non-intensive therapy is defined as a model of insulin replacement based on CSII or MDI aiming at mean blood glucose concentration and percentage of HbA1c above the values

	Intensive	Non-intensive
Fasting, pre-meal, bedtime blood glucose (mmol/l)	6.5–8.0	8.0–11.0
HbA1c* (%)	6.0–7.0	7.0–8.5

Note: * HPLC method, values in normal, non-diabetic subjects 3.8–5.5%

Table 22.1

Targets of blood glucose control in intensive as well as non-intensive management of Type 1 diabetes

indicated by the DCCT to prevent long-term complications (Table 22.1). For different reasons, special populations such as young children, adults with devastating, advanced complications, or T1DM above 65–70 years of age, should be treated with non-intensive, rather than intensive, therapy. For example, in very small children it is often not possible to achieve the glycaemic goals of intensive therapy. In adults with major advanced complications and in old patients, it is useless to aim at near-normoglycaemia because of expected benefits and because of greater risk for hypoglycaemia.

One concept should be clear: the difference between intensive and non-intensive therapy as defined in this article is limited to the glycaemic targets outlined in Table 22.1. Everything else described above in terms of therapy of T1DM (CSII or MDI model of insulin treatment, diet, blood glucose monitoring, education, etc.) in non-intensive therapy should be identical to intensive therapy. Thus, there is a fundamental difference between the non-intensive therapy of this article and the 'conventional' treatment of the Stockholm[68] and DCCT studies,[2] where 'conventional' is one or two daily injections of mixtures of insulins. The 'conventional' insulin treatment proposed by these studies[2,68] is no longer acceptable either for the patients for whom it is not possible, or for those in whom it is not convenient to aim at long-term near-normoglycaemia. The 'conventional' treatment results in excessively elevated HbA1c and high risk of hypoglycaemia. For example, in the DCCT study, the 'conventional' treatment resulted in a frequency of severe hypoglycaemia of ~0.20 episodes/100 patient-year, despite markedly elevated HbA1c (up to ~9.0%). The priority aim of non-intensive therapy is prevention of hypoglycaemia, while aiming at suboptimal glycaemic control. This can be solely achieved with the above-described CSII or MDI treatment combined with appropriate education.

Education

The time spent with the patient is the most valuable to decrease the percentage of HbA1c and frequency of hypoglycaemia. Unfortunately, there are many patients, and only a few real diabetologists. Diabetologists, busy in academia, are not the ideal professional people to take care of patients. Nurses, although very important in their job, cannot be fully delegated to assist with most of the patients' requirements.

The most important job that a diabetologist can do is instil in his/her patient the motivation and the enthusiasm to make intensive therapy a (nearly) life-long commitment. The patient should be reassured that he/she can have a normal lifestyle, can be nearly free from hypoglycaemia, and based on the DCCT data, free from long-term complications. Only if the patient develops a positive attitude towards his/her diabetes, and considers T1DM not as a disease but as a manageable, although sometimes tedious condition, will the diabetologist have succeeded in their job. Understandably, this is particularly important for the youngest patients.

Acknowledgements

This chapter is dedicated to the people who live and suffer in the Middle-East region of the world. Might justice, peace, fraternity and ultimately love triumph, and gather individuals from different ethnic, religious and country origins under similar ideals of living together.

References

1. Gerich J, Mokan M, Veneman T et al. Hypoglycemia unawareness. Endocr Rev 1991; 12: 356–71.

2. The Diabetes Control and Complications Trial Research Group. The effect of intensive treatment of diabetes on the development and progression of long-term complications in insulin-dependent diabetes mellitus. N Engl J Med 1993; 329: 977–86.

3. Shade DS, Santiago JV, Skyler JS, Rizza RA. Intensive insulin therapy. Excerpta Medica, Amsterdam, 1993.

4. Pampanelli S, Fanelli C, Lalli C et al. Long-term intensive insulin therapy: effects of HbA1c risk for severe and mild hypoglycaemia, status of counterregulation and unawareness of hypoglycaemia. Diabetologia 1996; 39: 677–86.

5. Amiel S, Archibald H, Chusney G et al. Ketone infusion lowers hormonal responses to hypoglycaemia: evidence for acute cerebral utilization of a non-glucose fuel. Clin Sci 1991; 81: 189–94.

6. Veneman T, Mitrakou A, Mokan M et al. Effect of hyperketonemia and hyperlactacidemia on symptoms, cognitive dysfunction and counter-regulatory hormone responses during hypoglycemia in normal humans. Diabetes 1994; 43: 1311–17.

7. Maran A, Cranston I, Lomas J et al. Protection by lactate of cerebral function during hypoglycaemia. Lancet 1994; 343: 16–20.

8. Fanelli C, Di Vincenzo A, Modarelli F et al. Post-hypoglycaemic hyperketonaemia does not contribute to brain metabolism during insulin-induced neuroglycopenia in humans. Diabetologia 1993; 36: 1191–7.

9. Wahren J, Ekberg K, Fernqvist-Forbes E, Nair S. Brain substrate utilisation during acute hypoglycaemia. Diabetologia 1999; 42: 812–18.

10. Bolli GB. From physiology of glucose counter-regulation to prevention of hypoglycaemia in Type 1 diabetes mellitus. Diabetes Nutr Metab 1990; 3: 333–49.

11. Mitrakou A, Ryan C, Veneman T et al. Hierarchy of glycemic thresholds for counter-regulatory hormone secretion, symptoms, and cerebral dysfunction. Am J Physiol 1991; 260: E67–E74.

12. Schwartz N, Clutter W, Shah S, Cryer P. Glycemic thresholds for activation of glucose counter-regulatory systems are higher than the thresholds for symptoms. J Clin Invest 1987; 79: 777–81.

13. Fanelli C, Pampanelli S, Epifano L et al. Relative roles of insulin and hypoglycaemia on induction of neuroendocrine responses to, symptoms of, and deterioration of cognitive function in, hypoglycaemia in humans. Diabetologia 1994; 37: 797–807.

14. Foster DW, Rubenstein AH. Hypoglycemia. In: Wilson JD, Braunwald E, Isselbacher KJ et al., eds. Harrison's Principles of Internal Medicine. New York: McGraw-Hill, Inc., 1991:1759.

15. Young CW, Karam JH. Hypoglycemic disorders. In: Greenspan FS, ed. Basic and Clinical Endocrinology. East Norwalk, Connecticut: Appleton & Lange, 1991: 651.

16. Bolli GB, Perriello G, Fanelli C, De Feo. Nocturnal blood glucose control in Type 1 diabetes mellitus. Diabetes Care 1993; Suppl. 3: 71–89.

17. Bolli GB, Dimitriadis GD, Pehling GB et al. Abnormal glucose counterregulation after subcutaneous insulin in insulin-dependent diabetes mellitus. N Engl J Med 1984; 310: 1706–11.

18. Fanelli C, Pampanelli S, Epifano L et al. Long-term recovery from unawareness, deficient counterregulation and lack of cognitive dysfunction during hypoglycaemia, following institution of a rational, intensive insulin therapy in IDDM. Diabetologia 1994; 37: 1265–76.

19. Mitrakou A, Fanelli C, Veneman T et al. Reversibility of unawareness of hypoglycemia in patients with insulinomas. N Engl J Med 1993; 329: 834–9.

20. Amiel S, Sherwin R, Simonson D, Tamborlane W. Effect of intensive insulin therapy on glycemic thresholds for counterregulatory hormone release. Diabetes 1988; 37: 901–7.

21. Fruehwald-Schultes B, Born J, Kern W et al. Adaptation of cognitive function to hypoglycemia in healthy men. Diabetes Care 2000; 23: 1059–66.

22. Veneman T, Mitrakou A, Mokan M et al. Induction of hypoglycemia unawareness by asymptomatic nocturnal hypoglycemia. Diabetes 1993; 42: 1233–7.

23. Mokan M, Mitrakou A, Veneman T, Ryan C et al. Hypoglycemia unawareness in IDDM. Diabetes Care 1994; 17: 1397–403.

24. Hvidberg A, Fanelli CG, Hersbey T, Cryer PE.

Impact of recent antecedent hypoglycemia on hypoglycemic cognitive dysfunction in nondiabetic humans. Diabetes 1996; 45: 1030–6.

25. Fanelli C, Paramore D, Hershey T et al. Impact of noctunal hypoglycemia on hypoglycemic cognitive dysfunction in Type 1 diabetes mellitus. Diabetes 1998; 47 Suppl. 1: A109.

26. Maran A, Lomas J, Macdonald IA, Amiel SA. Lack of preservation of higher brain function during hypoglycaemia in patients with intensively treated IDDM. Diabetologia 1995; 38: 1412–18.

27. Fanelli CG, Pampanelli S, Porcellati F, Bolli GB. Shift of glycaemic thresholds for cognitive function in hypoglycaemia unawareness in humans. Diabetologia 1998; 41: 720–3.

28. Amiel SA. Cognitive function testing in studies of acute hypoglycaemia: rights and wrongs? Diabetologia 1998; 41: 713–19.

29. Heller SR, Macdonald IA. The measurement of cognitive function during acute hypoglycaemia: experimental limitations and their effect on the study of hypoglycaemia unawareness. Diabet Med 1996; 13: 607–15.

30. Fanelli C, Epifano L, Rambotti AM et al. Meticulous prevention of hypoglycemia (near-) normalizes magnitude and glycemic thresholds of neuroendocrine responses to, symptoms of, and cognitive function during hypoglycemia in intensively treated patients with IDDM of short duration. Diabetes 1993; 42: 1683–9.

31. Cranston I, Lomas J, Maran A et al. Restoration of hypoglycaemia awareness in patients with long-duration insulin-dependent diabetes. Lancet 1994; 344: 283–7.

32. Dagogo-Jack S, Rattarasarn C, Cryer PE. Reversal of hypoglycemia unawareness, but not defective glucose counterregulation, in IDDM. Diabetes 1994; 43: 1426–34.

33. Heller S, Cryer P. Reduced neuroendocrine and symptomatic responses to subsequent hypoglycemia after one episodes of hypoglycemia in nondiabetic humans. Diabetes 1991; 40: 223–6.

34. Dagogo-Jack SE, Cryer PE. Hypoglycemia-associated autonomic failure in insulin-dependent diabetes mellitus. Recent antecedent hypoglycemia reduces autonomic responses to, symptoms of, and defense against subsequent hypoglycemia. J Clin Invest 1993; 91: 819–18.

35. Ovalle F, Fanelli CG, Paramore DS et al. Brief

twice-weekly episodes of hypoglycemia reduce detection of clinical hypoglycemia in Type 1 diabetes mellitus. Diabetes 1998; 47: 1472–9.

36. Fanelli C, Pampanelli S, Lalli C et al. Long-term intensive therapy of IDDM diabetic patients with clinically overt autonomic neuropathy: effects on awareness of, and counterregulation to hypoglycemia. Diabetes 1997; 46: 1172–81.

37. McCall A, Fixman L, Fleming N et al. Chronic hypoglycemia increases brain glucose transport. Am J Physiol 1986; 251: E442–E447.

38. McCall AL, Millington WR, Wurtman RJ. Metabolic fuel and aminoacid transport into the brain in experimental diabetes mellitus. Proc Natl Acad Sci USA 1982; 79: 5406–10.

39. Kumagai AK, Kang YS, Boado RJ, Pardridge WM. Upregulation of blood-brain barrier GLUT1 glucose transporter protein and mRNA in experimental chronic hypoglycemia. Diabetes 1995; 44: 1399–404.

40. Simpson IA, Appel NM, Hokari M et al. Blood-brain barrier glucose transporter: effects of hypo- and hyperglycemia revisited. J Neurochem 1999; 72: 238–47.

41. Uehara Y, Nipper V, McCall AL. Chronic insulin hypoglycemia induces GLUT-3 protein in rat brain neurons. Am J Physiol 1997; 272 4 Pt 1: E716–19.

42. Boyle PJ, Nagy RJ, O'Connor AM et al. Adaptation in brain glucose uptake following recurrent hypoglycemia. Proc Natl Acad Sci USA 1994; 91: 9352–6.

43. Boyle PJ, Kempers S, O'Connor AM, Nagy RJ. Brain glucose uptake and hypoglycemia unawareness in patients with insulin-dependent diabetes mellitus. N Engl J Med 1995; 333: 1726–31.

44. Segel SA, Fanelli CG, Dence CS et al. Blood-to-brain glucose transport, cerebral glucose metabolism, and cerebral blood flow are not increased after hypoglycemia. Diabetes 2001; 50: 1911–17.

45. Fanelli CG, Dence CS, Markham J et al. Blood-to-brain glucose transport and cerebral glucose metabolism are not reduced in poorly controlled Type 1 diabetes. Diabetes 1998; 47: 1444–50.

46. Cranston I, Reed LJ, Marsden PK, Amiel SA. Changes in regional brain (18)F-fluorodeoxyglucose uptake at hypoglycemia in Type

1 diabetic men associated with hypoglycemia unawareness and counter-regulatory failure. Diabetes 2001; 50: 2329–36.

47. Davis SN, Shavers C, Costa F, Mosqueda-Garcia R. Role of cortisol in the pathogenesis of deficient counterregulation after antecedent hypoglycemia in normal humans. J Clin Invest 1996; 98: 680–91.

48. Davis SN, Shavers C, Davis B, Costa F. Prevention of an increase in plasma cortisol during hypoglycemia preserves subsequent counter-regulatory responses. J Clin Invest 1997; 100: 429–38.

49. McGregor VP, Banarer S, Cryer PE. Elevated endogenous cortisol reduces autonomic neuroendocrine and symptom responses to subsequent hypoglycemia. Am J Physiol Endocrinol Metab 2002; 282: E770–7.

50. Evans SB, Wilkinson CW, Bentson K et al. PVN activation is suppressed by repeated hypoglycemia but not antecedent corticosterone in the rat. Am J Physiol Regul Integr Comp Physiol 2001; 281: R1426–36.

51. Horner HC, Packan DR, Sapolsky RM. Glucocorticoids inhibit glucose transport in cultured hippocampal neurons and glia. Neuroendocrinology 1990; 52: 57–64.

52. Guerin C, Wolff JE, Laterra J et al. Vascular differentiation and glucose transporter expression in rat gliomas: effects of steroids. Ann Neurol 1992; 31: 481–7.

53. Chipkin SR, van Bueren A, Bercel E et al. Effects of dexamethasone in vivo and in vitro on hexose transport in brain microvasculature. Neurochem Res 1998; 23: 645–52.

54. De Kloet, E, Ratka A, Reul J et al. Corticosteroid receptor types in brain regulation and putative function. Ann NY Acad Sci 1987; 512: 351–61.

55. Kirschbaum C, Wolf OT, May M et al. Stress- and treatment-induced elevations of cortisol levels associated with impaired declarative memory in healthy adults. Life Sci 1996; 58: 1475–83.

56. Elliott EM, Sapolsky RM. Corticosterone impairs hippocampal neuronal calcium regulation – possible mediating mechanisms. Brain Res 1993; 602: 84–90.

57. Berlin I, Grimaldi A, Payan C et al. Hypoglycemic symptoms and decreased beta-adrenergic sensitivity in insulin-dependent diabetic patients. Diabetes Care 1987; 10: 742–7.

58. Fritsche A, Stumvoll M, Grub M et al. Effect of hypoglycemia on beta-adrenergic sensitivity in normal and Type 1 diabetic subjects. Diabetes Care 1998; 21: 1505–10.

59. Fritsche A, Stefan N, Haring H et al. Avoidance of hypoglycemia restores hypoglycemia awareness by increasing beta-adrenergic sensitivity in Type 1 diabetes. Ann Intern Med 2001; 134 9 Pt 1: 729–36.

60. Ciofetta M, Lalli C, Del Sindaco P et al. Contribution of postprandial versus interprandial blood glucose to HbA1c in Type 1 diabetes on physiologic intensive therapy with lispro insulin at mealtime. Diabetes Care 1999; 22: 795–800.

61. Bolli GB, Di Marchi RD, Park GD et al. Insulin analogues and their potential in the management of diabetes mellitus. Diabetologia 1999; 42: 1151–67.

62. Bolli GB. Rationale for using combinations of short-acting insulin analogue and NPH insulin at mealtime in the treatment of Type 1 diabetes mellitus. J Pediatr Endocrinol Metab 1999; 12 Suppl. 3: 737–44.

63. Fanelli CG, Pampanelli S, Porcellati F et al. Administration of neutral protamine Hagerdon insulin at bedtime versus with dinner in Type 1 diabetes mellitus to avoid nocturnal hypoglycemia and improve control. A randomized, controlled trial. Ann Intern Med 2002; 136: 504–14.

64. Lepore M, Pampanelli S, Fanelli C et al. Pharmacokinetics and pharmacodynamics of subcutaneous injection of long-acting human insulin analog glargine, NPH insulin, and ultralente human insulin and continuous subcutaneous infusion of insulin lispro. Diabetes 2000; 49: 2142–8.

65. Ratner RE, Hirsch IB, Neifing JL et al. Less hypoglycemia with insulin glargine in intensive insulin therapy for Type 1 Diabetes. U.S. Study Group of Insulin Glargine in Type 1 Diabetes. Diabetes Care 2000; 23: 639–43.

66. Porcellati F, Rossetti P, Fanelli CG et al. Glargine vs NPH as basal insulin in intensive treatment of T1 DM given at meals: one year comparison. Diabetes 2002; 51 Suppl. 2: A53.

67. Rossetti P, Pampanelli S, Costa E et al. A three-month comparison between multiple daily NPH and once daily glargine insulin administration in intensive replacement of basal insulin in Type 1 diabetes mellitus. Diabetes 2002; 51 Suppl. 2: A53.

68. Reichard P, Nilsson BY, Rosenqvist U. The effect of long-term intensified treatment on the development of microvascular complications of diabetes mellitus. N Engl J Med 1993; 329: 304–9.

69. Bolli GB. Hypoglycaemia unawareness. Diabetes Metab 1997; 23 Suppl. 3: 29–35.

23

Combined therapy with oral hypoglycemics and insulin in Type 2 diabetes
Matthew C Riddle

Most common disorders are routinely treated with combinations of treatments for the best possible result with the fewest unwanted effects. In this way, Type 2 diabetes has differed from the rest. At one extreme is continued enthusiam for lifestyle change as the fundamental therapy,[1] at the other the view that insulin alone is the best treatment for Type 2 as for Type 1 diabetes.[2] Several forces have led to re-evaluation of the view that monotherapy of any kind will be effective for Type 2 diabetes. These include a growing demand for evidence-based protocols; epidemiologic observations and proof of the benefits of good glycemic control; clarification of the underlying pathophysiology; and especially the appearance of many new therapies, both new classes of oral agents and novel forms of insulin.

This chapter describes the theoretical and experimental basis for using combinations of oral agents with insulin, and also the clinical use of several of the more important combinations. This is a review of an ongoing process. That is, combinations of agents are already widely used, but with lack of consensus on the best way to deploy them between different kinds of patients and different stages of diabetes, and new agents continue to be introduced. However, about ten years have passed since the first widely tested combination, insulin with a sulfonylurea, began to gain acceptance, and a body of data has emerged that allows detailed analysis.

Progression of Type 2 diabetes and failure of monotherapy

Perhaps the most persuasive evidence of the progressive nature of Type 2 diabetes comes from a study of lifestyle intervention based in Belfast, Northern Ireland.[3] The investigators assigned 223 newly diagnosed patients to an intensive program of diet and exercise with extraordinary success. Over 70% of these patients lost a significant amount of weight and maintained this level for six years. The mean weight loss after a year of treatment was about 10 kg, and the clinical result was a decline of mean fasting glucose from 11 to 8 mmol/l. Despite maintenance of nearly normal weight, fasting glucose slowly rose over the next five years to 10 mmol/l. Subsequent analysis of glucose and insulin values by the HOMA method showed this loss of glycemic control was due to declining beta cell function rather than increasing insulin resistance.[4]

The same progression of Type 2 diabetes was evident in the United Kingdom Prospective Diabetes Study (UKPDS).[5,6] Recently diagnosed patients were randomized to continued lifestyle treatment, or treatment with a sulfonylurea, metformin, or insulin. Those assigned to lifestyle alone showed a steady rise of fasting glucose and HbA1c over subsequent years, at a rate quite similar to that seen in the Belfast study. Those starting oral agents or insulin had immediate improvement of control to a median HbA1c approaching 6%. After that, all the groups assigned to pharmacotherapy showed gradual increases of HbA1c over time at the same rate as the 'conventional treatment' group assigned to lifestyle alone. Beta cell function by HOMA analysis declined in all groups at similar rates.[5] Three years after assignment to these therapies, only about 50% of the subjects continued to have HbA1c below 7% with monotherapy.[6] After nine years less than 25% maintained this level of control with monotherapy. The obvious conclusion is that, for a typical patient to maintain good control, combination therapy will be needed by three to five years after diagnosis.

Insights into pathophysiology

These studies, along with others, show that progression of the pathophysiologic abnormalities underlying Type 2 diabetes forces a choice between accepting high levels of glycemia, or using combinations of therapies. In the past, allowing higher levels of glucose has been the usual choice for several reasons. Prior to the reports of the randomized comparison of conventional versus intensive treatments in the UKPDS, solid evidence that improved control could reduce complications in Type 2 diabetes was lacking, and the therapeutic tools available had not been proven equal to the task of keeping HbA1c close to 7%. Moreover, the pathophysiology of Type 2 diabetes has come to light only gradually. Prior to immunoassays for insulin in plasma, insulin deficiency was thought to be the main lesion. Later studies have consistently confirmed a defect in secretion of insulin,[7,8] but resistance to insulin action in peripheral tissues has also been documented by glucose-insulin clamp studies in

virtually all patients.[8–10] Studies of hepatic substrate patterns have shown the liver is relatively resistant to insulin as well,[10] and that hepatic glucose overproduction is a major cause of fasting hyperglycemia.[9] Quite recently, attention has shifted to the contribution of postprandial hyperglycemia to daily mean glucose elevations.[11] Each of these observations adds a piece to the rationale for combination therapy.

Because insulin deficiency is routinely present, a treatment that enhances the availability of insulin should be helpful for nearly all patients. Because insulin resistance is routinely present, a treatment that improves insulin sensitivity of muscle, adipose tissue, liver, or a combination of these should also benefit nearly all patients. Treatments that address just one of these basic defects are likely to work well only for some patients, and for a limited time. Moreover, neither insulin secretion nor insulin action is a simple process, and single-agent regimens may not adequately restore either of these two functions. Basal insulin secretion is normally regulated very accurately at low levels, and its replacement should be similarly regulated. After a meal, plasma levels of insulin normally rise rapidly up to ten-fold, then rapidly decline to baseline. Restoration of this pattern by drug therapy is difficult, and is an entirely different challenge from correcting basal insulin deficiency. Furthermore, changes of insulin resistance at various sites may not always be the same, and a treatment that improves sensitivity at muscle may have more effect on postprandial glucose than fasting glucose, while a treatment targeting hepatic sensitivity may have more effect on fasting hyperglycemia.

Given these complexities, therapy of Type 2 diabetes should strive to do several things at once. Both insulin deficiency and insulin resistance should be treated, and both basal and postprandial hyperglycemia should be addressed. Because no single agent can do all this, combinations will routinely be needed.

Pharmacologic aspects of treatment

New therapeutic agents

Opportunities for combination regimens have been enhanced by the appearance of new classes of therapeutic agents and new versions of older agents. While the widely used sulfonlyureas glibenclamide (glyburide), glipizide, and gliclazide work best when given twice daily, glimepiride[12] and extended-release glipizide[13] can be taken once daily with full effect. Evidence is accumulating that the longer-acting agents have less tendency to cause hypoglycemia than the others, especially glibenclamide.[14–16] Repaglinide[17] and nateglinide[18] are insulin secretagogues which, like sulfonlyureas, act by binding to the K_{ATP}-channel complex on beta cells, but they have more rapid onset and shorter duration of action than the sulfonylureas. Because of this difference they may have slightly more effect on postprandial hyperglycemia than sulfonylureas. The alpha-glucosidase inhibitors acarbose[19] and miglitol[20] delay absorption of dietary carbohydrate by blocking digestion of starches in the upper small intestine, and thereby reduce postprandial glycemic peaks. An extended-release form of metformin has been introduced, but data documenting its effectiveness with once daily dosing compared to twice daily conventional metformin are not yet published. The thiazolidinediones (glitazones) pioglitazone and rosiglitazone have various effects mediated at least in part by binding to PPAR-γ, forming a complex that alters expression of many genes affecting carbohydrate and lipid metabolism. The thiazolidinediones improve insulin sensitivity at fat, muscle, and to some extent liver, and thus can reduce both fasting and postprandial hyperglycemia.[21–24]

After 80 years of use, animal and human insulins seem on the verge of being replaced by analogs with small alterations of peptide sequence that markedly change their pharmacokinetics without changing their effectiveness in activating the insulin receptor.[25,26] The rapid-acting analogs aspart and lispro provide action profiles after subcutaneous injection that closely resemble those seen at mealtimes in persons without diabetes. Insulin glargine[27] has a prolonged, consistent, and nearly peakless action profile that permits basal insulin supplementation with a single daily injection.

Dose-response relationships

Fortunately, most of the various classes of agents listed above act through different mechanisms, and have additive effects on plasma glucose. Specifically, sulfonylureas and the other secretagogues improve delivery of endogenous insulin into the portal vein with first effect on the liver, injections of insulin deliver insulin to the peripheral circulation, metformin acts at the liver to improve the response to insulin, thiazolidinediones act mainly on fat with secondary effects in muscle and liver that result in better responses to insulin, and alpha-glucosidase inhibitors act only in the intestinal lumen. Also fortunately, the major side effects of these classes are not additive, except for hypoglycemia. Because of their diversity of actions, combinations of agents offer greater therapeutic power than monotherapy in most cases.

Beyond this advantage of combination therapy, however, lies another benefit that depends on the dose-response relationships of both desired and unwanted effects. The maximal dosage of agents suitable for clinical use can be determined either by efficacy or by side effects. Sulfonylureas and metformin can be used as examples. The dose-response relationship for glucose lowering by the sulfonylurea glimepiride is non-linear, with about 50–60% of the total therapeutic power provided by a 1 mg dose, only 25% of the fully effective 4 mg daily dose.[28] Side effects, other than potential hypoglycemia, are low throughout this range. Metformin has maximal clinical benefit at a dosage of 2000 mg daily, but increasingly frequent gastrointestinal symptoms above 1500 mg daily.[29,30] An apparent decline in clinical effectiveness of metformin at dosages above 2000 mg is probably related to reduced adherance due to side effects. Another version of the same problem is illustrated in the dose-response relationship for the thiazolidinedione pioglitazone.[31] The highest approved dosage is 45 mg daily, but this has not been shown to be maximally effective. Because development of this class of agents has been influenced by concern about various side effects,[32,33] notably fluid retention which presumably would be greater at higher dosages, the maximal permitted dosage is probably defined by side effects rather than efficacy.

Because of these relationships, submaximal dosages of two different agents might achieve equivalent (or better) glycemic control with fewer side effects (e.g. hypoglycemia from a sulfonylurea, or gastrointestinal symptoms from metformin) than a full dose of either alone. This concept has been directly tested and verified for a sulfonylurea with metformin.[34]

A similar rationale applies to combining insulin with oral agents. Theoretically, insulin has nearly unlimited therapeutic power. Practically, its effectiveness is limited by dosage-related hypoglycemia, which is most apparent when reduced food intake coincides with increased physical activity. If insulin dosage is not decreased when dietary intake declines hypoglycemia may occur, and exercise increases glucose uptake by muscle and speeds absorption of subcutaneously injected insulin, further increasing the risk of hypoglycemia.[35–37] People do not eat or exercise consistently, and are rarely able to adjust insulin to match day to day changes perfectly. Although the risk of insulin-induced hypoglycemia is lower in Type 2 than in Type 1 diabetes, severe hypoglycemia can occur and is the leading barrier to achieving target levels of control with insulin.[14]

Continuing oral agents after starting injections of insulin should, theoretically, reduce the risk of hypoglycemia at any given level of glycemic control. Any antihyperglycemic effect should reduce the total dosage of insulin needed, and this by itself should reduce the risk of hypoglycemia by limiting the pool of subcutaneous insulin available to be mobilized at an increased rate during or after exercise. Beyond this general effect, sulfonylureas, metformin, and thiazolidinediones each have specific effects in combination with insulin that have the potential to improve glycemic stability and thereby reduce the risk of hypoglycemia. These will be discussed later in this chapter.

Non-glycemic benefits of antihyperglycemic agents

Three proposed additional effects of agents used primarily to control glucose also are pertinent here. In some cases, desirable non-glycemic effects will enhance the value of an agent as part of a combination therapy regimen.

The best proven of these is the weight-control effect of metformin. In the UKPDS, metformin was the only agent that caused no more weight-gain than conventional therapy, which consisted mainly of diet and exercise.[38] Many smaller studies confirm this feature of metformin, some of them showing significant weight loss that may be associated with improved insulin sensitivity of peripheral tissues.[39] The mechanism of this effect is unknown, but seems independent of gastrointestinal side effects in many cases. Recently, three small studies with differing design but similar intent have shown that using metformin limits the weight gain usually seen when starting or intensifying insulin treatment.[40–42] Although medical outcome trials have not verified that this effect reduces cardiovascular events, the apparent cardiovascular benefits of metformin monotherapy in the UKPDS suggest a similar benefit when metformin is used with insulin.[38]

The proposed cardiovascular benefits of thiazolidinediones are more speculative, not because they lack a strong theoretical basis, but because data on medical outcomes are entirely lacking. Their clinical use is based on effects on glycemic control, but in addition they may suppress inflammatory processes leading to progression of vascular lesions.[43,44] However, these apparently favorable effects coexist with a tendency to cause weight-gain, fluid retention, or anemia. Studies assessing the net long-term results of therapy with these agents are underway.

Finally, insulin itself may have non-glycemic benefits. The Diabetes, Insulin, Glucose and Myocardial Infarction (DIGAMI) study strongly suggests that insulin treatment at the time of myocardial infarction can reduce short- and long-term mortality.[45,46] The most likely mechanism for this protection is suppression of high, stress-related levels of free fatty acids (FFA) by adequate levels of insulin in the systemic circulation.[47,48] Oral therapies may not sustain insulin levels during severe stress because beta cell function is suppressed,

permitting excessive release of FFA from adipose tissue. High plasma FFA concentrations may drive aerobic metabolism in ischemic myocardial tissue, leading to arrhythmias or greater damage to tissue. Further studies are needed to confirm the DIGAMI findings, and to test whether injected insulin can also protect patients with very high risk of infarction who have not yet experienced an acute event. Confirmation of this benefit would support use of insulin earlier in the course of diabetes, in preference to a second (or third) oral agent.

Dosing frequency and convenience

Physicians who care for patients with Type 2 diabetes are aware of the large numbers of both prescription and non-prescription agents many patients take daily. It is common for patients to take two drugs for glycemic control, two for blood pressure, one for hyperlipidemia, a multivitamin with folic acid, an aspirin tablet, an antihistamine, a sleeping remedy, and perhaps something for another illness such as an arrhythmia, a seizure disorder, a hormone deficiency, or arthritis. This comes to ten drugs prescribed for specific reasons, and to this list patients may add as many more unproven agents which they hope will improve their energy, mood, sexual vigor, or longevity, not to mention their diabetic control. With polypharmacy of this kind becoming usual, simplicity of the treatment for diabetes has a high priority.

The need for simplicity favors medications that are effective taken once daily. Once daily sulfonylureas, thiazolidinediones, and basal insulins are attractive in this way, while two or three daily doses of metformin, alpha-glucosidase inhibitors, or rapid-acting secretagogues are less attractive. Multiple injections of insulin, along with the increased frequency of glucose testing that usually accompanies them, are particularly unappealing. Many patients may prefer combining oral agents with a single injection of insulin if this regimen can postpone multiple injections and glucose tests.

Selection of combinations

With these considerations in mind, some principles for selecting a combination therapy regimen are apparent. An ideal regimen would address both insulin resistance and insulin deficiency, improve both fasting and postprandial hyperglycemia, and be as simple as possible. Additional cardiovascular benefits are of course highly desirable.

Early in Type 2 diabetes, the first combination used is usually lifestyle plus either metformin or a sulfonylurea. Lifestyle advice should include exercise and calorie restriction to reduce insulin resistance, and also multiple, moderate-sized meals each containing mixtures of foods, emphasizing carbohydrates that are gradually absorbed, to limit postprandial hyperglycemia. Either a once daily sulfonylurea or twice daily metformin adds therapeutic power to lifestyle efforts, mainly by improving fasting glucose levels. A sulfonylurea does this by enhancing the insulin response to basal hyperglycemia, while metformin improves the hepatic response to basal insulin levels. Once daily sulfonylurea is simpler, but twice daily metformin may help limit weight.

The next step is usually a sulfonylurea and metformin together. Because this advance to combination drug therapy is best done sooner rather than later, for the reasons described above, there seems little reason to debate strenuously which should be used first. In the relatively infrequent cases where hyperglycemia after meals (not to be confused with an oral glucose challenge) is much more prominent than fasting hyperglycemia, a rapid-acting secretagogue, a thiazolidinedione, or an alpha-glucosidase inhibitor might be used along with metformin, instead of (or in addition to) a sulfonylurea. Each of these three classes of agents can blunt postprandial hyperglycemia.

Viewing treatment for diabetes as a combination approach from the beginning should help prepare both the patient and the provider for the more difficult therapeutic challenge that lies ahead as insulin reserve dwindles. When two or more oral agents together fail to control glucose adequately, an oral agent plus insulin combination should be considered. At this time decisions must be made between adding basal insulin, a rapid-acting insulin, or both, and between stopping one or more oral agents or continuing them.

Adding insulin to oral agents

The simplest way to start insulin is with a single injection of intermediate or long-acting insulin. However, early success with a simple insulin regimen often depends on continuing oral therapy. If oral agents are discontinued when insulin is started, glycemic control deteriorates during the time of transition to insulin unless insulin dosage is rapidly titrated upward. Moreover, a simple insulin regimen used without oral agents is less likely to achieve glycemic control close to the HbA1c 7% target level. Two studies illustrate these points.

In one (Figure 23.1), 145 subjects proven to have poor glycemic control with full dosage of glimepiride began 70/30 (70% NPH/30% Regular) insulin once daily before the evening meal, accompanied by either placebo or continued glimepiride.[49] The dosage of insulin was titrated upward seeking fasting plasma glucose 7.8 mmol/l (equivalent to whole blood glucose 6.7 mmol/l). Both treatment groups reached this target, but a month sooner and with 35% less injected insulin with the combination regimen. Also, 15% of the insulin-alone

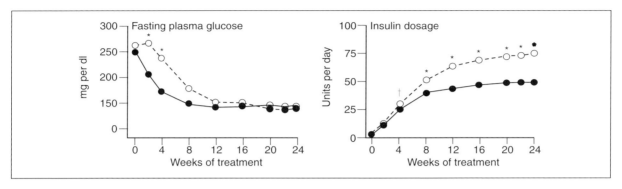

Figure 23.1

*Fasting plasma glucose and insulin dosage after human 70/30 insulin was started by patients who were previously taking full dosage of glimepiride, and the dosage adjusted seeking fasting plasma glucose 7.8 mmol/l (140 mg/dl). Means for a group randomized to insulin plus placebo (open circles and broken line) are compared with those for a group taking insulin plus continued glimepiride (solid circles and line). Notes: * signifies p <0.05 and † signifies p <0.001 between treatments. Source: adapted from Riddle et al.[49]*

subjects dropped out of the study, in most cases because of symptoms compatible with hyperglycemia in the first four weeks after starting insulin. More aggressive titration of insulin dosage might have been possible, but this would require more frequent glucose testing for safety.

The second study (Figure 23.2) differed from the first in its glycemic target. In this study, 30 patients not controlled by full dosage of glipizide were treated with bedtime NPH insulin plus placebo or insulin plus continued glipizide.[50] The dosage of insulin was increased gradually, seeking the lowest fasting glucose value possible without significant hypoglycemia. With insulin alone the mean fasting glucose achieved was 7.8 mmol/l and HbA1c was 7.8%, while with combined therapy mean fasting glucose was 6.3 mmol/l and HbA1c was 7.1%. Another small study with similar design, but using glyburide and suppertime 70/30 insulin, had very similar results.[51] Furthermore, review of many other studies with varying designs confirms there is usually an additional

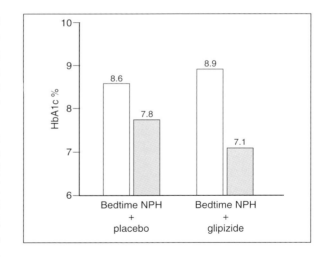

Figure 23.2

Hemoglobin A1c before (open bars) and six months after (solid bars) bedtime NPH insulin was started by 30 Type 2 diabetic patients who were previously taking glipizide. In the last three months insulin dosage was titrated seeking optimal glycemic control. Means for a group randomized to insulin plus placebo are compared to those for a group randomized to insulin plus continued glipizide. Source: data adapted from Shank et al.[50]

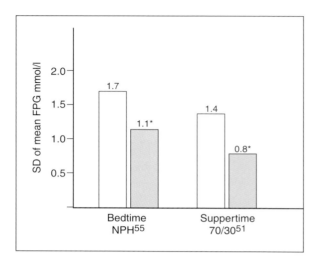

Figure 23.3
*Variability of sequential fasting plasma glucose (FPG) values after stabilization of insulin dosage in two studies of insulin–glyburide combination therapy. Means of standard deviations (SD) from the mean FPG for each subject are shown, comparing values with insulin plus placebo (open bars) with insulin plus glibenclamide (solid bars). Note: * signifies p <0.05 between treatments. Source: adapted from data from Riddle et al.[55] and Riddle et al.[51]*

glycemic benefit of combining a sulfonylurea with an insulin.[52–54]

Why enhancing endogenous insulin secretion with a sulfonylurea improves the control possible with injected insulin, which can be increased to any dosage, is not immediately obvious. The explanation probably lies in the ability of sulfonylureas to reduce glycemic variability. Further analyses from two insulin–sulfonylurea combination studies from our clinic support this hypothesis (Figure 23.3).[51,55] These analyses compare the standard deviations of sequential fasting plasma glucose values late in the studies when mean fasting values were stable over time. During combin-

ation therapy there was about 40% less variability of fasting glucose values. Most likely this was due to a greater contribution to glycemic control from endogenous insulin, which is regulated both upward and downward to dampen variations of glucose. In one of the studies a 118% increase of the fasting C-peptide to glucose ratio occurred during combination therapy, in contrast to no change from baseline during use of insulin alone.[55]

A large trial now underway suggests very good glycemic control is possible when basal insulin is added to one or two oral agents and systematically titrated seeking fasting plasma glucose as close to 5.6 mmol/l as possible. The main aim of the trial is to compare the effectiveness of bedtime NPH insulin versus insulin glargine, but the results of the randomized comparison are not yet available. However, a preliminary analysis of data from 401 subjects, with the two treatment groups pooled, showed reduction of mean fasting plasma glucose to 6.6 mmol/l, and reduction of mean HbA1c from 8.6 to 6.9% after 18 weeks of treatment.[56] Two-thirds (66%) of the subjects had values equal to or less than 7%.

Whether addition of mealtime insulin rather than basal insulin, in combination with continued oral therapy, can achieve equal or better results has not yet been rigorously tested. Two small trials have demonstrated improved glycemic control by adding three injections of a rapid-acting insulin analog to a sulfonylurea. In a four-month crossover trial, mealtime injections of lispro plus continued glibenclamide reduced HbA1c to 7.1% in comparison to 9.0% with glibenclamide alone.[57] In a three-month parallel comparison, mean HbA1c was 8.3% with glibenclamide plus metformin, 8.5% with glibenclamide plus bedtime NPH, and 7.7% with glibenclamide plus three injections of lispro.[58] These findings suggest that adding injections of rapid-acting insulin to oral therapy can improve control, but whether the inconvenience of multiple injections will be rewarded by better glycemic control, less hypoglycemia, or other benefits when compared with properly titrated basal insulin remains to be demonstrated.

Similarly, oral agents can be discontinued once the patient has become familiar with using insulin, and the regimen advanced to multiple injections of basal plus mealtime insulin. In general this more intensive use of insulin is no more effective than a single injection plus continued oral therapy at this stage of diabetes.[59] However, with waning of endogenous insulin over time, multiple injections of insulin will become necessary for many or most patients.

Oral agents with complex insulin regimens

Intensification of insulin therapy to provide both basal and mealtime insulin supplementation with multiple injections may be considered another form of combination therapy. This is especially true now that rapid-acting and long-acting analogs of insulin are available. While both human regular and NPH insulins can provide both basal and mealtime coverage to varying degrees, the new analogs are deployed for separate purposes and should be thought of as separate treatments.[26] Insulin glargine controls glycemia overnight and between meals, while aspart or lispro can prevent marked postprandial hyperglycemia. Together they have the power to reduce glucose in almost any patient, but the clinical effectiveness of this insulin–insulin combination is still limited by the risk of hypoglycemia.

Objective data on the benefits of continuing one or more oral agents while intensifying insulin therapy are still limited, but the rationale is quite strong. Whatever endogenous insulin secretion remains can still contribute to glycemic control, and presumably to glycemic stability, and insulin assisting agents should be able to enhance this contribution. The potential size of this contribution is illustrated by findings of an elegant physiologic study (Figure 23.4).[60] Small groups of patients with typical Type 2 diabetes, previously treated with insulin, were brought into excellent glycemic control by four weeks of insulin pump therapy. They were then given either metformin 850 mg twice daily or the thiazolidinedione troglitazone (which has subsequently been withdrawn from clinical use because of serious hepatic toxicity) 400 to 600 mg daily for seven weeks. The dosage of subcutaneously infused insulin, needed to maintain excellent control, was reduced by 31% by concurrent metformin therapy and by 53% by troglitazone. Endogenous insulin secretion, reflected by C-peptide profiles, was similar with and without the added oral agents. Plasma insulin profiles, shown in the figure, were reduced by about the same amount as was the dosage of exogenous insulin. Presumably the effectiveness of endogenous and exogenous insulin is increased by the same proportion as the requirement for injected insulin declined. In theory, enhancing the effect of endogenous insulin would decrease the risk of hypoglycemia, because insulin secretion can decline along with plasma glucose.

The best study published to date defines the limits of glycemic control that can be achieved in Type 2 diabetes with intensified insulin therapy combined with an insulin-assisting oral agent used metformin (Figure 23.5).[41] Forty-three patients were treated for six months with two or more injections of regular and NPH insulin alone or with metformin, starting with HbA1c about 9%. With insulin alone, mean HbA1c was reduced to 7.6%, while with the combination regimen HbA1c 6.5% was

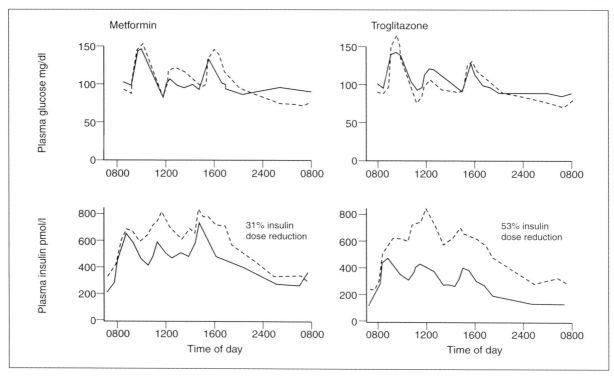

Figure 23.4

Plasma glucose and insulin profiles during intensive treatment of patients with Type 2 diabetes by continuous subcutaneous insulin infusion, both before (broken lines) and after (solid lines) addition of metformin (left) or troglitazone (right). The reductions of dosage required to maintain excellent glycemic control are similar to the reductions of plasma insulin levels over 24 hours with each treatment. Source: adapted from Yu et al.[60]

achieved. This study also illustrates the ability of metformin to prevent the weight-gain caused by intensifying insulin therapy. The patients using combination therapy gained only 0.5 kg, while those taking insulin alone gained a more typical mean of 3.2 kg.

Whether combining intensive insulin therapy with pioglitazone or rosiglitazone can produce similar results has not been tested, although physiologic studies suggest that both fasting and postprandial glycemic control may be enhanced by these agents. At present we are in a vexing position regarding clinical use of

thiazolidinediones. On the one hand, some patients show dramatic glycemic responses when pioglitazone or rosiglitazone is combined with other oral agents or insulin.[61–63] On the other hand, the safety of thiazolidinediones continues to be debated. Lack of evidence for significant hepatic toxicity with pioglitazone and rosiglitazone since their release in the United States has calmed fears they might share this hazard with troglitazone. However, weight-gain and fluid retention occur in some patients, especially when these agents are used with insulin, posing a risk of congestive heart

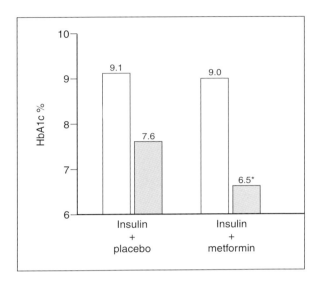

Figure 23.5
*Hemoglobin A1c before (open bars) and six months after (solid bars) intensified treatment with two to four injections of insulin in 43 Type 2 diabetic patients who were previously taking insulin. Means for a group randomized to insulin plus placebo are compared to those for a group randomized to insulin plus metformin. Note: * signifies p <0.05 between treatments. Source: data adapted from Aviles-Santa et al.[41]*

failure in vulnerable individuals. Objective evidence of how great this risk may be and which patients are most vulnerable is limited.

Only one large trial of pioglitazone or rosiglitazone used in combination with insulin has been published in a peer-reviewed form and thus can be evaluated confidently.[62] This trial's 319 patients were randomized in equal numbers to continued treatment with twice daily insulin plus placebo, 4 mg rosiglitazone, or 8 mg rosiglitazone. The placebo-adjusted HbA1c reduction was 1.2% with 8 mg rosiglitazone, despite a 12% reduction of insulin

dosage to limit hypoglycemia in some patients. At 26 weeks the mean HbA1c was 7.9%. Edema was reported in the groups taking placebo, 4 mg rosiglitazone, and 8 mg rosiglitazone at rates of 5, 13, and 16%, a two- to three-fold increase with rosiglitazone. Congestive heart failure was reported in one patient taking placebo, versus two with 4 mg and two with 8 mg rosiglitazone. The rates of heart failure (1, 2, and 2%) in the three groups were not statistically different. One of the two patients said to have developed heart failure in each of the rosiglitazone groups was known to have had the same condition prior to the trial. The results of a similar trial of pioglitazone in combination with insulin has not yet been published except in abstract.[63,64] It is noteworthy that, while rosiglitazone was tested at its maximally approved 8 mg dosage, the highest dosage used in the pioglitazone trial was 30 mg, not the 45 mg dosage that is often used in clinical practice.

These results call attention to fluid retention as a side effect, but they are not as alarming as has been feared. Patients with long-duration diabetes are known to be at risk for edema and heart failure, and should always be monitored for signs of these complications. The increased frequency of edema with rosiglitazone, relative to placebo, is no greater than that reported in trials of non-steroidal anti-inflammatory agents and vasodilating antihypertensive drugs in healthier populations. For example, in one set of studies rates of edema for placebo, rofecoxib, ibuprofen, and diclofenac were 1.1, 3.7, 3.8 and 3.4%, a three-fold increase for the anti-inflammatory agents.[65] For amlodipine, the frequency of edema has been reported to be 10.8% with a 10 mg dose versus 0.6% with placebo.[66] As with these other classes of drugs, which are widely used by insulin-taking patients with diabetes, problems related to fluid retention with thiazolidinediones can probably be minimized by appropriate caution and timely use of diuretics. The main issue, of course, is the risk to benefit ratio. Therefore, much better information is needed on the glycemic benefits and potential non-glycemic benefits and risks of the thiazolidinediones.

Treatment for a typical patient

To bring this body of information into clinical focus, it may be useful to describe the sequence of combination regimens we use for typical newly diagnosed patients with Type 2 diabetes in our own clinic. These commonly seen patients have Body Mass Index 28–34 kg/m², are about 50 years old, and have HbA1c in the 8 to 10% range at diagnosis. Lifestyle efforts are invoked for all patients and should be lifelong. In addition we advise starting oral therapy almost immediately, with either a low dose of a long-acting sulfonylurea (glimepiride 1 mg or extended-release glipizide 2.5 mg) or metformin 500 mg once or twice daily, and increasing the dosage as needed. Within a year or two we expect most patients will be taking both a sulfonylurea and metformin. Within five years many will need additional therapy, usually basal insulin added while these two oral agents are continued at previous dosages. In the past we used NPH at bedtime or 70% NPH/30% Regular premixed insulin before the evening meal, but now we more often use insulin glargine at bedtime. The starting dosage is 10 units, and the patient is advised to increase this weekly by increments that are individualized. When target HbA1c levels are not met or maintained, the sulfonylurea is usually stopped and either Regular human insulin or one of the rapid-acting analogs added before one or more meals, while basal insulin and metformin are continued. Most patients are on this full regimen by 10 years after diagnosis.

The most common variation of this sequence involves rosiglitazone or pioglitazone. Three situations may call for one of these. First, inability to use metformin due to renal insufficiency or gastrointestinal side effects favors adding a thiazolidinedione to a sulfonylurea. Secondly, concern about starting insulin because of a patient's limited self-care abilities or unusual aversion to injections may argue for adding a thiazolidine as the third agent with a sulfonylurea and metformin. Thirdly, failure of insulin plus metformin despite multiple injections of two kinds of insulin and a total dosage greater than 1 unit per kilogram suggests adding a thiazolidinedione. Of course, many other variations of combination therapy are possible, but situations that call for them are much less frequent.

Because patients are typically diagnosed near age 50, need insulin by 60, and may live beyond 80 years of age, the proportion of them using oral agents combined with insulin continues to rise. Therefore, better understanding of how to assign combination regimens to various groups of patients, and how to use future agents in combinations will be urgently needed.

References

1. Toumilehto J, Lindstrom J, Eriksson JG et al. The Finnish Diabetes Prevention Study Group. N Engl J Med 2001; 344: 1343–50.
2. Berger M, Jorgens V, Muhlhauser I. Rationale for the use of insulin therapy alone as the pharmacologic treatment of Type 2 diabetes. Diabetes Care 1999; 22 (Supp 3): C71–75.
3. Hadden DR, Blair ALT, Wilson EA et al. Natural history of diabetes presenting age 40–69 years: a prospective study of the influence of intensive dietary therapy. QJM 1986; 59: 579–98.
4. Rudenski AS, Hadden DR, Atkinson AB et al.

Natural history of pancreatic islet β-cell function in Type 2 diabetes mellitus studied over six years by homeostasis model assessment. Diabet Med 1988; 5: 36–41.

5. UK Prospective Diabetes Study 16: Overview of 6 years' therapy of type II diabetes: a progressive disease. Diabetes 1995; 44: 1249–58.

6. Turner RC, Cull CA, Frighi V, Holman RR. The UK Prospective Diabetes Study Group. Glycemic control with diet, sulfonylurea, metformin, or insulin in patients with Type 2 diabetes mellitus. Progressive requirement for multiple therapies (UKPDS 49). JAMA 1999; 281: 2005–12.

7. Polonsky KS, Sturis J, Bell G. Non-insulin-dependent diabetes mellitus – a genetically programmed failure of the beta cell to compensate for insulin resistance. N Engl J Med 1996; 334: 777–83.

8. DeFronzo RA. The triumvirate: β-cell, muscle, lever. A collusion responsible for NIDDM. Diabetes 1988; 37: 667–87.

9. Lilloija S, Mott DM, Spraul M et al. Insulin resistance and insulin secretory dysfunction as precursors of non-insulin-dependent diabetes mellitus: prospective studies of Pima Indians. N Engl J Med 1993; 329: 1988–92.

10. Groop LC, Bonadonna RC, DelPrato S et al. Glucose and free fatty acid metabolism in non-insulin-dependent diabetes mellitus. Evidence for multiple sites of insulin resistance. J Clin Invest 1989; 84: 205–13.

11. American Diabetes Association. Postprandial blood glucose. Diabetes Care 2001; 24: 775–8.

12. Rosenstock J, Samols E, Muchmore DB, Schneider J. The Glimepiride Study Group. Glimepiride, a new once-daily sulfonylurea. Diabetes Care 1996; 19: 1194–9.

13. Berelowitz M, Fischette C, Cefalu W et al. Comparative efficacy of a once-daily controlled-release formulation of glipizide and immediate-release glipizide in patients with NIDDM. Diabetes Care 1994; 17: 1460–4.

14. UK Prospective Diabetes Study (UKPDS) Group. Intensive blood-glucose control with sulphonylureas or insulin compared with conventional treatment and risk of complications in patients with Type 2 diabetes (UKPDS 33). Lancet 1998; 352: 837–53.

15. Holstein A, Plaschke A, Egberts E-H. Lower incidence of severe hypoglycemia in Type 2 diabetic patients treated with glimepiride versus glibenclamide. EASD Meeting Program, A40, Sept. 2000.

16. Riddle MC, McDaniel P, Bugos C. First-dose C-peptide response and risk of hypoglycemia are lower with glimepiride than glyburide. Diabetes 2001; 50 (Supp 1): A129.

17. Damsbo P, Clauson P, Marbury TC, Windfeld K. A double-blind randomized comparison of meal-related glycemic control by repaglinide and glyburide in well-controlled Type 2 diabetic patients. Diabetes Care 1999; 22: 789–94.

18. Hollander PA, Schwartz SL, Gatlin MR et al. Importance of early insulin secretion. Comparison of nateglinide and glyburide in previous diet treated patients with Type 2 diabetes. Diabetes Care 2001; 24: 983–8.

19. Coniff RF, Shapiro JA, Robbins D et al. Reduction of glycosylated hemoglobin and postprandial hyperglycemia by acarbose in patients with NIDDM. Diabetes Care 1995; 18: 817–24.

20. Segal P, Feig PU, Scherntaner G et al. The efficacy and safety of miglitol therapy compared with glibenclamide in patients with NIDDM inadequately controlled by diet alone. Diabetes Care 1997; 20: 687–91.

21. Henry RR. Thiazolidinediones. Endocrinol Clin NA. 1997; 26: 553–73.

22. Olefsky JM. Treatment of insulin resistance with peroxisome-proliferator-activated receptor γ agonists. J Clin Invest 2000; 106: 467–72.

23. Inzucchi SE, Maggs D, Spollet GR et al. Efficacy and metabolic effects of metformin and troglitazone in type II diabetes mellitus. N Engl J Med 1998; 338: 867–72.

24. Miyazaki Y, Mahankali A, Matsuda M et al. Improved glycemic control and enhanced insulin sensitivity in Type 2 diabetic subjects treated with pioglitazone. Diabetes Care 2001; 24: 710–19.

25. Lee WL, Zinman B. From insulin to insulin analogs: progress in the treatment of Type 1 diabetes. Diabetes Rev 1998; 6: 73–88.

26. Bolli GB, DiMarchi RD, Park GD et al. Insulin analogues and their potential in the management of diabetes mellitus. Diabetologia 1999; 42: 1151–67.

27. Lepore M, Pampanelli S, Fanelli C et al.

Pharmacokinetics and pharmacodynamics of subcutaneous injection of long-acting human insulin analog glargine, NPH insulin, and ultralente human insulin and continuous subcutaneous infusion of insulin lispro. Diabetes 2000; 49: 2142–8.

28. Goldberg RB, Holvey SM, Schneider J. The Glimepiride Protocol 201 Study Group. A dose-response study of glimepiride in patients with NIDDM who have previously received sulfonylurea agents. Diabetes Care 1996; 19: 849–56.

29. Garber AJ, Duncan TG, Goodman AM et al. Efficacy of metformin in type II diabetes: results of a double-blind, placebo-controlled, dose-response trial. Am J Med 1997; 102: 491–7.

30. Krentz AJ, Ferner RE, Bailey CJ. Comparative tolerability profiles of oral antidiabetic agents. Drug Safety 1994; 11: 223–41.

31. Aronoff S, Rosenblatt S, Braithwaite S et al. The Pioglitazone 001 Study Group. Pioglitazone hydrochloride monotherapy improves glycemic control in the treatment of patients with Type 2 diabetes. A 6-month randomized placebo-controlled dose-response study. Diabetes Care 2000; 23: 1605–11.

32. Riddle MC. Learning to use troglitazone (Editorial). Diabetes Care 1998; 21: 1389–90.

33. Gale EAM. Lessons from the glitazones: a story of drug development. Lancet 2001; 357: 1870–5.

34. Hermann LS, Schersten B, Bitzen P-O et al. Therapeutic comparison of metformin and sulfonylurea, alone and in various combinations. Diabetes Care 1994; 1100–9.

35. Minuk HL, Vranic M, Marliss EB et al. Glucoregulatory and metabolic response to exercise in obese noninsulin-dependent diabetes. Am J Physiol 1981; 240: E458–64.

36. Bogardus C, Thuillez P, Ravussin E, et al. Effect of muscle glycogen depletion in vivo on insulin action in man. J Clin Invest 1983; 72: 1605.

37. Koivisto V, Felig P. Effects of leg exercise on insulin absorption in diabetic patients. N Engl J Med 1978; 298: 77.

38. UK Prospective Diabetes Study (UKPDS) Group. Effect of intensive blood-glucose control with metformin on complications in overweight patients with Type 2 diabetes (UKPDS 34). Lancet 1998; 352: 854–65.

39. Johansen K. Efficacy of metformin in the treatment of NIDDM. Diabetes Care 1999; 22: 33–7.

40. Bergenstal R, Johnson M, Whipple D et al. Advantages of adding metformin to multiple dose insulin therapy in Type 2 diabetes. Diabetes 1998; 47 (Supp1): A47.

41. Aviles-Santa L, Sinding J, Raskin P. Effects of metformin in patients with poorly controlled insulin-treated Type 2 diabetes mellitus. Ann Intern Med 1999; 131: 182–8.

42. Yki-Jarvinen H, Ryysy L, Nikkila K et al. Comparison of bedtime insulin regimens in patients with Type 2 diabetes mellitus. Ann Intern Med 1999; 130: 389–96.

43. Bishop-Bailey D. Peroxisome proliferator-activated receptors in the cardiovascular system. Br J Pharmacol 2000; 129: 823–34.

44. Hsueh WA, Jackson S, Law RE. Control of vascular cell proliferation and migration by PPAR-γ. Diabetes Care 2001; 24: 392–7.

45. Malmberg K, the DIGAMI Study Group. Prospective randomized study of intensive insulin treatment on long term survival after acute myocardial infarction in patients with diabetes mellitus. BMJ 1997; 314: 1512–15.

46. Malmberg K, McGuire DK. Diabetes and acute myocardial infarction: the role of insulin therapy. Am Heart J 1999; 138: S381–6.

47. Apstein CS. Glucose-insulin-potassium for acute myocardial infarction. Remarkable results from a new prospective, randomized trial. Circulation 1998; 98: 2223–6.

48. Taskinen M-R, Sane T, Helve E et al. Bedtime insulin for suppression of overnight free-fatty acid, blood glucose, and glucose production in NIDDM. Diabetes 1989; 38: 580–8.

49. Riddle MC, Schneider J, and the Glimepiride Combination Group. Beginning insulin treatment of obese patients with evening 70/30 insulin plus glimepiride versus insulin alone. Diabetes Care 1998; 21: 1052–7.

50. Shank ML, DelPrato S, DeFronzo RA. Bedtime insulin/daytime glipizide. Effective therapy for sulfonylurea failures in NIDDM. Diabetes 1995; 44: 165–72.

51. Riddle MC, Hart J, Bingham P et al. Combined therapy for obese Type 2 diabetes: suppertime mixed insulin with daytime sulfonylurea. Am J Med Sci 1992; 303: 151–6.

52. Pugh JA, Wagner ML, Sawyer J, Ramirez G,

Tuley M, Friedberg SJ. Is combination sulfony-lurea and insulin therapy useful in NIDDM patients? Diabetes Care 1992; 15: 953–9.

53. Johnson JL, Wolf SL, Kabadi UM. Efficacy of insulin and sulfonylurea combination therapy in type II diabetes. A meta-analysis of the random-ized placebo-controlled trials. Arch Intern Med 1996; 156: 259–64.

54. Yki-Jarvinen H. Combination therapies with insulin in Type 2 diabetes. Diabetes Care 2001; 24: 758–67.

55. Riddle MC, Hart JS, Bouma DJ et al. Efficacy of bedtime NPH insulin with daytime sulfony-lurea for a subpopulation of Type II diabetes mellitus. Diabetes Care 1989; 12: 623–62.

56. Rosenstock J, Riddle M, Dailey G et al. Treatment to target study: feasibility of achiev-ing control with the addition of basal bedtime insulin glargine (Lantus) or NPH insulin in insulin-naive patients with Type 2 diabetes on oral agents. Diabetes 2001; 50 (Supp 1): A129.

57. Feinglos MN, Thacker CH, English J et al. Modification of postprandial hyperglycemia with insulin lispro improves glucose control in patients with Type 2 diabetes. Diabetes Care 1997; 20: 1539–42.

58. Bastyr EJ, Stuart CA, Brodows RG et al. The IOEZ Study Group. Therapy focused on lower-ing postprandial glucose, not fasting glucose, may be superior for lowering HbA1c. Diabetes Care 2000; 23: 1236–41.

59. Yki-Jarvinen H, Kaupilla M, Kujansuu E et al. Comparison of insulin regimens in patients with non-insulin-dependent diabetes mellitus. N Engl J Med 1992; 327: 1426–33.

60. Yu JG, Kruszynska YT, Mulford MI, Olefsky JM. A comparison of troglitazone and met-formin on insulin requirements in euglycemic intensively insulin-treated Type 2 diabetic patients. Diabetes 1999; 48: 2414–21.

61. Fonseca V, Rosenstock J, Patwardian R, Salzman A. Effect of metformin and rosiglitazone combi-nation therapy in patients with Type 2 diabetes mellitus. JAMA 2000; 283: 1695–702.

62. Raskin P, Rendell M, Riddle MC et al. For the Rosiglitazone Clinical Trials Study Group. A randomized trial of rosiglitazone therapy in patients with inadequately controlled insulin-treated Type 2 diabetes. Diabetes Care 2001; 24: 1226–32.

63. Rubin C, Egan J, Schneider R, the pioglitazone 014 study group. Combination therapy with pioglitazone and insulin in patients with Type 2 diabetes. Diabetes 1999; 48 (Supp 1): A110.

64. Aronoff SL. Adverse events with pioglitazone HCl. Diabetes 2000; 49 (Supp 1): A340.

65. Rofecoxib package insert, March 2000.

66. Amlodipine besylate (Norvasc) package insert, April 2000.

24

Oral and nasal insulin administration in diabetes

Hanoch Bar-On, Miriam Kidron, Ehud Ziv

Introduction

Since the discovery of insulin in 1922[1,2] and its use as a therapeutic agent to combat diabetes, many modalities to improve its delivery have been made.[3,4] Several directions have been taken in order to deliver this hormone in a more genuine and convenient form to the patient. Thus, from a crude animal-derived product as it was injected 80 years ago, insulin was extensively purified. Today it is administered not as an animal extract but as a totally humanized molecule.[5,6] Moreover, in order to fulfill the goals of treatment, new devices to facilitate the presentation of the drug to the body at requested time and site have been invented. Disposable syringes with tiny needles, infusers and pens are now available for patients' use. These measures make intensive therapy more realistic and better tolerated. Recently, the results of two big studies (DCCT and UKPDS) showed unequivocally that achieving near normoglycemia delays the onset and the progression of diabetic complications.[7,8]

Since it is a peptide, insulin could not be used non-parenterally to treat diabetics. This, however, did not deter clinicians as well as researchers to invest effort and resourcefulness to try to administer insulin in novel ways. A few months after the discovery of insulin, trials to introduce insulin into mucosal cavities were conducted without apparent success.[9,10] In these experiments, the rectal and oral routes (i.e. via the portal system) were preferable. The absorption of the drug through the liver mimics the physiological pathway, and makes the oral route more attractive. Although still debatable, the transport of insulin through the liver carries theoretical advantage.[11,12] At the outset of this chapter, it should be noted that dermal, nasal and pulmonary preparations are still being explored and none, including oral preparation, is as yet commercially available.

The oral route

Two obstacles had to be removed in order for insulin given orally to be able to penetrate the intestinal wall and reach the blood stream:[13] the mucosal barrier and the gastric and intestinal proteolytic enzymes, degrading macromolecules. To understand the many difficulties encountered in any effort to bring about the transport of macromolecules, such as insulin, through the intestinal wall, one must understand the nature of this important barrier. Intestinal epithelial cells, known as enterocytes, create an intact cell lines that obstructs the transport of macromolecules into the interstitial space of the intestinal wall.[14,15] The impermeable living cells and the tight junction between them causes the impediment. This tough association between the cells limits the free movement of proteins, lipids and polysaccharides from the gastrointestinal (GI) lumen into the blood circulation.[16] In spite of this, tiny amounts of particles or polypeptides may pass across this barrier, possibly through the enterocytes rather than between them.[17] This is true especially in the neonatal period.[18] Earlier studies showed that immunoglobulins from the milk secreted by the nursing mother can be detected in the blood of suckling young babies and animals.[19] It was concluded that breast-fed children are better protected against various infective agents by this passive immunization through a continuous enrichment of their plasma with antibodies originating from their mother's milk.[20] More recent studies revealed the transfer of a significant amount of insulin through the mammary gland.[21] This supply of insulin provided growth factor activity for the maturation of neonatal intestinal mucosa.[22] However, the transfer of biologically-active insulin (with a hypoglycemic effect) into the blood circulation, was negligible.

The first problem to be overcome, in order to bring the insulin intact to the absorption domain of the enterocyte surface, is the hostile acidic environment of the stomach, which would denature the peptides moving down the GI tract after being swallowed. In addition, the many luminal and intracellular enzymes which reside in the small intestine, and are destined to break down macromolecules, prevent the invasion and flooding of the blood with foreign substances coming from the intestinal lumen.[23] The digestion by these enzymes of any ingested food ingredients is a prerequisite to their absorption. This is true with polypeptides, polysaccharides and lipids consumed as nutritional products, or accidentally swallowed. The hydrolyzed substances released following digestive activity, as well as most small molecular drugs or vitamins, reach the blood circulation

through the cells (transcytotic process).[24] The process includes the attachment to the cell surface receptors, internalization, shuttling inside the cell (assisted by special transporters), and arrival at the basolateral cell membranes. From there, secretion/exocytosis into the interstitial space takes place and moves further on to the capillaries.[25,26]

To overcome the barrier effect created by the intestinal wall, the use of special surface-active delivery agents was initiated. In general, the delivery agents would alter the plasma membrane of the enterocyte. This would allow the intact peptide to be integrated into the cell membrane and be engulfed by intracellular vesicles.[27] The process of this transport was demonstrated morphologically by various models and methods. Using isotopic labeling of insulin (by protein A-gold immunocytochemical technique) and electron microscopy at high resolution, and at timed intervals following the application of insulin, it was shown that primarily a transcytotic transfer of insulin occurs, and only a minute amount of the peptide creeps between the cells.[28,29] Therefore, the main purpose of the surface-active agents is to associate the peptide to a receptor (or any other cellular factor), to generate an interaction between the delivery agent and the cell membrane phospholipid and to induce an invagination of the plasma membrane containing the insulin in the cell.[30]

One of the first attempts to facilitate insulin transfer through the enterocytes was to entrap the hormone within liposomes as carriers and to introduce them intracellularly.[31,32] The lipophility of the water-lipid bilayer liposomes permitted mucosal attachment and permeation of insulin into the cell, to be later extruded into the interstitial space. In addition, the liposomes were coated with polyethylene glycol (PEG) or mucin in order to further protect them.[33] This resulted in an increase in the potency of liposomes to deliver insulin into the blood circulation. Although it brought promising results initially, these modalities were later rejected since they could not be reproduced systematically, due to the degradation of the liposomes in the lumen of the GI tract. In addition, the methods to synthesize them were costly.

Further studies applying fatty acids, especially of medium-chain length, have been shown to facilitate absorption of peptides, probably by the same mechanisms ascribed to liposomes.[34]

Insulin-containing microspheres or nanospheres have also been tried and have proven to be effective in reducing blood glucose levels.[35,36] The mechanism of the absorption was not fully elucidated and the possibility of transport through Payer's patches was suggested.[37] Further improvement of the microencapsulation was achieved using biodegradable polymers.[38,39] The advantage of these nanospheres resides in their tiny size and mucoadhesiveness, thus allowing their contents (e.g. insulin) to be attached to the mucous surface for a longer period of time. However, the polymerization procedures of the different preparations called for highly skilled techniques and no further human studies have been published.

A system of oral preparations was developed that would release the insulin further down the GI tract into the colonic lumen, bypassing unaltered the small intestine hours after ingestion. Special coating of a peptide-carrying device, which was time-controlled, was slowly dissolved during the movement through the upper segments of the GI tract, without exposing the insulin-containing core.[40] Upon reaching the colon the insulin was released and became available for transport. Alternatively, insulin-containing particles were coated with a pH-sensitive form, so that they would not be dissolved in the low pH (gastric) or in the neutral pH (small intestine), but would release their contents when exposed to high pH, which prevails at the colonic mucosal site.[41] An additional method of coating the particles with polymers which are sensitive and easily degraded by colonic flora, was also introduced. It enabled the particles to reach the large intestine intact and spill their insulin core only there.[42]

These applications, to bring the insulin to the large bowel unaffected (through the small intestine), became feasible following rat and human studies, which have shown that rectal (namely colonic) administration of insulin is indeed effective. The rectal route bypasses the difficulty presented by gastric and small intestinal proteolytic enzymes, since the colon is devoid of these enzymes. The use of surfactants was also found necessary in the rectal studies. Naturally occurring surfactants of the bile salts family were the preferred delivery agents.[43–46] The advantage of these compounds emanated from the fact that certain concentrations of bile salts turn into micelles with a hydrophilic outer layer and lipophilic core, thus enabling absorption of 'with-in micelles' trapped insulin, probably transcellularly. Bile salts also exerted their activity by changing the tight junctions and opening transient pores between the cells, through their chelating effect. Therefore, cholic acid, deoxycholic acid, sodium glycocholate, sodium taurocholate and cheno-deoxy cholate were applied as the surface acting molecules. The use of these agents rendered the mucosal lining of these cavities penetrable by peptides, like insulin. Insulin-containing mixtures which included bile salts were introduced into the rectal sac by microenemata or by suppositories.[47,48] Insulin was effectively absorbed by the colonic mucosa and the plasma glucose concentrations were lowered. It was also demonstrated that both increasing amounts of sodium

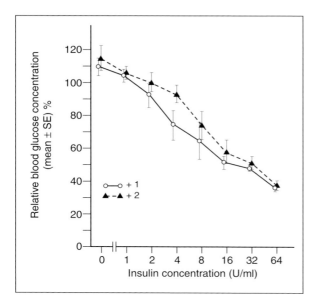

Figure 24.1
Relative blood glucose concentrations one and two hours following rectal administration of mixtures of sodium cholate and increasing doses of insulin.

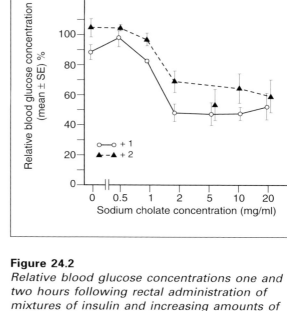

Figure 24.2
Relative blood glucose concentrations one and two hours following rectal administration of mixtures of insulin and increasing amounts of sodium cholate.

cholate and increasing amounts of insulin resulted in a drop of plasma glucose levels in a dose-response curve fashion (Figures 24.1 and 24.2). Human studies were also performed and proved efficacious (Figures 24.3 and 24.4).[49]

The feasibility of insulin absorption through the small intestinal wall was also demonstrated through studies using the rat and dog models. The design was to bypass the hostile environment of the stomach by applying the insulin-containing mixture directly into the small intestines of these animals.[50] Besides the surface-active materials, protease inhibitors were added as well (see below). This was performed in the rat by a surgical cut of the abdominal wall and the exposure of the intestinal lumen, through which the drug was applied. In the case of the dog, a special cannula was inserted percutaneously into the duodenal space. Through this cannula the mixture was introduced. A lowering of glucose levels was demonstrated (Tables 24.1 and 24.2). In another study, a solid formulation of insulin was prepared in microtablets and administered per-oral to the dogs. With this method it was demonstrated that blood glucose concentrations decreased, preceded by an increment of plasma insulin levels (Figure 24.5).[50]

Any surface-active substance used that facilitated the transfer of peptides transcytotically, may damage the integrity of the cell when applied chronically.[51] Therefore, agents that would modify the tight junction were proposed. A compound which was derived from a bacillus cholera array of toxins, named

Table 24.1

	Glucose		Insulin		
	% Decrease at minimum level	Time of minimum level (min)	Value at peak μIU/ml	Time of peak (min)	n
Non-coated capsule[a]	25 ± 3.4	37 ± 2.9	42 ± 14.5	25 ± 2.9	14
Microtablets					
1.2 g, S-1233	23 ± 3.2	57 ± 6.1	21 ± 2.8	33 ± 5.3	8
3.0 g, S-1302	24 ± 3.4	54 ± 6.8	26 ± 2.3	32 ± 2.0	5

Notes: [a]Containing insulin, 150 IU; SBTI, 40 mg; and sodium cholate, 100 mg

Plasma glucose and insulin characteristics in non-diabetic dogs following enteral administration of insulin

Table 24.2

	Glucose		Insulin			Glucose level at 0 time (mg/dl)
	% Decrease at minimum level	Time of minimum level (min)	Value at peak μIU/ml	Time of peak (min)	n	
Non-diabetic						
5.0 g, S-1233	18 ± 1.6	144 ± 12.0	36 ± 8.0	108 ± 23.0	4	77 ± 3.3 (n = 19)
6.0 g, S-1302	25 ± 5.2	150 ± 5.6	18 ± 1.9	123 ± 18.0	6	
Partially diabetic						
5.0 g, S-1233	27 ± 7.8	63 ± 5.1	17 ± 4.3	44 ± 7.1	6	84 ± 5.6 (n = 11)
6.0 g, S-1302	29 ± 5.0	81 ± 8.7	16 ± 2.6	52 ± 7.3	5	
Diabetic						
5.0 g, S-1233	42 ± 14.2	123 ± 8.8	100 ± 37.0	73 ± 6.0	3	265 ± 42 (n = 9)
6.0 g, S-1302	33 ± 6.4	126 ± 18.0	16 ± 7.2	88 ± 16.0	5	

Plasma glucose and insulin characteristics in diabetic and non-diabetic dogs after oral administration of insulin in enterocoated microtablets

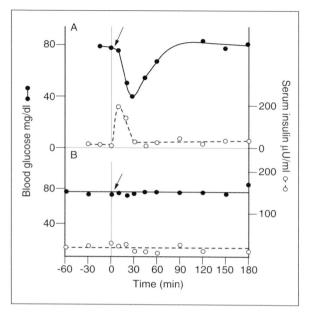

Figure 24.3
Rectal administration of insulin to non-diabetic human volunteers. Closed circles represent blood glucose levels; open circles represent plasma insulin levels. (A) Microenema, 2.5 ml, containing 150 μ insulin and 20 mg/ml sodium cholate, (B) Microenema 2.5 ml, containing 150 μ insulin without sodium cholate. Arrows indicate time of drug administration.

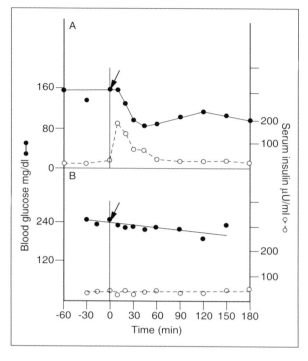

Figure 24.4
Rectal administration of insulin to non-insulin-dependent diabetic volunteers. Closed circles represent blood glucose levels; open circles represent plasma insulin levels. (A) Microenema, 2.5 ml, containing 150 μ insulin and 20 mg/ml sodium cholate. (B) Microenema, 2.5 ml, containing 150 μ insulin without sodium cholate. Arrows indicate time of drug administration.

Zonula occludens toxin (Zot) was tried with some success.[52,53] The possibility of the transfer of undesirable materials from the GI tract was raised. Fortunately, Zot was found to be active only in the small intestine and not in the large bowel, where most of these foreign substances might be found.

In order for the intact peptide hormone to be biologically effective upon being ingested, it has to be protected from both the hostile acidic conditions in the stomach and from digestion by enzymes of the small intestine.[54] A pharmaceutical design of enterocoating using pH-responsive hydrogels following loading of insulin into micropheres was applied.[55] Another approach promoted the use of enzyme inhibitors which were found to partially defend the peptides (e.g. insulin) against proteolysis.[56] The proteases which are secreted by the stomach, pancreas and the intestinal wall, should be inhibited to protect the peptides (like insulin) and preserve it intact and biologically

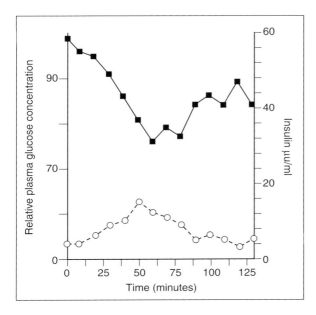

Figure 24.5
Changes in plasma glucose and insulin levels after oral administration of 5.0 g of enterocoated microtablets (S-1233) to partially pancreatectomized dog: (■) glucose, (○) insulin. Each 1.0 g contains 125 IU of insulin, 40 mg of SBTI and 123 mg of sodium cholate (n = 6).

enzyme. Furthermore, the matrices in which the hormone is embedded, could be built to release insulin at timed intervals according to the share of the polymers in the matrix. This characteristic was favorable compared to the non-controlled release of a peptide drug from a capsule.

Recently, a new technology to promote oral peptide and polysaccharide absorption has brought the discovery of modified complex amino acids.[60] These alpha and non-alpha amino acids were found to increase absorption of proteins and polysaccharides from the GI tract. The exact mechanism by which these agents enhance the absorption has not as yet been fully elucidated. In theory, a non-covalent reversible bonding of the compound with the peptide, which is better attained with increasing concentrations of both solutes in the mixtures, facilitates the transepithelial transport. It is also believed that an intermolecular association takes place, which is mandatory for the absorption activity of the compounds. By partial unfolding of the protein, induced by the delivery agent, conformational changes that occur allow the protein to be more readily transferable across the lipid bilayer mucosal barrier of the GI tract.[61]

Studies were conducted in animals[62] and human non-diabetic volunteers using one of these amino acid analogs – SNAC (sodium N-[8{2-hydroxybenzoyl}amino]caprylate). A satisfactory response was achieved when this delivery agent was added to insulin and administered per-orally.[63] The nadir of plasma glucose ranged between 20 and 40% of the initial levels, according to the amounts of insulin given, as described in a dose-response curve. In each case, the decrease in glucose concentrations was preceded by a peak of plasma insulin, detected between 15 and 30 min following the administration of the mixture. The early appearance of plasma

active. Therefore, the use of antiproteases was applied. They were comprised of naturally occurring substances like soybean trypsin inhibitor (SBTI) and also aprotinin.[56,57] Chitosan, a derivative of chitin, a cellulose-like natural product, was found to display two features, namely a protecting effect towards the proteinases and an absorption enhancing capacity.[58]

Another avenue of research brought the discovery of an insulin-carrier matrix of an artificial nature which resulted in the creation of polymer inhibitor conjugates (the inhibitors used were Bowman-Birk-SBTI and CMC-elastinal).[59] Each one of these inhibitors effectively protected the hormone against a specific insulin, concomitant with the elevation of plasma SNAC levels, indicated the necessary presence of both the carrier and insulin at the absorption site in the gut, probably in its upper part (possibly even in the stomach). Parallel to the elevation of plasma insulin, the plasma C-peptide levels were reduced, indicating the absorption of exogenous insulin, which suppresses the endogenous secretion of the hormone. SNAC was found to be a safe delivery agent and no adverse effects were noted.[64] Further trials are being conducted using these novel amino acid analogs (such as [4-(2-hydroxybenzoyl)aminophenyl]butyric acid (SABA)) as delivery agents. The main benefit of these modified amino acids is in the fact that while most of the previous enhancers exerted their effect on the mucosal barrier of the GI tract, the new promoters reversibly modify the peptide itself, rendering it absorbable across the transepithelial barrier. This feature makes these agents more attractive for long-term use, since the enterocytes would be free from chronic unfavorable stimulation induced by the other surface-acting agents.

The nasal route

Several months after the discovery of insulin, and its successful use to treat diabetic children, attempts were already being made to introduce it intranasally.[10] Since the mucosal lining of the nose is highly vascular and the total area of the mucous membranes is quite large, it became an attractive route for administration of this hormone. Encouragement to adopt this route for insulin was recently obtained, after the accomplishment of commercializing other peptides for nasal administration, namely vasopressin and calcitonin.[65] Insulin alone does not penetrate the mucosal barrier, mainly because of its high molecular weight.

Enzymatic activity capable of protein hydrolysis is scarce at the level of the epithelial nasal mucosa.[66] Thus, the need to use absorption enhancers was evident, without the use of enzyme inhibitors. Many promoting agents became available and systematic evaluation in animal models and human studies was launched.

The initial studies employed saponin and glycol. Their efficacy was quite impressive,[67,68] however nasal congestion and irreproducibility of the hypoglycemic effect, accompanied by the need for high doses of insulin, precluded further investment in this field. In the late 1950s, insulin-embedded nasal tampons were tried with an even higher success rate than previously[69], but were abandoned due to their uncomfortable application, and the high inter- and intra-individual variations of the absorption rate.

The new era in the employment of nasal insulin started with the use of bile salts and their derivatives. As in the rectal and oral routes, various salts, esters and conjugates of bile acids were examined. These include: taurocholate, cholate, deoxycholate, glycocholate, chenodeoxycholate, and sodium taurodihydroxyfusidate. The mixtures of insulin with a variety of these compounds in different concentrations, were the basis of many clinical studies with a broad range of absorption rates.[70–72] In most cases, rapid uptake and release into the blood circulation was exhibited, and a hypoglycemic effect has been shown. Comparison of the metabolic effect of these preparations with the subcutaneous injections in Type 1 and Type 2 diabetics proved their acceptable efficacy.[73] Nasal sprays were developed and novel delivery devices were introduced.[74,75] However, long-term application of bile salts and their derivatives produced adverse effects. Some of these side effects include congestion and damage to the nasal epithelium as demonstrated by pathological examinations.[76] Decreased ciliary activity, though beneficial in increasing the residence time of the hormone in the nasal space, seemed unacceptable.[77]

Further attempts to promote insulin absorption through the nasal route were intensified and the search for new delivery agents never ceased. The pharmacological arena and the pharmaceutical industry are continuously being offered novel enhancers encompassing various chemicals. These include chelators (e.g. EDTA, aspirin[78,79]), surfactants other than bile salts (e.g. Laureth-9, sodium lauryl-sulfate[80]), fatty acids and derivatives (e.g. caprylate, lecithin, lysolecithin[81]), dextrines (e.g. dodecylmaltoside[82]), dimethyl-beta-cyclodextrin[83]), chitosan nanospheres[84]), enzyme inhibitors (aprotinin, bestatin[85]) and bioadhesive delivery systems (e.g. carbopol,[86] carboxy-methylcellulose[87]). Most of these delivery agents have shown an effective absorption capacity through the nasal mucosa ranging from 8–18%.[88] However, in spite of the maximal efforts exerted to bring a valid and authentic nasal insulin device, no commercial end product is currently available. While short-term trials were partially successful in many of the above-mentioned delivery agents, chronic administration failed to establish safety, freedom from side effects and consistent and reproducible results.

out that the oral insulin and nasal insulin achieve about 10% efficiency. The need to use 10–15 times more insulin in the preparation would appear to be commercially prohibitive. Owing to the rather low efficacy and questionable therapeutic accomplishment of these oral and nasal routes, clinical application to Type 1 insulin-dependent diabetics may not be feasible at the present time. However, Type 2 diabetics who do not require strict control, and would need only adjunct treatment (with insulin), beyond diet and oral agents, might benefit from the alternative route of oral and/or nasal insulin. These Type 2 diabetic subjects who become insulin-requiring may otherwise avoid taking the injections because of the stigma as well as the pain involved.

The low bioavailability of the insulin and the difficulties encountered in the dose reproducibility, raise some uncertainties regarding the future outcome of oral or nasal delivery systems. In contrast to this skeptical view, the accelerated development and extensive research in this field, which we have witnessed in the last few years, should convey hope for an improvement. Experts in this pharmaceutical sphere claim that a future formulation, which would provide 25–30% insulin absorption efficiency, could become a medical miracle in the life of many diabetic patients. This goal must be pursued.

Conclusions

After reviewing many animal and human studies, we have demonstrated that by applying various measures to protect insulin and to enhance its absorption through mucous membranes, oral insulin and nasal insulin are feasible and within close reach. Experimental modalities have been tried with different rates of success. Most of the reports have pointed

References

1. Banting FG, Best CH. The internal secretion of the pancreas. J Lab Clin Med 1922; 7: 251–6.
2. Bliss M. The Discovery of Insulin. Chicago: The University of Chicago Press, 1982.
3. Hagedorn HC, Hensen BN, Krarup NB, Woodstrup I. Protamine insulinate. JAMA 1936; 106: 177–80.
4. Hallas-Mueller K, Jersild M, Peterson K, Schlichtrull J. Zinc insulin preparations for

single daily injections. JAMA 1952; 150: 1667–71.

5. Goeddel DV, Kleid DG, Bolivar F et al. Expression in escherichia coli of chemically synthesized genes for human insulin. Proc Natl Acad Sci USA 1979; 76: 106–10.

6. Saudek CD. Novel forms of insulin delivery. Endocrinol Metab Clin North Am 1997; 26: 599–610.

7. The Diabetes Control and Complications Trial Research Group. The effect of intensive insulin treatment of diabetes on the development and progression of long-term complications in insulin-dependent diabetes mellitus. N Engl J Med 1993; 329: 977–86.

8. UK Prospective Diabetes Study (UKPDS) Group. Intensive blood-glucose control with sulphonylureas or insulin compared with conventional treatment and risk of complications in patients with type 2 diabetes (UKPDS 33). Lancet 1998; 352: 837–53.

9. Harrison GA. Insulin in alcoholic solution by mouth. BMJ 1923; 18: 1204–5.

10. Woodyat RT. The clinical use of insulin. J Metab Res 1922; 2: 793–801.

11. Sindelar DK, Balcom JH, Chu C et al. A comparison of the effects of selective increases in peripheral or portal insulin on hepatic glucose production in the conscious dog. Diabetes 1996; 45: 1594–604.

12. Davis S, Gelho B, Tate D et al. The effects of HDV-insulin on carbohydrate metabolism in type 1 diabetic patients. J Diabetes Complications 2001; 15: 227–33.

13. Kidron M, Krausz MM, Raz I et al. The absorption of insulin. Tenside Surf Det 1989; 26: 352–4.

14. Bendayan M. Functional properties of the intestinal wall: novel aspects and recent avenues. Microsc Res Tech 2000; 49: 325–8.

15. Mayes PA. Digestion and absorption. In: Murray RK, Granner DK, Mayes PA, Rodwell VW, eds. Harper's Biochemistry, 25th edn. Stamford: Lange, 2000: 662–74.

16. Farquar MG, Palade GE. Junctional complexes in various epithelia. J Cell Biol 1963; 17: 375–412.

17. Warshaw AL, Walker WA, Cornell R, Isselbacher KJ. Small intestinal permeability to macromolecules: transmission of horseradish peroxidase into mesenteric lymph and portal blood. Lab Invest 1971; 25: 675–84.

18. Udall JN, Pang K, Fritze L et al. Development of gatrointestinal mucosal barrier. 1. The effect of age on intestinal permeability to macro-molecules. Pediatr Res 1981; 15: 241–5.

19. Mostov KE. Transepithelial transport of immunoglobulins. Ann Rev Immunol 1994; 12: 63–84.

20. Xanthou M, Bines J, Walker WA. Human milk and intestinal host defense in newborns: an update. Adv Pediatr 1995; 42: 171–208.

21. Shehadeh N, Gelertner L, Blazer S et al. The importance of insulin content in infant diet: suggestion for a new infant formula period. Acta Paediatr 2001; 90: 92–5.

22. Shulman RJ. Oral insulin increases small intestinal mass and disaccaridase activity in the newborn miniature pig. Pediatr Res 1990; 28: 171–5.

23. Guyton AC. Digestion and absorption in the gastrointestinal tract; gastrointestinal disorders. In: Human Physiology and Mechanism of Disease, 5th edn. Philadelphia: WB Saunders, 1992: 500–9.

24. Ross MH, Romrell LJ, Kaye GI. Digestive system II: small intestine. In: Ross, Romrell and Kaye, eds. Histology, 3rd edn. Baltimore: Williams & Wilkins, 1995: 453–64.

25. Silk DB. Peptide absorption in man. Gut 1974; 15: 494–501.

26. Smyth D. Glucose absorption. Gastroenterology 1962; 42: 76–9.

27. Lee VHL, Yamamoto A, Kompella UB. Mucosal penetration enhancers for facilitation of peptide and protein drug absorption. Crit Rev Ther Drug Carrier Syst 1991; 8: 91–192.

28. Bendayan M, Ziv E, Ben-Sasson R et al. Morpho-cytochemical and biochemical evidence for insulin absorption by the rat ileal epithelium. Diabetologia 1990; 33: 197–204.

29. Bendayan M, Ziv E, Gingras D et al. Biochemical and morpho-cytochemical evidence for the intestinal absorption of insulin in control and diabetic rats: comparison between the effectiveness of duodenal and colon mucosa. Diabetologia 1994; 37: 119–26.

30. Ziv E, Lior O, Kidron M. Absorption of protein via the intestinal wall. A quantitative model. Biochem Pharmacol 1987; 36: 1035–9.

31. Patel HM, Stevenson RW, Parsons JA, Ryman BE. Use of liposomes to aid intestinal absorption of entrapped insulin in normal and diabetic dogs. Biochem Biophys Acta 1982; 716: 188–93.

32. Spangler RS. Insulin administration via liposomes. Diabetes Care 1990; 13: 911–22.

33. Iwanaga K, Ono S, Narioka K et al. Application of surface-coated liposomes for oral delivery of peptide: effects of coating the liposome's surface on the GI transit of insulin. J Pharm Sci 1999; 88: 248–52.

34. Muranushi N, Mack E, Kim SW. The effects of fatty acids and their derivatives on the intestinal absorption of insulin in rat. Drug Ind Pharm 1993; 19: 929–41.

35. Damge C, Vranckx H, Balschmidt P, Convreur P. Poly(alkyl cyanoacrylate) nanospheres for oral administration of insulin. J Pharm Sci 1997; 86: 1403–9.

36. Carino GP, Jacobs JS, Mathiowitz E. Nanosphere based oral insulin delivery. J Control Release 2000; 65: 261–9.

37. Carr KE, Hazzard RA, Reid S, Hodges GM. The effect of size on uptake of orally administered latex micro-particles in the small intestine and transport to mesenteric lymph nodes. Pharm Res 1996; 13: 1205–9.

38. Mathiowitz E, Jacobs YS et al. Biologically erodable microspheres as potential oral drug delivery systems. Nature 1997; 286: 410–14.

39. Okada H, Toguchi H. Biodegradable microspheres in drug delivery. Crit Rev Ther Drug Carrier Syst 1995; 12: 1–99.

40. Lowman AM, Morishita M, Kajita M et al. Oral delivery of insulin using pH-responsive complexation gels. J Pharm Sci 1999; 88: 933–7.

41. Tozaki H, Komoike J, Tada C et al. Chitosan capsules for colon-specific drug delivery: improvement of insulin absorption from the rat colon. J Pharm Sci 1997; 86: 1016–20.

42. Saffran M, Kumar GS, Savariar C et al. A new approach to the oral administration of insulin and other peptide drugs. Science 1986; 233: 1081–4.

43. Ziv E, Bendayan M, Gingras D et al. Mechanism of insulin absorption by the intestinal mucosa: a morph-cytochemical and biochemical study. J Pharm Sci 1993; 82: 868–72.

44. Zic E, Kidron M, Teitelbaum, Bar-On H. Role of bile salts in macromolecular absorption from the gatrointestinal tract. J Pharm Sci 1989; 78: 890–2.

45. Bar-On H, Berry EM, Eldor A et al. Enteral administration of insulin in the rat. Br J Pharmac 1981; 73: 21–4.

46. Hosny EA, Ghilzai NM, Elmazar MM. Promotion of oral insulin absorption in diabetic rabbits using pH-dependent coated capsules containing sodium cholate. Pharma Acta Helv 1997; 72: 203–7.

47. Ziv E, Kidron M, Berry E, Bar-On H. Bile salts promote the absorption of insulin from the rat colon. Life Sci 1981; 29: 803–9.

48. Shichiri M, Yamasaki Y, Kawamori R et al. Increased intestinal absorption of insulin: an insulin suppository. J Pharmacol 1978; 30: 806–8.

49. Raz I, Kidron M, Bar-on H, Ziv E. Rectal administration of insulin. Isr J Med Sci 1984; 20: 173–5.

50. Ziv E, Kidron M, Raz I et al. Oral administration of insulin in solid form to nondiabetic and diabetic dogs. J Pharm Sci 1994; 83: 792–4.

51. Rafter JJ, Eng VWS, Furrer R et al. Effects of calcium and pH on the mucosal damage produced by deoxycholic acid in the rat colon. Gut 1986; 27: 1320–9.

52. Fasano A, Uzzau S. Modulation of intestinal tight junctions by zonula occludens toxin permits enteral administration of insulin and other macromolecules in an animal model. J Clin Invest 1997; 99: 1158–64.

53. Fasano A. Novel approaches for oral delivery of macromolecules. J Pharm Sci 1998; 87: 1351–6.

54. Bernkop-Schnurch A. The use of inhibitory agents to overcome the enzymatic barrier to perorally administered therapeutic peptides and proteins. J Control Release 1998; 52: 1–16.

55. Lowman AM, Morishita M, Peppas NA, Nagai T. Novel bioadhesive complexation networks for oral protein drug deliver. In: McCulloch I, Shalaby SW, eds. Materials for Controlled Released Applications. Washington DC: Chemical Society, 1998: 156–64.

56. Yamamoto A, Taniguchi T, Rikyuu K et al. Effects of various protease inhibitors on the intestinal absorption and degradation of insulin in rats. Pharm Res 1994; 11: 1496–500.

57. Woodley JF. Enzymatic barriers for GI peptide and protein delivery. Crit Rev Ther Drug 1994; 11: 61–95.

58. Bernkop-Schnurch A, Krajicek ME. Mucosadhesive polymers for peroral peptide delivery: synthesis and evaluation of chitosan-EDTA conjugates. J Control Release 1998; 50: 215–23.

59. Bernkop0-Schnurch A, Pasta M. Intestinal peptide and protein delivery: novel bioadhesive drug-carrier matrix shielding from enzymatic attack. J Pharm Sci 1998 87: 430–4.

60. Leone-Bay A, Paton DR, Freeman J et al. Synthesis and evaluation of compounds that facilitate the gastrointestinal absorption of heparin. J Med Chem 1998; 41: 1163–71.

61. Leone-Bay A, Leipold H, Baton DR et al. Oral delivery of rhGHL preliminary mechanistic considerations. Drug News Perspect 1996; 9: 586–90.

62. Kidron M, Mizrachi Y, Bar-On H, Variano B. New oral formulation of human insulin (abstract #1833). Diabetes 2001; 50: A439–98.

63. Kidron M, Menachem Y, Variano B et al. A novel per-oral insulin formulation: Stage 1 study in non-diabetic subjects. In press.

64. Rivera T, Leone-Bay A, Paton D. Oral delivery of heparin in combination with sodium N-[8-(2-hydroxybenzoyl)amino]caprylate: pharmacological considerations. Pharm Res 1997; 14: 1830–3.

65. Morimoto K, Yamaguchi H, Iwakura et al. Effects of viscous hyaluronate sodium solutions on the nasal absorption of vasopressin and an analogue. Pharm Res 1991; 8: 471–4.

66. Hirai S, Yashiki T, Mima H. Mechanisms for the enhancement of the nasal absorption of insulin by surfactants. Int J Pharm 1981; 9: 173–84.

67. Collens WS, Goldzieher MA. Absorption of insulin by nasal mucous membranes. Proc Soc Exp Biol Med 1932; 29: 756–9.

68. Major RH. The intranasal application of insulin, experimental and clinical experiences. Am J Med Sci 1936; 192: 257–63.

69. Hankiss J, Hadhazy CS. Resorption von insulin und asthmolysin von der nasenschleimhaut. Acta Med Hung 1958; 12: 107–14.

70. Hirai S, Ikenaga T, Matsuzawa T. Nasal absorption of insulin in dogs. Diabetes 1978; 27: 296–9.

71. Hirai S, Yashiki T, Mima H. Effect of surfactants on the nasal absorption of insulin rats. Int J Pharm 1981; 9: 165–72.

72. Aungst BJ, Rogers NJ, Shefter E. Comparison of nasal, rectal, buccal, sublingual and intramuscular insulin efficacy and the effects of a bile salt absorption promoter. J Parmacol Exp Ther 1988; 244: 23–7.

73. Lalej-Bennis D, Boillot J, Bardin C et al. Efficacy and tolerance of intranasal insulin administered during 4 months in severely hyperglycaemic Type 2 diabetic patients with oral drug failure: a cross-over study. Diabet Med 2001; 18: 614–18.

74. Lalej-Bennes D, Boillot J, Bardin C et al. Six month administration of gelified intranasal insulin in 16 type 1 diabetic patients under multiple injections: efficacy vs. subcutaneous injections and local tolerance. Diabetes Metab 2001; 27: 372–7.

75. Mitra R, Pezron I, Chu WA, Mitra AK. Lipid emulsions as vehicles for enhanced nasal delivery of insulin. Int J Pharm 2000; 205: 127–34.

76. Ennis RD, Borden L, Lee WA. The effects of permeation enhancers on the surface morphology of the rat nasal mucosa: a scanning electron microscopy study. Pharm Res 1990; 7: 468–75.

77. Hermens WAJJ, Hooymans PM, Verhoef JC, Merkus FWHM. Effect of absorption enhancers on human nasal tissue ciliary movement in vitro. Pharm Res 1990; 7: 144–6.

78. Uchida N, Maitani Y Machida Y et al. Influence of bile salts on the permeability through the nasal mucosa of rabbits of insulin in comparison with dextran derivaties. Drug Dev Ind Pharm 1991; 17: 1625–34.

79. Aungst BJ, Rogers NJ. Site dependence of absorption-promoting actions of laureth-9, sodium salicylate, disodium EDTA, and aprotinin on rectal, nasal and buccal insulin delivery. Pharm Res 1988; 5: 305–8.

80. Salzman R, Manson JE, Griffing GT. Intranasal aerosolized insulin. Mixed-meal studies and long-term use in type 1 diabetes. N Engl J Med 1985; 312: 1078–84.

81. Stafford RE, Dennis EA. Lysophospholipids as biosurfactants. Colloids Surfaces 1988; 30: 47–64.

82. Yoshida A, Arima H, Uekama K, Pitha J. Pharmaceutical evaluation of hydroxyalkyl ethers of B-cyclodextrins. Int J Pharm 1988; 46: 217–22.

83. Shao Z, Krishnamoorthy R, Mitra AK. Cyclodextrins as nasal absorption promoters of insulin: mechanistic evaluation. Pharm Res 1992; 9: 1157–63.

84. Schipper NGM, Olsson S, Hoogstraate JA et al. Chitosans as absorption enhancers for poorly soluble drugs 2: Mechanism of absorption enhancement. Pharm Res 1997; 14: 923–9.

85. Hewlett G. Apropos aprotinin: a review. Biotechnology 1990; 6: 565–8.

86. Morimoto K, Morisaka K, Kamanda A. Enhancement of nasal absorption of insulin and calcitonin using polyacrylic acid gel. J Pharm Pharmacol 1985; 37: 134–6.

87. Junginger HE. Bioadhesive polymer systems for peptide delivery. Acta Pharm Technol 1990; 36: 110–26.

88. Hinchcliffe M, Illum L. Intranasal insulin delivery and therapy. Adv Drug Delivery Rev 1999; 35: 199–234.

25

Evidence-based care of Type 2 diabetes

Michael Berger†, Ingrid Mühlhauser, Bernd Richter

Introduction

With the worldwide rise of its incidence and prevalence rates, Type 2 diabetes is becoming a major public health problem. Any rational approach to the problem needs to consider the demographic and pathophysiological heterogeneity of the disease. Depending on its severity and duration, the clinical presentation of Type 2 diabetes may be described in three major categories:

(1) as a risk status due to non-symptomatic hyperglycaemia (and associated other risks as part of the metabolic syndrome X) for macro- and microvascular disease;
(2) as a disease state with hyperglycaemia- and hypoinsulinaemia-derived symptoms; and
(3) as a (multi-) morbid state due to vascular late complications of the disease.

Primary therapeutic objectives for the treatment of Type 2 diabetes are to maintain a quality of life as little affected by the disease as possible, the prevention of its acute complications, its hyperglycaemia-induced symptoms and therapeutic collateral effects and the prevention of excess cardiovascular morbidity and mortality, as well as microangiopathic organ damage. Lamentably, there are no systematic reviews or Cochrane Reviews available on the treatment of Type 2 diabetes. With excess mortality due to macroangiopathy being the principal clinical problem of Type 2 diabetes, it is surprising that only two studies have ever attempted to demonstrate an effect of treatments to lower glycaemia upon the incidence of cardiovascular morbidity and mortality.[1,2] Only four randomized controlled trials were ever conducted to document the effects of attempts to normalize blood glucose on incidence and progression of microangiopathy in Type 2 diabetes.[1-4]

With the diagnosis of Type 2 diabetes, the patient's individual disease state is to be assessed and, if at all possible together with the patient, his/her individual therapeutic goals are to be defined. With advancing age and a shorter remaining life expectancy, the therapeutic objective to achieve freedom from diabetes-related symptoms and acute complications will become more central as a therapeutic objective – whereas the lowering of glycaemia to prevent microangiopathic late complications will become less urgent. In this context, it is of note that in central and northern Europe the majority of patients with Type 2 diabetes belong to the geriatric age range.

Some 100,000 publications can be retrieved that deal with pharmacological agents to lower elevated levels of glycaemia. A multitude of therapeutic strategies is being advocated as consensus recommendations and guidelines. Often, these documents are based on majority opinions of (a self-appointed gremium of) experts or on the application of delphi techniques involving so-called opinion leaders. In addition, the pharmaceutical industry is launching increasing numbers of sophisticated and expensive products to combat the endemic growth of Type 2 diabetes and its complications. In order to review the various therapeutic strategies, we suggest focusing on the patient-oriented outcome goals of Type 2 diabetes treatment,[5] applying the principles of evidence-based medicine.

Sackett et al.[6] have called for the implementation of evidence-based medicine as the integration of best research evidence with clinical expertise and patient values. Unfortunately, the recent volume on *Evidence-based Diabetes Care* edited by Gerstein and Haynes does not focus adequately on patient-oriented outcomes in the treatment of Type 2 diabetes.[7] Physicians today face tremendous problems in integrating the results of vast amounts of published trials in their everyday care. Narrative reviews should no longer be used as guidance for decision making due to their often subjective and unsystematic approach. Systematic reviews and meta-analyses rank among the highest levels of evidence and could have a profound impact on diabetes care.[8] The 'Cochrane Metabolic and Endocrine Disorders Group' as part of the Cochrane Collaboration Movement is about to publish several systematic reviews on diabetes care with particular focus on patient-oriented outcomes.[9] In this chapter we shall comment on the impact of scientific evidence and patient preferences on the definition of a rational treatment of Type 2 diabetes mellitus.

Non-drug therapy as the basis for the treatment of Type 2 diabetes

Newly diagnosed Type 2 diabetes mellitus is being treated with non-drug therapy as long as the individually defined therapeutic goals can be achieved. Such treatment consists of lifestyle modification, e.g. nutrition therapy to normalize body weight and to avoid fast absorbable carbohydrates as well as advice to increase physical activity. In many cases therapeutic success can be achieved: hyperglycaemia-related symptoms may disappear and glucose homoeostasis may be reinstalled, at least for some time.

Several authors have reported the particular success of non-drug therapy during the initial phases of Type 2 diabetes.[10–13] In the UKPDS, the initial three months' diet therapy resulted in a mean weight loss of approximately 4 kg and a mean reduction of HbA1c values of 1.7%; only in 15% of 3044 patients was primary diet failure diagnosed.[2,14–16]

The burden associated with this lifestyle modification phase of the treatment, as perceived by the patients, differs individually, but the risk of negative side effects is usually limited to a decrease of quality of life associated with the behaviour modification involved.

Several educational programmes for non-drug therapy of Type 2 diabetes mellitus have been published with various short-term success rates; medium- or long-term evaluations have rarely been performed, as recently presented in a systematic review on self-management training in Type 2 diabetes.[17] An important aspect for the possible success of any patient education, however, is its integration into the treatment programme.[18] Based upon the recommendations of a flexible hypocaloric nutrition and systematic glucosuria self-monitoring as the basis for non-drug therapy by Bouchardat[19] and Davidson,[11] we have developed and evaluated a structured group treatment and teaching programme for Type 2 diabetic patients in general practice based on a one-year controlled trial directed to medium-term outcomes.[20] Following 1991, this programme was officially implemented as a reimbursable therapeutic strategy in the routine health care system in Germany,[21] and it has sucessfully been used in other countries and health care systems.[22–25]

If the individual therapeutic goals can no longer be achieved by non-drug therapy and lifestyle intervention, the second phase of Type 2 diabetes management must be initiated, i.e. drug therapy.

Anti-hyperglycaemic drug therapy in Type 2 diabetes mellitus

Relevant scientific evidence has to be sought from patient-centred clinical research into the efficacy and safety of therapeutic and preventive regimens. Thus, we shall focus on data from randomized controlled trials directed at clinically relevant end points of Type 2 diabetes, i.e. cardiovascular morbidity and mortality and hyperglycaemia-associated organ damage, rather than on surrogate markers, such as indices of glycaemia.

Prevention of macroangiopathy

With regard to the incidence of macroangiopathy (cardiovascular morbidity and mortality), neither of the randomized controlled trials (RCTs)[1,2] directed at this end point were able to detect significant improvements as a result of blood glucose lowering, with the exception of a positive effect of metformin monotherapy in overweight Type 2 diabetic patients on diabetes-related vascular complications and death, as well as on total mortality.[26] In the feasibility phase of the Veteran's Affairs Cooperative Study on Diabetes Mellitus,[4] there was a tendency for a negative effect of intensified blood glucose control (using a complex protocol which included insulin and sulfonylurea drugs) on the incidence of macroangiopathy which almost reached statistical significance. The number of macroangiopathic

events that occured during the six years of the Kunamoto study on the effects of intensified insulin therapy in Type 2 diabetes was too small to draw any conclusions.[3]

Based on the data of both the UGDP and the UKPDS, there was no indication that the treatment with exogenous insulin might lead to a progression of macroangiopathy and/or atherosclerotic organ damage.[1,2]

Data from the UGDP study carried out in the 1960s had indicated that the blood glucose-lowering sulfonylurea drug tolbutamide was associated with increased cardiovascular mortality in Type 2 diabetic patients.[27] Whilst the validity of this finding became the centre of an unprecedented controversy,[28,29] it was compatible with observational findings collected at the Joslin Clinic patient cohort by Kanarek.[30] It was not until some 25 years later, that a pathophysiological plausibility of these earlier findings was described[31] as sulfonylurea-induced blockage of ATP-dependent K-channels in cardiocytes may possibly interfere with the concept of hypoxic preconditioning in coronary artery disease. We have hypothesized that the clinical relevance of this pathomechanism may actually be compatible with the findings of the DIGAMI study.[32] Even though respective negative cardiovascular side effects by the sulfonylurea glibenclamide have not been observed in the UKPDS,[2] earlier concerns about the possible cardiotoxic effects of sulfonylureas in the treatment of patients with Type 2 diabetes and coronary heart disease (as supported by recent pathophysiological data[33]), remain[34] because patients with clinically significant coronary artery disease were excluded from the UKPDS.[15] (At the most, those 2% of patients included in the study who have had a myocardial infarction prior to 12 months before being recruited may have to be considered coronary artery disease patients.) On the basis of these safety concerns, we suggest not

	Blood glucose control		
	Intensive (n = 2729 median HbA1c over 10 years: 7.0%)	Conventional (n = 1138 median HbA1c over 10 years: 7.9%)	
Any diabetes related end point (ADREP)			
Events per 1000 patient-years*	40.9		46
ARR/ARI		5.1	
NNT/NNH (95% CI)		19.6 (10–500)	
p value		0.029	
RR (95% CI)		0.88 (0.79–0.99)	
RRR/RRI		12% (1–21%)	
Microvascular complications			
Events per 1000 patient-years*	8.6		11.4
ARR/ARI		2.8	
NNT/NNH		35.7	
p value		0.0099	
RR (95% CI)		0.75 (0.60–0.93)	
RRR/RRI		25% (7–40%)	

Notes: ARR/ARI absolute risk reduction/absolute risk increase
NNT/NNH number needed to treat/number needed to harm
RR relative risk
CI confidence interval
RRR/RRI relative risk reduction/relative risk increase
* persons with events per 1000 person-years
Sources: refs 2, 56

Table 25.1
Reduction of vascular complications and organ damage by intensive versus conventional blood glucose control in the UK Prospective Diabetes Study

to use sulfonylurea drugs in Type 2 diabetic patients with coronary artery disease outside formal clinical trials.

When aiming to reduce the excessive cardiovascular morbidity and mortality in Type 2 diabetes, it appears evidence-based to normalize arterial blood pressure using certain cardioselective β-blockers, diuretics and/or ACE-inhibitors, to use simvastatin in case of hypercholesterolaemia,[35] to stop smoking, to take aspirin,[5] and, possibly independent of its antihypertensive effects, to prescribe ramipril.[36]

Prevention of microangiopathy

Compatible with the concept of the causal relationship between hyperglycaemia and diabetic microangiopathy[37] and with the results of the Diabetes Control and Complications Trial[38] and other studies in Type 1 diabetic patients, lowering of blood glucose levels by intensified therapy decreased the incidence and progression of microangiopathic organ damage in Type 2 diabetic patients.[2,3] Table 25.1 depicts the effects of intensive blood glucose control during the 10-year study period of the UKPDS[2] on absolute risk reduction and numbers needed to treat (NNT) for the aggregate study end points *microangiopathy* and *any diabetes-related end point (ADREP)*.

In those Type 2 diabetic patients with arterial hypertension, antihypertensive treatment with atenolol or captopril had a significant effect in preventing microangiopathic organ damage (absolute risk reduction 7.2%; $NNT_{8\ years} = 14$).[39]

When hyperglycaemia was lowered by insulin treatment, a significant reduction of microangiopathic organ damage was demonstrated in two randomized controlled trials.[2,3] A comparable benefit was achieved when glibenclamide was used to improve glycaemic control in the UKPDS.[2] Even though comparably effective with regard to lowering HbA1c levels, chlorpropamide – a first generation sulfonylurea drug – did not improve microvascular outcomes, but was associated with an increase in blood pressure.

Insulin therapy

Subcutaneous insulin therapy aiming at normalizing glycaemic control, results in significant reductions of the incidence and the progression of diabetic microangiopathy; there is no indication that it leads to a worsening of macroangiopathy or to the development of atherosclerosis.

The particular strategy of insulin therapy varied between (and within) the randomized controlled studies in Type 2 diabetic patients[1–3] – circumstances which are known to result in differences concerning the associated weight gain, incidence of mild and severe hypoglycaemia and related interference with quality of life. It is conceivable that these negative aspects of insulin treatment in Type 2 diabetic patients

may be ameliorated by a strategy of preprandial regular insulin (supplementary insulin) treatment.[40] Unfortunately, there are no randomized controlled studies to compare effectivity and safety of various insulin treatment strategies in Type 2 diabetes.

In elderly patients with Type 2 diabetes requiring insulin treatment, a conventional insulin therapy with two daily injections of a combination insulin (e.g. pre-mixed solutions of 30% regular and 70% NPH human insulin) is preferably used in this part of Europe. A respective structured group treatment and teaching programme has been developed, evaluated for surrogates and patient-oriented end points based on long-term follow-up up to ten years[41,42] and implemented into the routine health care system in Germany.[43,44]

Numerous attempts have been made to compare different types of strategies combining insulin therapies and oral antidiabetic agents concerning surrogate outcomes (body weight) or at best secondary end points (incidence of hypoglycaemia, HbA1c levels) during short-term studies of up to one or two years.[45] No evidence for a positive effect on patient-oriented outcomes exists for the whole array of such combination therapies using insulin injections in parallel with various oral antidiabetic agents.

Oral antidiabetic agents

Based on the UKPDS, glibenclamide is an evidence-based alternative to insulin as the first-line pharmacological treatment of younger patients with newly manifest Type 2 diabetes free of coronary artery disease. To extrapolate from glibenclamide to a uniformly beneficial 'class effect' of sulfonylureas or to other β-cytotropic drugs that exert their β-cytotropic action via the blockage of ATP-dependent K-channels is not justified.[5] In fact, the differences between tolbutamide, glibenclamide and chlorpropamide underscore the need to establish efficacy and safety for each oral antidiabetic agent seperately. This basic requirement has still not been fulfilled for any other sulfonylurea drug, including the recently most popular glimepiride.[46]

Concern is often raised about the increase of body weight in Type 2 diabetes during glibenclamide (or insulin) treatment. However, previous epidemiological data[47,48] have indicated that overweight in Type 2 diabetes is not necessarily associated with a negative prognosis. When comparing the control groups of 1138 normal-weight (BMI 27.8 ± 5.5 kg/m²) and 411 overweight (BMI 31.8 ± 4.9 kg/m²) Type 2 diabetic patients, the 10-year UKPDS data have indicated no hazard of obesity with regard to any single or combined end point analyzed in the study.[2,26] In any case, concerns about therapy-associated weight gain are to be considered secondary to the focus on patient-oriented outcomes.

With regard to acarbose[49,50] and the group of glitazones,[51] no data exist to support their role in the achievement of patient-oriented outcomes in Type 2 diabetes, and there is concern about various aspects of their safety.

Whereas phenformin was associated with increased cardiovascular mortality in the UGDP study[52] and subsequently taken off the US market,[29] metformin has always remained part of the oral antidiabetic armamentarium in many European countries. Beginning in the late 1980s, marketing activities promoted a worldwide 'renaissance of metformin'. Even though not a single patient-oriented outcome benefit had been documented, metformin was introduced on the US market in 1995. In 1998 the UKPDS provided, for the first time, some data to evaluate effectivity and safety of metformin with regard to end point objectives.[26] In relatively young (mean age 53 years; newly manifest) Type 2 diabetic patients with overweight of >120% ideal body weight (corresponding to a mean BMI of 31.8 ± 4.9 kg/m²) the use of metformin monotherapy to achieve the goals of intensive glycaemic control (i.e. a medium HbA1c value of 7.4% during 10 years) was associated with a significant reduction of *any diabetes-related end point*, of diabetes-related and total mortality (Table 25.2). However, there was no positive effect with regard to microvascular complications.[26]

These findings have been criticized on methodological grounds – especially since the combination treatment of sulfonylurea plus metformin (in normal weight and overweight patients) was associated with a statistically significant increase of total mortality[53] (Table 25.2). Whilst controversy prevails concerning this particular part of the UKPDS data, any combination therapy between glibenclamide and metformin in the treatment of Type 2 diabetes must presently be discouraged.

In conclusion, only glibenclamide has been proven to be effective and safe for the subgroup of Type 2 diabetic patients studied in the UKPDS study. Efficacy and safety of sulfonylurea drugs need to be proven for every single drug – a beneficial class effect is non-existent. There is indirect evidence for a cardiotoxic effect of sulfonylureas in patients with coronary heart disease. Until respective data have been accumulated by appropriate long-term studies, sulfonylurea treatment should be withheld from patients with coronary heart disease. Metformin appears to be effective in monotherapy of obese people with Type 2 diabetes, if the long list of contraindications is observed and the patients' glycaemia can be well controlled on metformin monotherapy. Following the principles of evidence-based medicine, any other oral antidiabetic drug should not be used outside clinical trials.

	Overweight patients (n = 753)		Combined group (n = 537)	
	Conventional (n = 411)	Metformin (n = 342)	Sulfonylurea (n = 269)	Sulfonylurea plus metformin (n = 268)
Any diabetes-related end point (ADREP)				
Events per 1000 patient-years*	43.3	29.8	58.4	60.5
ARR/ARI	13.5		2.1	
NNT/NNH	7.4			
p value	0.0023		0.78	
RR (95% CI)	0.68 (0.53–0.87)		1.04 (0.77–1.42)	
RRR/RRI	32% (13–47%)		4% (-0.13–42%)	
Diabetes-related death				
Events per 1000 patient-years*	12.7	7.5	8.6	16.8
ARR/ARI	5.2		8.2	
NNT/NNH	19.2		12.2	
p value	0.017		0.039	
RR (95% CI)	0.58 (0.37–0.91)		1.96 (1.02–3.75)	
RRR/RRI	42% (9–63%)		96% (2–275%)	
Total mortality				
Events per 1000 patient-years*	20.6	13.5	19.1	30.3
ARR/ARI	7.1		11.2	
NNT/NNH	14.1		8.9	
p value	0.011		0.041	
RR (95% CI)	0.64 (0.45–0.91)		1.60 (1.02–2.52)	
RRR/RRI	36% (9–55%)		60% (2–152%)	
Microvascular complications				
Events per 1000 patient-years*	9.2	6.7	12.1	10.1
ARR/ARI	2.5		2	
NNT/NNH	40			
p value	0.19		0.62	
RR (95% CI)	0.71 (0.43–1.19)		0.84 (0.43–1.66)	
RRR/RRI	29% (-19–57%)		-16% (-0.57–166%)	

Notes: ARR/ARI absolute risk reduction/absolute risk increase
NNT/NNH number needed to treat/number needed to harm
RR relative risk
CI confidence interval
RRR/RRI relative risk reduction/relative risk increase
* persons with events per 1000 person-years
Sources: refs 2, 26, 56

Table 25.2
Reduction of vascular complications and organ damage by metformin in the UK Prospective Diabetes Study

The integration of patient values by evidence-based patient information and decision-making

Sackett et al.[6] call for the integration of patient values, preferences, concerns and expectations into clinical decisions as a basic element in their concept of evidence-based medicine. Obviously, the patients' preferences must be based on informed decision-making processes, as recently described in detail by the UK's General Medical Council.[54] This document calls for specific and detailed information of the patient with regard to therapeutic options, their quantitative risks and their uncertainties as well as revelation of potential conflicts of interests involved in the process; it is specifically stated that a possibility/probability that the patient may decide not to opt for a recommended procedure/treatment must not be a reason for withholding any information. We have recently tried to adapt such recommendations for Type 2 diabetic patients about to undergo antidiabetic therapy.[55] As long as the treatment is to focus on the amelioration of diabetes-related symptoms, the definition of therapeutic goals will usually present little difficulty. If the treatment is to reduce the risks of long-term complications in symptom-free individuals, the process to enable the patient to make an informed decision is certainly more complex. Such an attempt requires a method to present the quantitative analysis of the randomized controlled trials[1-3] available in this area of clinical medicine to the patient in an unbiased and balanced manner.

First, the patient needs to know that there is no evidence that their primary clinical problem, i.e. their excess cardiovascular morbidity and mortality, can be successfully addressed by antihyperglycaemic therapy. Alternative preventive interventions to combat macro-angiopathy need to be presented in order to facilitate respective decisions by the patient.

With regard to the possibility to reduce the risk of microangiopathic organ damage, the actual data of the relevant studies need to be presented. In quantitative terms, the much heralded benefit on microvascular disease achieved by intensive blood glucose treatment in the UKPDS was rather modest[2,56] (see Table 25.1). The exceptional efforts on the part of the patients and the medical system to lower medium HbA1c levels by 0.9% throughout a decade resulted in a 25% relative reduction of microvascular end points; the absolute risk reduction, however, amounted to a mere 2.8%, i.e. the number needed to treat in order to prevent the occurrence of the aggregate end point microvascular complications in one patient was $NNT_{10 \text{ years}} = 36$.[56]

In addition, a comprehensive estimate of the potential benefit–harm relationship would have to include information on secondary effects and quality-of-life aspects. In this context, the patient would be informed what his/her personal extra contribution/effort would have to be, for example, to maintain a median HbA1c of 7.0% versus a median value of 7.9% over a period of ten years. This effort would include sustained extra efforts concerning drug/insulin therapy, blood glucose self-monitoring, therapeutic side effects and inconveniences. On the other hand, avoidance of hospitalizations and of diagnostic and therapeutic procedures (e.g. laser therapy for retinopathy) attributed to diabetes-related complications should be presented in quantitative terms.

Similar consequences evolve from the analysis of the aggregate end point *any diabetes-related end point* (Table 25.1).

It is this type of evidence-based analysis of the UKPDS data which is required to explain the complex sets of data to the patients. After all, it is up to the patient to decide whether it is worth her/his efforts during a period of 10 years to keep HbA1c levels at 7.0%, rather than at 7.9%, if the $NNT_{10\ years}$ – indicative of the probability of a benefit for their own case – is in the magnitude of 20 (for *any diabetes-related end point*, with a 95% confidence interval of 10–500). That means, out of 100 newly diagnosed Type 2 diabetic patients with intensive therapy, 95 have no benefit over the next 10 years (when compared with conventional therapy) since they would not have a diabetes-related end point (ADREP) with conventional therapy (54 patients) or they will have such an end point despite intensive therapy (41 patients).

Even though it is generally felt to be justified to extrapolate from these data to the even greater benefit that may be achievable when initially much higher HbA1c levels are lowered by appropriate therapy, it is noteworthy that hard data, based on randomized controlled trials, are only available for relatively young, early manifest Type 2 diabetic patients in relatively good (controls, median HbA1c 7.9%) compared with very good (intensive therapy, median HbA1c 7.0%) glycaemic control as followed for a period of 10 years. Also, it is uncertain whether the benefit in risk reductions achieved will increase, remain or decrease if the therapeutic efforts go beyond 10 years. Finally, it can only be speculated if the preventive benefits will increase if median HbA1c levels are reduced even below 7.0%. This may possibly improve outcome data, but will certainly increase the efforts on the part of the patients and their health care system as well as the problems derived from therapeutic side effects.

On the other hand, it must be assumed that at HbA1c levels of above 9.0–9.5% an improvement of glycaemic control is justified and opted for by the informed patient because of the resulting improvement of the patient's well-being and a reduction of a variety of hyperglycaemia- and hypoinsulinaemia-induced sequelae and symptoms.

Conclusions

Following the principles of evidence-based medicine, it will eventually be up to the patients to decide on their own HbA1c target level, depending on the risks (concerning diabetes-related end points) they are prepared to take and the efforts (lifestyle changes, nutrition, metabolic self control, drug/insulin treatment) they are prepared to make. In order to achieve these therapeutic goals, a step-wise approach, including non-drug therapy, insulin therapy and treatment with glibenclamide and metformin monotherapy as options for subgroups of patients, is justified by adequate evidence from randomized controlled trials. Furthermore, the efficacy of a multifactorial intervention in slowing the progression of vascular organ damage in Type 2 diabetes merits consideration.[57] In fact the person with Type 2 diabetes should be enabled to choose individual target levels not only for HbA1c values, but likewise for blood pressure control, blood lipids, body weight etc., as to their (sequential) priorities and to what extent he/she wants to employ various self-monitoring strategies and non-drug or drug treatments to reach these objectives.

Enabling the patients to enter into such a decision-making process will require innovative methodological approaches in the area of patient education and communication, which do not yet seem to be available. The systematic integration of patients' preferences on therapeutic goals and strategies based on informed decision-making processes with the scientific evidence from patient-centred clinical research forms the basis of a treatment of Type 2 diabetes mellitus according to the principles of evidence-based medicine.

References

1. The University Group Diabetes Program (UGDP). Effects of hypoglycemic agents on vascular complications in patients with adult-onset diabetes. VIII. Diabetes 1982; 31 Suppl 5: 1–81.
2. UK Prospective Diabetes Study (UKPDS) Group. Intensive blood-glucose control with sulphonylureas or insulin compared with conventional treatment and risk of complications in patients with Type 2 diabetes (UKPDS 33). Lancet 1998; 352: 837–53.
3. Ohkubo Y, Kishikawa H, Araki E et al. Intensive insulin therapy prevents the progression of diabetic microvascular complications in Japanese patients with non-insulin-dependent diabetes mellitus: a randomized prospective 6-year study. Diabetes Res Clin Pract 1995; 28: 103–17.
4. Abreira C, Colwell JA, Nuttal FQ et al. Veterans Affairs Cooperative Study on glycemic control in Type II diabetes. (VACSDM) Diabetes Care 1995; 18: 1113–23.
5. Berger M, Mühlhauser I. Diabetes care and patient-oriented outcomes. JAMA 1999; 281: 1676–8.
6. Sackett DL, Strauss SE, Richardson WS et al. Evidence-based Medicine. How to Practise and Teach EBM, 2nd Edn. Edinburgh: Churchill Livingstone, 2000.
7. Gerstein HC, Haynes RB, eds. Evidence-based Diabetes Care. London Canada: BC Decker, Hamilton, 2001.
8. Richter B, Clar C, Berger M. The Cochrane Collaboration and its possible impact on diabetes care. Diabetres Care 2000; 23: 1217–18.
9. Cochrane Metabolic and Endocrine Disorders Group. http://www.uni-duesseldorf.de/WWW/MedFak/MDN/Cochrane/ccset.htm
10. Davidson JK, Delcher HK, Englund A. Spin off cost/benefit of expanded nutritional care. J Am Diet Assoc 1979; 75: 250–7.
11. Davidson JK. The Grady Memorial Diabetes Programme. In: Mann JI, Pyörälä K, Teuscher A, eds. Diabetes in Epidemiological Perspective. Edinburg/UK: Churchill Livingstone, 1983: 332–41.
12. Hadden DR, Blair ALT, Wilson EA et al. Natural history of diabetes presenting age 40–69 years: a prospective study of the influence of intensive dietary therapy. QJM 1986; 59: 579–98.
13. Ratzmann KP, Ilius A. Erfahrungen mit einem strukturierten Diät-Schulungsprogramm an frisch manifestierten insulinunabhängigen (Typ II) Diabetikern. Z klin Med 1986; 41: 289–91.
14. United Kingdom Prospective Diabetes Group. Response of fasting plasma glucose to diet therapy in newly presenting Type 2 diabetic patients (UKPDS 7). Metabolism 1990; 39: 905–12.
15. United Kingdom Prospective Diabetes Group. Study design, process and performance (UKPDS 8). Diabetologia 1991; 34: 877–90.
16. United Kingdom Prospective Diabetes Group. A nine-year update of a randomized, controlled trial on the effect of metabolic control on complications in non-insulin-dependent diabetes mellitus (UKPDS 17). Ann Intern Med 1996; 124 (1, pt 2): 136–45.
17. Norris SL, Engelgau MN, Narayan KMV. Effectiveness of self-management training in Type 2 diabetes. Diabetes Care 2001; 24: 561–97.
18. Assal JP, Mühlhauser I, Pernet A et al. Patient education as the basis for diabetes care in clinical practice and research. Diabetologia 1985; 28: 602–13.
19. Bouchardat A. De la Glycosurie ou Diabète Sucré. Paris: Librairie Germer Baillière, 1875.
20. Kronsbein P, Jörgens I, Mühlhauser I et al. Evaluation of a structured treatment and teaching programme on non-insulin dependent diabetes. Lancet 1988; 2: 1407–11.
21. Berger M, Jörgens V, Flatten G. Health care for persons with non-insulin-dependent diabetes: the German experience. Ann Intern Med 1996; 124 (1, pt 2): 153–5.
22. Pieber TR, Holler A, Siebenhofer A et al. Evaluation of a structured teaching and treatment programme for Type 2 diabetes in general practice in a rural area of Austria. Diabet Med 1995; 12: 349–54.
23. Domenech MI, Assad D, Mazzei ME et al. Evaluation of the effectiveness of an ambulatory teaching/treatment programme for non-insulin dependent (Type 2) diabetic patients. Acta Diabetol 1995; 32: 143–7.
24. Gagliardino JJ, Etchegoyen G for the PEDNID-

LA Research Group. A model education program for people with Type 2 diabetes. Diabetes Care 2001; 24: 1001–7.

25. Trento M, Passera P, Tomalino M et al. Group visits improve metabolic control in Type 2 diabetes. Diabetes Care 2001; 24: 995–1000.

26. United Kingdom Prospective Diabetes Study. Effect of intensive blood glucose control with metformin on complications in overweight patients with Type 2 diabetes (UKPDS 34). Lancet 1998; 352: 854–65.

27. The University Group Diabetes Program. A study on the effects of hypoglycemic agents on vascular complications in patients with adult-onset diabetes. I. Diabetes 19 Suppl 2: 474–830, 1970.

28. Kolata GB. Controversy over study on diabetes drugs continues for nearly a decade. Science 1979; 203: 986–90.

29. Berger M, Richter B. Oral agents in the treatment of diabetes mellitus. In: Davidson JK, ed. Diabetes Mellitus, a Problem Oriented Approach, 3rd Ed. New York: Thieme-Stratton, 2000; 415–36.

30. Kanarek PH. Assessing survival in a diabetic population. PhD Thesis, Boston, Mass: Harvard School of Public Health, 1973.

31. Leibovitz G, Cerasi E. Sulfonylurea treatment of NIDDM patients with cardiovascular disease: a mixed blessing? Diabetologia 1996; 39: 503–14.

32. Malmberg K for the DIGAMI Study Group. Prospective randomized study of intensive insulin treatment on long-term survival after acute myocardial infarction in patients with diabetes mellitus. BMJ 1997; 314: 1512–15.

33. Engler RL, Yellon DM. Sulfonylurea KATP blockade in Type 2 diabetes and preconditioning in cardiovascular disease: time for reconsideration. Circulation 1996; 94: 2297–2301.

34. Berger M, Mühlhauser I, Sawicki PT. Possible risk of sulfonylureas in the treatment of non-insulin-dependent diabetes mellitus with coronary heart disease (letters). Diabetologia 1997; 40: 1492–3; Diabetologia 1998; 41: 744.

35. Pyörälä K, Pedersen TR, Kekshus MJ et al. Cholesterol lowering with simvastatin improves prognosis of diabetic patuents with coronary heart disease. A subgroup analysis of the Scandinavian Simvastatin Survival Study. Diabetes Care 1997; 20: 614–20.

36. Heart Outcomes Prevention Evaluation (HOPE) Study Investigators. Effects of ramipril on cardiovascular and macrovascular outcomes in people with diabetes mellitus: results of the HOPE study and MICRO-HOPE sub-study. Lancet 2000; 355: 253–9.

37. Cahill DF Jr, Etzwiler DD, Freinkel N. 'Control' and diabetes. New Engl J Med 1976; 294:1004–5.

38. The DCCT Research Group. The effect of intensive treatment of diabetes on the development and progression of long-term complications in insulin-dependent diabetes mellitus. New Engl J Med 1993; 329: 977–86.

39. United Kingdom Prospective Diabetes Group. Tight blood pressure control and risk of macrovascular and microvascular complications in Type 2 diabetes (UKPDS 38). BMJ 1998; 317: 705–13.

40. Kalfhaus J, Berger M. Insulin treatment with preprandial injections of regular insulin in middle-aged type-2 diabetic patients. A two years observational study. Diabetes Metab 2000; 26: 197–201.

41. Mühlhauser I, Keim U, Hemmann D et al. Qualitätskontrolle der Langzeittherapie von älteren, insulinpflichtigen Diabetikern nach Teilnahme an einem stationären Diabetes-Behandlungs- und Schulungs-Programm. Z klin Med 1989; 44: 1221–7.

42. Spraul M, Schönbach AM, Mühlhauser I, Berger M. Amputationen und Mortalität bei älteren, insulinpflichtigen Patienten mit Typ 2–Diabetes. Zentralbl Chir 1999; 124: 25–31.

43. Müller UA, Müller R, Hunger-Dathe W et al. Should insulin therapy be started on an outpatient basis? Results of a prospective controlled trial using the same treatment and teaching programme in ambulatory care and a university hospital. Diabète Metab 1998; 24: 251–5.

44. Grüsser M, Hartmann P, Schlottmann N, Jörgens V. Structured treatment and teaching programme for Type 2 diabetic patients on conventional insulin treatment: evaluation of reimbursement policy. Pat Educ Counsell 1996; 29: 123–30.

45. Cheng AYY, Zinman B. Insulin for treating Type 1 and Type 2 diabetes. In: Gerstein HC, Haynes RB, eds. Evidence-based Diabetes Care. London Canada: BC Decker, Hamilton, 2001: 323–43.

46. Richter B, Berger M. Randomized controlled trials remain fundamental to clinical decision making in Type 2 diabetes mellitus: a comment to the debate on randomized controlled trials. Diabetologia 2000; 43: 254–8.

47. Klein R, Klein BE, Moss SE. Is obesity related to microvascular and macrovascular complications in diabetes? Arch Intern Med 1997; 157: 650–6.

48. Fuller JH, Chaturvedi N and the WHO Multinational Study Group. Obesity and mortality in people with non-insulin-dependent diabetes (NIDDM) in three ethnic groups. Perspectives on Epidemiology in Europe, Abstracts from the IEA Regional Meeting, 27–30 August 1995, Abs. No. 49.

49. Berger M, Köbberling J, Windeler J. Appraisal of effectiveness and potential therapeutic benefit of acarbose: a non-consensus conference. Diabetologia 1996; 39: 873–4.

50. Holman RR, Turner RC, Cull CA on behalf of the UKPDS Study Group. A randomized double-blind trial of acarbose in Type 2 diabetes shows improved glycemic control over 3 years (UKPDS 44). Diabetes Care 1999; 22: 960–4.

51. Gale EAM. Lessons from the glitazones: a story of drug development. Lancet 2001; 357: 1870–5.

52. University Group Diabetes Program V. Evaluation of phenformin therapy. Diabetes 1975; 24 (suppl. 1): 65–184.

53. Nathan DM. Some answers, more controversy from UKPDS. Lancet 1998; 352: 832–3.

54. General Medical Council. Protecting patients, guiding doctors. Seeking patients' consent: the ethical considerations. London: General Medical Council, 1999.

55. Mühlhauser I, Berger M. Evidence-based patient information in diabetes. Diabet Med 2000; 17: 823–9.

56. Mühlhauser I. UKPDS-Darstellung nach Evidence-based Medicine Kriterien. Stoffwechsel und Ernährung 1998; 7: 267–73.

57. Gaede P, Vedel P, Parving HH, Pedersen O. Intensified multifactorial intervention in patients with Type 2 diabetes mellitus and microalbuminuria: the Steno Type 2 randomised study. Lancet 1999; 353: 617–22.

26

Oxidative stress and glycation: mechanisms and prevention in diabetes

Including the use of glycation and antioxidant modalities

Matthew D Oldfield, Mark E Cooper

Introduction

Oxidative stress and subsequent tissue damage occurs as a by-product of normal metabolism, but to an exaggerated degree in a number of chronic diseases including atherosclerosis, rheumatoid arthritis and diabetes. It represents an imbalance between increased pro-oxidant generation and/or decreased antioxidant defences, both of which are detrimentally affected by diabetes. The benefits for improving antioxidant function continue to accumulate in experimental models, in particular with agents that inhibit the formation of advanced glycation products; however the benefits in human disease remains elusive.

The DCCT and UKPDS trials have established the ostensibly obvious premise that hyperglycaemia is a risk factor for the development of diabetic complications; in particular the evidence is strongest for a reduction in the risk of microvascular complications. There are a number of equally tenable pathogenic mechanisms believed to underlie hyperglycaemia-mediated tissue damage. Substantial experimental evidence supports roles for increased accumulation of advanced glycation end-products (AGEs), increased flux through the polyol pathway, protein kinase C activation, increased carbonyl and reductive stress and altered lipoprotein metabolism. The numerous metabolic derangements overlap and interact with one another. It has been suggested that the generation of ROS links all these perturbations.[1] In particular the processes of advanced glycation and oxidative stress are inextricably intertwined, the formation of AGEs is accompanied by oxidative, radical generating reactions and represents a major source of oxygen-free radicals under hyperglycaemic conditions.[2] Further reactive oxygen species are generated by AGE-receptor binding. Critically the creation of a strongly oxidant microenvironment also increases the rate of AGE formation resulting in a positive feedback cycle of oxidant generation. Increased flux through the polyol pathway generates sorbitol which is further metabolized by sorbitol dehydrogenase to produce fructose, a powerful reducing sugar that enters the Maillard pathway and increases AGE formation[3] (Figure 26.1).

Although hyperglycaemia is clearly an important primary target for the treatment and prevention of diabetic complications, diabetic complications are likely to remain a chronic problem, particularly since restoration of normoglycaemia appears to be very difficult in the present clinical environment. Appreciation of the role glycoxidation and carbonyl stresses play in diabetic complications and their

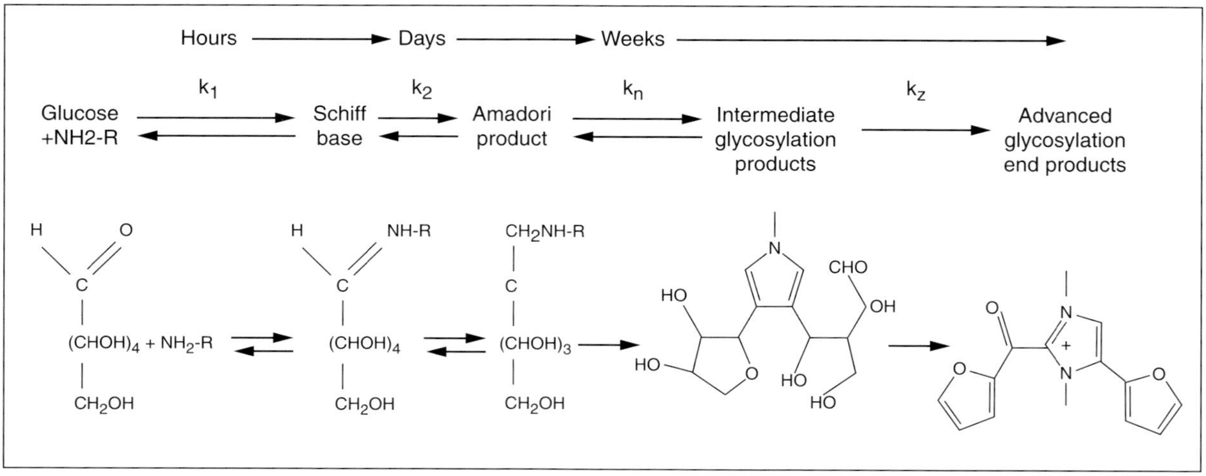

Figure 26.1
The Maillard reaction. Schema showing the classical pathway of AGE formation. Reproduced from Raj et al. 2000,[102] with permission from WB Saunders.

importance in the order of changes may allow modulation of the multiple steps that occur between hyperglycaemia and complications.

Advanced glycation end product formation

The spontaneous and non-enzymatic reaction between reducing sugars and the free amino groups of proteins, lipoproteins and nucleic acids is a ubiquitous process, and as such, AGEs accumulate during the physiological ageing process. In the presence of high substrate, or a pro-oxidative environment such as occurs in the diabetic microenvironment, AGE accumulation occurs at an accelerated rate. Indeed, tissue levels of AGE correlate with serum levels of glucose, fructoselysine and glycated haemoglobin implying a close relationship to the degree of hyperglycaemia. Despite the structural heterogeneity of AGEs, they share

a number of characteristics, including the formation of brown substances with the ability to form cross-links between proteins and fluorescence at typical excitation and emission spectra. Such compounds identified as AGEs initially and ultimately isolated are typified by pentosidine. More recently a number of other AGE forms have been chemically identified which do not display the characteristic properties such as fluorescence, originally described for AGE moieties. These include carboxymethyl-lysine (CML), believed to represent a major immunological AGE epitope in tissues, pyralline and imidazolium salts.

In the classical Maillard pathway of AGE formation, the early generation of Schiff bases is followed by rearrangements forming still reversible Amadori products. This group includes the clinically useful glycated-haemoglobin (HbA1c) and fructoselysine. Subsequent complex dehydration and condensation reactions occur that, via a series of highly

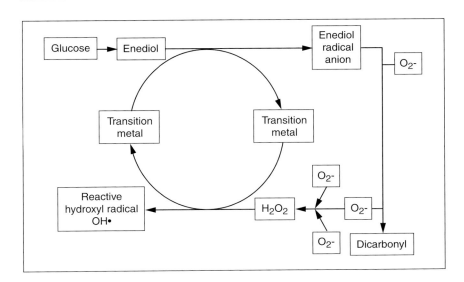

Figure 26.2
Transitional metals such as copper are able to catalyze the auto-oxidation of glucose to protein-reactive dicarbonyls, in parallel with the formation of superoxide (O_2^-). These reactive molecules can then generate reactive hydroxyl radicals via dismutation to hydrogen peroxides. Adapted from Bierhaus et al.[103] with permission from Elsevier Science.

reactive dicarbonyl compounds such as 1- and 3-deoxyglucosone, ultimately result in AGE formation. It is these latter steps, associated with the generation of reactive dicarbonyls and free-radicals, that are believed to contribute to the oxidative stress load of tissues in diabetes.

It has also become apparent recently that progression through the ordered series of steps in the Maillard reaction is not essential for the formation of AGE modifications. Work by Wolff et al. demonstrated that AGE compounds were generated from metal catalyzed auto-oxidation of glucose, and suggested that this may be the major route for AGE accumulation in the tissues in diabetes.[4,5] Baynes, Fu and co-workers also demonstrated that CML could be formed through the peroxidation of lipids as well as by glycoxidation. Furthermore metabolic intermediates have been shown to generate AGE proteins.[6]

Oxidative versus carbonyl stress

Carbonyl stress represents an increase in the reactive carbonyl compounds generated in association with the formation of AGEs, glucose auto-oxidation and lipoxidation reactions. The distinction between oxidative and carbonyl stress centres on whether cellular damage occurs as a consequence of oxidative or non-oxidative processes, and has received considerable interest. Methylglyoxyl, imidazolone and 3-deoxyglucosone are examples of toxic dicarbonyl compounds that do not require oxidation in their production and can form from hydrolysis and rearrangement, or β-eliminations of Amadori products.[7-9] An excess of reactive carbonyls leads to increased chemical modification of biomolecules and tissue damage, in part through the generation of oxidative stress.

The tendency for oxidation to occur appears to be increased in diabetes, both in experimental models and in human subjects.[9-13] This increase may be a function of decreased antioxidant defences as well as augmented generation of free-radicals.

In the context of hyperglycaemia free-radicals may arise from multiple sources in addition to those already mentioned. Aortic endothelial cells incubated in 30 mM glucose

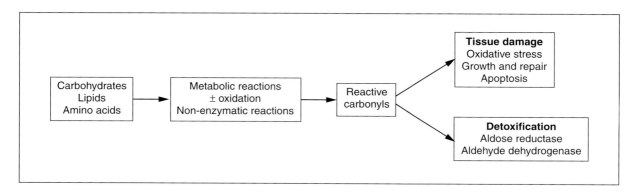

Figure 26.3

Carbonyl stress. Schema representing the generation of reactive carbonyls from both enzymatic and non-enzymatic reactions. This process may or may not require oxygen for formation and results in a range of responses including apoptosis as well as cellular growth and remodelling. The concentration of these species depends upon both formative and detoxification systems. From Baynes and Thorpe, 1999; 48: 1–9,[21] with permission from American Diabetes Association © 1999.

increase ROS formation by over 200%.[14] Hydrogen peroxide can be generated from the oxidation of Amadori products, and superoxide (O_2^-) can form as a consequence of mitochondrial oxidation of NADPH[3]. The major defences against the superoxide anion radical are the superoxide dismutases (SODs). Three forms exist and exert protective roles in separate compartments, as O_2^- crosses membranes poorly. Little evidence as to their role in diabetic complications has been described. ApoE mice, deficient in extracellular SOD, show no difference in their atherosclerotic lesions.[15]

A central role for ROS as secondary mediators or activators of several interdependent processes in diabetic complications has been recently postulated.[1] It was demonstrated that hyperglycaemia-dependent increases in ROS activated a number of metabolic mechanisms purported to be relevant to the genesis of diabetic complications, namely the accelerated formation of AGEs, aldose reductase activation and protein kinase C stimulation. In addition, normalizing mitochondrial levels of ROS prevented glucose-induced activation of all three apparently separate pathways.

The processes of oxidation and the generation of reactive dicarbonyl compounds are now viewed as interrelated mechanisms that contribute to ongoing protein damage that involves both glycation modification of protein moieties and free-radical damage. Indeed the two processes are inextricably intertwined. In the context of hyperglycaemia, AGE accumulation is proportional not just to the degree of glycaemia but also to the pro-oxidative nature of the microenvironment. It has been suggested that the set point for oxidative stress within individuals may determine that person's risk for the development of complications.

Defence mechanisms for carbonyl stress

The diabetic state has been demonstrated to compromise natural antioxidant defence systems. Tissue glutathione levels are lower, as

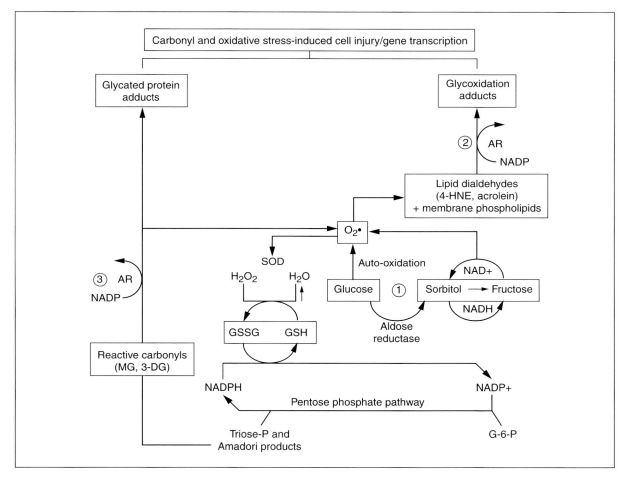

Figure 26.4

Schema showing the importance of aldose reductase and its paradoxical roles in both exacerbating and relieving oxidative stresses. (1) The accelerated conversion of glucose into sorbitol and thence to fructose leads to decreased GSH availability, increased O_2^- production and the generation of reactive carbonyls via the pentose phosphate pathway. However, aldose reductase (AR) also alleviates stress through the detoxification of reactive carbonyls (2) and lipid dialdehydes (3). From Dunlop, 2000,[3] with permission from Blackwell Publishers.

are levels of vitamin C, vitamin E and anti-oxidant enzymes, and a number of studies have demonstrated beneficial effects due to anti-oxidant modalities in a number of animal models.[16–19]

Reactive carbonyls can be detoxified through their conversion to less reactive metabolites.

This can happen in a number of ways and involves either reduction to alcohols, oxidation to carboxylic acids or a glutathione-catalyzed rearrangement to hydroxyacids. Diabetes-induced shifts in redox potential (pseudohypoxia, increased NADH/NAD+ ratio) may compromise the ability of these pathways to

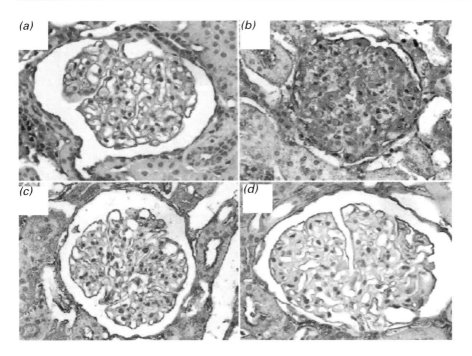

Figure 26.5
Immunohistochemical staining for advance glycation end products (AGEs) in the kidney is shown for (a) control, (b) diabetic, (c) diabetic + aminoguanidine and (d) diabetic + a novel AGE inhibitor, ALT 946. From Forbes et al. 2001,[58] with permission from © Springer-Verlag.

adequately detoxify these reactive compounds.[20] In the hyperglycaemic state, increased flux through the polyol pathway competes for reduced glutathione and NADPH. In cells in which aldose reductase activity is sufficient to deplete glutathione, oxidative stress due to hyperglycaemia is augmented through effects on NADPH requiring pathways. The ability of aldose reductase-catalyzed detoxification of aldehydes to inactivate alcohols is impaired as is the regeneration of reduced glutathione by glutathione reductase which requires adequate levels of NADPH.

A failure to detoxify dicarbonyl compounds may be as important as increased formation in providing an explanation for the observed increase in steady state dicarbonyl compounds observed in diabetes.[21]

Several researchers feel that oxidative stress in diabetes may not represent an early event, and may only occur as a late rise when tissue damage is essentially irreversible.[21] This is an important concept for reasons that become apparent when looking at the contradictory evidence for benefits of antioxidant supplementation. Intervention in a primary process may be expected to prevent complications; however application of antioxidant therapy to a downstream or delayed event may only be expected to ameliorate change. Indeed, as is discussed below, the nature of antioxidant function may result in later intervention being detrimental.

Advanced glycation-binding proteins

AGE moieties represent a post-translational modification of proteins, and in common with other damaged molecules, such as oxidized LDL, specific receptors have been described that may play roles in the removal and detoxification of such altered proteins. The best

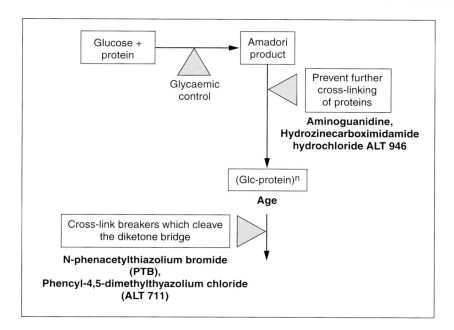

Figure 26.6
Schema showing treatment strategies aimed at blocking the formation of AGE-proteins and preventing AGE-mediated complications. Adapted from Raj et al. 2000,[102] with permission from WB Saunders.

characterized of these binding proteins has been termed the receptor for advanced glycation end products (RAGE) and is a 35 kDa member of the immunoglobulin family of cell surface receptors. RAGE has been identified on a wide variety of cell types that may have roles in the development of diabetic complications, such as mesangial cells, smooth muscle cells and macrophages.[22] Surprisingly RAGE has also been identified upon cerebral neurones, where it appears to play a role in neurite outgrowth and neuronal development.[23] Binding of AGE to RAGE has been shown to result in the formation of intracellular reactive oxygen species[22] that induce an oxidative stress response with activation of the free-radical sensitive transcription factor NF-κB and induction of tissue factor expression.[24]

Some controversy now exists as regards this view of AGE–RAGE generation of oxidative stress since compounds generated by the *in vitro* method of AGE preparation have been

identified, for example the superoxide generator dihydroxyphenylalanine, which may mediate the observed increase in oxidative stress when AGE and RAGE interact.[25]

The role of these receptors in AGE removal and catabolism awaits clarification. *In vivo* the removal of naturally occurring advanced glycated LDL is not efficient, nor is the half-life of diabetic erythrocytes significantly shortened.[26] In contrast AGE–LDL prepared *in vitro* exhibits highly efficient binding to RAGE and the scavenger receptor. Furthermore, the decrease in serum AGE that occurs following renal transplantation exhibits kinetics consistent with normal rates of protein turnover. Conversely, Vlassara and colleagues have suggested that AGE-R1, an endocytosis mediating AGE-binding protein, may play a role in the removal of AGEs from the circulation.[27]

The AGE–RAGE interaction clearly plays a significant pathogenic role in diabetic complications. In an elegant study, Yamamoto and co-workers created a transgenic mouse that over-expressed human RAGE in vascular cells.[28] This strain was crossbred with another transgenic line that develops insulin-deficient diabetes soon after birth. The double transgenic mice demonstrated enlargement of the kidneys, albuminuria, mesangial expansion, an increased serum creatinine and advanced glomerulosclerosis. These changes of an advanced phenotype of diabetic nephropathy could be largely prevented through the administration of the AGE inhibitor OPB-9195, establishing the AGE–RAGE system as a promising target for amelioration of clinical disease.

Other AGE-receptors have been correlated with the degree of complications occurring in diabetic subjects. This evidence suggests that regardless of the true role for these AGE-receptors, such interactions have significant implications for diabetes and its complications.

Atherosclerosis

Macrovascular disease represents the major complication affecting the burgeoning numbers of Type 2 diabetic subjects,[29] however its pathogenesis is not well understood. The earliest lesions in atherosclerosis appear to be due to dysfunction of the vascular endothelium[30] and appear to be causally related to modifications of lipoproteins and oxidative stress.[31] It has been shown that incubation of macrophages in the presence of high LDL concentrations failed to cause cholesterol accumulation.[32] However, modification of LDL-lysine moieties caused the macrophages to take up lipids via scavenger receptors and undergo subsequent foam cell transformation, a hallmark of early atherosclerotic lesions.[32,33] Cultured smooth muscle and endothelial cells from artery walls demonstrate an ability to oxidise LDL to a form that is recognized by macrophage scavenger receptors.[34,35]

Additional support for the concept of modified LDL comes from the observations that levels of autoantibodies to oxidized LDL correlate with the progression of vascular disease,[36] and that LDL isolated from atherosclerotic lesions, both in animal and in human studies, shows evidence of oxidative damage.[37]

Glycation of lipoproteins

Oxidation and glycoxidation both increase the atherogenic potential of LDL and other lipoproteins such as lipoprotein(a), Lp(a).[38–40] Like other proteins, lipoproteins are modified by non-enzymatic glycation at accelerated rates in the context of hyperglycaemia and pro-oxidative stress, conditions present in the vessel wall in areas of atherosclerosis. It has also been demonstrated that circulating AGEs react with lipoproteins and prevent their recognition by tissue receptors.[26] In addition AGE–LDL prepared *in vitro*, to the same degree of modification as found *in vivo*, exhibited markedly impaired clearance kinetics when injected into mice transgenic for the human LDL receptor.

These chemical modifications are favoured by circumstances of hyperglycaemia and attenuated oxidant defence[41] and are considered to contribute to the development of glomerulosclerosis.[42] The implication for the diabetic subject of LDL and Lp(a) modification, whether by oxidation or glycoxidation, is an alteration in LDL uptake and disposal. Altered forms of LDL are 'diverted' to receptor scavenger pathways on macrophages where they accumulate as foam cells, an important and continuing event in the genesis of vascular lesions.

Hyperglycaemia-dependent mechanisms in macrovascular disease

Hyperglycaemia per se is an independent cardiovascular risk factor, independent of hypertension and hyperlipidaemia.[43] Both AGEs and RAGE have been detected at the sites of atherosclerotic lesions.[44,45] Experiments using AGEs prepared *in vitro* have suggested possible roles for AGEs in the pathogenesis of atherosclerosis. AGEs have been shown to decrease vascular barrier function and enhance the expression of factors promoting coagulation and vasoconstriction, effects largely mediated through binding to cellular receptors on the endothelium.[46,47] *In vivo* models of accelerated atherosclerosis, such as ApoE-deficient mice made diabetic by streptozotocin administration, demonstrate increased AGE and RAGE staining in association with accelerated atherosclerotic disease.[48] Administration of soluble RAGE, a truncated form of the receptor which interrupts AGE–RAGE binding, reduced lesion formation to baseline in these animals.[48] Interestingly, levels of AGEs detected within the tissues were also reduced. This is consistent with a reduction of AGE–RAGE generated ROS ameliorating oxidation-induced AGE formation. In another study the expression of vascular cell adhesion molecule (VCAM-1),[49] a molecule highly expressed in areas of atherosclerosis, could also be reduced by blocking RAGE.[50]

Inhibitors of advanced glycation end product formation

The importance of the role that AGE modifications may play in atherosclerosis has been supported by use of inhibitors of AGE formation. Aminoguanidine, a hydrazine-derived compound, prevents progression of the Maillard reaction by binding to reactive compounds formed early post-Amadori product formation. The initial studies confirmed the ability of this agent to reduce aortic AGE accumulation.[51] It is also apparent that aminoguanidine acts as a general carbonyl scavenger, trapping both oxidative and non-oxidative AGE precursors, as well as lipid peroxidation intermediates.

Oxidative modification of LDL involves the modification of apo B lysine moieties by reactive aldehydes. Aminoguanidine was demonstrated to both prevent this modification and to ameliorate oxidation-dependent increases in LDL binding to the scavenger receptor.[52] This was due in large part to its binding to reactive aldehydes formed during oxidation. Aminoguanidine had a beneficial effect of retarding the development of atherosclerosis in euglycaemic cholesterol-fed rabbits.[53] In addition, aminoguanidine decreased circulating levels of LDL in the sera of diabetic patients by 28%. Benefits *in vitro* and in experimental models of diabetic complications have led to clinical trials of aminoguanidine, focused on a role in diabetic nephropathy. Although the findings of these studies are as yet unpublished, preliminary analysis has revealed a reduction in albuminuria, a secondary end point of the study. However, time to doubling of creatinine, the major primary end point was unaffected. Interestingly, there were also beneficial effects on retinopathy and lipid levels.

Pyridoxamine has also been demonstrated to inhibit AGE accumulation, acting at a similar stage to aminoguanidine, post-Amadori product formation,[54] and has been shown to retard the development of nephropathy in STZ-diabetic rats.[55] Pyridoxamine may have more specific antioxidant benefits. During copper catalyzed oxidation of LDL and in a lipid-protein model pyridoxamine was shown to inhibit potently the modification of lysine moieties.[56] These observations suggest a future role for pyridoxamine in inhibiting chemical modification of proteins, both in diabetes and uraemia.

Newer inhibitors of AGE formation, such as ALT 946 and OPB-9195 have shown *in vivo* benefits in ameliorating diabetes-induced increases in cytokine production[57] and in diabetes-dependent structural and functional changes.[28,58]

Agents that can cleave the carbon–carbon bonds mediated by AGE modifications on long lived matrix proteins have been shown to reduce AGE accumulation and ameliorate diabetic complications,[59,60] presumably by allowing degradation and removal of AGE fragments. One of the newer compounds, 3-phenyacyl-4,5-dimethylthiazolium chloride, ALT 711, has entered clinical trials and has been successful in the reduction of abnormal vascular compliance and systemic vascular resistance occurring in aged humans.[61] These agents hold promise for the treatment of abnormal vascular stiffening seen in diabetes.

Antioxidant modalities

Vitamins E, C and α-lipoic acid

Vitamin E is a powerful hydrophilic scavenger molecule that interrupts lipid peroxidation by scavenging peroxyl radical intermediates.[62] This reaction converts vitamin E into a relatively unreactive tocopherol radical of low oxidation potential that undergoes inactivation through combination with another tocopherol radical or a lipid peroxyl radical. Co-antioxidants such as vitamin C also scavenge the tocopherol radical

and in the process regenerate vitamin E. It is important to recognize that vitamin E has other potent effects on monocytes and macrophages, as well as on smooth muscle cells and platelets, separate from its function as an antioxidant.[63,64] The availability of co-antioxidants may be critical; there is evidence that the tocopherol radical may act as a pro-oxidant when incorporated into lipoproteins and promote lipid peroxidation.[65] The physiological relevance of this is not yet known.

Alpha-lipoic acid is a multifunctional antioxidant and a naturally occurring co-enzyme in the pyruvate dehydrogenase and α-ketoglutarate dehydrogenase mitochondrial enzyme complexes.[66] α-Lipoic acid or its reduced form are able to quench a number of free-radical species, chelate transitional metals and prevent membrane lipid peroxidation via reactions with vitamin C and glutathione.[66] It has been demonstrated to prevent AGE-mediated activation of the transcription factor NF-κB.[67]

Microvascular complications

The complications of diabetic neuropathy, nephropathy and retinopathy are believed to be consequent upon dysfunction of the microvasculature. Endothelium-dependent vasodilation is impaired in animal models and humans with diabetes and involves the generation of free-radicals.[68,69] Non-diabetic subjects made acutely hyperglycaemic through infusion of dextrose, display similarly abnormal vascular responses that are prevented by the administration of vitamin C.[70] Similarly diabetes-dependent impaired vasodilation responses can be improved by vitamin C administration in Type 1 and Type 2 diabetic subjects.[68,71]

Hyperglycaemia-induced generation of ROS in rat vascular tissue has been shown to subsequently activate protein kinase C and reduce NO.[72] Administration of vitamin E prevented these changes and restored normal vascular function. A similar finding has been described in the retina, where vitamin E prevented diabetes-induced abnormalities in retinal blood flow, via normalization of diacylglycerol and PKC activity.[73] In addition, pericyte drop-out and the number of acellular capillaries were reduced in diabetic rats that received either vitamin C and E or a multioxidant diet that also contained n-acetyl cysteine, β-carotene and selenium.[74]

Dietary deficiency of vitamin E has been reported to lead to renal injury. Significantly higher levels of lipid peroxides (LPO) have been found in the plasma and urine of STZ-diabetic rats,[75] and these have been correlated with the degree of renal enlargement. The administration of vitamin E and probucol both reduced urinary lipophilic aldehydes and renal enlargement.[75] However the administration of vitamin E (100 mg/day) had no effect on LPO measurements in another study. Vitamin C and vitamin E supplementation had beneficial effects, preventing diabetes-dependent increases in plasma and liver lipid peroxidation in STZ-diabetic rats;[76] additional benefits on the activity of glutathione peroxidase and glutathione-s-transferase were also observed.

Dietary supplementation with α-lipoic acid has recently been reported to ameliorate diabetes-dependent early glomerular changes of increased albuminuria, glomerular TGF-β content and cortical glutathione content.[77] Our own group has compared the effects of antioxidants such as butylated hydroxytoluene (BHT) and probucol to aminoguanidine.[78] All treatments reduced renal AGE accumulation, consistent with these AGEs being glycoxidation products. However, aminoguanidine was more effective at retarding the development of albuminuria.

In neurones, reductions in nerve conduction velocity, nerve growth factor and substance P levels were observed in diabetic neuropathy and could be reproduced by the generation of oxidative stress using primaquine.[79] Restoration of normal neuronal parameters was achieved by administration of a diester of α-lipoic acid and γ-linoleic acid in these animals. Interestingly only minor changes of neuronal function were seen in vitamin E-deficient animals.[79]

Other studies have also demonstrated that the antioxidants probucol, vitamin E and glutathione have some benefits in preventing or reversing diabetes-induced nerve dysfunction.[80,81] α-Lipoic acid has been in clinical use for a number of years in the treatment of diabetic neuropathy.[82]

Antioxidant therapy and lipoprotein modification in macrovascular disease

Considerable experimental support as discussed above exists for the role of LDL modification as a mechanism for atherosclerosis. Many structurally unrelated antioxidants have been shown to retard atherosclerosis in animal models. Indeed such evidence may represent some of the strongest support for the role of LDL oxidation in the genesis of atherosclerosis.[83] Probucol inhibits LDL oxidation *in vitro* and retards the progression of atherosclerotic disease in diet-induced hypercholesterolaemic rabbits and primates,[84,85] although the effect in the latter group was only of borderline significance. The effects of antioxidants on events that are known to occur in human disease, such as the rupture of atherosclerotic plaques, have been much less studied.

In a recent 4-year prospective study of nearly 20,000 people in the UK, vitamin C levels were shown to correlate with cardiovascular mortality, independently of diabetic status.[86] The lowest quintile of vitamin C level displayed double the risk of dying from a cardiovascular event than those with the highest levels. The administration of vitamin C has been shown to restore coronary microcirculation in smokers.[87] In diabetic subjects, hyperglycaemia-induced deficiency of vitamin C may well promote endothelial dysfunction and the development of atherosclerosis.[88] The benefits of vitamin C supplementation for diabetic subjects, whilst attractive, are not yet proven.

The role of vitamin E in atherosclerosis remains controversial. Doses of vitamin E insufficient to reduce cholesterol levels have not shown consistent inhibition of atherosclerosis in hypercholesterolaemic animals.[89] A modest increase in atherosclerosis was seen in a genetically vitamin E-deficient mouse model.[90] Possessing a serum level of vitamin E <10% of the wild type, these mice developed 30% more atherosclerosis and had evidence of a two-fold increase in tissue markers of lipid oxidation. The detrimental effects seen in this model may, however, reflect other documented influences of vitamin E on monocyte, smooth muscle cell and platelet function.[89] Interestingly, vitamin E, perhaps through modulation of ROS, has been shown to decrease AGE formation in diabetic subjects.[91]

Two studies in the apo E deficient mouse model of accelerated atherosclerosis have demonstrated that vitamin E supplementation significantly reduced the development of atherosclerosis.[92,93] Importantly the dose of vitamin E administered (0.2% of the diet) was demonstrated to be sufficient to inhibit lipid peroxidation.

Problems with antioxidant therapies

Human cells generally function in a reduced state, however local oxidation is a requirement for normal cellular function. For example, cellular proliferation requires the activation of gene transcription factors which require oxidation for their function. Indeed, there is evidence that whole organs, such as the kidney, operate in a state of precarious oxidative stress as a consequence of normal function.

In certain circumstances antioxidants may, paradoxically, worsen oxidative damage depending on the stage of the pathogenic process. Effective antioxidants are in effect reducing agents and, as such, may potentiate the damage caused by metal catalyzed free-radicals, released as a consequence of oxidative damage.[94] This may explain the paradox seen in the effects of vitamin C administration on paraquat toxicity.[95] If vitamin C is administered before administration of paraquat, oxidative damage is preventable. However, if vitamin C is given after injury, damage is potentiated. This dichotomous effect has also been seen in concurrent smokers. Indeed there is a suggestion that the protective cardiovascular benefits of aspirin administration are due to sequestration of these transitional-metal ions, in addition to anticoagulation.

Statins

The benefits for cerebrovascular and renal disease of the statin class of medications has suggested roles beyond their actions on cholesterol. One of these may be an action against oxidant stress. Fluvastatin, though not pravastatin or simvastatin, demonstrated strong protective effects in an *in vitro* system assessing ROS damage to DNA.[96] Furthermore, mutagenesis was significantly reduced.

Clinical studies of vitamin E

Large-scale clinical trials have examined the apparent benefits of consumption of a Mediterranean-style diet. Epidemiological studies have shown associations between the consumption of a diet rich in fresh fruit, vegetables and red wine and a reduced incidence of atherosclerosis and malignancy. However, dietary supplementation has in the main been unsuccessful in human studies. Indeed a number of paradoxes exist. Diets rich in fruit and vegetables result in an increased level of β-carotene in the blood and an association with a reduced incidence of cancer. However, supplementation results in no benefit. In fact increased rates of malignancy are observed in smokers. Similar dietary intakes have been shown to decrease free-radical damage to DNA. However, most studies fail to show that supplements of vitamins C, E and β-carotene have any benefit, and may actually increase DNA damage from ROS.

There are several possible reasons for this apparent paradox. It is important to recognize that *in vivo* experimental models have generally used doses of antioxidants in the order of 1% of dietary intake. Consequently levels of antioxidants within the tissues are achieved in animal trials that are not matched by trials in man. In addition there is little evidence that effective suppression of oxidation in humans has occurred. GISSI-prevenzione used one of the lower doses of vitamin E; however this was equivalent to 100 gm of fatty fish per day and represents a 50-fold increase over current recommended daily intakes.

GISSI-prevenzione and HOPE included significant numbers of diabetic subjects (15 and 38% respectively) and as such, findings from these trials are broadly applicable for diabetic patients.

The Cambridge Heart Antioxidant Outcome Study (CHAOS) administered 400–800 IU/day to 2000 subjects in a prospective, double blind, randomized secondary prevention study over six years. Results were encouraging and demonstrated an 80% reduction in the risk of non-fatal myocardial infarction. More recent results have been less supportive. The Gruppo Italiano per lo Studio della Sopravvivenza nell'Infarto Miocardico (GISSI) secondary prevention trial administered 300 IU/day with no statistical reduction in reinfarction rates.[97] However it has been suggested that the data analysis of this study was inappropriate and in fact α-tocopherol supplementation had resulted in a significant 20% reduction in cardiovascular death.[98,99]

Dietary supplementation with 400 IU/ day in the HOPE trial in high cardiovascular risk also demonstrated no benefits for vitamin E supplementation. In the HOPE substudy, Study to Evaluate Carotid Ultrasound Changes in Patients Treated with Ramipril and Vitamin E (SECURE), vitamin E also failed to show a benefit on carotid disease.[100]

One primary prevention trial, the Alpha-tocopherol, Beta-carotene Cancer Prevention trial, also failed to demonstrate a benefit of vitamin E supplementation on vascular outcomes. This was consistent with another primary prevention study including 20% diabetic subjects showing a neutral effect of vitamin E supplementation.[101] However the recent Secondary Prevention with Antioxidants of Cardiovascular disease in Endstage Renal Disease (SPACE) reported a dramatic 50% reduction in cardiovascular events in patients with pre-existing cardiovascular disease and renal failure due to the administration of 800 IU/ day.

From the available evidence the use of lower doses of vitamin E cannot be recommended for the reduction of cardiovascular disease in either a primary or secondary preventative role. Further studies need to be performed with the higher doses of vitamin E used in the SPACE and CHAOS trials, to assess whether these doses offer effective antioxidant effects in subjects. For diabetic subjects, the evidence for benefits from vitamin E supplementation remain limited.

Conclusions

The benefits of a diet rich in antioxidants are widely accepted as being self evident, yet the evidence for benefits in human trials has been disappointing and has not upheld initial positive findings from animal models. Indeed there is evidence *in vitro* and in experimental models that antioxidant modalities may actually be harmful if administered late in the pathogenic process. However use of other modalities such as α-lipoic acid have definite roles; inhibitors of the process of advanced glycation and experimental data particularly with vitamin C offer significant promise for the future. A greater understanding of the role that oxidative and glycoxidative processes play in the pathogenesis of diabetic complications is still required. In particular, further clinical trials are needed of vitamin E supplementation in doses sufficient to inhibit *in vivo* lipid peroxidation in humans.

References

1. Nishikawa T, Edelstein D, Du XL et al. Normalizing mitochondrial superoxide production blocks three pathways of hyperglycaemic damage. Nature 2000; 404: 787–90.
2. Mohamed AK, Bierhaus A, Schiekofer S et al. The role of oxidative stress and NF-kappaB activation in late diabetic complications. Biofactors 1999; 10: 157–67.
3. Dunlop M. Aldose reductase and the role of the polyol pathway in diabetic nephropathy. Kidney Int 2000; 58 Suppl. 77; S3–12.
4. Wolff SP, Dean RT. Glucose autoxidation and protein modification. The potential role of 'autoxidative glycosylation' in diabetes. Biochem J 1987; 245: 243–50.
5. Wolff SP, Jiang ZY, Hunt JV. Protein glycation and oxidative stress in diabetes mellitus and ageing. Free Radical Biol Med 1991; 10: 339–52.
6. Fu MX, Requena JR, Jenkins AJ et al. The advanced glycation end product, Nepsilon-(carboxymethyl)lysine, is a product of both lipid peroxidation and glycoxidation reactions. J Biol Chem 1996; 271: 9982–6.
7. Beck J, Ledl F, Sengl M, Severin T. Formation of acids, lactones and esters through the Maillard reaction. Z Lebensm Unters Forsch 1990; 190: 212–6.
8. Lal S, Randall WC, Taylor AH et al. Fructose-3-phosphate production and polyol pathway metabolism in diabetic rat hearts. Metabolism 1997; 46: 1333–8.
9. Laaksonen DE, Atalay M, Niskanen L et al. Increased resting and exercise-induced oxidative stress in young IDDM men. Diabetes Care 1996; 19: 569–74.
10. Mezzetti A, Cipollone F, Cuccurullo F. Oxidative stress and cardiovascular complications in diabetes: isoprostanes as new markers on an old paradigm. Cardiovasc Res 2000; 47: 475–88.
11. Maytin M, Leopold J, Loscalzo J. Oxidant stress in the vasculature. Curr Atheroscler Rep 1999; 1: 156–64.
12. Velazquez E, Winocour PH, Kesteven P et al. Relation of lipid peroxides to macrovascular disease in type 2 diabetes. Diabet Med 1991; 8: 752–8.
13. Sato Y, Hotta N, Sakamoto N et al. Lipid peroxide level in plasma of diabetic patients. Biochem Med 1979; 21: 104–7.
14. Ha H, Lee HB. Reactive oxygen species as glucose signaling molecules in mesangial cells cultured under high glucose. Kidney Int 2000; 58 Suppl. 77: S19–25.
15. Sentman ML, Brannstrom T, Westerlund S et al. Extracellular superoxide dismutase deficiency and atherosclerosis in mice. Arterioscler Thromb Vasc Biol 2001; 21: 1477–82.

16. Karasu C, Dewhurst M, Stevens EJ, Tomlinson DR. Effects of anti-oxidant treatment on sciatic nerve dysfunction in streptozotocin-diabetic rats; comparison with essential fatty acids. Diabetologia 1995; 38: 129–34.

17. Wohaieb SA, Godin DV. Alterations in free radical tissue-defense mechanisms in streptozocin-induced diabetes in rat. Effects of insulin treatment. Diabetes 1987; 36: 1014–18.

18. Loven D, Schedl H, Wilson H et al. Effect of insulin and oral glutathione on glutathione levels and superoxide dismutase activities in organs of rats with streptozocin- induced diabetes. Diabetes 1986; 35: 503–7.

19. van Dam PS, van Asbeck BS, Bravenboer B et al. Nerve function and oxidative stress in diabetic and vitamin E-deficient rats. Free Radical Biol Med 1998; 24: 18–26.

20. Williamson JR, Chang K, Frangos M et al. Hyperglycemic pseudohypoxia and diabetic complications. Diabetes 1993; 42: 801–13.

21. Baynes JW, Thorpe SR. Role of oxidative stress in diabetic complications: a new perspective on an old paradigm. Diabetes 1999; 48: 1–9.

22. Schmidt AM, Hori O, Cao R et al. RAGE: a novel cellular receptor for advanced glycation end products. Diabetes 1996; 45 Suppl 3: S77–80.

23. Hori O, Brett J, Slattery T et al. The receptor for advanced glycation end products (RAGE) is a cellular binding site for amphoterin. Mediation of neurite outgrowth and co-expression of rage and amphoterin in the developing nervous system. J Biol Chem 1995; 270: 25752–61.

24. Bierhaus A, Illmer T, Kasper M et al. Advanced glycation end product (AGE)-mediated induction of tissue factor in cultured endothelial cells is dependent on RAGE. Circulation 1997; 96: 2262–71.

25. Fu S, Fu MX, Baynes, JW et al. Presence of dopa and amino acid hydroperoxides in proteins modified with advanced glycation end products (AGEs): amino acid oxidation products as a possible source of oxidative stress induced by AGE proteins. Biochem J 1998; 330: 233–9.

26. Bucala R, Makita Z, Vega G et al. Modification of low density lipoprotein by advanced glycation end products contributes to the dyslipidemia of diabetes and renal insufficiency. Proc Natl Acad Sci USA 1994; 91: 9441–5.

27. He CJ, Zheng F, Stitt A et al. Differential expression of renal AGE-receptor genes in NOD mice: possible role in nonobese diabetic renal disease. Kidney Int 2000; 58: 1931–40.

28. Yamamoto Y, Kato I, Doi T et al. Development and prevention of advanced diabetic nephropathy in RAGE-overexpressing mice. J Clin Invest 2001; 108: 261–8.

29. Pyorala K, Laakso M, Uusitupa M. Diabetes and atherosclerosis: an epidemiologic view. Diabetes Metab Rev 1987; 3: 463–524.

30. Ross R. The pathogenesis of atherosclerosis: a perspective for the 1990s. Nature 1993; 362: 801–9.

31. Watts GF, Playford DA. Dyslipoproteinaemia and hyperoxidative stress in the pathogenesis of endothelial dysfunction in non-insulin dependent diabetes mellitus: an hypothesis. Atherosclerosis 1998; 141: 17–30.

32. Fogelman AM, Shechter I, Seager J et al. Malondialdehyde alteration of low density lipoproteins leads to cholesteryl ester accumulation in human monocyte-macrophages. Proc Natl Acad Sci USA 1980; 77: 2214–18.

33. Goldstein JL, Ho YK, Basu SK, Brown MS. Binding site on macrophages that mediates uptake and degradation of acetylated low density lipoprotein, producing massive cholesterol deposition. Proc Natl Acad Sci USA 1979; 76: 333–7.

34. Steinbrecher UP, Parthasarathy S, Leake DS et al. Modification of low density lipoprotein by endothelial cells involves lipid peroxidation and degradation of low density lipoprotein phospholipids. Proc Natl Acad Sci USA 1984; 81: 3883–7.

35. Heinecke JW, Rosen H, Chait A. Iron and copper promote modification of low density lipoprotein by human arterial smooth muscle cells in culture. J Clin Invest 1984; 74: 1890–4.

36. Holvoet P, Collen D. Oxidation of low density lipoproteins in the pathogenesis of atherosclerosis. Atherosclerosis 1998; 137 Suppl: S33–8.

37. Yla-Herttuala S, Palinski W, Rosenfeld ME et al. Evidence for the presence of oxidatively modified low density lipoprotein in atherosclerotic lesions of rabbit and man. J Clin Invest 1989; 84: 1086–95.

38. Numano F, Tanaka A, Makita T, Kishi Y. Glycated lipoprotein and atherosclerosis. Ann

NY Acad Sci 1997; 811: 100–13, discussion 113–14.

39. Steinberg D, Parthasarathy S, Carew TE et al. Beyond cholesterol. Modifications of low-density lipoprotein that increase its atherogenicity. N Engl J Med 1989; 320: 915–24.

40. Palinski W, Rosenfeld ME, Yla-Herttuala S, Gurtner GC et al. Low density lipoprotein undergoes oxidative modification in vivo. Proc Natl Acad Sci USA 1989; 86: 1372–6.

41. Galle J, Wanner C. Modification of lipoproteins in uremia: oxidation, glycation and carbamoylation. Miner Elec Metab 1999; 25: 263–8.

42. Grone EF, Walli AK, Grone HJ et al. The role of lipids in nephrosclerosis and glomerulosclerosis. Atherosclerosis 1994; 107: 1–13.

43. Kannel WB, McGee DL. Diabetes and cardiovascular disease. The Framingham study. JAMA 1979; 241: 2035–8.

44. Palinski W, Koschinsky T, Butler SW et al. Immunological evidence for the presence of advanced glycosylation end products in atherosclerotic lesions of euglycemic rabbits. Arterioscler Thromb Vasc Biol 1995; 15: 571–82.

45. Brownlee M. Advanced protein glycosylation in diabetes and aging. Annu Rev Med 1995; 46: 223–34.

46. Esposito C, Gerlach H, Brett J et al. Endothelial receptor-mediated binding of glucose-modified albumin is associated with increased monolayer permeability and modulation of cell surface coagulant properties. J Exp Med 1989; 170: 1387–407.

47. Wautier JL, Zoukourian C, Chappey MP et al. Receptor-mediated endothelial cell dysfunction in diabetic vasculopathy. Soluble receptor for advanced glycation end products blocks hyperpermeability in diabetic rats. J Clin Invest 1996; 97: 238–43.

48. Park L, Raman KG, Lee KJ et al. Suppression of accelerated diabetic atherosclerosis by the soluble receptor for advanced glycation endproducts. Nat Med 1998; 4: 1025–31.

49. Kasper HU, Schmidt A, Roessner A. Expression of the adhesion molecules ICAM, VCAM, and ELAM in the arteriosclerotic plaque. Gen Diagn Pathol 1996; 141: 289–94.

50. Schmidt AM, Hori O, Chen JX et al. Advanced glycation endproducts interacting with their endothelial receptor induce expression of vascular cell adhesion molecule-1 (VCAM-1) in cultured human endothelial cells and in mice. A potential mechanism for the accelerated vasculopathy of diabetes. J Clin Invest 1995; 96: 1395–403.

51. Brownlee M, Vlassara H, Kooney A et al. Aminoguanidine prevents diabetes-induced arterial wall protein cross-linking. Science 1986; 232: 1629–32.

52. Picard S, Parthasarathy S, Fruebis J, Witztum JL. Aminoguanidine inhibits oxidative modification of low density lipoprotein protein and the subsequent increase in uptake by macrophage scavenger receptors. Proc Natl Acad Sci USA 1992; 89: 6876–80.

53. Panagiotopoulos S, O'Brien RC, Bucala R et al. Aminoguanidine has an anti-atherogenic effect in the cholesterol-fed rabbit. Atherosclerosis 1998; 136: 125–31.

54. Khalifah RG, Todd P, Booth AA et al. Kinetics of nonenzymatic glycation of ribonuclease A leading to advanced glycation end products. Paradoxical inhibition by ribose leads to facile isolation of protein intermediate for rapid post-Amadori studies. Biochemistry 1996; 35: 4645–54.

55. Stadtman ER, Berlett BS. Reactive oxygen-mediated protein oxidation in aging and disease. Drug Metab Rev 1998; 30: 225–43.

56. Onorato JM, Jenkins AJ, Thorpe SR, Baynes JW. Pyridoxamine, an inhibitor of advanced glycation reactions, also inhibits advanced lipoxidation reactions. Mechanism of action of pyridoxamine. J Biol Chem 2000; 275: 21177–84.

57. Tsuchida K, Makita Z, Yamagishi S et al. Suppression of transforming growth factor beta and vascular endothelial growth factor in diabetic nephropathy in rats by a novel advanced glycation end product inhibitor, OPB-9195. Diabetologia 1999; 42: 579–88.

58. Forbes JM, Soulis T, Thallas V et al. Renoprotective effects of a novel inhibitor of advanced glycation. Diabetologia 2001; 44: 108–14.

59. Cooper ME, Thallas V, Forbes J et al. The cross-link breaker, N-phenacylthiazolium bromide prevents vascular advanced glycation end-product accumulation. Diabetologia 2000; 43: 660–4.

60. Vasan S, Zhang X, Kapurniotu A et al. An agent cleaving glucose-derived protein crosslinks in vitro and in vivo. Nature 1996; 382: 275–8.

61. Kass DA, Shapiro EP, Kawaguchi M et al. Improved arterial compliance by a novel advanced glycation end-product crosslink breaker. Circulation 2001; 104: 1464–70.

62. Burton GW, Ingold KU. Vitamin E as an in vitro and in vivo antioxidant. Ann NY Acad Sci 1989; 570: 7–22.

63. Jialal I, Traber M, Devaraj S. Is there a vitamin E paradox? Curr Opin Lipidol 2001; 12: 49–53.

64. Jialal I, Devaraj S, Kaul N. The effect of alpha-tocopherol on monocyte proatherogenic activity. J Nutr 2001; 131: 389S-94S.

65. Stocker R. The ambivalence of vitamin E in atherogenesis. Trends Biochem Sci 1999; 24: 219–23.

66. Packer L, Witt EH, Tritschler HJ. alpha-Lipoic acid as a biological antioxidant. Free Radical Biol Med 1995; 19: 227–50.

67. Bierhaus A, Chevion S, Chevion M et al. Advanced glycation end product-induced activation of NF-kappaB is suppressed by alpha-lipoic acid in cultured endothelial cells. Diabetes 1997; 46: 1481–90.

68. Ting HH, Timimi FK, Boles KS et al. Vitamin C improves endothelium-dependent vasodilation in patients with non-insulin-dependent diabetes mellitus. J Clin Invest 1996; 97: 22–8.

69. Pieper GM, Gross GJ. Oxygen free radicals abolish endothelium-dependent relaxation in diabetic rat aorta. Am J Physiol 1988; 255: H825–33.

70. Beckman JA, Goldfine AB, Gordon MB, Creager MA. Ascorbate restores endothelium-dependent vasodilation impaired by acute hyperglycemia in humans. Circulation 2001; 103: 1618–23.

71. Timimi FK, Ting HH, Haley EA et al. Vitamin C improves endothelium-dependent vasodilation in patients with insulin-dependent diabetes mellitus. J Am Coll Cardiol 1998; 31: 552–7.

72. Ganz MB, Seftel A. Glucose-induced changes in protein kinase C and nitric oxide are prevented by vitamin E. Am J Physiol Endocrinol Metab 2000; 278: E146–52.

73. Kunisaki M, Bursell SE, Clermont AC et al. Vitamin E prevents diabetes-induced abnormal retinal blood flow via the diacylglycerol-protein kinase C pathway. Am J Physiol 1995; 269: E239–46.

74. Kowluru RA, Tang J, Kern TS. Abnormalities of retinal metabolism in diabetes and experimental galactosemia. VII. Effect of long-term administration of antioxidants on the development of retinopathy. Diabetes 2001; 50: 1938–42.

75. Kim SS, Gallaher DD, Csallany AS. Vitamin E and probucol reduce urinary lipophilic aldehydes and renal enlargement in streptozotocin-induced diabetic rats. Lipids 2000; 35: 1225–37.

76. Garg MC, Bansal DD. Protective antioxidant effect of vitamins C and E in streptozotocin induced diabetic rats. Indian J Exp Biol 2000; 38: 101–4.

77. Melhem MF, Craven PA, Derubertis FR. Effects of dietary supplementation of alpha-lipoic acid on early glomerular injury in diabetes mellitus. J Am Soc Nephrol 2001, 12: 124–33.

78. Soulis-Liparota T, Cooper ME, Dunlop M, Jerums G. The relative roles of advanced glycation, oxidation and aldose reductase inhibition in the development of experimental diabetic nephropathy in the Sprague-Dawley rat. Diabetologia 1995; 38: 387–94.

79. Hounsom L, Corder R, Patel J, Tomlinson DR. Oxidative stress participates in the breakdown of neuronal phenotype in experimental diabetic neuropathy. Diabetologia 2001; 44: 424–8.

80. Bravenboer B, Kappelle AC, Hamers FP et al. Potential use of glutathione for the prevention and treatment of diabetic neuropathy in the streptozotocin-induced diabetic rat. Diabetologia 1992; 35: 813–17.

81. Kishi Y, Schmelzer JD, Yao JK et al. Alpha-lipoic acid: effect on glucose uptake, sorbitol pathway, and energy metabolism in experimental diabetic neuropathy. Diabetes 1999; 48: 2045–51.

82. Ziegler D, Hanefeld M, Ruhnau KJ et al. Treatment of symptomatic diabetic peripheral neuropathy with the anti- oxidant alpha-lipoic acid. A 3-week multicentre randomized controlled trial (ALADIN Study). Diabetologia 1995; 38: 1425–33.

83. Diaz MN, Frei B, Vita JA, Keaney JF., Jr. Antioxidants and atherosclerotic heart disease. N Engl J Med 1997; 337: 408–16.

84. Sasahara M, Raines EW, Chait A et al. Inhibition of hypercholesterolemia-induced atherosclerosis in the nonhuman primate by probucol. I. Is the extent of atherosclerosis related to resistance of LDL to oxidation? J Clin Invest 1994; 94: 155–64.

85. Sparrow CP, Doebber TW, Olszewski J et al. Low density lipoprotein is protected from oxidation and the progression of atherosclerosis is slowed in cholesterol-fed rabbits by the antioxidant N,N'-diphenyl-phenylenediamine. J Clin Invest 1992; 89: 1885–91.

86. Khaw KT, Bingham S, Welch A et al. Relation between plasma ascorbic acid and mortality in men and women in EPIC-Norfolk prospective study: a prospective population study. European Prospective Investigation into Cancer and Nutrition. Lancet 2001; 357: 657–63.

87. Kaufmann PA, Gnecchi-Ruscone T, di Terlizzi M et al. Coronary heart disease in smokers: vitamin C restores coronary microcirculatory function. Circulation 2000; 102: 1233–8.

88. Price KD, Price CS, Reynolds RD. Hyperglycemia-induced ascorbic acid deficiency promotes endothelial dysfunction and the development of atherosclerosis. Atherosclerosis 2001; 158: 1–12.

89. Heinecke JW. Is the emperor wearing clothes? Clinical trials of vitamin E and the LDL oxidation hypothesis. Arterioscler Thromb Vasc Biol 2001; 21: 1261–4.

90. Terasawa Y, Ladha Z, Leonard SW et al. Increased atherosclerosis in hyperlipidemic mice deficient in alpha- tocopherol transfer protein and vitamin E. Proc Natl Acad Sci USA 2000; 97: 13830–4.

91. Ceriello A, Giugliano D, Quatraro A et al. Vitamin E reduction of protein glycosylation in diabetes. New prospect for prevention of diabetic complications? Diabetes Care 1991; 14: 68–72.

92. Thomas SR, Leichtweis SB, Pettersson K et al. Dietary cosupplementation with vitamin E and coenzyme Q(10) inhibits atherosclerosis in apolipoprotein E gene knockout mice. Arterioscler Thromb Vasc Biol 2001; 21: 585–93.

93. Pratico D, Tangirala RK, Rader DJ et al. Vitamin E suppresses isoprostane generation in vivo and reduces atherosclerosis in ApoE-deficient mice. Nat Med 1998; 4: 1189–92.

94. Halliwell B. The antioxidant paradox. Lancet 2000; 355: 1179–80.

95. Kang SA, Jang YJ, Park H. In vivo dual effects of vitamin C on paraquat-induced lung damage: dependence on released metals from the damaged tissue. Free Radical Res 1998; 28: 93–107.

96. Imaeda A, Aoki T, Kondo Y et al. Protective effects of fluvastatin against reactive oxygen species induced DNA damage and mutagenesis. Free Radical Res 2001; 34: 33–44.

97. Dietary supplementation with n-3 polyunsaturated fatty acids and vitamin E after myocardial infarction: results of the GISSI-Prevenzione trial. Gruppo Italiano per lo Studio della Sopravvivenza nell'Infarto miocardico. Lancet 1999; 354: 447–55.

98. Jialal I, Devaraj S, Huet BA, Traber M. GISSI-Prevenzione trial. Lancet 1999; 354: 1554, discussion 1556–7.

99. Salen P, de Lorgeril M. GISSI-Prevenzione trial. Lancet 1999; 354: 1555, discussion 1556–7.

100. Lonn E, Yusuf S, Dzavik V et al. Effects of ramipril and vitamin E on atherosclerosis: the study to evaluate carotid ultrasound changes in patients treated with ramipril and vitamin E (SECURE). Circulation 2001; 103: 919–25.

101. de Gaetano G. Low-dose aspirin and vitamin E in people at cardiovascular risk: a randomized trial in general practice. Collaborative Group of the Primary Prevention Project. Lancet 2001; 357: 89–95.

102. Raj DS, Choudhury D, Welbourne TC, Levi M. Advanced glycation end products: a nephrologist's perspective. Am J Kidney Dis 2000; 35: 365–80.

103. Bierhaus A, Hofmann MA, Ziegler R, Nawroth PP. AGEs and their interaction with AGE-receptors in vascular disease and diabetes mellitus. I. The AGE concept. Cardiovasc Res 1998; 37: 586–600.

27

Progression of insulin resistance to beta-cell failure and overt diabetes: inevitable or preventable?

Mary Ann Banerji

Introduction: natural history of Type 2 diabetes

The pathogenesis of Type 2 diabetes has been attributed variably to defects in insulin action or to defects in insulin secretion and it is likely that both defects are usually involved.[1] A more important question centers on the timing and extent of each defect. Indeed, the dominant defect in Type 2 diabetes may differ in different populations.

In the development of diabetes, obesity and insulin resistance usually precede beta-cell failure and insulin deficiency. Beta-cell failure and hyperglycemia are generally thought to constitute an inevitable downhill spiral, requiring continually escalating treatment. There is a convincing body of literature suggesting that under the correct circumstances, euglycemia may be restored with recovery and preservation of beta-cell function.[2]

Insulin resistance and the beta-cell – a synchronized interplay

The inability of beta-cells to produce sufficient insulin results in hyperglycemia and diabetes. The etiology of beta-cell dysfunction may be structural or functional. Structural defects in human islet cells are poorly understood and may take the form of excessive amyloid deposition and decreased beta-cell mass.[3] Defects in beta-cell function are better understood and may be measured in several ways, including decreased response to oral glucose, glucose-specific decreases in first phase insulin response to intravenous glucose, delays in early insulin response to oral glucose, or impairment in pulsatility of beta-cell insulin secretion. That some of these abnormalities may be reversed suggests that beta-cell defects in Type 2 diabetes may be functional in nature.

Our understanding of the interrelationship of insulin resistance and beta-cell function comes from various models and methods including observational, cross-sectional and longitudinal studies in persons with impaired or diabetic glucose tolerance as well as in individuals with normal glucose tolerance predisposed to developing diabetes. Observational studies show that Type 2 diabetes is a progressive disorder associated with worsening of either insulin action or insulin secretion or both, and with increasing microvascular and macrovascular complications.[1,4–6] Cross-sectional studies show that longer durations of diabetes are associated with progressively increasing requirements of insulin replacement therapy in order to control blood sugar.[5,6] This finding suggests that beta-cell function gradually deteriorates over time and is supported by the United Kingdom Prospective Diabetes Study (UKPDS).[7]

The UKPDS was a large-scale longitudinal study designed to test the hypothesis that excellent glycemic control improved microvascular and macrovascular complications;[7] newly diagnosed patients with Type 2 diabetes assigned to conventional treatment were compared with patients under intensive glycemic treatment. The study succeeded in demonstrating the inverse relationship of glycemic control to rates of vascular complication; numerous secondary observations also emerged.[8,9] First, beta-cell function was already only 50% of normal at the time of diagnosis.

Second, both glycemic control and beta-cell function (as measured using the HOMA model) deteriorated over time in both intensive and conventional treatment groups.[7]

A major limitation of the UKPDS was its inability to maintain optimum glycemic control over long periods of time. It was also not designed to measure changes in beta-cell function. The deterioration of beta-cell function over time and how and when the decline begins is better addressed by following metabolic changes as these evolve during the progression from normal to impaired to diabetic glucose tolerance. Such a longitudinal study, by Weyer et al. among insulin-resistant Pima Indians,[10,11] demonstrated that the development of hyperglycemia was associated with

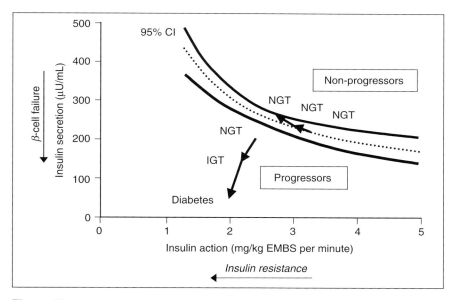

Figure 27.1
The relationship between insulin secretion and insulin action during a 40 mu/kg/m² euglycemic insulin clamp in a population with normal glucose tolerance is shown by the three curved lines (a dotted line flanked by two black lines). The longitudinal changes in those who remained with normal glucose tolerance are superimposed on the normal population data and are the non-progressors. The longitudinal changes in insulin action and insulin secretion as glucose tolerance develops from normal to impaired to diabetic glucose tolerance are shown as progressors. In the people who progressed, the acute insulin response was already well below normal levels while glucose tolerance remained normal. Source: Used with permission from Weyer et al.[10]

both a marked deterioration of beta-cell function as measured by the acute insulin response to intravenous glucose, and a small deterioration in insulin action as measured using the euglycemic insulin clamp (Figure 27.1). Individuals who did not develop hyperglycemia experienced a similar decline in insulin action but with a compensatory increase in insulin secretion; i.e. without the deterioration of beta-cell function. This implies that in insulin-resistant individuals, the failure of compensatory insulin secretion sparks the transition from normal to diabetic glucose tolerance. Similar data among Japanese also implicate low insulin secretion in the development of diabetes.[12] Further analysis of these data and others suggests that individuals with the most insulin resistance and least insulin secretion are at greatest risk for developing Type 2 diabetes.[11,13]

The question then arises as to whether this same process occurs in insulin-sensitive Type 2 diabetes patients. While such patients are less common than insulin-resistant subjects, they provide an important conceptual counterpoint in understanding the pathogenesis of diabetes.[14–17] A small longitudinal study among insulin-resistant and insulin-sensitive African–American patients with Type 2 diabetes,[15] found that, similar to Weyer's findings in Pima Indians, the transition from near-normoglycemia to hyperglycemia in the insulin-resistant subtype was characterized by a decrease in insulin secretion with little change in insulin action. In contrast, there was a decrease in both insulin secretion *and* insulin action in the insulin-sensitive subtype. This suggests that the original underlying defect in Type 2 diabetes may vary between patients.

This heterogeneity is corroborated by Pimenta et al.'s cross-sectional study.[18] Individuals with normal oral glucose tolerance and with diabetic first degree relatives (a predisposition to diabetes), had either decreased insulin response (first or second phase) to intravenous glucose or decreased insulin action. Defects in insulin secretion were more prevalent than defects in insulin action, but both were present. Neither abnormality was present in individuals not predisposed to diabetes. In addition, beta-cell defects were also present in persons with impaired glucose tolerance.[19,20] Thus, we see that defects in either insulin secretion or action may be present very early in the pathogenesis of Type 2 diabetes.

In summary, deterioration in beta-cell function may be demonstrated very early in the diabetic progression of susceptible patients, even when glucose tolerance is normal, and continues to deteriorate through the onset of hyperglycemia and clinical diabetes under usual suboptimal treatment conditions.

Insulin resistance

Insulin resistance, or decreased insulin-mediated glucose disposal, characterizes the majority of individuals with Type 2 diabetes. It is also an integral feature of the metabolic syndrome which includes obesity, dyslipidemia, impaired glucose tolerance, increased atherosclerosis and hypercoagulability, some forms of hypertension, and polycystic ovary syndrome[1,21–25] and is found in 85% of persons with Type 2 diabetes.[26] While insulin resistance, as well as obesity, is associated with diabetes, not all insulin resistant or obese individuals develop diabetes. In non-diabetic individuals, higher insulin resistance is accompanied by greater insulin secretion in response to all levels of glycemic stimuli.[27,28] Thus, although insulin resistance is a common feature of diabetes, it does not necessarily lead to glucose intolerance and diabetes if insulin secretion is commensurate with insulin requirements. When insulin secretion is sufficient to meet insulin requirements, whether large or small, normal glucose homeostasis will be maintained and glucose intolerance will be avoided.

An interesting question to consider is why both insulin resistance and insulin deficiency often occur together and whether there might be a common cause. An area of active research in cell culture and transgenic mouse models suggests that abnormalities in the insulin receptor signaling pathway, in both pancreatic beta-cells and muscle cells, may be involved.[29–31]

Interventions in the progression of Type 2 diabetes: primary prevention and secondary beta-cell recovery and preservation

There are several approaches to maintaining optimal glycemic control and normal glycohemoglobin. Traditionally, hyperglycemia is treated once it manifests clinically.[32] Achieving and maintaining long-term intensive glycemic control at this stage is typically arduous and is frequently unsuccessful at stemming the progressive worsening of hyperglycemia. An alternative and promising approach is prevention of the development of Type 2 diabetes in susceptible individuals through diet, exercise or pharmacological agents. Several trials have either been completed or are in progress.[33–38] Finally, re-institution of glucose homeostasis and the recovery and preservation of beta-cell function present a novel and intriguing approach to glycemic control.

Primary prevention of hyperglycemia in Type 2 diabetes

Methods of prevention of Type 2 diabetes include diet, exercise, and pharmacological interventions. One of the earliest observations of the effect of hypocaloric diets on the development of Type 2 diabetes comes from the Dutch famine during the Second World War.[39] During this period of food rationing, the development of new diabetes was markedly reduced. More recent observational studies in women in the Nurses Study associated increased physical activity with a significant decrease in the development of diabetes.[33] The Chinese Da Qing study also demonstrated an effect of diet and increased physical activity in decreasing diabetes.[34] The Finnish Diabetes Prevention study showed that a weight-reducing, reduced-fat diet and increased physical activity prevented the development of diabetes by 58%.[35] These findings were supported by the Diabetes Prevention Trial which showed that diet and exercise decreased the development of diabetes by approximately 58% while metformin decreased it by 31%.[36] Among women with a history of gestational diabetes, treatment with the thiazolidinedione troglitazone compared with placebo showed a 60% decrease in the development of diabetes (TRIPOD study).[37] Other large-scale studies using pharmacological agents to prevent the development of diabetes include STOP NIDDM, using acarbose, studies using a combination of an angiotensin-converting enzyme inhibitor and insulin sensitizers (ramipril and rosiglitazone, DREAM study) as well as an angiotensin receptor blocker and an insulin secretagogue (valsartan and nateglinide, Navigator study).[38,40] Secondary analyses of lipid-lowering studies have shown that the 'statins' may also decrease the development of diabetes by 30%,[41] possibly by reducing inflammation. Thus, it appears that numerous approaches including diet, exercise and pharmacological agents working at various metabolic sites, including insulin action, insulin secretion and inflammation, may decrease the development of diabetes.

Secondary remission of hyperglycemia: beta-cell recovery and preservation

Remission, or the recovery of glucose homeostasis, has been described in several different populations, including African–American, Japanese and European (Table 27.1).[2,42–53] This unusual phenomenon, occurring in individuals presenting with severe hyperglycemia, is the recovery of glucose homeostasis and maintenance of normal glyco-hemoglobin levels over prolonged periods of time without significant weight loss or continued use of pharmacological agents. Remission is defined as a fasting blood glucose less than 126 mg/dl and HbA1c within normal limits for three months in a patient with Type 2 diabetes who has discontinued active pharmacological treatment.

Banerji and Lebovitz have described remission among African–Americans with newly diagnosed Type 2 diabetes.[2] For the 79 reported cases, patients presented with acute, symptomatic hyperglycemia, requiring treatment with insulin and fluids and generally hospitalization.[2,53] Following discharge, they received intensive blood glucose control. Over several months, antidiabetic pharmacological agents were gradually withdrawn and, although no significant weight loss occurred, blood glucose levels remained normal.

Ilkova et al. described 9 out of 13 (68%) newly diagnosed European Type 2 diabetes patients who were treated with continuous subcutaneous insulin infusion for two weeks and discontinued insulin and remained euglycemic for 9–50 months (median ± SE 26 ± 4.8 months).[44] Even when five of the nine patients relapsed, a second course of treatment re-established glycemic control in four cases. At the time of the report, 6 of the 13 patients (46%) continued to have glycemic control

without pharmacological agents (median ± SEM, 45.5 ± 6.6 months). As with Banerji's series, weight loss was not a factor.

Kayashima et al. reported that 15 out of 21 (68%) Japanese patients, with poorly controlled or new onset diabetes achieved good glycemic control after intensive subcutaneous insulin treatment.[45] Umpierrez et al. described recovery of glucose homeostasis among African–Americans presenting with markedly elevated blood glucose who were treated with insulin.[43] However, unlike the others' data, only 20% were normoglycemic without pharmacological agents at six months after the initial withdrawal of insulin treatment. Finally, remission has been described by Rendell et al.[47] using insulin or sulfonylurea treatment, and by Lev-Ran[48] and Singer and Hurwitz[49] using sulfonylurea treatment, and sporadically as case reports.[50–52] The presence of remission in such diverse populations, as well as in animal models[48–50] suggests that the phenomenon may be universal.

Clinical features

Remission may occur within one year of the diagnosis of diabetes; Banerji et al. reported the clinical and metabolic features associated with this phenomenon.[2,16,47] In a group of 79 patients, the median presenting plasma glucose was 37.8 ± 19.3 mmol/l (680 ± 347 mg/dl) and the mean duration of intensive treatment before remission was eight months; treatment included insulin (28%), sulfonylureas (34%), both insulin and sulfonylureas (34%) and diet only (4%). While in remission (normal fasting glucose and HbA1c), 17% had normal glucose tolerance, 33% had impaired and 50% had diabetic glucose tolerance.[47] Both insulin-sensitive and insulin-resistant individuals developed remission and weight loss was not significant. However, those who developed normal glucose tolerance lost more weight and

Author	Race	No.	Age (years)	BMI (kg/m²)	Male: Female ratio	Plasma glucose (mg/dl)	HbA1c % Initial/in remission
Banerji 1996	African–American and Caribbean	79	45 ± 10	28.8 ± 3.7 (22–46)	51:28	680 ± 347#	NA/ 5.98 ± 0.6
McFarlaneπ 2001	African–American and Caribbean	14	48.4 ± 10	29.2 ± 2.8	8:3	655 ± 291#	9.3 ± 0.6/5.9 ± 0.2
Banerji 1990	African–American and Caribbean	33	45 ± 9.6	27.9 ± 3.4	22:11	700 ± 200	NA/5.2 ± 0.49
Kayashima* 1995	Japanese	15	55.3 ± 12	21.2 ± 2.1	10:5	244 ± 42x 338 ± 59@	11.3 ± 1.7/6.4 ± 0.8
Ilkova+ 1997	European	9	50.6 ± 3 (34–67)	26.9 ± 0.8 (24–34)	11:2	216 ± 19x 304 ± 32@	11.2 ± 0.9/6.1 ± 0.5
Umpierrez 1997	African–American	20	45.3 ± 3	38 ± 2	20:15	630 ± 36	13 ± 0.6/6.8 ± 0.15
Rendall§ 1981	Unknown (N. American)	11	40–70	1.35+0.21^ (1.04–1.66)	9:2	855 ± 434#	NA
Pirart and Lauvaux 1971	Unknown (European)	280	20–>60	38% <120%^ 45% 120–150% 16% >150%	138:142	94% <300# 6% >300	NA

Table 27.1
Clinical characteristics and frequency of remission

Notes: Data are mean ± SD except where noted; numbers in parentheses denote ranges; §Observational study; 29% presented with ketoacidosis (pH, 7.3); #presenting plasma glucose. All were GAD negative; πConsecutive, unselected new onset within two weeks, selected if presenting glucose >300 mg/dl; *Previously diagnosed with mean duration of diabetes 3.9 years; non-obese, drug naïve, selected if FPG >150 mg/dl after five days of strict diet; +New onset selected if FPG >160 and PPG >200 mg/dl following 3–6 weeks of diet and exercise. Data are mean ± SEM xFasting plasma glucose; @Postprandial glucose; ^Ideal body weight (IBW). BMI of 25 for women and 27 for men = 120% of IBW; §5/11 with ketoacidosis, pH 7.3–7.35; 6/11 with precipitating events; ¶Subset of 67 patients (ref. 61).

Duration of diabetes at time of presentation	Duration of experiment until remission	Duration of remission (months)	Type of treatment (%)		Frequency of developing remission
New onset	8.1 ± 10 mo§	40 median follow-up 12 yrs	Insulin Sulfonylurea (SU) Insulin and SU Diet	(36) (30) (28) (1)	Not available
New onset℥	83 ± 60 days (31–239)	11 ± 2.7 follow-up 1.3 yrs	Insulin Sulfonylurea Insulin and SU Diet	(70) (19) (8) (3)	11/26 (42%)
New onset	30% <90 days 64% <180 days 85% <365 days	16 follow-up 8 yrs	Insulin Sulfonylurea Insulin and SU Diet	(28) (34) (34) (3)	20/67 (30%)¶
3.9 ± 3.1 yrs Drug naive	24.1 ± 6.4 days (12–37)	6	Insulin 4 x daily	(100)	15/22 (68%)
New onset	14 days	26 ± 4.8 follow-up 4 yrs	Continuous SC insulin infusion x 2 weeks	(100)	9/13 (69%)
New onset	61 ± 7 days	8 median follow-up 2 yrs	Insulin and SU		13/21 (60%)
New onset 63%	1 day–24 mo	3–17 mo	Insulin	(91)	Not available
<1 yr (49%) >1 yr (51%)	73% <12 mo	50% <1 yr 37% 1–5 yrs 13% >5 yrs	Insulin OHA/diet	(26) (74)	Not available

Table 27.1 (cont.)

were more insulin-sensitive as a group than those whose glucose tolerance was not normalized.[2] Long-term follow-up of 71 patients over eight years showed that relapse to hyperglycemia occurred among 27 of 71 patients.[47]

A relapse was defined as a fasting plasma glucose of over 150 mg/dl with symptoms, or on three successive occasions without symptoms of hyperglycemia. Weight gain was not a prominent feature in relapse. Relapse was characterized by a loss of insulin secretion: insulin-resistant subjects had a 50% decline in insulin secretion without any change in insulin-mediated glucose disposal, similar to insulin-resistant Pima Indians who developed hyperglycemia.[10] In contrast, insulin-sensitive Type 2 diabetic patients sustained a 75% loss of insulin secretion as well as a decrease in insulin-mediated glucose disposal when hyperglycemia developed.

Duration of remission

Is remission a clinically durable phenomenon or is it evanescent, like the 'honeymoon' phase of Type 1 diabetes, which typically lasts for less than a year? Based on longitudinal data, it appears that, once re-established, glucose homeostasis is substantial and enduring.[37,39] In a group of 71 African–American patients in remission, followed for over eight years, the median duration of remission was 39 months (Figure 27.2), similar to the 26–46 months reported by Ilkova in Europeans.[38] Duration of remission ranged up to 12 years.[47]

Significance of remission

The ability to induce remissions could be a very potent strategy in the treatment of Type 2 diabetes, especially because traditional treatment does not result in such normal HbA1c levels. The fact that normal HbA1c levels are not typically achieved on pharmacological agents was demonstrated in the UKPDS.[6] The level of glycemic control achieved in remission exceeds various internationally recognized goals for glycemic control including the American Diabetes Association goal of HbA1c <7.0%, the European Association for the Study of Diabetes and the American Association of Clinical Endocrinologists goal of HbA1c <6.5%.[32,54]

The clinical significance of remission of diabetes, or a period of normal glycohemoglobin levels, comes from the Epidemiology of Diabetes Interventions and Complications (EDIC) trial, the four-year follow-up report of the Diabetes Control and Complications Trial (DCCT).[55] In the DCCT, intensive versus conventional treatment of Type 1 diabetes resulted in a 60–70% decrease in the development of microvascular complications. Four years after the trial ended, the improved rates of complications persisted, even though glycemic control no longer differed between the two groups. This suggests that the normal HbA1c levels achieved in remission could decrease complication rates well beyond the immediate period of remissions.

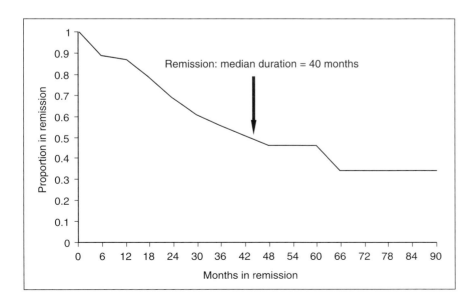

Figure 27.2
Kaplan–Meier survival curve of the duration of remission in 71 patients followed for eight years. The median time of remission or the time patients maintained normal HbA1c while remaining off pharmacologic agents was 40 months. Source: Used with permission from Banerji and Lebovitz.[2]

While the role of glycemic control in macrovascular disease is not as well established, the epidemiological analysis of the UKPDS suggests that lower HbA1c is associated with fewer macrovascular complications.[9] Similarly, among non-diabetic populations, the EPIC-Norfolk study showed that lower HbA1c levels (<5.0%) are associated with lower cardiovascular mortality among men after adjusting for other risk factors.[56,57] Although current treatment focuses on decreasing HbA1c levels to reduce mortality in the diabetic population,[57,58] similar interventions might also be valuable in non-diabetic but 'dysglycemic' populations, as small reductions in blood glucose levels may translate into substantial health benefits for the much larger non-diabetic population.

Causes of Remission

What might be involved in the development of remission? Obvious possibilities include weight loss, a misclassification as 'honeymoon' of Type 1 diabetes, removal of stress, and potential reversal of glucose or lipotoxicity.

Weight loss is an extremely attractive hypothesis, because it has been shown to be associated with the reversal of hyperglycemia in Type 2 diabetes. However, weight loss not only is difficult to sustain but also must be quite significant in order to be effective in controlling Type 2 diabetes.[58,59] In contrast, patients who developed remission usually did not lose significant amounts of weight.[37–41]

It is well known that newly diagnosed Type 1 diabetes may be associated with a 'honeymoon' period, generally lasting less than one year. Patients in remission have clearly not been misdiagnosed with Type 1 diabetes because antibodies to islet cell or glutamic acid decarboxylase are absent and thus a 'honeymoon' is not a possible explanation.

Medical or surgical stress was strikingly absent among the patients making it unlikely to be an important feature of remission. Importantly, during remission, neither medical nor surgical stress perturbed glucose homeostasis.[2,45]

Lastly, intensive glycemic control was considered as a possible explanation: most patients were enrolled in an intensive diabetes management policy, including weekly diabetes education classes and case management. Indeed, 30% of patients who attended more than two classes developed remission compared with those who attended one or fewer classes, who developed remission at a rate of 6%.[61]

Prolonging remission: beta-cell preservation

The question was then addressed of whether remissions could be prolonged using pharmacological treatment. Patients in remission were treated with placebo or low dose glipizide for 3.5 years.[62] Patients on low dose glipizide (1.25 to 2.5 mg) remained in remission significantly longer than patients on placebo. When glipizide was discontinued at the end of the study, patients remained normoglycemic for several months. At baseline, there were no metabolic differences between the glipizide group or the placebo group in terms of BMI, insulin sensitivity or insulin response to oral glucose stimuli. Using a slightly different approach, Umpierrez treated newly diagnosed, severely hyperglycemic African–American patients with intensive insulin therapy, followed by low doses of sulfonylurea treatment or placebo.[43] Sulfonylurea treatment maintained euglycemia longer than placebo treatment.

The mechanism whereby sulfonylureas prolong remission is not known; however, the mechanism for meal-related insulin secretion involves the sulfonylurea receptor (SUR1), a K^+_{ATP} channel, on the beta-cell.[63] Since the

SUR1 receptor is an integral part of the normal insulin secretory mechanism, it is possible that functional defects in this mechanism may be present in Type 2 diabetes.[64] In this case, chronic administration of low doses of sulfonylureas may be instrumental in prolonging remission.

Inducing remission: beta-cell recovery

Because of the potential benefits of re-establishing long-term glucose homeostasis, we must consider the following question: can remission and recovery of beta-cell function be induced in a systematic fashion, and if so, how? In a proof-of-concept study, 26 consecutive new-onset patients were treated intensively within one day of diagnosis. Most received multiple doses of insulin but a few received sulfonylureas.[65] Within a median of 2.5 months, 42% of patients discontinued

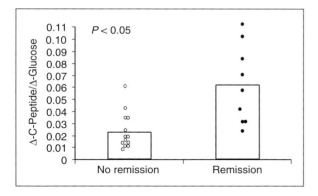

Figure 27.3

The C-peptide response to oral glucose at 57–112 days was significantly higher in those who developed remission compared with those who did not (p <0.05). The C-peptide response is expressed as the change or delta C-peptide to delta glucose areas over basal during an oral glucose tolerance test. Source: Used with permission from McFarlane et al.[65]

their pharmacological agents and developed remission. There were no differences between those developing and those not developing remission in terms of initial body weight, weight change with treatment, or presenting plasma glucose. It could not be determined whether greater intrinsic beta-cell abnormalities or a longer duration of preclinical hyperglycemia contributed to lack of remission. In order to determine a possible mechanism for remission, patients serially underwent oral glucose tolerance tests with plasma C-peptide determination to assess the role of the beta-cell in remission. Remission was associated with a greater increase in plasma C-peptide response to oral glucose compared with non-remission (Figure 27.3). Data from Umpierezz et al., Ilkova et al. and Koyashima et al.[43–45] are consistent with these data and demonstrate that intensive treatment of newly diagnosed Type 2 diabetes results in remission within a relatively short time. Although the emphasis has been on inducing remission initially after diagnosis, it is likely that remissions can be re-established once a patient has relapsed, as demonstrated by Ilkova et al. Thus, remission and recovery of beta-cell function can be induced with appropriate interventions.

Banerji and Lebovitz, Umpierezz et al., and Ilkova et al. all suggest that remission occurs in new onset and not in previously diagnosed patients.[2,43,44] Both Kayashima et al. and Banerji and Lebovitz note that patients whose diabetes is of long duration were unlikely to develop remission.[2,45] The reason for this is not understood, but may be related to the development of fixed islet cell defects such as amyloid deposition or a marked reduction in beta-cell mass. It is unclear how soon intensive treatment must begin in order to induce remission, but earlier intervention is more likely to lead to remission.

Mechanisms of beta-cell recovery – lipotoxicity and glucose toxicity

Recovery of glucose homeostasis seems to be associated with a critical recovery of beta-cell function and insulin secretion. The fact that beta-cell function may be restored suggests that the primary defect affecting insulin secretion is functional rather than structural. The fundamental question then becomes why beta-cell function declines in the first place. Glucose toxicity and lipotoxicity may be possible explanations in the presence of some as yet undefined genetic predisposition.[66–70] Intensive metabolic control may lessen both glucose toxicity and lipotoxicity and thus restore glucose homeostasis.

Glucose toxicity

Early studies showed that rats that had been made hyperglycemic had decreased insulin secretion and action.[68] In the presence of intensive metabolic control, islets from streptozotocin diabetic mice can be shown to regenerate.[66] Indeed, streptozotocin, which is used to destroy beta-cells and create a model of insulin-deficient diabetes in rodents, is itself a glucose analog and its action mimics glucose toxicity.

Elevated glucose is thought to result in increased beta-cell apoptosis; although the mechanism for this effect is not clear, there are several studies in humans which address this concept. An early study showed that, regardless of the approach to treatment – diet, sulfonylureas or insulin, intensively lowering blood glucose in Type 2 diabetes resulted in increased insulin response to oral glucose.[60] Using a different model to address the idea of glucose toxicity, Boden et al. exposed non-diabetic subjects to several days of progressively increasing hyperglycemia.[71] Insulin secretion decreased by the third day of glucose infusions of 12.6 mM (220 mg/dl). Similarly, incubation of non-diabetic cultured human islets in high concentrations of glucose resulted in the expression of the Fas receptor on the surface of beta-cells.[72] The Fas receptor is associated with cell death or apoptosis. Initial proliferation of beta-cells was followed by a prolonged decline and apoptosis. Interestingly, addition of Fas antibody abolished the deleterious effect of glucose, suggesting that apoptosis and impaired proliferation is caused by the interaction of the Fas ligand and its glucose-induced up-regulated Fas receptor.

Lipotoxicity

The role of lipotoxicity in human diabetes is limited, interesting and appears to depend on the chronicity of exposure to lipids.[73] Boden et al. showed that a four-hour infusion of intralipids in lean subjects was associated with a decrease in oxidative and non-oxidative glucose disposal and increased hepatic glucose output.[74] Subsequently, Schulman's work demonstrated that decreased insulin action resulted from decreased Glut-4-mediated glucose uptake across muscle membranes.[75]

The role of lipids or fatty acids on beta-cell insulin secretion is unclear. In animal models, a 5- to 10-fold increase in islet fat content as seen in the pre-diabetic phase of the obese Zucker rat is associated with beta-cell hyperplasia, while an increase in islet fat to 50% of normal causes a decrease in beta-cell number and diabetes.[76] Prolonged exposure to free fatty acids results in a decrease in insulin secretion in the Zucker diabetic fatty rat. In this model of diabetes, free fatty acid-mediated induction of inducible nitric oxide synthase (iNOS) and increased intracellular nitric oxide (NO) have been proposed as a mediator of beta-cell apoptosis.[76] Whether humans can accumulate an amount of fat equivalent to that of a Zucker rat, or whether this mechanism is operative in humans is not known. Free fatty acid infusions acutely increase insulin secretion in humans (as in animals),[77] but chronic lipid infusions (48 hours) result in decreased insulin release in response to graded glucose infusions.[78] The effect of free fatty acids on insulin secretion appears to be complex and is likely to be related to both the type and duration of free fatty acid exposure as well as to the individual's metabolic state.

Summary

Numerous studies suggest that beta-cell dysfunction is the key in the final step leading to hyperglycemia in diabetes. It appears that a progressive loss of glucose homeostasis and beta-cell dysfunction does not necessarily accompany diabetes. Remission or restoration of glucose homeostasis may occur under the right conditions of intensive metabolic treatment. This approach is probably most effective if intensive glycemic control is instituted early in the course of Type 2 diabetes. Remission or the recovery of glucose homeostasis is associated with recovery of insulin secretion and relapse is associated with the loss of insulin-secretion capabilities. Weight loss is not a major requirement for remission, and beta-cell recovery and preservation occur in both lean and obese individuals with Type 2 diabetes, in diverse ethnic groups, in both cell culture and animal models. Restoration of beta-cell function and preservation of glucose homeostasis may be prolonged through pharmacological treatment and may be crucial in reducing diabetic complications.

References

1. Lebovitz HE. Type 2 diabetes. An overview. Clinical Chem 1999; 48: 1339–45.
2. Banerji MA, Lebovitz HE. Remission in non-insulin-dependent diabetes mellitus: clinical characteristics of remission and relapse in black patients. Medicine 1990; 69: 176–85.
3. Hoppener JWM, Ahren B, Lips CJM. Islet amyloid and Type 2 diabetes mellitus. New Engl J Med 2000; 343: 411–19.
4. Wingard DL, Barrett-Connor E. Heart disease and diabetes. In: National Diabetes Data Group, eds. Diabetes in America. NHANES, Bethesda MD, 1995: 429–48.
5. Fertig BJ, Simmons DA, Martin DB. Therapy for diabetes. In: National Diabetes Data Group, eds. Diabetes in America. NHANES, Bethesda MD, 1995: 519–39.
6. Turner RC, Cull CA, Frighi V, Holman RR for the United Kingdom Prospective Diabetes Study (UKPDS) Group. Glycaemic control with diet sulphonylurea, metformin, or insulin in patients with Type 2 diabetes mellitus. Progressive requirement for multiple therapies. JAMA 1999; 281: 2005–12.
7. UK Prospective Diabetes Study group. UK Prospective diabetes study 16: overview of 6 years' therapy of Type 2 diabetes. A progressive disorder. Diabetes 1995; 44: 1249–58.
8. United Kingdom Prospective Diabetes (UKPDS) Group. Intensive blood glucose control with sulphonylureas or insulin compared with conventional treatment and risk of complications inpatients with Type 2 diabetes (UKPDS 33). Lancet 1998; 3562: 837–53.
9. Stratton IM, Adler AI, Neil HAW et al. Association of glycaemia with macrovascular and microvascular complication of Type 2 diabetes UKPDS 350: prospective observational study. BMJ 2000; 321: 405–12.
10. Weyer CJ, Bogardus C, Mott DM, Prateley RE. The natural history of insulin secretory dysfunction and insulin resistance in the pathogenesis of Type 2 diabetes mellitus. J Clin Invest 1999; 104: 787–94.
11. Weyer CJ, Bogardus C, Mott DM, Prateley RE. Insulin resistance and insulin secretory dysfunction are independent predictors of worsening glucose tolerance during each stage of Type 2

diabetes development. Diabetes Care 2001; 24: 89–94.

12. Kadowaki T, Miyake Y, Hagura R et al. Risk factors for worsening to diabetes in subjects with impaired glucose tolerance. Diabetologia 1984; 26: 44–9.

13. Haffner SM, Miettien H, Gaskill SP, Stern MP. Decreased insulin secretion and increased insulin resistance are independently related to the 7 year risk of NIDDM in Mexican Americans. Diabetes 1995; 44: 1386–91.

14. Gerich JE. Insulin resistance is not necessarily an essential component of Type 2 diabetes. J Clin Endocrinol Metab 2000; 85: 2113–15.

15. Banerji MA, Lebovitz HE. Insulin action in black Americans with NIDDM. Diabetes Care 1992; 15: 1295–302.

16. Chaiken RL, Banerji MA, Pasmantier RM et al. Patterns of glucose and lipid abnormalities in Black NIDDM subjects. Diabetes Care 1991; 14: 1036–42.

17. Arner P, Pollare T, Lithell H. Different aetiologies of Type 2 (non-insulin dependent) diabetes mellitus in obese and non-obese subjects. Diabetologia 1991; 34: 483–7.

18. Pimenta W, Korytkowski M, Mitrkou A et al. Pancreatic beta-cell dysfunction as a primary genetic lesion in NIDDM: Evidence from studies in normal glucose tolerant individuals with a first degree NIDDM relative. JAMA 1995; 273: 1855–61.

19. O'Meara NM, Sturis J, Van Cauter E, Polonsky KS. Lack of control by glucose of ultradian insulin secretory oscillations in impaired glucose tolerance and in non-insulin-dependent diabetes mellitus. J Clin Invest 1993; 92: 262–71.

20. O'Rahilly S, Turner RC, Mathews DR. Impaired pulsatile secretion of insulin in relatives of patients with non-insulin dependent diabetes. New Engl J Med 1988; 318: 1225–30.

21. Bonaro E, Kiechl S, Williet J et al. Prevalence of insulin resistance in metabolic disorders. The Bruneck study. Diabetes 1998; 47: 1643–9.

22. Banerji MA, Lebovitz HE. Insulin sensitive and insulin resistant variants in NIDDM. Diabetes 1989; 38: 784–801.

23. Reaven GM. The role of insulin resistance in human disease. Diabetes 1988; 37: 1595–607.

24. McFarlane SI, Banerji MA, Sowers JR. Insulin resistance and cardiovascular risk. J Clin Endocrinol Metab 2001; 86: 713–18.

25. Ferrannini E. Insulin resistance vs insulin deficiency in non-insulin-dependent diabetes mellitus, problems and prospects. Endocrinol Rev 1998; 19: 477–90.

26. Ford J. American Medical Association, 2002.

27. Kahn SE, Prigeon RL, McCulloch DK et al. Quantification of the relationship between insulin sensitivity and beta-cell function in human subjects. Evidence for a hyperbolic function. Diabetes 1993; 42: 1663–72.

28. Jones CNO, Pei D, Staris P et al. Alterations in the glucose stimulated insulin secretory dose-response curve and in insulin clearance in non-diabetic insulin-resistant individuals. J Clin Endocrinol Metab 1997; 82: 1834–8.

29. Sreenan SK, Zhou YP, Otani K et al. Calpains play a role in insulin secretion and action. Diabetes 2001; 50: 2013–20.

30. Kulkarni RN et al. Tissue specific knock-out of the insulin receptor in pancreatic beta-cells causes an insulin secretory defect similar to that in Type 2 diabetes. J Clin Invest 1999; 104: R69–R75.

31. Sesti G, Federici M, Hribal ML et al. Defects of the insulin receptor substrate (IRS) system in human metabolic disorders. FASEB J 2001; 15: 2099–111.

32. Anonymous. American Diabetes Association: Clinical practice recommendations. Diabetes Care 2002; 25: 51–147.

33. Hu FB, Sigal RJ, Rich-JW et al. Diabetes in women. A prospective study. JAMA 1999; 282: 1433–9.

34. Pan X, Li G, Hu Y et al. Effect of diet and exercise in preventing NIDDM in people with impaired glucose tolerance: The Da Qing IGT and Diabetes Study. Diabetes Care 1997; 20: 537–44.

35. Tuomilehto J, Lindstrom J, Eriksson JG et al. Prevention of Type 2 diabetes by changes in lifestyle among subjects with impaired glucose tolerance. N Engl J Med 2001; 244: 1343–50.

36. Diabetes Prevention Program Research Group. Reduction of the incidence of Type 2 diabetes with lifestyle intervention or metformin. New Engl J Med 2002; 346: 393–403.

37. Buchanan TA, Kahn S. Thiazolidinediones should/should not be used for the prevention of Type 2 diabetes. Diabetes 2002;(suppl) abstract.

38. Chiasson JL, Gomis R, Hanefeld M et al. The STOP-NIDDM Trial. An international study on

the efficacy of an alpha glucosidase inhibitor to prevent Type 2 diabetes in a population with impaired glucose tolerance; rationale, design and preliminary screening data. Diabetes Care 1998; 21: 1720–5.

39. Dutch Famine 1943–1944.

40. Baron AD. Impaired glucose tolerance as a disease. Am J Cardiol 2001; 88(Suppl): 16H-19H.

41. Freeman DJ et al. Pravastatin and the development of diabetes: evidence for a protective treatment effect in the West of Scotland Coronary Prevention Study. Circulation 2001; 103: 357–62.

42. Pirart J, Lauvaux JP. Remission in diabetes. In: Pfeiffer E, ed. Handbook of Diabetes Mellitus. Munchen: JF Lehman Verlag, 1971: Vol II 443–502.

43. Umpierrez G, Clark WS, Steen M. Sulfonylurea treatment prevents recurrence of hyperglycemia in obese African-American patients with a history of hyperglycemic crises. Diabetes Care 1997; 20: 479–83.

44. Ilkova H, Glaser B, Tunckale A et al. Induction of long term glycemic control in newly diagnosed Type 2 diabetic patients by transient intensive insulin treatment. Diabetes Care 1997; 20: 1353–6.

45. Kayashima T, Yamaguchi K, Konno Y et al. Effects of early introduction of intensive insulin therapy on the clinical course in non-obese NIDDM patients. Diabetes Res Clin Pract 1995; 28: 119–25.

46. Singer DL, Hurwitz D. Long term experience with sulphonylureas and placebo. N Engl J Med 1967; 277: 450–6.

47. Rendell M, Zariello J, Drew HM et al. Recovery from decompensated non-insulin dependent diabetes mellitus: Studies of C-peptide secretion. Diabetes Care 1981; 4: 354–9.

48. Lev-Ran A. Trial of placebo in long term chlorpropamide treated diabetics. Diabetologia 1974; 10: 197–200.

49. Singer DL, Hurwitz D. Long term experience with sulphonylureas and placebo. N Engl J Med 1967; 277: 450–6.

50. Genuth SM. Clinical remission in diabetes mellitus. Studies of insulin secretion. Diabetes 1970; 19: 116–21.

51. Cheng TO, Jahraus RC, Traut EF. Extreme hyperglycemia and severe ketosis with sponta-neous remission of diabetes mellitus. JAMA 1953; 152: 1531–3.

52. Peck FB Jr, Kirtley WR, Peck FB Sr. Complete remission of severe diabetes. Diabetes 1958; 7: 93–7.

53. Banerji MA, Chaiken RL, Lebovitz HE. Long term remission in NIDDM in Blacks. Diabetes 1996; 45: 337–41.

54. American College of Endocrinology Consensus Statement on guidelines for glycemic control. Endocr Pract 2001; 8(Suppl 1): 5–11.

55. Anonymous. Retinopathy and nephropathy in patients with Type 1 diabetes for four years after a trial of intensive therapy. The Diabetes Control and Complications Trial/Epidemiology of Diabetes Interventions and Complications research group. New Engl J Med 2000; 342: 381–8.

56. Khaw K-T, Wareham N, Luben R et al. Glycated haemoglobin, diabetes and mortality in men in Norfolk cohort of European Prospective Investigation of Cancer and Nutrition (EPIC-Norfolk). BMJ 2001; 322: 15–18.

57. Donahue RP, Abbott RB, Reed DM, Katsuhiko Y. Post challenge glucose concentration and coronary heart disease in men of Japanese ancestry. Honolulu heart program. Diabetes 1987; 36: 689–92.

58. Newburgh LH. Control of the 'hyperglycemia of obese diabetics' by weight reduction. Ann Intern Med 1942; 17: 935–42.

59. Turner RC. Ineffectiveness of diet in Type II diabetes. Quantitation of weight loss needed to induce basal normoglycemia. Diabetes Res Clin Prac 1988; 5(Suppl 1): S325.

60. Kosaka K Kuzuya T, Akanuma Y, Hagura R. Increase in insulin response after treatment of overt maturity onset diabetes is independent of the mode of treatment. Diabetologia 1980; 18: 23–8.

61. Hirsch S, Norton M, Harrington P. Education increases rate of near normoglycemic remission in newly diagnosed NIDDM. Diabetes 1995; Suppl 142, 25A (abstract).

62. Banerji MA, Chaiken RC, Lebovitz HE. Prolongation of near-normoglycemic remission in black NIDDM subjects with chronic low-dose sulfonylurea treatment. Diabetes 1995; 44: 466–70.

63. Lebovitz HE. Insulin secretagogues: old and new. Diabetes Rev 1999; 7: 139–53.

64. Grimber A, Ferry RJ Jr, Kelly A et al. Dysregulation of insulin secretion in children with congenital hyperinsulinemia due to sulfonylurea receptor mutations. Diabetes 2001; 50: 322–8.

65. McFarlane SI, Chaiken RL, Hirsch S et al. Near normoglycemic remission in African–Americans with Type 2 diabetes mellitus is associated with recovery of beta-cell function. Diabetic Medicine 2001; 18: 10–16.

66. Guz Y, Nasir I, Teitelman G. Regeneration of pancreatic beta-cells from intra-islet precursor cells in an experimental model of diabetes. Endocrinology 2001; 142: 4956–68.

67. Leahy JR, Cooper HE, Deal DA, Weir G. Chronic hyperglycemia is associated with impaired glucose influence on insulin secretion: a study in normal rats using chronic in vivo glucose infusion. J Clin Invest 1986; 77: 908–15.

68. Rosetti L, Schulman GI, Zawalich W, DeFronzo RA. Effect of acute and chronic hyperglycemia on in vivo insulin secretion in partially pancreatectomized rats. J Clin Invest 1987; 80: 1037–40.

69. Yki-Jarvinen H. Glucose toxicity. Endocrin Rev 1992; 13: 415–31.

70. Leibowitz G, Yui M, Donath MY et al. Beta-cell glucotoxicity in the *Psammomys obesus* model of Type 2 diabetes Diabetes 2001; Suppl 1.: S113–17.

71. Boden G, Ruiz J, Kim C-J, Chex X. Effects of prolonged glucose infusion on insulin secretion, clearance and action in normal subjects. Am J Physiol 1996; 270: E251–8.

72. Maedler K, Spinas GA, Lehman R et al. Glucose induces beta beta-cell apoptosis via up regulation of the Fas receptor in human islets Diabetes 2001; 50: 1683–90.

73. McGarry JD. What if Minkowski had been ageusic? An alternative angle on diabetes. Science 1992; 258: 766–70.

74. Boden G et al. Effects of fat on insulin stimulated carbohydrate metabolism in normal men. J Clin Invest 1991; 88: 960–6.

75. Schulman GI. Cellular mechanisms of insulin resistance. J Clin Invest 2000; 106: 171–6

76. Shimabukuro M, Zhou Y-T, Levi M, Unger RH. Fatty acid induced beta-cell apoptosis: A link between obesity and diabetes. Proc Natl Acad Sci USA 1998; 95: 2498–502.

77. Maedler K, Spinas GA, Dyntar D et al. Distinct effects of saturated and monounsaturated fatty acids on beta-cell turnover and function Diabetes. 2001; 50: 69–76.

78. Carpentier A, Mittleman SD, Lamarche B et al. Acute enhancement of insulin secretion by FFA in humans is lost with prolonged FFA elevation. Am J Physiol 1999;276. Endocrinol Metab 1999; 39: E1055–E1066.

28

New treatments for prevention of insulin resistance and diabetes complications: PKC involvement

Judith RC Jacobs, Net Daş-Evcimen, George L King

Many different factors participate in the development of diabetic complications and insulin resistance. Hyperglycemia has been shown to be responsible for the development and progression of microvascular diseases involving the retina, glomeruli and neuronal tissues in both Type 1 and Type 2 diabetes.[1,2] The Diabetes Control and Complications Trial (DCCT) demonstrated that intensive insulin therapy, to achieve near euglycemia, can delay the onset and retard the progression of diabetic retinopathy, nephropathy, neuropathy and, potentially, cardiac abnormalities.[1] The UK Prospective Diabetes Study (UKPDS) showed that intensive blood glucose control in Type 2 diabetes decreased the risk of microvascular end points associated with the retina and kidney.[2] The molecular mechanisms for the development of vascular dysfunction due to hyperglycemia are being intensively studied. Several mechanisms have been proposed to explain the adverse effects of elevated glucose levels, including the polyol pathway, oxidative stress, non-enzymatic glycation and the diacylglycerol protein kinase C (DAG–PKC) activation. In addition, insulin resistance and the associated hyperinsulinemia have been reported to be independent risk factors for cardiovascular diseases.[3–5]

In this chapter we will primarily focus on the hyperglycemia-induced DAG–PKC pathway activation in the pathogenesis of complications in diabetes mellitus.

Protein kinase C (PKC) is a family of structurally and functionally related proteins derived from multiple genes or, in the case of PKC isoforms βI and βII, from alternative splicing of a single mRNA transcript.[6,7] Members of the PKC superfamily are involved in a variety of physiological processes, including protein synthesis, transcriptional regulation, cell growth, differentiation and apoptosis.[8–10] PKC is a single polypeptide with an amino-terminal regulatory domain and a carboxyl-terminal catalytic region. The kinase can be divided into four conserved domains (C1–C4) with five variable regions (V1–V5). The regulatory domain consists of the C1 and C2 regions, whereas the C3 and C4 regions belong to the catalytic domain (Figure 28.1). The C1 region, containing two cysteine-rich zinc finger-like regions, binds DAG and phorbol esters. The C2 region is involved in the Ca^{2+}-dependent membrane binding. The C3 region, part of the catalytic domain, is responsible for ATP binding and the C4 region keeps the enzyme in an inactive state during the absence of activators and co-factors.[11]

Differences in the structure and substrate requirements of the PKC family members divide the different PKC isoforms into three groups:[12–17]

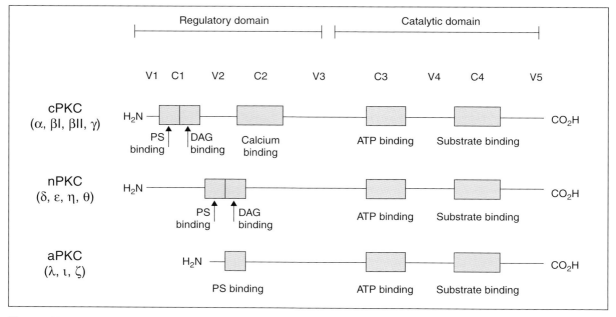

Figure 28.1
Structure of PKC isoforms according to their subgroups. Regulatory and catalytic domains are displayed. The four conserved (C1 to C4) and five variable (V1 to V5) regions are indicated. PS, phosphatidylserine; DAG, diacylglycerol; ATP, adenosine tri-phosphate.

(1) The conventional or cPKCs include the PKC isoforms α, βI, βII and γ, are calcium- and phospholipid-dependent, and can be activated by phosphatidylserine (PS), Ca^{2+} and DAG.

(2) The novel or nPKCs include the PKC isoforms δ, ε, η, and θ, are calcium-independent. They lack the C2 region and one of the zinc finger-like cysteine-rich motifs in the C1 region as well.

(3) The atypical or aPKCs, including the PKC isoforms ζ and ι/λ, do not require Ca^{2+} or DAG for activation, but PS is able to regulate the activity.

PKC isoforms are widely distributed in mammalian tissues, but possess tissue-specific expression patterns. For example PKC γ is expressed mainly in the central nervous system and spinal cord. PKC β is present in pancreatic islet cells, monocytes, brain and in many vascular tissues including retina, kidney and heart, and PKC θ is mainly present in skeletal muscle and hematopoietic cells.[8,12,14,18,19] Besides the variation in distribution, there is a difference in activation patterns depending on the intracellular localization. For example, PKC α isoform is observed mainly in the plasma membrane when activated, whereas PKC βI and βII are located in perinuclear regions.[20]

Regulation of PKC

Biochemical and biophysical studies have revealed that PKC activity is regulated by different lipid co-factors,[9,17] by phosphorylation events[17] or by specific binding proteins.[17,21] PKC

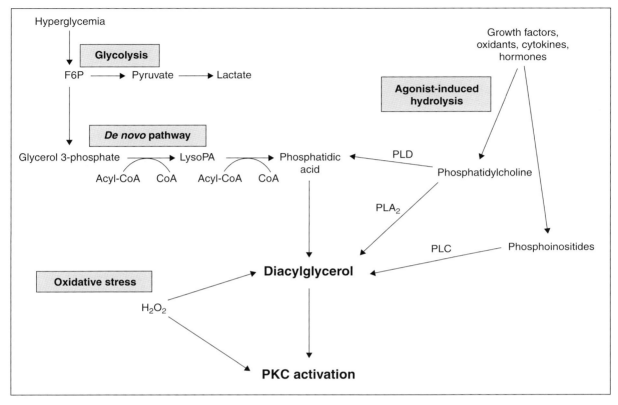

Figure 28.2
Pathways leading to DAG-PKC activation. Hyperglycemia induces DAG increases mainly by de novo synthesis and possibly from phosphatidylcholine by activation of PLC and PLD. F6P, fructose-6-phosphate; acyl-CoA, acyl-coenzyme A; CoA, coenzyme A; PLD, phospholipase D; PLA$_2$ phospholipase A$_2$; PLC, phospholipase C.

isoforms are typically activated at the plasma or nuclear membrane by forming a complex with DAG and different phospholipids, which lead to a conformational change.[8,9] This change in PKC structure will remove the pseudosubstrate sequence from the C4 region and subsequently allow the enzyme to bind its protein substrate.[22] Intracellular release of DAG, resulting in PKC activation, can be derived from different sources. As shown in Figure 28.2, phospholipase C (PLC)-mediated hydrolysis of phosphoinositides, phospholipase D (PLD)-mediated hydrolysis of phosphatidylcholine, conversion by phospholipase A$_2$ (PLA$_2$) and *de novo* synthesis from phosphatidic acid increases the DAG turnover.

The activation of calcium-dependent PKC isoforms induces receptor-mediated activation of PLC and results in generation of DAG and inositol-(1,4,5)-triphosphate (IP3) from membrane-associated phosphatidyl inositol-(4,5)-biphosphate. The formed IP3 stimulates the release of intracellular calcium, which then binds to the C2 region of the PKC enzyme and promotes its translocation from the cytosol to the plasma membrane.[8]

Co-factor regulation within each PKC isoform is similar, suggesting that other regulatory mechanisms are involved in the differential modulation of the multiplicity of isoform function. Phosphorylation processes might play a role, as phosphoinositide-dependent protein kinase-1 (PDK-1) can phosphorylate and thereby directly activate the PKC isoform. This transphosphorylation by PDK-1 is followed by autophosphorylation at two additional serine/threonine residues specific for the PKC isoform.

Some PKC isoforms can also be activated through tyrosine phosphorylation within the regulatory domain such as in response to H_2O_2, a non-receptor-coupled mechanism that has been shown to tyrosine phosphorylate and activate PKC δ.[23] However the role of tyrosine phosphorylation in PKC activation is still unclear. Another mechanism to regulate PKC activity within a cell is the use of receptors for activated C kinase (RACKs). These receptors are specific binding proteins and are isoform selective; there might be different RACKs for each PKC isoform, which provides another mode to regulate PKC activities.

Glucose-induced PKC activity

Many *in vivo* and *in vitro* studies have shown increased DAG and PKC levels in tissues of

	DAG	PKC	Species	Reference
Cultured cells				
Aortic endothelial	↑	↑	Rat, bovine	28
Aortic smooth muscle	↑	↑	Rat, human	28, 29, 135
Retinal endothelial	↑	↑	Bovine	66
Retinal pericytes	ND	↑	Bovine	66
Renal mesangial	↑	↑	Rat	34, 43
Tissues				
Aorta	↑	↑	Rat, canine	26, 27, 29, 137
Heart	↑	↑	Rat, human	27
Retina	↑	↑	Rat, canine	19, 26
Renal glomeruli	↑	↑	Rat	24, 25, 36 38, 138
Liver	↑	↑	Rat, human	39
Monocytes	ND	↑	Human	41
Granulation tissue	↑	ND	Rat	152
Brain	↔	↔	Rat	19
Peripheral nerve	↔,↓	↑,↓,↔	Rat	44, 45, 46, 47, 48, 143

↑ = increase, ↓ = decrease, ↔ = unchanged, ND = not determined in references cited

Table 28.1
Summary of alterations in DAG levels and PKC activity in cultured vascular cells exposed to high glucose concentrations and in vascular tissues from diabetic patients and animals

diabetic animals and patients including the retina,[19,24–26] aorta,[27–29] heart,[27,29–32] renal glomeruli,[25,33–38] liver,[39,40] skeletal muscle[40] and monocytes.[41] (see Table 28.1) Vascular cell culture studies showed that the causal role of increased DAG levels is hyperglycemia. Glucose elevation in cell culture from 5.5 to 22 mmol/l for up to 3–5 days increased DAG in retinal endothelial cells,[19] aortic endothelial cells, smooth muscle cells[27] and in renal mesangial cells.[42,43] Xia et al. reported that DAG levels were elevated in the aorta of diabetic rats and dogs after 2–4 months of diabetes and even after 5 years of disease.[26] Inoguchi et al. demonstrated that euglycemic control by islet cell transplantation for three weeks reversed

the increased DAG and PKC levels in the heart, but not in the aorta of the diabetic rats.[27] These results clearly suggest that the activation of DAG and PKC can be sustained chronically, but may be difficult to reverse.

Hyperglycemia-induced PKC activity appears to be tissue specific and PKC isoform specific. No consistent alteration in PKC activity was found in the central nervous system or in peripheral nerves. Studies performed in peripheral nerves showed conflicting results, as one study reported an increase in PKC activity, whereas other studies showed a decrease or no alteration in PKC activity.[44–48] The DAG levels are decreased in nerves of diabetic rats. As shown in Table 28.2, there seems to be a

Tissue and cultured cell type	PKC isoforms detected in normal tissue	PKC isoforms activated by high glucose/diabetes	References
Rat aorta	α, βII	βII	27
Rat aortic smooth muscle cells	α, βII	βII	28, 29
Rat heart	α, βII	βII	27
	α, β, δ, ε, γ	α>δ	30
	α, β, δ, ε, ζ	α	31
Rat cardiac myocytes	δ, ε	ε	32
Rat retina	α, βI, βII, ε	βII>ε>α>βI	19
Bovine retinal endothelial cells	α, βI, βII, δ, ε, ζ	δ>βII>α>βI	66
Rat kidney	α, βI, βII, δ, ε, ζ	α, ε	31
Rat glomeruli	α, βI, βII, δ, ε	α=βI	136
	α, βII, δ, ε	βII	24
	α, βII, δ, ε	ε>δ>α	35
Rat mesangial cells	α, δ, ε, ζ	ζ>α	37
Rat corpus cavernosum	α, βI, βII, δ, ε	βII	151
Rat sciatic nerve	α, βI, βII, δ, ε	No difference	45
	α, βI, βII, γ	α	47

Table 28.2
Summary of PKC isoforms, detected by immunoblot, in cultured vascular cells and vascular tissues in healthy conditions and in high glucose concentrations or in the diabetic state

preferential increase of PKC isoforms β and δ in diabetic vascular tissues and in vascular cells exposed to high glucose levels. However other isoforms, like PKC α, ε and ζ, were also reported to be increased in some vascular tissues of diabetic animals.

Elevation of DAG levels can be derived from different pathways (Figure 28.2). However the increase in DAG levels by hyperglycemia has been shown to be caused by *de novo* synthesis and phospholipase D activation. DAG can be synthesized *de novo* from glycolytic intermediates by acetylation of glucose by glycerol-3-monoacyl-phosphate acyltransferase and glycerol-3-monoacylglycerol-3-phosphate acyltransferase. Metabolic labeling studies have shown that glucose incorporates into the glycerol backbone of DAG,[26,27,49] and that this process is increased during exposure to high glucose. Activation of phospholipase D, which metabolizes phosphotidylcholine into phosphatidic acid, can also result in an increase in DAG levels.[50] Both mechanisms may be increased in diabetes. The third possible mechanism for increasing DAG levels in diabetes is the result of glyco-oxidation production. Oxidants like H_2O_2 can also activate PKC by increasing the DAG production via the activation of PKC γ.[23,51]

PKC activation in diabetes

Many biochemical, biological, and pathological manifestations of diabetic complications have been associated with increased PKC activation (Figure 28.3). Some of these changes include vascular contractility, blood flow alterations, basement membrane thickening and extracellular matrix expansion, vascular permeability, angiogenesis, cell growth and enzymatic activity alterations such as Na+-K+-ATPase, cPLA₂, and MAP kinases.

Vascular contractility and blood flow alteration

The most prominent features occurring early in the course of diabetes are hemodynamic changes such as blood flow and vascular contractility changes. Hemodynamic changes have been reported in many organs including the kidney, retina, skin, arteries and peripheral nerves in the diabetic state. The relaxation phase in large peripheral arteries after acetylcholine stimulation is delayed or blunted in diabetic patients.[52,53] This impaired vascular relaxation can be mimicked by phorbol ester and restored by PKC inhibitors,[54,55] suggesting an important role for PKC activation in causing these hemodynamic abnormalities. In the following, PKC-induced changes in specific tissues of clinical relevance to diabetes will be discussed.

Retina

Many studies have reported that retinal blood flow is altered in diabetes. The changes appear to be dependent on duration of the disease.[56-60] In patients with a short duration of diabetes, the retinal blood flow is decreased without a dilation of major arteries. With longer duration of diabetes and presence of clinical retinopathy, retinal blood flow velocity becomes faster and results in a transition from negative to normal retinal blood flow. The mechanisms of these alterations are beginning to emerge.

Intra-vitreal injection of phorbol ester, a PKC activator, reduced retinal blood flow in normal rats.[19] Streptozotocin-induced diabetic rats develop decreased retinal blood flow in parallel with increases in PKC activation. Intra-vitreal or oral administration of PKC inhibitors, including the PKC β specific inhibitor LY333531, decreased retinal PKC activity, and the retinal mean circulation time with normalization of retinal blood flow in diabetic rats (Figure 28.3).[61]

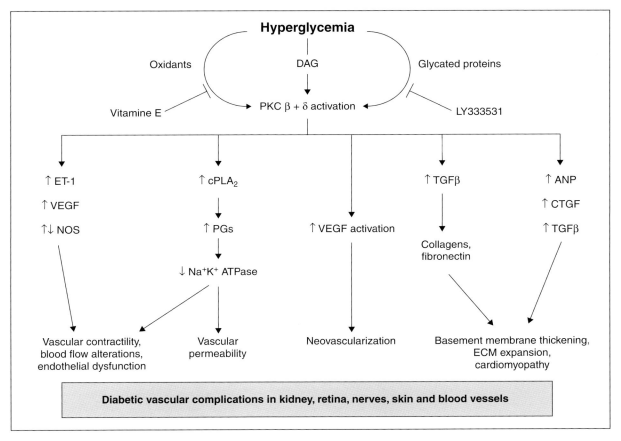

Figure 28.3
Cellular and physiological effects of DAG-PKC activation induced by hyperglycemia and the potential sites of action for vitamin E and PKCβ isoform inhibitor LY333531. DAG, diacyl glycerol; ET-1, endothelin-1; VEGF, vascular endothelial growth factor; NOS, nitric oxide synthase; cPLA₂ cytosolic phospholipase A₂; PGs, prostaglandins; TGFβ, transforming growth factor beta; ANP, atrial natriuretic peptide; CTGF, connective tissue growth factor; ECM, extracellular matrix.

Alterations in vasotropic factors like vascular endothelial growth factor (VEGF), endothelin-1 (ET-1) and nitric oxide (NO) are likely to be involved in PKC-mediated blood flow changes in diabetes. VEGF is an angiogenic growth factor, which increases endothelial cell proliferation, and permeability. In retinal ischemic diseases, like diabetic retinopathy, VEGF expression is increased which can increase capillary permeability and induces intra-ocular neovascularization.[62] The newly formed vessels in the retina are fragile, which can lead to macula edema, even hemorrhaging and eventually fibrosis. PKC activation has also been implicated both in the expression and signaling of VEGF's effects on capillary permeability and angiogenic actions.

ET-1 is a potent vasoconstrictor, secreted mainly by endothelial cells, and mediates many of its effects through PKC activation. Increased expression of ET-1 has been reported in the retina and other tissues from diabetic rats.[63,64] Diabetic rats exhibit decreased retinal blood flow after one month of diabetes, and the reduced blood flow was prevented by bosentan, an endothelin receptor antagonist.[63] Furthermore, intra-vitreal injection of ET-1 causes prolongation of retinal circulation times and retinal artery constriction in normal rats. This response to ET-1 was blunted in diabetic rats.[65] Exposure of capillary bovine retinal endothelial cells and bovine retinal pericytes to high glucose levels increased membranous PKC activity and ET-1 expression, which were reduced by the PKC inhibitor GF109203X.[66]

Multiple groups have reported that vasodilation induced by NO production is blunted in the diabetic state due to either decreases in NO production or being neutralized by oxidants.[67–70] Inhibition of PKC enabled the reduced NO production or effects to be normalized. Thus, PKC activations can either inhibit NO actions or production by decreasing eNOS expressions or activities. A dose-dependent reduction of NO synthesis occurred in cultured retinal microvascular endothelial cells exposed to high glucose. Co-incubation with PKC inhibitors, calphostin and staurosporine, increased NO synthesis, suggesting that PKC activation can inhibit eNOS expression or activities in retinal microvascular endothelial cells.[71] Inoguchi et al. reported that PKC inhibitors prevent the effect of high glucose levels on activation of NAD(P)H oxidase in vascular cells, suggesting PKC activation can also enhance O- products to neutralize NO.[72]

Kidney
In early stages of diabetic nephropathy in the presence of hyperglycemia, glomerular filtration rate is increased in both diabetic patients and animal models of diabetes.[73–75] Since the increase in renal plasma flow is rather small,

the increased glomerular filtration might be related to changes in arteriolar resistance of the afferent and efferent arterioles.[76] The involvement of several mechanisms has been proposed in diabetes-induced glomerular hyperfiltration, and PKC activity appears to be involved in many of these pathophysiological pathways. Activation of PKC in renal glomeruli of multiple animal species has been reported in spontaneously occurring or chemically-induced diabetes. Furthermore PKC activation has also been implicated in increasing permeability of endothelial cells to albumin, and stimulates matrix protein synthesis in mesangial cells. Vasoactive factors like prostaglandins (PGs) E_2, I_2, and F_2-α are increased in diabetic rats and might play a role in increasing vascular permeability.[77,78] In cultured glomerular mesanglial cells, PG E_2, F_2-α and, in some studies, thromboxane levels also, were increased when exposed to high glucose.[77,79] Furthermore arachidonic acid release is increased in diabetes by the increased cytosolic enzyme phospholipase A_2 ($cPLA_2$). PKC activation may be involved since PKC can phosphorylate serine residues of $cPLA_2$.[80] Besides PKC activation, hyperglycemia itself can increase $cPLA_2$ by activating p38 MAP kinase, which has been shown to activate $cPLA_2$.[81] PKC inhibitors, H-7, staurosporine and LY333531 have all been reported to prevent hyperglycemia-induced increases in arachidonic acid release and prostaglandin production.[79,82]

The vasodilator NO may also contibute to the increases of blood flow and glomerular hyperfiltration in diabetes. NO synthesis may be increased in renal tissues of diabetes, as measured by the reduction in NO2-/NO3- levels in the urine and plasma of diabetic rats. NO synthesis inhibitor nitro-L-arginine reduced renal blood flow and glomerular filtration rate,[83] suggesting that NO may contribute to glomerular hyperfiltration in diabetes. Another pathway to increase NO synthesis in diabetes is through cytokines. Enhanced expressions of inducible NO synthase (iNOS) and NO^{2-} production were observed in cytokine-stimulated glomerular mesanglial cells exposed to high glucose levels.[84] PKC inhibitors, H-7 and staurosporine, decreased NO^{2-} in cytokine-stimulated cells exposed to high glucose, indicating that PKC is involved in cytokine-inducible process of NO formation.[61] On the other hand, NO production and cyclic GMP generation in response to cholinergic stimuli could be impaired in glomeruli of diabetic rats.[85-87] PKC inhibition partly restored the decreased cyclic GMP response in the glomeruli from diabetic rats, suggesting PKC activation can suppress constitutive NO-mediated cyclic GMP responses.[85] Further-more, a decrease in neuronal constitutive NOS (cNOS) mRNA was observed in juxta-glomerular macula dense cells of diabetic rats.[88] The decreased cNOS can inhibit renin secretion and thereby induce glomerular hyperfiltration.[89,90] Another group showed a reduction in NO production in the early stage of streptozotocin-induced diabetes in rats. Total NOS activity in the renal cortex was reduced starting 30 hours after the induction of diabetes, and was associated with decreased levels of neuroneal NOS activity and protein in the macula densa.[91]

These studies show that both increased NO synthesis and decreased NO synthesis are involved in the regulation of renal hemodynamics, and glucose-induced PKC activation is at least partly involved in these pathways. Further studies need to clarify the apparently conflicting results on NO-induced glomerular filtration rates in diabetic animals, which could be due to tissue differences in the regulation of NO production.

Nerves

Abnormalities in hemodynamics such as decreased endoneural blood flow and possibly ischemia have been documented in diabetic neuropathy. Furthermore, decreases in axonal transport, nerve conduction velocity and impaired axon regeneration are observed in experimental diabetic neuropathy.

Different studies have reported conflicting results regarding PKC activities in neuronal tissues from diabetic animals (Table 28.1). It has been proposed that increases in polyol pathway flux may cause changes in the phosphoinositide turnover, leading to reduction of DAG levels resulting in a decreased PKC activity in diabetes. Decreases in the neuronal PKC activity may reduce the Na^+-K^+-ATPase phosphorylation leading to deficits in nerve conduction and nerve degeneration. According to this theory, PKC inhibition should promote the nerve defects. However, recent studies, using PKC β inhibitor, have reported improvement in peripheral nerve function in diabetic animals. Thus it is likely that high glucose can activate PKC activities in the vasa nervorum, which secondarily can increase contractile responsiveness and diminish blood flow. PKC inhibition could then be useful to enhance perfusion and improve nerve dysfunction in the vasa nervorum. Animal studies have reported that streptozotocin-induced diabetic rats develop delayed motor nerve conduction velocity, reduced sciatic nerve blood flow and prolonged peak latencies of oscillatory potentials. PKC activities in diabetic animals have reported no change or decreases in total PKC activities in the peripheral nerves. These functional abnormalities were reduced by LY333531 treatment, a PKC β specific inhibitor,[48] which suggests a potential role of PKC β in diabetes-induced neuropathy. Diabetic rats treated with WAY151003, a non-isoform specific PKC inhibitor, have also shown improvement to motor nerve conduction velocity, correct decreased nerve blood flow and partially improve Na+-K+-ATPase activity.[44] The benefits of WAY151003 on blood flow and conduction velocity were blocked by a nitric oxide synthase inhibitor;[44] this suggests that PKC contributes to diabetic neuropathy by a neurovascular mechanism.

Extracellular matrix change and thickening of basement membrane

In early diabetes, the most prominent structural abnormalities of vasculature or mesangium are capillary basement thickening and extracellular matrix (ECM) expansion. These changes are associated with altered vascular permeability, cellular adhesion, proliferation, differentiation and gene expression. Multiple studies have shown that changes in the basement membrane, including increases in collagens Type IV and VI, fibronectin and decreases in proteoglycans, can be caused by high glucose levels.[42,92–94] PKC agonists are capable of stimulating collagen Type I and IV expression and fibronectin accumulation *in vitro* and PKC inhibitors are able to reduce ECM production, locating a possible causal role in these abnormalities of the basement membrane to PKC.[43,95]

Furthermore, growth factors play a key role in basement membrane thickening and increasing ECM. For example, transforming growth factor β (TGF-β) and connective tissue growth factor (CTGF) are important in these processes since they increase collagen, fibronectin and laminin synthesis. PKC activation is involved in hyperglycemia-induced increased expression of TGF-β by stimulating AP-1 binding sites on the transcription factors c-fos and c-jun. Promotor regions of TGF-β, fibronectin and laminin contain the AP-1 binding consensus sequences, therefore PKC can regulate the transcription of genes expressing these growth factors (see Figure 28.3).

Vascular permeability, cell growth and angiogenesis

Increases in vascular permeability to different circulating small or macromolecules in all vessels is one of the earliest and most consistent findings in diabetic animals and patients. For example increased permeation of Evan's blue dye, fluorescens, albumin and other labeled molecules have been reported in the eye, sciatic nerve, aorta and kidney.[96] PKC activator, PMA, can also increase the permeability of endothelial and epithelial cells to macromolecules including albumin, whereas PKC inhibition reduced the increased permeability.[97] In another study, rat skin chamber granulation tissue exposed to high glucose or phorbol esters increased microvascular clearance, and this effect was restored by the PKC inhibitor staurosporine.[98] Human dermal endothelial cells overexpressing PKC βI increased the endothelial permeability, measured by transendothelial albumin clearance rate.[99] Another group showed the involvement of PKC α activation in glucose-induced increases in cell permeability in porcine aortic endothelial cells using a specific antisense oligonucleotide against PKC α.[100] These studies have indicated that at least the activation of PKC α and β are involved in diabetes-induced increased vascular permeability, which might lead to diabetic macula edema and nephropathy (See Figure 28.3).

The causal mechanisms are not clear, but it has been suggested that PKC activation can stimulate the contractile apparatus of endothelial cells, which phosphorylates the specific cytoskeletal proteins forming the tight junctions such as caldesmon, vimentin, talin and vinculin. Phosphorylation of these proteins can lead to vascular permeability. Another mechanism of diabetes-induced vascular permeability is the overexpression or dysregulation of various growth factors, e.g. vascular endothelial growth factor (VEGF) or vascular permeability factor (VPF). VEGF stimulates cell growth, vascular permeability and hypoxia-induced angiogenesis. Diabetic patients with retinopathy have increased levels of VEGF in their ocular fluid, suggesting that VEGF contributes to neovascularization in diabetic retinopathy.[62] Furthermore, in human aortic smooth muscle cells exposed to high glucose, increased VEGF expressions have been reported, which can be prevented by PKC inhibitors.[101] VEGF administration to rats caused an increase in membrane translocation of PKC isoforms α, βII and δ,[102] indicating that these isoforms are activated. PKC isoforms α, βII and δ are involved in VEGF-induced neovascularization in diabetes. In both retina and glomerula, VEGF mRNA expressions are increased in diabetic rats. In contrast, VEGF mRNA expression is decreased in the myocardium in the diabetic or insulin resistance state. Treatment with PKC β selective inhibitor compound LY333531 in diabetic rats normalized the actions of VEGF in retina and renal tissues rather than reducing VEGF expression, but LY333531 had no effect in the myocardium.[103] Furthermore, VEGF can mediate its mitogenic and vascular permeability-inducing effect by activating PKC β through tyrosine phosphorylation of phospholipase C (PLC). The PKC β selective PKC inhibitor LY333531 prevented VEGF-induced endothelial proliferation, angiogenesis and permeability both *in vitro* and *in vivo*.[102]

Na+-K+-ATPase activity change

The levels of Na+-K+-adenosine triphosphate, an essential component of the sodium pump, are decreased in cardiovascular and neuronal tissues of both diabetic patients and animals. The sodium pump plays an important role in cellu-

lar functions including cell contractility, growth and differentiation. During hyperglycemia, PKC activity and cytosolic phospholipase A_2 (cPLA$_2$) activity increases, resulting in the elevation of arachidonic acid release, prostaglandin E_2 (PGE$_2$) production and inhibition in Na+-K+-ATPase activity.[82] Glucose-induced Na+-K+-ATPase inhibition can be prevented by cPLA$_2$ inhibitors and PKC inhibitors, suggesting that PKC activation is involved in the diabetes-induced decrease in Na+-K+-ATPase activity. In some tissues, PKC can regulate Na+-K+-ATPase levels by phosphorylation and dephosphorylation processes of its α-subunit.

However, studies have revealed some conflicting data regarding the role of PKC on Na+-K+-ATPase activity. The paradoxic results could be explained by the use of phorbol ester in some experiments. Phorbol ester, which is not a physiological PKC activator, activates many PKC isoforms with a five- to ten-fold increase. In contrast, the pathophysiological hyperglycemia-induced PKC activation is a PKC isoform selective process and is restricted to a two-fold increase in PKC activity. Therefore, the results derived from experiments using phorbol esters should be interpreted with some caution.

Insulin resistance and PKC

PKC activation has been reported to influence insulin production, insulin signaling pathways and insulin actions. Some groups claim that PKC can activate insulin actions, whereas other groups reported a PKC-induced decrease in insulin signaling (see Considine and Caro[104]), Figure 28.4. This apparent contradiction is probably the result of PKC isoforms, which may play different roles in insulin actions. However, it is still unknown which isoforms are mainly causing changes of insulin actions in different

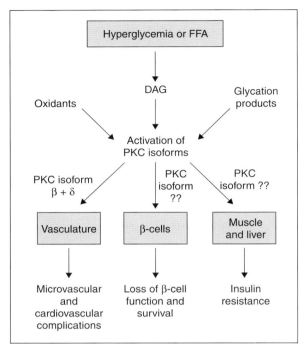

Figure 28.4
Effects of nutritional-induced activation of DAG-PKC pathway on insulin secretion, insulin action and diabetic complications.

cell types. After insulin binds to the α-subunit of the insulin receptor, the β-subunit of the insulin receptor activates and undergoes autophosphorylation. The insulin receptor substrate (IRS) binds, and different signaling pathways are activated, including the PI3-kinase/Akt pathway, which is important for eNOS production in the vasculature, glucose uptake and protein synthesis in muscle, fat and liver.

Bollag et al.[105] showed that PKC can phosphorylate the solubilized insulin receptor resulting in a reduction of receptor tyrosine kinase activity. Takayama et al. reported that the insulin receptor is a substrate for PKC in a hepatoma cell line and that increased serine phosphorylation caused by phobol esters,

reduced insulin-induced tyrosine kinase activity *in vivo* and *in vitro*.[106] Koshio et al.[107] and Lewis et al.[108] identified threonine 1336 of insulin's β-subunit to be phosphorylated by PKC. These studies clearly indicate that PKC activation can disturb the insulin cascade by phosphorylating specific residues. PKC inhibitors were able to prevent glucose-induced insulin receptor tyrosine kinase inactivation.[109] It appears that different PKC isoforms are involved in the inactivation of insulin signaling cascade. For example PKC βI and βII were reported to phosphorylate the β-subunit of the insulin receptor, thereby inhibiting the insulin cascade.[110] Experiments in cultured human kidney embryonic cells (HEK 293) overexpressing different PKC isoforms demonstrated that PKC isoforms α, δ and θ require insulin receptor substrate-1 to inhibit the tyrosine kinase activity.[111] The same group showed that PKC θ and βII could phosphorylate serine residues 994 and 1023/25 of the insulin receptor which inhibit the insulin-induced insulin receptor autophosphorylation.[112] Others have reported that activation of PKC will stimulate an unknown kinase, which can phosphorylate IRS-1 at serine 612 in HEK 293 cells, resulting in inhibition of the insulin signaling cascade.[54]

PKC activation is also able to influence insulin signaling molecules downstream from IRS. The PKC-phosphorylated IRS proteins inhibited insulin-stimulated PI3-kinase and Akt activation, whereas PKC θ activation inhibited insulin-stimulated PI3-kinase activation. And PKC ζ impaires insulin signaling by IRS-1 phosphorylation accompanied by impaired IRS-1-associated PI3-kinase activation.[113] Overexpression of PKC ε in HEK 293 cells, resulted in both down-regulation of the insulin receptor and reduction in insulin-induced phosphorylation of Akt.[114] Furthermore the atypical PKC isoforms ζ and λ are able to reduce both Akt and PI3-kinase activities of the insulin signaling.

In *ex vivo* studies, rat soleus muscle pre-incubated with phorbol ester, a PKC activator, showed translocation of PKC α, βI, θ, ε and probably βII from cytosol to membranes, which correlated with the inhibition of insulin-stimulated activation of the insulin receptor tyrosine kinase and phosphorylation of Akt and glycogen synthase kinase-3.[115] The PKC β specific inhibitor, LY333531, was able to restore the blunted insulin-induced phosphorylation of Akt in the aorta of insulin resistant Zucker fa/fa rats (Naruse et al., unpublished data) suggesting that PKC β isoform activation is involved in the reduced insulin signaling of vascular tissues in the insulin resistant state.

Insulin resistance

PKC activation has been implicated in inducing insulin resistance in the presence of hyperglycemia or elevation of free fatty acids several models of insulin resistance. Increased PKC activity has been reported in association with insulin resistance in the liver[39] and muscle[116] from diabetic humans and rats. Insulin resistance caused by obesity,[117] aging,[118,119] muscle denervation, high fat diet[120] or high fructose diet[121] is associated with hyperglycemia-induced activation of DAG-PKC pathway in the liver, muscle and adipose tissues. High fat or high fructose diets are reported to activate PKC θ and PKC ε in muscle of rats.[120,121] High fat diet combined with an antilipolytic compound improved insulin sensitivity and reversed the increased expression of the two novel PKCs,[122] suggesting that activation of PKC isoforms θ and ε are involved in fat-induced insulin resistance. The sand rat, a nutritionally-induced diabetes animal model, which develops hyperinsulinemia, followed by hyperglycemia and finally diabetes, has a reduced insulin-induced activation of muscle insulin receptor tyrosine kinase, in association with overexpression of PKC ε.[116,123] This overexpression and translocation of PKC ε to the membrane was already present prior to the development of hyperinsulinemia, suggesting that PKC ε might be involved in the progression of nutritionally-induced diabetes.[114]

It has been suggested that PKC activation plays a role in the 'glucose toxicity'-induced insulin resistance by increasing serine phosphorylation of the insulin receptor.[124] Enhanced flux through the hexosamine biosynthesis pathway, another signaling cascade overexpressed during hyperglycemia, inhibits glucose transport in a PKC-mediated manner. Furthermore, the tumor necrosis factor-α (TNF-α), a pro-inflammatory cytokine-induced insulin resistance is reported to be mediated by PKC ε, β and ζ activation.[125–127]

Glucose transporters (GLUT) have also been reported to be targets of PKCs. Translocation of GLUT 4, an insulin sensitive glucose transporter, to both plasma membrane and T-tubules was impaired in muscle of rats on a high fat diet, and associated with elevated PKC ζ and λ activities.[125] Insulin action on regulating glycogen synthase (GS) activation has also been reported to be affected by PKC activation. PKC can phosphorylate GS directly, which stabilizes the GS in the inactive phosphorylated form and thereby reduces insulin's effect.[129] In the liver, PKC isoforms α, β and γ can phosphorylate glycogen synthase kinase-3β, an important GS regulating hepatic kinase,[130] and affect insulin's action indirectly. The role of PKC activation is unclear, since data to test directly the role of specific PKC isoforms in producing severe classical insulin resistance and diabetes *in vivo* have not been reported. All the results are correlations or produced in transformed cells, which makes the interpretation of the available data to a pathophysiological state questionable.

PKC inhibitors

Owing to the accumulating evidence that PKC activation has a substantial role in causing insulin resistance and complications in diabetes, a great deal of effort has been made in developing PKC inhibitors. Non-isoform specific PKC inhibitors have proven to be toxic, which is not surprising since PKC is an important family of kinases, involved in many different cellular processes. Thus, isoform specific inhibition is critical for *in vivo* studies, unless PKC inhibition is indirect such as with the use of vitamin E. At present most of the available data on PKC inhibitors in human diseases are focused on the treatment of cancer and diabetes complications. Very few studies are available with regard to insulin resistance since it is not clear which PKC isoforms are consistently involved in liver, muscle and fat. For vascular complications in diabetes, increased PKC β and δ isoform activities are consistently shown to be present in vascular tissues in the diabetic state (see Figure 28.4). In the following section, several PKC inhibitors will be discussed.

Rottlerin or mallotoxin, a natural product derived from *Mallotus philippinesis*, is an ATP-binding inhibitor, which has higher affinity for PKC δ (IC_{50}: 3–6 μM) but inhibits other PKC isoforms (IC_{50}: > 30 μM), protein kinase A (IC_{50}: 78 μM) and calmodulin (IC_{50}: 5,3 μM) as well. Staurosporine-derived compounds, such as indolocarbazole and bisindolylmaleimides, show better selectivity for PKC isoforms, in comparison with staurosporine. So far, all of these compounds have exhibited potent effect for non-PKC serine and threonine kinases, thus inducing too much toxicity for chronic use.

Another way to inhibit PKC activity is by decreasing PKC expression at genetic level. The principle of antisense oligonucleotides in PKC isoform inhibition is the sequence specific binding of an antisense oligonucleotide to the mRNA of the PKC isoform, resulting in the prevention of translation of that specific PKC isoform. Potentially, this method can be used for selective inhibition. Different human PKC isoforms have been used in cell culture studies and shown to be effective. The only agent used in humans to date is the compound ISIS3521, an oligonucleotide to human PKC α mRNA. In a Phase 1 trial, after intermittent intravenous infusion, it showed effective antitumor activity with only mild toxicity in patients with advanced cancer.[131]

Inhibition of PKC translocation is possible by PKC-binding proteins, like receptors for activated C kinases (RACKs). The PKC–RACK interaction for cPKC is partly mediated by the C2 region, therefore peptide inhibitors of PKC β translocation are derived from this domain.[132]

In the area of diabetes complications, only vitamin E and PKC β isoform selective inhibitor LY333531 have been extensively studied.

Vitamin E

Oxidative stress is suggested to be one of the underlying causes of diabetic vascular complications. Vitamin E (d-α-tocopherol) is an antioxidant and has therefore been of great interest with respect to the potential ability to ameliorate diabetic complications. Besides its antioxidant property, vitamin E has inhibitory effects on the DAG–PKC pathway in vascular tissues and cultured vascular cells exposed to elevated levels of glucose. DAG levels were decreased and PKC levels were normalized in retinal vascular endothelial cells and in rat aortic smooth muscle cells exposed to high glucose when treated with d-α-tocopherol at 10–50 μM.[29,133] This is different from the effect of direct PKC inhibitor which will not reduce DAG. Intraperitoneal injection of 40 mg/kg d-α-tocopherol decreased the membranous PKC activity and total DAG level in retina, aorta, heart and renal glomeruli of diabetic rats.[133–135] Vitamin E normalized retinal blood flow and ameliorated the glomerular filtration of diabetic rats in parallel with the inhibitory effects on DAG and PKC activation. Furthermore increased albuminuria was prevented by 40 mg/kg body weight vitamin E in diabetic rats.[136]

The mechanism of vitamin E's action on PKC inhibition is unclear since it requires concentrations at micromolar range which are much greater than needed for antioxidant actions. In addition the effect of vitamin E on PKC activity is indirect, because d-α-tocopherol did not inhibit purified PKC α or βII isoform activation *in vitro*.[133] Activation of DAG kinase by d-α-tocopherol has been suggested to be the site of action to increase the metabolic breakdown of DAG to phosphatidyl acid with decreased DAG levels and decreased PKC activity as a result.[136–138]

In a clinical study at the Joslin Diabetes Center,[139] 36 Type 1 diabetic patients, average duration of diabetes 4.3 ± 2.7 years with no evidence of clinical retinopathy, received a daily dose of 1800 IU (1350 mg) d-α-tocopherol for four months. Vitamin E significantly increased retinal blood flow (88% normalization) and normalized the renal hyperfiltration as measured by renal creatinine clearance levels. These effects occurred without any changes in Hb1Ac or fasting glucose levels. Plasminogen activator inhibitor-1 (PAI-1) plasma levels, which have been associated with vascular complications, also decreased in diabetic

patients during vitamin E supplementation. This study suggests that a high dose vitamin E treatment can normalize retinal blood flow and renal creatinine clearance in the early stages of diabetes, which could subsequently reduce the risk of developing pathological vascular complications of diabetes. In addition, the need for high doses of vitamin E also indicates that its effect is more than just neutralizing oxidants. Thus, doses of vitamin E that only neutralize oxidants would probably be ineffective.

This idea is supported by the results of the Heart Outcomes Prevention Evaluation (HOPE)[140] study which reported no beneficial effects on cardiovascular death in a high risk patient group, after a daily vitamin E intake of 400 IU for five years. Vitamin E administration at high doses could have preventative effects to reduce vascular complications in diabetes. More research is necessary to find the optimal dosage, time and duration of vitamin E treatment, and to find out which diabetic patient groups would benefit from vitamin E supplementation.

LY333531

As described above, preferential activation of PKC β isoform occurs in many vascular cells exposed to high glucose levels or vascular tissues of diabetic animals. LY333531 ((S)-13-[(dimethylamino)methyl]-10,11,14,15–tetrahydro-4,9:16,21-dimetheno-1H,13H-dibenzo[e,k] pyrrolo[3,4-h][1,4,13]oxadiazacyclohexadecene-1,3(2H)-dione) is a competitive inhibitor of ATP binding, presumably by interacting at the ATP binding site (see Figure 28.3).[141] This compound shows selectivity for PKC βI and βII, over PKC α and γ, the novel and atypical PKC isoforms, and is effective in the nanomolar concentration range. The half-maximal inhibitory constant (IC$_{50}$) of LY333531 to inhibit PKC βI and βII are respectively 4.5 and

5.9 nM, whereas the IC_{50} to inhibit other PKC isoforms is 250 nM or greater.[138] LY333531 shows selective inhibition of PKC over other ATP dependent kinases, including calcium calmodulin (1060-fold selective) and src tyrosine kinase (2200-fold selective).[141]

The PKC β selective inhibitor LY333531 reversed several high glucose-induced changes in cultured cells. Rat and human mesangial cells treated with LY333531 (20–200 nM) had a lower glucose-induced increase in PKC activity, arachidonic acid release and PGE_2 production and LY333531 treatment normalized Na^+-K^+-ATPase activity.[25] In addition, LY333531 significantly decreased elevated PKC activity in membrane fractions of failed human hearts, suggesting that selective inhibition of PKC β could be a suitable therapy for the prevention and treatment of heart failure.[142]

Ishii et al. reported that oral administration of 0.1–10 mg/kg body weight LY333531 in diabetic rats for up to 10 weeks reduced the elevated glomerular filtration rate, increased albumin excretion and decreased retinal mean circulation time (MCT).[24] No adverse side effects of the drug at these doses were observed in the animals. Intra-vitreal administration of 5 nM LY333531 decreased retinal PKC activity, decreased retinal MCT and increased blood flow in diabetic rats.[61] Another study showed normalization of diabetes-induced reductions in both Na^+-K^+-ATPase and Ca^{2+}-ATPase activity in the retina of diabetic rats by LY333531.[143] Furthermore, LY333531 attenuate the diabetes-induced disturbances in retinal microcirculatory flow involving the entrapment of leukocytes.[144] Animal models for ischemia-induced retinal disorders showed the potential effectiveness of LY333531 treatment in ischemia-induced complications.[145] Oral treatment of 50 mg/kg LY333531 in diabetic rats prevented decreased motor nerve conduction velocity and sciatic nerve blood flow, which

may be mediated by the reduction of ischemia in the endoneural microvasculature.[48] Reduced Na^+-K^+-ATPase activity in the glomeruli was also normalized, and increased levels of TGFβ, fibronectin and collagen IV in the glomeruli were reduced by 10 mg/kg LY333531 in diabetic rats for four weeks.[25]

Experiments in db/db mice, an animal model of Type 2 diabetes, showed a reduction in albumin excretion and amelioration of mesangial expansion after a long-term (16 weeks) LY333531 treatment (10 mg/kg).[38] Mice overexpressing PKC βII in the myocardium develop morphological and functional characteristics similar to cardiomyopathy. LY333531 treatment improved these histological and functional pathological changes.[146,147]

Outcomes of clinical studies using LY333531 are limited at this time. The first results of LY333531 treatment in humans are very promising. Aiello et al.[148,149] showed that LY333531 was well tolerated in a double-masked, randomized, placebo-controlled study for one month. A total of 29 Type 1 or 2 diabetic patients with no or minimal retinopathy and a disease duration of less than 10 years, received LY333531 orally up to 16 mg twice a day. The retinal blood flow and MCT were ameliorated in a dose-responsive manner. These observations, in the absence of altered fasting blood glucose or Hb1Ac, suggest that LY333531 treatment might be an effective intervention for retinopathy in diabetes. This study confirmed that PKC activation, especially the PKC β isoform, contributes to the pathogenesis of diabetic complications. Further clinical studies have been initiated to observe potential effects of the PKC β specific inhibitor LY333531 on diabetic neuropathy, and other vascular diseases.

In a recent study, Beckman et al. have shown that the impaired endothelium-dependent vasodilation caused by six hours of hyper-

29

Antioxidants in diabetic complications and insulin resistance

Joseph L Evans, Betty A Maddux, Ira D Goldfine

Introduction

Increased oxidative stress is associated with a variety of pathological conditions including diabetes, atherosclerosis and cardiovascular disease, and neurodegenerative diseases.[1–3] Oxidative stress is likely to play a causative role in the tissue and cellular damage in these diseases.[1,2] In particular, diabetes mellitus is strongly associated with increased oxidative stress, which could be a consequence of either increased production of free radicals, or reduced antioxidant defenses.[2,4]

In both Type 1 and Type 2 diabetes, late diabetic complications in nerve, vascular endothelial, and kidney arise from chronic elevations of glucose and other metabolites including free fatty acids (FFA). Recent evidence suggests that chronic activation of common stress-activated signaling pathways such as transcription factor nuclear factor-κB (NF-κB), p38 MAP kinase (MAPK), and the NH_2-terminal Jun kinases (JNK/SAPK) plays a major role in the etiology of these late diabetic complications. In addition, in Type 2 diabetes, there is evidence that the activation of these same stress pathways by glucose and FFA leads to both impaired insulin secretion and insulin resistance. Thus, we propose a unifying hypothesis whereby hyperglycemia and FFA-induced activation of NF-κB, p38 MAPK, and

JNK/SAPK stress pathways, along with the additional stress pathways, plays a key role in causing late complications in Type 1 and Type 2 diabetes, along with insulin resistance and impaired insulin secretion in Type 2 diabetes (Figure 29.1).[5] Studies with antioxidants such as α-lipoic acid (LA), vitamin E, and others suggest that new strategies may become available to treat these conditions.

Hyperglycemia and oxidative stress

A number of processes have been described to explain how hyperglycemia mediates its toxic effects both intra- and extracellularly.[6–9] A widely recurring theme is increased oxidative stress, defined as a persistent imbalance between the production of highly reactive molecular species (chiefly oxygen and nitrogen) and antioxidant defenses, leading to potential tissue damage. Many, though not all, experimental and clinical studies have found evidence of increased oxidative stress in diabetes.[2,4,10,11] Oxidative stress can result from either increased production of reactive oxygen species (ROS), or their inadequate removal (or both). Examples of ROS include charged species such as superoxide, hydroxyl radical, and uncharged species such as hydrogen peroxide (Table 29.1).

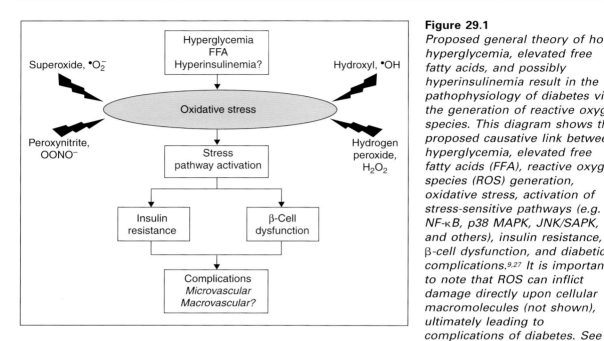

Figure 29.1
Proposed general theory of how hyperglycemia, elevated free fatty acids, and possibly hyperinsulinemia result in the pathophysiology of diabetes via the generation of reactive oxygen species. This diagram shows the proposed causative link between hyperglycemia, elevated free fatty acids (FFA), reactive oxygen species (ROS) generation, oxidative stress, activation of stress-sensitive pathways (e.g. NF-κB, p38 MAPK, JNK/SAPK, and others), insulin resistance, β-cell dysfunction, and diabetic complications.[9,27] It is important to note that ROS can inflict damage directly upon cellular macromolecules (not shown), ultimately leading to complications of diabetes. See text for details.

Type	Free-radicals	Non-radicals
Reactive oxygen species (ROS)	Superoxide, $\cdot O_2^-$ Hydroxyl, $\cdot OH$ Peroxyl, $\cdot RO_2^-$ Hydroperoxyl, $\cdot HO_2^-$	Hydrogen peroxide, H_2O_2 Hydrochlorous acid, HOCl
Reactive nitrogen species (RNS)	Nitric oxide, $\cdot NO$ Nitrogen dioxide, $\cdot NO_2^-$	Peroxynitrite, OONO- Nitrous oxide, HNO_2

Notes: Reactive oxygen and nitrogen species (ROS, RNS) are defined as highly reactive molecules including charged species such as superoxide, hydroxyl radical, and nitric oxide and uncharged species such as hydrogen peroxide. *Source:* Adapted from Rösen et al.[2]

Table 29.1
Selected examples of biologically important reactive species

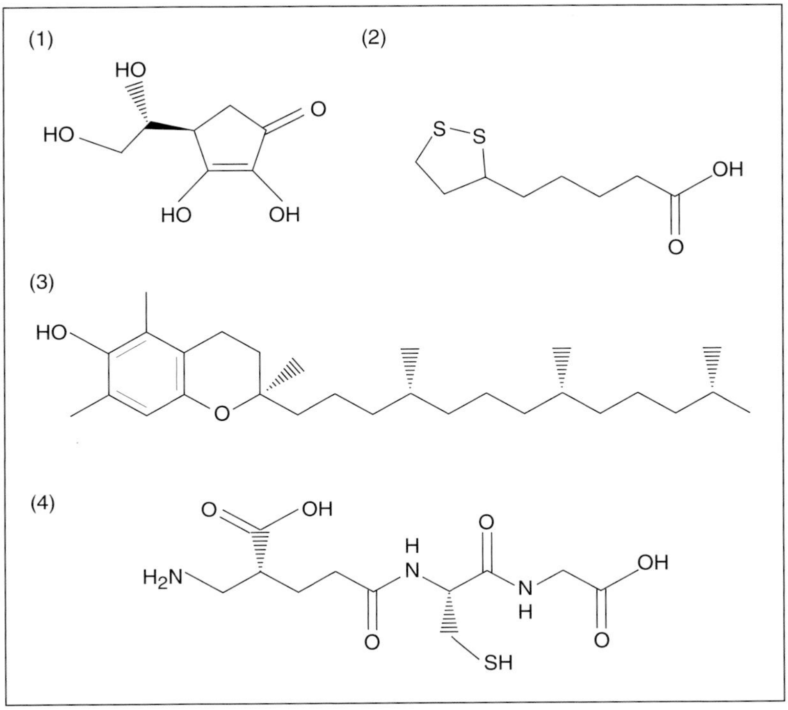

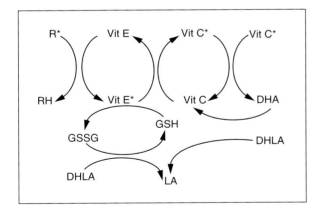

Figure 29.2
Chemical structures of vitamin C, α-lipoic acid, vitamin E, and glutathione. (1) Vitamin C, (2) α-lipoic acid, (3) Vitamin E (α-tocopherol), (4) Glutathione (γ-glutamylcysteinylglycine; reduced form, GSH).

Figure 29.3
Regeneration of vitamin E by α-lipoic acid (LA), dihydrolipoic acid (DHLA), vitamin C, and glutathione. The regeneration of vitamin E (Vit E) occurs through a cooperative set of reactions that can involve several antioxidants and other substances (e.g. NADH, NADPH).[13,14] Shown here is a highly simplified example of how dihydrolipoic acid (DHLA; bottom right), the reduced form of α-lipoic acid (LA), is able to convert dihydroascorbate (DHA) to vitamin C (Vit C), which is able to regenerate Vit E from Vit E*. In addition, DHLA (bottom left) is able to provide reducing equivalents to facilitate the conversion of glutathione, the major intracellular antioxidant, from its oxidized form (GSS) to its reduced form (GSH). GSH is also able to regenerate Vit E from Vit E*. Reducing equivalents for the conversion of LA to DHLA are provided by NADH or NADPH (not shown). Notes: R*, Vit C*, Vit E* = charged species. Source: figure reprinted with permission from Evans JL et al. Diabetes Technol Therapeut *2000; 2: 401–13.[69]*

There is considerable evidence to show that ROS formation is a direct consequence of hyperglycemia; more recent studies have suggested that ROS formation also results from increased FFA. Excessive production of ROS, or their inadequate neutralization by antioxidants, leads to the damage of proteins, lipids, and DNA.[12] In the absence of an appropriate compensatory response from the endogenous antioxidant network, the system becomes overwhelmed (redox imbalance). A major cellular antioxidant system is reduced glutathione (GSH), which is regenerated by vitamins C and E, LA and other antioxidants (Figures 29.2 and 29.3).[13,14] LA is a naturally occurring antioxidant and co-factor in the pyruvate dehydrogenase complex, and participates in establishing a cellular antioxidant network by raising intracellular glutathione levels.[15] LA has been shown to:

(1) quench free-radicals;
(2) prevent singlet oxygen induced DNA damage;
(3) chelate metals;
(4) reduce lipid peroxidation;
(5) increase intracellular glutathione levels; and
(6) prevent glycation of serum albumin.[13,14]

When the endogenous antioxidant network fails to provide a sufficient compensatory response to restore cellular redox balance, oxidative stress ensues.

In addition to their ability to directly inflict damage upon cellular macromolecules, ROS play a significant role in regulating gene expression. ROS activate multiple stress-sensitive intracellular signaling pathways such as NF-κB, p38 MAPK, JNK/SAPK, PKC, AGE/RAGE, sorbitol, and others. The consequence is the production of an array of gene products[14] that, in turn, cause cellular damage

and are ultimately responsible for the late complications of diabetes.

Hyperglycemia and stress-activated pathways

Hyperglycemia activates several major well characterized biochemical pathways that play a significant role in the development of diabetic complications, including AGE/RAGE,[17] PKC,[7] and the polyol pathway.[18] More recently, hyperglycemia has been implicated in the activation of additional biochemical pathways that appear to promote the development of the late complications of diabetes, along with exerting a negative influence on insulin action and insulin secretion. These pathways include the hexosamine pathway,[19-22] and the stress-activated signaling pathways including NF-κB, JNK/SAPK, and p38 MAP kinase pathways.[23,24]

The most extensively studied intracellular target of hyperglycemia and oxidative stress is the transcription factor nuclear factor-κB (NF-κB).[25] NF-κB plays a critical role in mediating immune and inflammatory responses, and apoptosis. NF-κB regulates the expression of a large number of genes, including growth factors (e.g. vascular endothelial growth factor; VEGF), pro-inflammatory cytokines (e.g. TNF-α, II-1β), the receptor for advanced glycation end products (RAGE), adhesion molecules (e.g. VCAM-1), and others. Many products of the genes regulated by NF-κB also, in turn, activate NF-κB (e.g. VEGF, TNF-α, II-1β, RAGE). The aberrant regulation of NF-κB is associated with a number of chronic diseases including diabetes and atherosclerosis. NF-κB is activated through a common pathway, which involves the phosphorylation-induced, proteasome-mediated degradation of the inhibitory subunit, IκB.[26] IκB is phosphorylated by the upstream serine kinase, IKKβ, which is phosphorylated and activated by additional upstream serine kinases.

Hyperglycemia leads to mitochondrial dysfunction and activation of NF-κB and other stress pathways

Compelling evidence demonstrating the importance of ROS generation in mediating hyperglycemia-induced cellular damage was recently provided.[27] In bovine endothelial cells, exposure to hyperglycemia initially increased the production of intracellular ROS and activated NF-κB. Subsequently, PKC activity, AGE, and sorbitol levels increased. Disruption of mitochondrial ROS production was achieved using several different approaches including:

(1) treatment with CCCP (carbonyl cyanide m-chlorophenylhydrazone), a small molecule uncoupler of mitochondrial oxidative phosphorylation;
(2) overexpression of UCP-1, a protein uncoupler; or
(3) overexpression of manganese superoxide dismutase, the mitochondrial antioxidant enzyme.

Each of these approaches blocked the hyperglycemia-induced increase in ROS production. As a consequence, the hyperglycemia-induced effects on NF-κB, PKC, AGEs, and sorbitol were also suppressed. Moreover, the effects of hyperglycemia on ROS formation and NF-κB activation preceded the stimulation of the other systems, indicating that activation of NF-κB was an initial and crucial signaling event leading to the activation of additional stress-sensitive pathways (Figure 29.1).

Hyperglycemia-dependent NF-κB activation in patients with diabetes mellitus

When patients with diabetes mellitus were studied, a positive correlation of NF-κB activation in peripheral blood mononuclear cells was found with the quality of glycemic control (indicated by HbA1c).[28,29] Moreover, a significant correlation between mononuclear NF-κB binding activity and the severity of albuminuria was observed in diabetic patients with renal complications.[29] When patients with diabetes were treated with the antioxidant LA, a significant suppression of NF-κB activation as well as of plasma markers for lipid oxidation was observed.[28,29] These observations further support the idea that hyperglycemia-induced late diabetic complications result from a cycle of oxidative stress-mediated cellular damage, which further exacerbates the condition of increased oxidative stress.

Antioxidants and complications of diabetes

In addition to an increase in reactive ROS, a decrease in antioxidant capacity occurs in diabetes mellitus.[2] A decline in important cellular antioxidant defense mechanisms, including the glutathione redox system, vitamin C – vitamin E cycle, and the LA/dihydrolipoic acid (DHLA) redox pair (Figures 29.2 and 29.3), significantly increases susceptibility to oxidative stress. Thus, attempts have been made to reduce oxidative stress-dependent cellular changes in patients with diabetes by supplementation with naturally occurring antioxidants, especially LA, vitamin E, and vitamin C.[30-34] The major goals of antioxidant treatment have been to reduce oxidative stress with the expectation of:

(1) preventing;
(2) delaying the progression; or
(3) reversing (i.e. improving) the late microvascular and/or macrovascular complications of diabetes.

α-Lipoic acid

In patients with diabetes, LA levels are reduced.[14,35] LA has been prescribed in Germany for over 30 years for the treatment of diabetic neuropathy, a major microvascular complication of diabetes.[30] There have been four recent controlled clinical studies evaluating LA for the treatment of diabetic neuropathy, and one study for the treatment of autonomic neuropathy. The overall conclusions are:

(1) three-week treatment with i.v. LA (600 mg) reduced the main symptoms of diabetic polyneuropathy;

(2) the effect is accompanied by an improvement in neuropathic deficits;

(3) oral treatment with LA (800–1800 mg) for four to seven months appears to improve neuropathic deficits and autonomic neuropathy;

(4) preliminary data also suggest an improvement in motor and sensory function in lower limbs;

(5) LA has an excellent safety profile at oral doses up to 1800 mg/day.

A pivotal multicenter trail, NATHAN (Neurological Assessment of Thioctic Acid in Neuropathy) Study, is in process in Europe and North America to evaluate the ability of oral LA to slow the progression of diabetic neuropathy.[30] This study is using the most rigid statistical design and quantitative indices of efficacy of any trial performed to date. If efficacy is demonstrated, LA could become the first approved treatment for diabetic neuropathy in the USA. Results from a recent study indicated that treatment with LA improved endothelial function in patients with diabetes.[36]

Vitamin E

Cardiovascular disease is the leading cause of morbidity and mortality in the Western world, and the major macrovascular complication of diabetes.[37] It is associated with increased oxidative stress,[3] and studies, both *in vitro* and *in vivo* have provided the rationale for numerous prospective clinical studies evaluating the effects of vitamin E (α-tocopherol) on cardiovascular events in different populations.[38,39] A review of these data by Jialal and colleagues has led to the overall conclusion that four of the five major prospective trials have reported a beneficial effect on cardiovascular end points, including cardiovascular death, non-fatal myocardial infarction, ischemic stroke, peripheral vascular disease, and others.[39] The one major study (HOPE Study[40]) that was negative for all end points had several limitations.[39] It was terminated early due to the overwhelming positive effects of the angiotensin-converting enzyme ramipril, its lack of data on the dietary intake of other antioxidants, and its evaluation of synthetic vitamin E (a mixture of tocopherols and tocotrienols) and not α-tocopherol, the most potent and effective tocopherol. In a study in patients with Type 2 diabetes evaluating the effects of vitamin E on biochemical risk factors for the development of cardiovascular disease, vitamin E treatment significantly reduced low-density lipoprotein oxidizability and soluble cell adhesion molecules.[41] Taken together the evidence suggests a beneficial effect of vitamin E in patients with pre-existing cardiovascular disease, and in those who are at a greater risk for its development.

Oral vitamin E treatment appears to be effective in normalizing abnormalities in retinal hemodynamics, and improving renal function in patients with Type 1 diabetes of short (disease) duration.[31] Vitamin E was beneficial in those individuals with poorest glycemic control and the most impaired retinal blood flow (Figure 29.4).[31] In a well controlled study, short-term (four weeks) supplementation of patients with Type 2 diabetes with persistent micro/macroalbuminuria with both vitamins E and C significantly lowered their urinary albumin excretion rate.[42] Four months' treatment of patients with Type 2 diabetes with autonomic neuropathy with vitamin E improved the ratio of cardiac sympathetic to parasympathetic tone coincident with lowering of several indices of oxidative stress.[43] Interestingly, the study also reported a lowering of glycated hemoglobin, insulin, norepinephrine, and the homeostatic model assessment index, indicative of increased insulin sensitivity and glycemic control. These data suggest that vitamin E and perhaps other antioxidant supplementation may provide a benefit in the treatment of microvascular complications of diabetes including diabetic retinopathy or nephropathy.

Vitamin C

The normal functions of vascular endothelial tissue include regulation of vasomotor tone, inhibition of platelet activity, and regulation of recruitment of inflammatory cells into the vasculature.[44] A damaged endothelium ('endothelial dysfunction') is a key event in the development of diabetic macroangiopathy, and is associated with the oxidative stress-mediated blunting of nitric oxide action.[45,46] Endothelial dysfunction has been documented in individuals who are insulin-resistant, and in those at risk for developing Type 2 diabetes.[47] Acute treatment with vitamin C improved endothelial function in obese subjects,[48] and in patients with Type 1, Type 2, and gestational diabetes.[49–51]

In patients with cardiovascular disease, including endothelial dysfunction, both acute (single dose, 2 g) and chronic treatment with vitamin C (30 days, 500 mg/d) reverses the vasomotor defect, as judged by increased

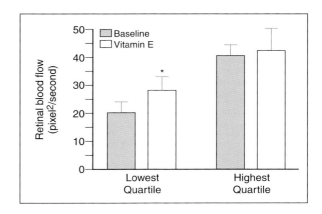

Figure 29.4

*Vitamin E treatment increases retinal blood flow in patients with Type 1 diabetes. An eight-month randomized double blind placebo-controlled crossover trial evaluated 36 patients with Type 1 diabetes and nine non-diabetic control subjects.[31] Subjects were randomly assigned to receive either 1800 IU vitamin E/day or placebo for four months and followed, after treatment crossover, for an additional four months. Retinal blood flow (RBF) was measured at baseline, and at months four and eight using video fluorescein angiography (details of procedure provided in reference). In diabetic patients at baseline, RBF (29.1 ± 7.5 pixel²/s) was significantly ($p < 0.03$) reduced compared with non-diabetic controls (35.2 ± 6.4 pixel²). After four months' treatment with vitamin E, RBF (34.5 ± 7.8 pixel²/s) in patients with diabetes was significantly increased ($p < 0.002$), and normalized compared with non-diabetic controls. Subsequent analyses were performed on diabetic patients grouped into quartiles based on baseline RBF. Patients in the lowest quartile (shown above) exhibited the largest increase in RBF (9.4 ± 3.2 pixel²/s) after treatment with vitamin E (19.9 ± 3.5 to 28.9 ± 3.0 pixel²/s). The increases in RBF in response to vitamin E treament were progressively less in the higher quartiles (quartile 2, 6.0 ± 6.6 pixel²/s, $p < 0.03$ (data not shown); quartile 3, 6.0 ± 6.1 pixel²/s, $p < 0.02$ (data not shown); and quartile 4 (highest; shown above), 1.1 ± 5.3 pixel²/s, not significant). Notes: *, $p < 0.003$ (compared to baseline). All values are mean $\pm$ SD. Source: figure redrawn with modifications from Bursell S-E et al.[31]*

flow-mediated dilation of the brachial artery.[52,53] All of the above studies involved relatively small populations (<75) and used acute treatment except one, which was for 30 days.[53] Nonetheless, the persistent finding of a beneficial effect of antioxidant treatment on endothelial function (flow-mediated dilation) in individuals with demonstrated endothelial dysfunction is encouraging. It is likely that these results will stimulate additional clinical studies of larger size and longer duration to evaluate the efficacy of vitamin C and perhaps other antioxidants.

Antioxidants and insulin resistance

Oxidative stress not only is associated with complications of diabetes, but also has been linked to insulin resistance *in vitro* and *in vivo*.[54–58] Both insulin resistance and decreased insulin secretion are major features of Type 2 diabetes.[59,60] Insulin resistance most often precedes the onset of Type 2 diabetes by many years, is present in a large segment of the general population, and is multifactorial.[59,60] Clearly, insulin resistance has a genetic component.[59,61,62] Insulin resistance also is caused by acquired factors such as obesity, sedentary lifestyle, pregnancy, and hormone excess.[59] Initially, insulin resistance is compensated for by hyperinsulinemia, thus preserving normal glucose tolerance. Reaven and others have presented data that show at least 25% of non-diabetic individuals have insulin resistance that is in the range of that seen in patients with Type 2 diabetes.[60] Deterioration into impaired glucose tolerance occurs when either insulin resistance increases or the insulin secretory responses decrease, or both.

When glucose and FFA increase, they cause oxidative stress along with activation of stress-sensitive signaling pathways. Activation of these pathways, in turn, worsens both insulin action and secretion leading to overt Type 2 diabetes.[63] Furthermore, insulin-resistant patients, with and without Type 2 diabetes, are at increased risk for developing the Metabolic Syndrome, a major cause of heart disease, hypertension and dyslipidemia.[60] Thus, treatment aimed at reducing the degree of oxidative stress and activation of oxidative stress signaling pathways would appear to warrant consideration for inclusion as part of the treatment program for patients with Type 2 diabetes.

Antioxidants and insulin sensitivity: clinical studies

α-Lipoic acid

Studies in animal models of diabetes indicate that antioxidants, especially LA, improve insulin sensitivity.[64] A number of studies have found that the antioxidants LA, glutathione, vitamin E, and vitamin C increase insulin sensitivity in patients with insulin resistance, Type 2 diabetes, and/or cardiovascular disease. In patients with Type 2 diabetes, both acute and chronic administration of LA improves insulin resistance as measured by both the euglycemic-hyperinsulinemic clamp and the Bergman minimal model (Figure 29.5).[65–70] In addition, the short-term (six-week) oral administration of a novel controlled release formulation of LA lowered plasma fructosamine levels in patients with Type 2 diabetes.[71]

Glutathione

In patients with Type 2 diabetes, there is a significant inverse correlation between fasting plasma FFA concentration and the ratio of reduced/oxidized glutathione (a major endogenous antioxidant).[57] In healthy subjects, infusion of FFA (as Intralipid) causes increased

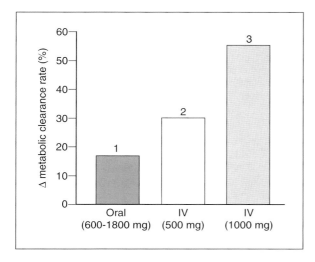

Figure 29.5

α-Lipoic acid increases insulin-stimulated glucose metabolism in patients with Type 2 diabetes. Oral and intravenous (IV) administrations of α-lipoic acid are able to significantly increase insulin sensitivity (as judged by % change (Δ) in metabolic clearance rate (MCR)) in patients with Type 2 diabetes. Effect is greater after IV administration. Each study employed the euglycemic-hyperinsulinemic clamp for assessment of insulin sensitivity.[70] (1) Oral administration of LA enhanced insulin-stimulated glucose disposal in patients with Type 2 diabetes.[67] In a randomized, placebo-controlled, multicenter study, LA (600, 1200, or 1800 mg per day) was administered to 74 patients with Type 2 diabetes for four weeks. Subjects were well controlled by diet alone, or diet combined with other antihyperglycemic medications. Subjects in each arm of the study had a similar degree of hyperglycemia and insulin sensitivity at baseline. Compared to the placebo group, a greater percentage of patients who received LA treatment exhibited an increase in MCR (insulin sensitivity). No differences were observed among groups receiving the different doses of LA. Thus, patients from each arm were combined into a single group for comparison with those who received the placebo tablet. Overall, insulin sensitivity improved approximately 17% following LA treatment (p <0.05). Fasting plasma glucose did not change, but there was a trend toward reduced fasting insulin. (2) Repeated parenteral administration of 500 mg LA (daily infusions for ten days) enhanced insulin-stimulated glucose disposal in patients with Type 2 diabetes.[66] Study subjects (n = 20) were well controlled by diet alone, or diet combined with glibenclamide and/or acarbose. After treatment with LA for 10 days, MCR (insulin sensitivity) was significantly increased by approximately 30% (p <0.05). (3) Acute intravenous infusion of 1000 mg of LA significantly improved insulin-stimulated metabolic clearance rate (MCR) and insulin sensitivity in patients with Type 2 diabetes.[63] Study subjects (n = 13) were well controlled by diet alone, or diet combined with glibenclamide. After LA treatment, the glucose infusion rate increased 47% (p <0.05), and MCR increased 55% (p <0.05). No improvement was seen in the saline-treated control group. Source: figure reprinted with permission from Evans JL, et al. Diabetes Technol Therapeut 2000; 2: 401–13.[69]

oxidative stress as judged by increased malondialdehyde levels and a decline in the plasma reduced/oxidized glutathione ratio.[58] Malondialdehyde, a highly toxic by-product generated in part by lipid oxidation and ROS, is increased in diabetes mellitus.[72] In both healthy individuals and in subjects with Type 2 diabetes, restoration of redox balance by infusing glutathione improves insulin sensitivity along with β-cell function.[73]

Vitamin E

Initial reports of a positive effect of vitamin E on insulin action in insulin-resistant patients with Type 2 diabetes were published almost 10 years ago.[74,75] Twenty-five patients with Type 2 diabetes were treated with vitamin E (d-α-tocopherol; 900 mg/d) or placebo for three months in a double blind, crossover design.[75] There was a trend in the reduction of plasma glucose, along with significant reductions in

HbA1c levels (7.8 versus 7.1), triglycerides, free fatty acids, total cholesterol, low-density lipoprotein cholesterol, and apoprotein B.[73] The β-cell response to glucose was unaffected. These intriguing results prompted additional evaluations by Paolisso and colleagues using a more sensitive technique to measure insulin sensitivity, the euglycemic-hyperinsulinemic clamp.

Ten healthy subjects and 15 patients with Type 2 diabetes underwent an oral glucose tolerance test and euglycemic-hyperinsulinemic clamp before and after vitamin E supplementation (900 mg/d for 4 mo).[76] In patients with Type 2 diabetes, vitamin E supplementation significantly increased both whole-body glucose disposal (i.e. insulin sensitivity) by approximately 50%, and non-oxidative glucose disposal by approximately 60%. Vitamin E also improved insulin action in the healthy subjects.

Vitamin E also improved insulin action in elderly people.[77] Twenty elderly, non-obese subjects with normal glucose tolerance were submitted to the euglycemic-hyperinsulinemic clamp in a double blind, crossover, and randomized study after four months' treatment with either vitamin E (900 mg/d) or placebo. Whole-body glucose disposal was significantly potentiated by vitamin E compared to placebo. Furthermore, plasma vitamin E concentrations were correlated with net changes in insulin-stimulated whole-body glucose disposal.

In a four-week, double blind, randomized study of vitamin E administration (600 mg/d) versus placebo in 24 hypertensive patients, whole-body glucose disposal was measured by the euglycemic-hyperinsulinemic clamp.[78] In hypertensive subjects, vitamin E administration significantly increased whole-body glucose disposal, along with the ratio of reduced glutathione/oxidized glutathione in plasma.

Four months' treatment of patients with Type 2 diabetes with cardiac autonomic neuropathy with vitamin E lowered glycated hemoglobin, insulin, norepinephrine, and the homeostatic model assessment index, was indicative of increased insulin sensitivity and improved glycemic control.[43]

Vitamin C

In addition to playing a major role in the etiology of diabetic macroangiopathy, endothelial dysfunction could promote insulin resistance.[47] It is possible that oxidative stress-mediated blunting of nitric oxide action indirectly affects insulin sensitivity (e.g. reduced peripheral blood flow, increased peroxynitrite formation) consequently reducing insulin-stimulated glucose transport in skeletal muscle.

Cigarette smoking impairs endothelial function, and is one of the major risk factors for hypertension, atherosclerosis, and coronary heart disease. The effects of vitamin C (infusion) on insulin sensitivity and endothelial function (measured by flow-mediated dilation of brachial artery; FMD) were evaluated in smokers, non-smokers with impaired glucose tolerance, and non-smokers with normal glucose tolerance.[79] Both insulin sensitivity and FMD were blunted in smokers and non-smokers with IGT, compared with controls. In smokers and in non-smokers with impaired glucose tolerance, vitamin C significantly improved FMD, increased insulin sensitivity, and decreased plasma thiobarbituric acid-reactive substances, an index of oxidative stress. In contrast, vitamin C had no effect on these parameters in non-smokers with normal glucose tolerance. In patients with coronary spastic angina and endothelial dysfunction, vitamin C infusion augmented FMD and increased insulin sensitivity.[80] In contrast, vitamin C had no effect in healthy controls.

It is important to note that these trials have been relatively small and of short duration. Although consistent and very encouraging, these results need to be confirmed in larger, double blind, placebo-controlled studies. Ideally, these trials would include the measurement of multiple indices of oxidative stress, plasma levels of antioxidants, and measures of insulin sensitivity and glycemic control. Nonetheless, the beneficial effects on insulin action reported following treatment with the antioxidants LA, vitamin E, and vitamin C clearly support the idea that there is an interaction between oxidative stress and insulin action. This area of research certainly merits further and more detailed investigation, with a particular focus on identifying molecular mechanisms along with the sites of antioxidant action.

Antioxidants and insulin sensitivity: possible sites of action

Protection against inhibition of insulin signal transduction mediated by activation of stress-kinases and increased serine phosphorylation

As discussed previously, oxidative stress leads to the activation of multiple serine kinase cascades, including p38 MAPK, JNK/SAPK, and IKKβ/NF-κB.[81–83] There are a number of potential targets of these kinases in the insulin signaling pathway, including the insulin receptor and the insulin receptor substrate (IRS) family of proteins. Increased phosphorylation of the insulin receptor or IRS on discrete serine or threonine sites decreases the extent of their tyrosine phosphorylation, and is consistent with impaired insulin action including protein kinase B activation, and glucose transport.[84–89] There is growing evidence *in vitro* that activation of each of these pathways can render cells insulin resistant. When activation of these pathways is prevented, insulin action is restored (Figure 29.6).

Recently, it has been reported that activation of IKKβ, which activates NF-κB, inhibits

insulin action.[90] Salicylates, which inhibit IKKβ activity,[91] restore insulin sensitivity both *in vitro* and *in vivo*.[90,92] Treatment with aspirin and salicylates alter the phosphorylation patterns of the IRS proteins, resulting in decreased serine phosphorylation and increased tyrosine phosphorylation.[90,92] Preliminary clinical evidence implicating IKKβ in insulin resistance has also been recently provided. Treatment of nine patients with Type 2 diabetes for two weeks with high-dose aspirin (7 g/day) resulted in reduced hepatic glucose production, fasting hyperglycemia, and increased insulin sensitivity.[93] Taken together, these data support a role for activation of IKKβ and NF-κB in the pathogenesis of insulin resistance, and suggest that it might be an attractive pharmacological target to increase insulin sensitivity.

Antioxidants and prevention of NF-κB activation *in vitro*

Activation of NF-κB *in vitro* can be blocked by several thiol-containing antioxidants including LA,[94] a positively charged analog of LA with increased potency,[95] N-acetyl-L-cysteine (NAC),[96] and the glutathione precursor L-2-oxothiazolidine-4-carboxylic acid.[97] Other clinically available antioxidants reported to have anti-inflammatory, antioncogenic, and/or antiatherogenic properties that have been shown to block the activation of NF-κB include resveratrol,[97,99] (-)-epicatechin-3-gallate,[100] pycnogenol,[101] silymarin,[102] and curcumin.[103] IRFI-042, a novel vitamin E analog, inhibited the activation of NF-κB, and reduced the inflammatory response in myocardial ischemia-reperfusion injury.[104] Melatonin is another example of an antioxidant that inhibits NF-κB activation.[105]

Alpha-phenyl-tert-butylnitrone (PBN), an effective spin-trapping agent that reacts with and stabilizes free-radical species,[106] significantly reduced the severity of hyperglycemia in

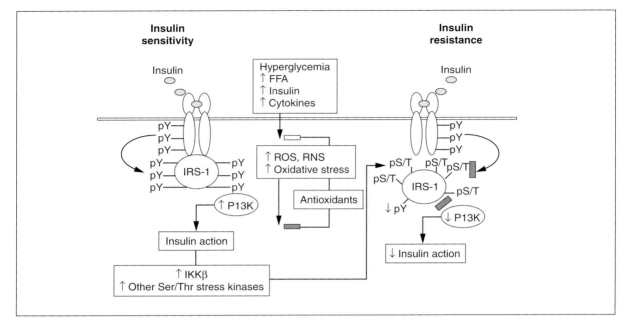

Figure 29.6
Possible sites of action to account for the protective effects of antioxidants against oxidative stress-induced insulin resistance. A variety of stimuli including hyperglycemia, elevated free fatty acids (FFA), hyperinsulinemia, cytokines, and other agents increase ROS production and oxidative stress. This results in the activation of multiple stress-sensitive serine/threonine kinase signaling cascades such as IKKβ and others. Once activated, these kinases are able to phosphorylate multiple target proteins including the insulin receptor and the insulin receptor substrate (IRS) proteins. Increased phosphorylation of the insulin receptor or IRS proteins on discrete serine or threonine sites (pS/T) decreases the extent of their tyrosine phosphorylation (pY).[82–87] Consequently, the association and/or activities of downstream signaling molecules (e.g. phosphatidylinositol 3-kinase; PI3K) are decreased resulting in decreased insulin action (insulin resistance).[85–87] The protective effects of α-lipoic acid (LA) and other antioxidants on oxidative stress-induced insulin resistance may relate to their ability to preserve the intracellular redox balance (neutralizing ROS), or by directly preventing the activation of redox-sensitive kinases (e.g. IKK β).

both alloxan- and streptozotocin (STZ)-induced diabetes, coincident with inhibiting both alloxan- and STZ-induced activation of NF-κB.[107] Inhibiting the activation of NF-κB prevents the activation and the transcription of genes under NF-κB control, including VEGF and others.[108] These studies are consistent with the suggestion that one site of action of antioxidants might be in the NF-κB pathway. With the exception of LA, little attention has been afforded other antioxidants that block NF-κB activation with respect to their potential impact on insulin action. An important goal of future studies in this area will be the determination of which antioxidants are the most effective at preventing NF-κB activation, whether they affect insulin action, and the identification of their molecular sites of action.

Conclusions and implications

The molecular mechanisms whereby oxidative stress causes diabetic complications are undefined. In a variety of tissues, hyperglycemia and elevated FFA result in the generation of ROS and RNS, leading to increased oxidative stress. In the absence of an appropriate compensatory response from the endogenous antioxidant network, the system becomes overwhelmed (redox imbalance), leading to the activation of stress-sensitive signaling pathways, such as NF-κB, p38 MAPK, JNK/SAPK, PKC, AGE/RAGE, sorbitol, and others. The consequence is the production of gene products such as VEGF and others that cause cellular damage, and are ultimately responsible for the long-term complications of diabetes. In addition, activation of the same or similar pathways appears to mediate insulin resistance and impair insulin secretion. It is our view that there appears to be a common biochemical basis that involves oxidative stress-induced activation of stress-sensitive signaling pathways. Thus, the use of antioxidants may be very important in preventing activation of these pathways. Moreover, identification of the molecular basis for the protection afforded by a variety of antioxidants against oxidative-induced damage might lead to the discovery of pharmacological targets for novel therapies to prevent, reverse, or delay the onset of the resultant pathologies.

Acknowledgements

This work was supported, in part, by the American Diabetes Association, and the following Mt Zion funds: Jay Gershow, MH Fishbon, Lee K Schwartz.

References

1. Halliwell B, Gutteridge JM, Free Radicals in Biology and Medicine. Oxford: Oxford University, 1989.
2. Rösen P, Nawroth PP, King G et al. The role of oxidative stress in the onset and progression of diabetes and its complications: A summary of a Congress Series sponsored by UNESCO-MCBN, the American Diabetes Association and the German Diabetes Society. Diabetes Metab Res Rev 2001; 17: 189–212.
3. Paolisso G, Esposito R, D'Alessio MA, Barbieri M. Primary and secondary prevention of atherosclerosis: is there a role for antioxidants? Diabetes Metab 1999; 25: 298–306.
4. West IC. Radicals and oxidative stress in diabetes. Diabet Med. 2000; 17: 171–80.
5. Evans JL, Goldfine ID, Maddux BA, Grodsky GM. Oxidative stress and stress-activated signaling pathways: a unifying hypothesis of type 2 diabetes. Endrocr Rev 2002; 23: 599–622.
6. Giardino I, Brownlee M. The biochemical basis of microvascular disease. In: Pickup JC, Williams G, eds. Textbook of Diabetes. 2nd ed. Oxford: Blackwell Science; 1997: 859–866.
7. Koya D, King GL. Protein kinase C activation and the development of diabetic complications. Diabetes 1998; 47: 859–66.
8. Nadler JL, Natarajan R. Oxidative stress, inflammation, and diabetic complications. In: LeRoith D, Taylor SI, Olefsky JM, eds. Diabetes Mellitus. 2nd ed. Philadelphia: Lippincott Williams & Wilkins; 2000: 1008–1016.
9. Nishikawa T, Edelstein D, Brownlee M. The missing link: a single unifying mechanism for diabetic complications. Kidney Int 2000; 58: 26–30.
10. Giugliano D, Ceriello A, Paolisso G. Diabetes mellitus, hypertension, and cardiovascular disease: which role for oxidative stress? Metabolism 1995; 44: 363–8.
11. Baynes JW, Thorpe SR. Role of oxidative stress in diabetic complications: a new perspective on an old paradigm. Diabetes 1999; 48: 1–9.
12. Shigenaga MK, Hagen TM, Ames BN. Oxidative damage and mitochondrial decay in aging. Proc Natl Acad Sci USA 1994; 91: 10771–8.
13. Biewenga GP, Haenen GR, Bast A. The pharmacology of the antioxidant lipoic acid. Gen Pharmacol 1997; 29: 315–31.

14. Packer L, Witt EH, Tritschler HJ. alpha-Lipoic acid as a biological antioxidant. Free Radical Biol Med 1995; 19: 227–50.
15. Han D, Handleman G, Marcocci L et al. Lipoic acid increases de novo synthesis of cellular glutathione by improving cystine utilization. BioFactors 1997; 6: 321–38.
16. Allen RG, Tresini M. Oxidative stress and gene regulation. Free Radical Biol Med 2000; 28: 463–99.
17. Brownlee M. Advanced protein glycosylation in diabetes and aging. Annu Rev Med 1995; 46: 223–34.
18. Stevens MJ, Obrosova I, Feldman EL, Greene DA. The sorbitol-osmotic and sorbitol-redox hypothesis. In: LeRoith D, Taylor SI, Olefsky JM, eds. Diabetes Mellitus. 2nd ed. Philadelphia: Lippincott Williams & Wilkins; 2000: 972–983.
19. Marshall S, Garvey WT, Traxinger RR. New insights into the metabolic regulation of insulin action and insulin resistance: role of glucose and amino acids. FASEB J 1991; 5: 3031–6.
20. McClain DA, Crook ED. Hexosamines and insulin resistance. Diabetes 1996; 45: 1003–9.
21. Boden G, Chen X, Ruiz J et al. Mechanisms of fatty acid-induced inhibition of glucose uptake. J Clin Invest 1994; 93: 2438–46.
22. Schleicher ED, Weigert C. Role of the hexosamine biosynthetic pathway in diabetic nephropathy. Kidney Int 2000; 58 (Suppl. 77): S13–S18.
23. Lewis TS, Shapiro PS, Ahn NG. Signal transduction through MAP kinase cascades. In: Woude GFV, Klein G, eds. Advances in Cancer Research, Vol 74. San Diego: Academic Press Inc; 1998: 49–139.
24. Obata T, Brown GE, Yaffe MB. MAP kinase pathways activated by stress: the p38 MAPK pathway. Crit Care Med 2000; 28: N67–N77.
25. Barnes PJ, Karin M. Nuclear factor-kappaB: a pivotal transcription factor in chronic inflammatory diseases. N Engl J Med 1997; 336: 1066–71.
26. Karin M, Ben Neriah Y. Phosphorylation meets ubiquitination: the control of NF-κB activity. Annu Rev Immunol 2000; 18: 621–63.
27. Nishikawa T, Edelstein D, Du XL et al. Normalizing mitochondrial superoxide production blocks three pathways of hyperglycaemic damage. Nature 2000; 404: 787–90.
28. Hofmann MA, Schiekofer S, Kanitz M et al. Insufficient glycemic control increases nuclear factor-kappa B binding activity in peripheral blood mononuclear cells isolated from patients with Type 1 diabetes. Diabetes Care 1998; 21: 1310–16.
29. Hofmann MA, Schiekofer S, Isermann B et al. Peripheral blood mononuclear cells isolated from patients with diabetic nephropathy show increased activation of the oxidative-stress sensitive transcription factor NF-kappaB. Diabetologia 1999; 42: 222–32.
30. Ziegler D, Reljanovic M, Mehnert H, Gries FA. Alpha-lipoic acid in the treatment of diabetic polyneuropathy in Germany: current evidence from clinical trials. Exp Clin Endocrinol Diabetes 1999; 107: 421–30.
31. Bursell SE, Clermont AC, Aiello LP et al. High-dose vitamin E supplementation normalizes retinal blood flow and creatinine clearance in patients with Type 1 diabetes. Diabetes Care 1999; 22: 1245–51.
32. Bursell SE, King GL. Can protein kinase C inhibition and vitamin E prevent the development of diabetic vascular complications? Diabetes Res Clin Pract 1999; 45: 169–82.
33. Price KD, Price CS, Reynolds RD. Hyperglycemia-induced ascorbic acid deficiency promotes endothelial dysfunction and the development of atherosclerosis. Atherosclerosis 2001; 158: 1–12.
34. Packer L, Rösen P, Tritschler H et al. Antioxidants and Diabetes Management. New York: Marcel Dekker; 2000.
35. Shigeta Y, Hiraizumi G, Wada M et al. Study on the serum level of thioctic acid in patients with various diseases. J Vitaminol 1961; 7: 48–52.
36. Heitzer T, Finckh B, Albers S et al. Beneficial effects of alpha-lipoic acid and ascorbic acid on endothelium-dependent, nitric oxide-mediated vasodilation in diabetic patients: relation to parameters of oxidative stress. Free Radical Biol Med 2001; 31: 53–61.
37. Pyorala K, Laakso M, Uusitupa M. Diabetes and atherosclerosis: an epidemiologic view. Diabetes Metab Rev.1987; 3: 463–524.
38. Devaraj S, Jialal I. Antioxidants and vitamins to reduce cardiovascular disease. Curr Atheroscler Rep 2000; 2: 342–51.

39. Jialal I, Traber M, Devaraj S. Is there a vitamin E paradox? Curr Opin Lipidol 2001; 12: 49–53.

40. Yusuf S, Dagenais G, Pogue J et al. Vitamin E supplementation and cardiovascular events in high-risk patients. The Heart Outcomes Prevention Evaluation Study Investigators. N Engl J Med 2000; 342: 154–60.

41. Devaraj S, Jialal I. Low-density lipoprotein postsecretory modification, monocyte function, and circulating adhesion molecules in Type 2 diabetic patients with and without macrovascular complications: the effect of alpha-tocopherol supplementation. Circulation 2000; 102: 191–6.

42. Gaede P, Poulsen HE, Parving HH, Pedersen O. Double-blind, randomised study of the effect of combined treatment with vitamin C and E on albuminuria in Type 2 diabetic patients. Diabet Med 2001; 18: 756–60.

43. Manzella D, Barbieri M, Ragno E, Paolisso G. Chronic administration of pharmacologic doses of vitamin E improves the cardiac autonomic nervous system in patients with Type 2 diabetes. Am J Clin Nutr 2001; 73: 1052–7.

44. Levine GN, Keaney JF Jr, Vita JA. Cholesterol reduction in cardiovascular disease. Clinical benefits and possible mechanisms. N Engl J Med 1995; 332: 512–21.

45. Cai H, Harrison DG. Endothelial dysfunction in cardiovascular diseases: the role of oxidant stress. Circ Res 2000; 87: 840–4.

46. Laight DW, Carrier MJ, Anggard EE. Antioxidants, diabetes and endothelial dysfunction. Cardiovasc Res 2000; 47: 457–64.

47. Baron AD, Quon MJ. Insulin action and endothelial function. In: Reaven GM, Laws A, eds. Insulin Resistance: The Metabolic Syndrome X. Totowa: Humana Press; 1999: 247–263.

48. Perticone F, Ceravolo R, Candigliota M et al. Obesity and body fat distribution induce endothelial dysfunction by oxidative stress: protective effect of vitamin C. Diabetes 2001; 50: 159–65.

49. Timimi FK, Ting HH, Haley EA et al. Vitamin C improves endothelium-dependent vasodilation in patients with insulin-dependent diabetes mellitus. J Am Coll Cardiol 1998; 31: 552–7.

50. Ting HH, Timimi FK, Boles KS et al. Vitamin C improves endothelium-dependent vasodilation in patients with non-insulin-dependent diabetes mellitus. J Clin Invest 1996; 97: 22–8.

51. Lekakis JP, Anastasiou EA, Papamichael CM et al. Short-term oral ascorbic acid improves endothelium-dependent vasodilatation in women with a history of gestational diabetes mellitus. Diabetes Care 2000; 23: 1432–4.

52. Levine GN, Frei B, Koulouris SN et al. Ascorbic acid reverses endothelial vasomotor dysfunction in patients with coronary artery disease. Circulation 1996; 93: 1107–13.

53. Gokce N, Keaney JF, Jr., Frei B et al. Long-term ascorbic acid administration reverses endothelial vasomotor dysfunction in patients with coronary artery disease. Circulation 1999; 99: 3234–40.

54. Rudich A, Tirosh A, Potashnik R et al. Lipoic acid protects against oxidative stress induced impairment in insulin stimulation of protein kinase B and glucose transport in 3T3–L1 adipocytes. Diabetologia 1999; 42: 949–57.

55. Maddux BA, See W, Lawrence JC et al. Protection against oxidative stress-induced insulin resistance in rat L6 muscle cells by micromolar concentrations of α-lipoic acid. Diabetes 2001; 50: 404–10.

56. Paolisso G, D'Amore A, Volpe C et al. Evidence for a relationship between oxidative stress and insulin action in non-insulin-dependent (type II) diabetic patients. Metabolism 1994; 43: 1426–9.

57. Paolisso G, Giugliano D. Oxidative stress and insulin action: is there a relationship? Diabetologia 1996; 39: 357–63.

58. Ceriello A. Oxidative stress and glycemic regulation. Metabolism 2000; 49: 27–9.

59. DeFronzo RA. Pathogenesis of Type 2 diabetes: metabolic and molecular implications for identifying diabetes genes. Diabetes Rev 1997; 5: 177–269.

60. Reaven GM. Insulin resistance and its consequences: Type 2 diabetes mellitus and coronary heart disease. In: LeRoith D, Taylor SI, Olefsky JM, eds. Diabetes Mellitus: A Fundamental and Clinical Text, 2nd ed. Philadelphia: Lippincott Williams & Wilkins; 2000: 604–615.

61. Froguel P, Velho G. Genetic determinants of Type 2 diabetes. Recent Prog Horm Res 2001; 56: 91–105.

62. Kahn CR, Vicent D, Doria A. Genetics of non-insulin-dependent (type-II) diabetes mellitus. Annu Rev Med 1996; 47: 509–31.

63. Evans JL, Goldfine ID, Maddux BA and Grodsky GM. Are oxidative stress-activated signaling pathways mediators of insulin resistance and β-cell dysfunction? Diabetes 2003; in press.

64. Henriksen EJ. Oxidative stress and antioxidant treatment: effects on muscle glucose transport in animal models of Type 1 and Type 2 diabetes. In: Packer L, Rösen P, Tritschler HJ, King GL, eds. Antioxidants in Diabetes Management, 1st ed. New York: Marcel Dekker; 2000: 303–317.

65. Jacob S, Henriksen EJ, Schiemann AL et al. Enhancement of glucose disposal in patients with Type 2 diabetes by alpha-lipoic acid. Arzneimittel-Forschung 1995; 45: 872–4.

66. Jacob S, Henriksen EJ, Tritschler HJ et al. Improvement of insulin-stimulated glucose-disposal in Type 2 diabetes after repeated parenteral administration of thioctic acid. Exp Clin Endocrinol Diabetes 1996; 104: 284–8.

67. Jacob S, Ruus P, Hermann R et al. Oral administration of RAC-alpha-lipoic acid modulates insulin sensitivity in patients with Type 2 diabetes mellitus: a placebo-controlled pilot trial. Free Radical Biol Med 1999; 27: 309–14.

68. Konrad T, Vicini P, Kusterer K et al. Alpha-lipoic acid treatment decreases serum lactate and pyruvate concentrations and improves glucose effectiveness in lean and obese patients with Type 2 diabetes. Diabetes Care 1999; 22: 280–7.

69. Evans JL, Goldfine ID. α-Lipoic acid: a multi-functional antioxidant that improves insulin sensitivity in patients with Type 2 diabetes. Diabetes Technol Therap 2000; 2: 401–13.

70. Ferrannini E, Mari A. How to measure insulin sensitivity. J Hypertens 1998; 6: 895–906.

71. Evans JL, Heymann CJ, Goldfine ID, Gavin LA. Pharmacokinetics, tolerability, and fructos-amine-lowering effect of a novel, controlled release formulation of α-lipoic acid. Endocr Pract 2002; 8: 29–35.

72. Slatter DA, Bolton CH, Bailey AJ. The importance of lipid-derived malondialdehyde in diabetes mellitus. Diabetologia 2000; 43: 550–7.

73. Paolisso G, Di Maro G, Pizza G et al. Plasma GSH/GSSG affects glucose homeostasis in healthy subjects and non-insulin-dependent diabetics. Am J Physiol 1992; 263: E435–E440.

74. Caballero B. Vitamin E improves the action of insulin. Nutr Rev 1993; 51: 339–40.

75. Paolisso G, D'Amore A, Galzerano D et al. Daily vitamin E supplements improve metabolic control but not insulin secretion in elderly type II diabetic patients. Diabetes Care 1993; 16: 1433–7.

76. Paolisso G, D'Amore A, Giugliano D et al. Pharmacological doses of vitamin E improve insulin action in healthy subjects and non-insulin-dependent diabetic patients. Am J Clin Nutr 1993; 57: 650–6.

77. Paolisso G, Di Maro G, Galzerano D et al. Pharmacological doses of vitamin E and insulin action in elderly subjects. Am J Clin Nutr 1994; 59: 1291–6.

78. Barbagallo M, Dominguez LJ, Tagliamonte MR et al. Effects of vitamin E and glutathione on glucose metabolism: role of magnesium. Hypertension 1999; 34: 1002–6.

79. Hirai N, Kawano H, Hirashima O et al. Insulin resistance and endothelial dysfunction in smokers: effects of vitamin C. Am J Physiol 2000; 279: H1172–H1178.

80. Hirashima O, Kawano H, Motoyama T et al. Improvement of endothelial function and insulin sensitivity with vitamin C in patients with coronary spastic angina: possible role of reactive oxygen species. J Am Coll Cardiol 2000; 35: 1860–6.

81. Cohen P. Dissection of protein kinase cascades that mediate cellular response to cytokines and cellular stress. Adv Pharmacol 1996; 36: 15–27.

82. Kyriakis JM, Avruch J. Sounding the alarm: protein kinase cascades activated by stress and inflammation. J Biol Chem 1996; 271: 24313–6.

83. Adler V, Yin Z, Tew KD, Ronai Z. Role of redox potential and reactive oxygen species in stress signaling. Oncogene 1999; 18: 6104–11.

84. Paz K, Hemi R, LeRoith D et al. A molecular basis for insulin resistance. Elevated serine/threonine phosphorylation of IRS-1 and IRS-2 inhibits their binding to the juxtamembrane region of the insulin receptor and impairs their ability to undergo insulin-induced tyrosine phosphorylation. J Biol Chem 1997; 272: 29911–18.

85. Kellerer M, Mushack J, Seffer E et al. Protein kinase C isoforms alpha, delta and theta require insulin receptor substrate-1 to inhibit the tyrosine kinase activity of the insulin receptor in human kidney embryonic cells (HEK 293 cells). Diabetologia 1998; 41: 833–8.

86. Li J, DeFea K, Roth RA. Modulation of insulin receptor substrate-1 tyrosine phosphorylation by an Akt/phosphatidylinositol 3-kinase pathway. J Biol Chem 1999; 274 : 9351–6.

87. Qiao LY, Goldberg JL, Russell JC, Sun XJ. Identification of enhanced serine kinase activity in insulin resistance. J Biol Chem 1999; 274: 10625–32.

88. Griffin ME, Marcucci MJ, Cline GW et al. Free fatty acid-induced insulin resistance is associated with activation of protein kinase C theta and alterations in the insulin signaling cascade. Diabetes 1999; 48: 1270–4.

89. Aguirre V, Uchida T, Yenush L et al. The c-jun NH(2)-terminal kinase promotes insulin resistance during association with insulin receptor substrate-1 and phosphorylation of Ser(307). J Biol Chem 2000; 275: 9047–54.

90. Yuan M, Konstantopoulos N, Lee J et al. Reversal of obesity- and diet-induced insulin resistance with salicylates or targeted disruption of IKKβ. Science 2001; 293: 1673–7.

91. Rossi A, Kapahi P, Natoli G et al. Anti-inflammatory cyclopentenone prostaglandins are direct inhibitors of IkappaB kinase. Nature 2000; 403: 103–8.

92. Kim JK, Kim YJ, Fillmore JJ et al. Prevention of fat-induced insulin resistance by salicylate. J Clin Invest 2001; 108: 437–46.

93. Hundal RS, Mayerson AB, Petersen KF et al. Potential for a novel class of insulin sensitizing agents by inhibition of IKKβ activity. Diabetes 2001; 50 Suppl. 2: A117.

94. Zhang WJ, Frei B. Alpha-lipoic acid inhibits TNF-alpha-induced NF-kappaB activation and adhesion molecule expression in human aortic endothelial cells. FASEB J 2001; 15: 2423–32.

95. Sen CK, Tirosh O, Roy S et al. A positively charged alpha-lipoic acid analogue with increased cellular uptake and more potent immunomodulatory activity. Biochem Biophys Res Commun 1998; 247: 223–8.

96. Oka S, Kamata H, Kamata K et al. N-acetyl-cysteine suppresses TNF-induced NF-kappaB activation through inhibition of IκB kinases. FEBS Lett 2000; 472: 196–202.

97. Iimuro Y, Bradford BU, Yamashina S et al. The glutathione precursor L-2-oxothiazolidine-4-carboxylic acid protects against liver injury due to chronic enteral ethanol exposure in the rat. Hepatology 2000; 31: 391–8.

98. Manna SK, Mukhopadhyay A, Aggarwal BB. Resveratrol suppresses TNF-induced activation of nuclear transcription factors NF-kappa B, activator protein-1, and apoptosis: potential role of reactive oxygen intermediates and lipid peroxidation. J Immunol 2000; 164: 6509–19.

99. Holmes-McNary M, Baldwin AS, Jr. Chemopreventive properties of trans-resveratrol are associated with inhibition of activation of the IkappaB kinase. Cancer Res 2000; 60: 3477–83.

100. Shi X, Ye J, Leonard SS et al. Antioxidant properties of (-)-epicatechin-3-gallate and its inhibition of Cr(VI)-induced DNA damage and Cr(IV)- or TPA-stimulated NF-kappaB activation. Mol Cell Biochem 2000; 206: 125–32.

101. Peng Q, Wei Z, Lau BH. Pycnogenol inhibits tumor necrosis factor-alpha-induced nuclear factor kappa B activation and adhesion molecule expression in human vascular endothelial cells. Cell Mol Life Sci 2000; 57: 834–41.

102. Manna SK, Mukhopadhyay A, Van NT, Aggarwal BB. Silymarin suppresses TNF-induced activation of NF-kappa B, c-Jun N-terminal kinase, and apoptosis. J Immunol 1999; 163: 6800–9.

103. Pan M, Lin-Shiau S, Lin J. Comparative studies on the suppression of nitric oxide synthase by curcumin and its hydrogenated metabolites through down-regulation of IkappaB kinase and NFkappaB activation in macrophages. Biochem Pharmacol 2000; 60: 1665–76.

104. Altavilla D, Deodato B, Campo GM et al. IRFI 042, a novel dual vitamin E-like antioxidant, inhibits activation of nuclear factor-kappaB and reduces the inflammatory response in myocardial ischemia-reperfusion injury. Cardiovasc Res 2000; 47: 515–28.

105. Gilad E, Wong HR, Zingarelli B et al. Melatonin inhibits expression of the inducible isoform of nitric oxide synthase in murine macrophages: role of inhibition of NFkappaB activation. FASEB J 1998; 12: 685–93.

106. Thomas CE, Ohlweiler DF, Carr AA et al. Characterization of the radical trapping activity of a novel series of cyclic nitrone spin traps. J Biol Chem 1996; 271: 3097–3104.

107. Ho E, Chen G, Bray TM. Alpha-phenyl-tert-butylnitrone (PBN) inhibits NFkappaB activation offering protection against chemically induced diabetes. Free Radical Biol Med 2000; 28: 604–14.

108. Redondo P, Bandres E, Solano T et al. Vascular endothelial growth factor (VEGF) and melanoma. N-acetylcysteine downregulates VEGF production in vitro. Cytokine 2000; 12: 374–8.

30

Outlook of diabetes treatment possibilities with vanadium and other metal salts

Sonia Brichard

Introduction

Much effort has been devoted to novel therapeutic approaches to Type 2 diabetes and other insulin-resistant states. Besides compounds that increase insulin sensitivity (i.e. thiazolidinediones), those that mimic actions of insulin through alternative signalling pathways are of considerable interest. Vanadium derivatives have been the most extensively characterized insulin mimickers (for reviews see refs 1–4). This chapter will mainly focus on their insulin-like properties and antidiabetic value. Properties of other related metal salts will also be briefly tackled.

Vanadium (V) was discovered in 1831 by Sefström who was struck by the rich colours of V crystals and solutions and named the element after *Vanadis*, the Scandinavian goddess of youth and beauty.

V is a transition metal widely distributed in nature. It is the twenty-first most abundant element in the earth's crust. In mammals, V is present as an ultratrace element. In man, the total body pool of V amounts to ~100–200 μg with tissue concentrations ranging from 1–140 ng/g, the serum concentration is ~1 ng/ml or even less, and the daily intake varies between 10–60 μg.[5] As yet, there is no conclusive demonstration that V is an essential requirement for man.

The chemistry of V is complex.[6] Under physiological conditions, in the +5 oxidation state (V^V), it predominantly exists in an anionic form that resembles phosphate, namely metavanadate (VO_3^-) or orthovanadate ($H_2VO_4^-$) (Figure 30.1). In the +4 oxidation state (V^{IV}), vanadium exists in a cationic form, vanadyl (VO^{2+}), and resembles Mg^{2+} (Figure 30.1).

Vanadate, the major form of the element in plasma, enters cells by an anion transport and is then reduced to vanadyl. This appears to be mediated at least in part by intracellular glutathione to which vanadyl can bind.[5,7]

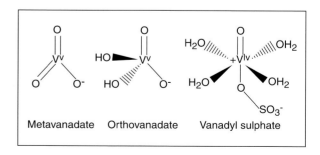

Metavanadate   Orthovanadate   Vanadyl sulphate

Figure 30.1
Chemical structure of the most widely used vanadium salts which exhibit insulin-like properties.

The first demonstration that V could influence a biological system dates back to 1977 when vanadate was discovered to be a potent *in vitro* inhibitor of the Na[+]/K[+]-transporting ATPase.[8] Vanadium salts were subsequently shown to inhibit other transport ATPases.[5] However, evidence that the element was a physiological regulator of these ion pumps has not been provided.

The insulin-like properties of vanadium in vitro

A series of landmark studies in 1979 and 1980 have shown that V salts stimulate glucose transport and metabolism in insulin target tissues or cells.[9–11] These insulin-like effects of V (i.e. observed in the absence of insulin) were rapidly confirmed and dissociated from its ability to inhibit the Na[+]/K[+]-ATPase. Since then, V has been found to mimic most biological effects of insulin in various cell types.

In isolated adipocytes, V compounds stimulate glucose transport by recruiting insulin-sensitive glucose transporters to the plasma membrane,[12] and promote oxidation of the sugar. They also activate lipogenesis, inhibit lipolysis and increase the release of lipoprotein lipase activity from rat adipose tissue.[13]

In hepatocytes, V accelerates glycolysis and is generally found to increase glycogen deposition. Concomitantly, V lowers gene expression of phosphoenolpyruvate carboxykinase, the rate limiting enzyme of gluconeogenesis and potently inhibits glucose-6-phosphatase,[14] the terminal enzyme of gluconeogenesis and glycogenolysis, thereby reducing glucose production by perfused rat liver.[15]

In muscles, vanadium and insulin produce qualitatively similar changes in glucose metabolism. However, unlike insulin, V does not modify protein synthesis or degradation[16]

and has controversial effects on amino acid transport in muscle.[17,18]

Insulin-like effects were also observed with other transition metals (molybdenum, tungsten etc.[19,20]) and with selenium[21] whose oxidized forms exhibit, like vanadate, a spatial configuration which closely resembles phosphate.

The major mechanisms by which vanadium and related metals promote their insulin-like effects involve inhibition of protein-phosphotyrosine phosphatases (PTP)[22] and resultant indirect stimulation of tyrosine phosphorylation (review in ref. 2). Accordingly, unreduced intracellular vanadate, which is a more potent inhibitor of PTP than vanadyl, could be the most relevant insulinomimetic species in intact cells.[7,23] Although V may enhance tyrosine phosphorylation of the insulin receptor[24] (Figure 30.2), this phenomenon is not consistently observed and inhibition of the insulin receptor tyrosine kinase does not abolish a number of effects on glucose metabolism.[1,25] This suggests that V may operate via insulin-independent pathways and/or act at step(s) distal to the insulin receptor. In adipocytes, some insulin-like effects of V (i.e. lipogenesis, glucose oxidation) were found to be mediated by activation of a cytosolic, insulin-independent, tyrosine kinase,[26] while plasma membrane events (i.e. antilipolysis, glucose transport) resulted from stimulation of a non-receptor membranous tyrosine kinase[27] (Figure 30.2). V may also directly stimulate signals downstream of the insulin receptor and its substrates (IRS-1/2) such as mitogen-activated protein (MAP) kinase or phophatidylinositol 3– (PI 3–) kinase (Figure 30.2). PI 3-kinase appears to be essential for virtually all metabolic effects of insulin. However, glucose transport and antilipolysis induced by V were shown to be independent of PI 3-kinase activation.[28–30] Taken together, these findings suggest that V may by-pass some events of the insulin

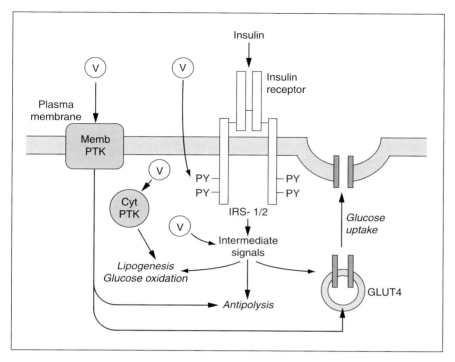

Figure 30.2
Putative sites of vanadium (V) action and insulin signal transduction pathways. Insulin signal transduction proceeds via receptor autophosphorylation on tyrosine residues (PY). This is followed by phosphorylation of insulin receptor substrates (IRS-1 and/or IRS-2) and subsequent activation of intermediate signals, among which PI 3-kinase plays an essential role in the metabolic responses to the hormone (in italics). In muscle and fat cells, these metabolic responses include translocation of GLUT4 glucose transporters from an intracellular pool to the plasma membrane, thereby allowing rapid uptake of glucose by these tissues. V may increase the phosphorylation of the insulin receptor or act at post-receptor sites. V may also activate insulin-independent membranous (Memb) or cytosolic (Cyt) protein tyrosine kinases (PTK). V activation of Memb PTK would allow stimulation of glucose uptake or the antilipolytic effect of the element while activation of Cyt PTK would stimulate lipogenesis or glucose metabolism.

signalling cascade and/or use alternative (insulin-independent) pathways. This raises the possibility that the element might be able to influence glucose metabolism, even when the insulin transduction pathway is not functioning correctly.

Because of poor permeation of vanadium into cells, most of the insulin-like effects require high concentrations of the salts (0.5–1 mM), except when long-term effects are studied using cultured cells. However, in addition to its insulin-like properties, V also increases the sensitivity of target cells to insulin and prolongs the biological effects of the hormone. These 'insulin-sensitizing' effects may be observed at lower concentrations of the salts (10–200 µM).[31] Moreover, the ability of V to inhibit PTP and stimulate glucose transport

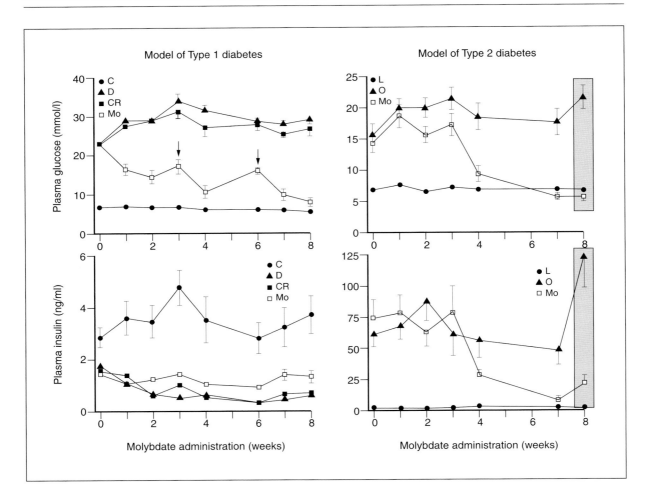

Figure 30.3

Time course of molybdate treatment on plasma glucose and insulin levels in animal models of Type 1 and Type 2 diabetes. (Left panels) rats were made insulin-deficient and diabetic by streptozotocin (Type 1 diabetes): a group of diabetic rats was untreated (D), another group received Na₂MoO₄ in drinking solutions and food (Mo), and a last group was mildly calorie restricted (CR) to ensure a body weight gain similar to that of Mo rats. Diabetic animals were compared to untreated non-diabetic control (C) ones. (Right panels) obese, hyperinsulinemic and diabetic ob/ob *mice (Type 2 diabetes) were either untreated (O) or treated with oral molybdate (Mo). Obese mice were compared to untreated lean (L) mice. The initial concentrations of Mo was increased after three, then six weeks of treatment (first and second arrows) (left panels) or progressively over the first month (right panels). Values are the mean ± SEM for 6–10 rats in each group (left panels) or 13–16 mice in each group (right panels). All measurements were made between 0830 and 0900 h except those in the grey area (0200–0400 h). Source: data from Ozcelikay et al.[34] and Reul et al.[53]*

may be enhanced in hyperglycaemia-induced insulin-resistant states, a situation of oxidative stress as V action may be modulated by the cellular redox state.[7]

The antidiabetic properties of vanadium and other metal salts in animal studies

The properties of vanadium described above prompted investigations of the antidiabetic activity of the compound in the animal. The demonstration of its efficacy by Heyliger et al.[32] in 1985 was at the origin of numerous studies in animal models of Type 1 and Type 2 diabetes. Other metal salts, more particularly molybdate (Mo) and tunstgate (W), were subsequently tested.

Insulin-deficient rats

The most spectacular effects of vanadium or related elements are seen in rats made insulin-deficient and diabetic by injection of strepto-zotocin (STZ), a drug which destroys pancreatic B-cells (models of Type 1 diabetes). Oral administration of V (vanadate or vanadyl),[32,33] Mo[34] or W[35] causes a fall in blood glucose levels which usually occurs within the first week (Figure 30.3, left panels; Mo shown as an example). A similar beneficial effect was also observed after selenate treatment.[36,37] A comparison study between these elements has not yet been performed. The efficacy of these agents appears to be inversely related to the severity of diabetes and persists for up to one year.[38,39] Their antihyperglycaemic effect does not result from a rise in circulating insulin levels which remain low[32–36] (Figure 30.3, left panels). It can also not be ascribed to the lower food intake usually caused by the treatment

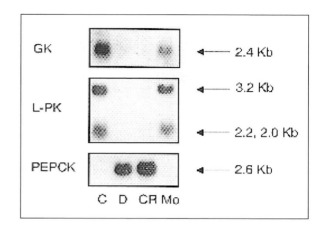

Figure 30.4
Northern-blot analysis of two glycolytic enzymes (glucokinase, GK and L-type pyruvate kinase, L-PK) and of the key gluconeogenic enzyme (phosphoenolpyruvate carboxykinase, PEPCK) in liver from diabetic rats treated with molybdate. C, D, CR and Mo rats were the same as those described in the left panels of Figure 30.3. This blot is representative from 6–10 different rats in each group. Kb, kilobase. Source: adapted from Ozcelikay et al.[34]

(via taste aversion and possibly a central effect on the appetite)[1] as no glucose-lowering effect was detected in untreated diabetic rats which were merely calorie-restricted[34,36] (Figure 30.3, left panels).

Chronic treatment of diabetic rats with the insulin-like compounds restored the blunted mRNA and activity of glycolytic enzymes (glucokinase and L-type pyruvate kinase) and decreased to normal phosphoenolpyruvate carboxykinase values in liver, thereby inducing a shift of the predominating gluconeogenic flux, which contributes to hepatic glucose overproduction, into a glycolytic flux (Figure 30.4).[34,36,39–41] Moreover, impaired hepatic glycogen synthase activity and glycogen reserves were normalized.[34,39,42–44] The ability of insulin to stimulate glucose disposal by muscles was also restored by the treatment, through correction of the decreased amounts of glucose transporter GLUT4 and of the low activity of glycogen synthase.[45–47] The effects of insulin-like compounds on adipose tissue are less clear. A reduction of the high rate of lipolysis has been observed,[48] but the blunted expression and activity of lipogenic enzymes were not modified.[34,49]

These *in vivo* studies have thus established that these elements play a determinant role in the improvement of glucose homoeostasis via an action on insulin target tissues. However, the underlying molecular mechanisms are still unclear. The tyrosine kinase activity of insulin receptors in tissues from treated diabetic rats has indeed been found to be increased[50] or unchanged.[34,45,46] It also remains unclear whether these compounds act *in vivo* as insulin mimickers or increase the effect of the residual amounts of circulating insulin, or both.[1,3,51]

Insulin-resistant animals

The antidiabetic effects of these agents have also been investigated in genetically obese, hyperinsulinaemic and insulin-resistant mice and rats (models of Type 2 diabetes).[1,51–54]

Vanadate and Mo improved glucose homoeostasis in *ob/ob* and *db/db* mice in which an extreme insulin resistance leads to overt diabetes in spite of very high plasma insulin levels.[53,55,56] Marked and sustained decreases in glycaemia and insulinaemia were observed during treatment (Figure 30.3, right panels; Mo in *ob/ob* mice as an example). This resulted in part from attenuation of liver insulin resistance.[53] Moreover, this antihyper-glycaemic effect partly prevented the exhaustion of pancreatic insulin stores that otherwise occurs in some of these animals when they become older.

In genetically obese and only mildly glucose-intolerant *fa/fa* rats, oral vanadate had little effect on basal glycaemia but improved the tolerance to glucose loads, and markedly lowered plasma insulin levels (Table 30.1, basal glycaemia and insulinemia as an example).[52] This was mainly due to correction of the poor sensitivity to insulin in peripheral tissues, more particularly muscles.[57,58] This beneficial effect occurred via post-receptor events which were likely to involve a functional improvement of GLUT4.[58]

Importantly, unlike thiazolidinediones,[59] V compounds did not upregulate adipose tissue metabolism or differentiation *in vivo*[53,57,58] and, as mentioned earlier, did not induce hyperphagia (in some cases, they did actually reduce food intake). Thus, V compounds did not accelerate weight gain in animals prone to develop obesity and even restrained the development of adiposity in some studies (Table 30.1).

Trials with vanadium in man

The first report suggesting that vanadium salts can influence glucose metabolism is probably that of Lyonnet et al. who, in 1899, observed that oral V decreased the glucosuria in two out of three diabetic patients.[60]

Recently, six reports from four different groups have examined the effects of metavana-date ($NaVO_3$) or vanadyl sulphate (VS) admin-istered to diabetic patients for a period of two to six weeks (Table 30.2).[61–66] The doses used were ~10- to 75-fold lower than those given in most animal studies. However, beneficial effects were observed.

In Type 1 diabetic patients, no consistent influence on the glycaemic control could be detected, but daily insulin requirements were decreased by 14%.[61] In Type 2 diabetic

	Vanadate	Pioglitazone
	% of control fa/fa rats	
Body weight gain	20*	177*
Basal plasma levels		
Glucose	86*	86*
Insulin	50*	37*
White adipose tissue		
Basal glucose uptake	60	294*
GLUT4 mRNA	140	~400*
FAS mRNA	ND	600*
Adipocyte differentiation	ND	+++

Table 30.1
Comparison between vanadate and pioglitazone treatments of obese fa/fa *rats*

Notes: Sodium vanadate (25 mg/kg/d) was administered for 8 to 14 weeks (compiled data from refs 52, 57, 58) and Pioglitazone (10 mg/kg/d) for 4 weeks (from ref. 59) to obese hyperinsulinemic *fa/fa* rats. Treatment-induced changes were expressed as percentages of values obtained in respective control (i.e. untreated) *fa/fa* rats. FAS, fatty acid synthase (a key lipogenic enzyme); ND, not done; *$p < 0.05$ or less versus respective control *fa/fa* rats.

patients, fasting plasma glucose levels were decreased by 14–20% and HbA1c by 6–8%. Insulin sensitivity increased during V treatment. This improvement resulted from a greater inhibition of hepatic glucose production and a greater stimulation of peripheral (predominantly muscular) glucose disposal (Table 30.2). Besides its effects on glucose metabolism, V also affected the lipid profile and exerted a cardiovascular benefit by reducing total and LDL cholesterol[61,64,66] in agreement with reports from the early 1960s.[67] It is interesting to note that some of these effects were sustained for up to two weeks following cessation of the treatment.[62]

After V treatment, plasma vanadium concentrations were around 100 ng/ml, that is, two orders of magnitude higher than in untreated subjects (Table 30.2). In these therapeutic trials or in the few control studies in which vanadium was given orally, no marked perturbations of biochemical parameters were detected on the screening laboratory profiles.

The most common side-effect was a mild gastrointestinal intolerance whose incidence may be lowered by gradual titration of V doses.[66] In rats, administration of V for up to one year at high doses had no significant toxicity on various organs. However, the long-term repercussions of a marked elevation of plasma V in humans remain unknown. The effects of V on tyrosine kinases, which are involved in cell growth and differentiation, deserve attention as they raise the potential carcinogenicity of these compounds. Further evaluation of the long-term safety of vanadium compounds (i.e. carcinogenicity and potential for body accumulation) in humans is therefore mandatory.

New compounds and perspectives

The clinical studies reported so far have used simple naturally occurring inorganic vanadium salts. Attempts are being made to develop

Treatment and patients studied (n)	Goldfine et al.[61]	Cohen et al.[62]	Boden et al.[63]	Cusi et al.[66]
	NaVO$_3$ (125 mg/d) – 2 weeks (n = 5)[a]	VOSO$_4$ (100 mg/d) – 3 weeks (n = 6)[b]	VOSO$_4$ (100 mg/d) – 4 weeks (n = 8)	VS (150 mg/d) – 6 weeks (n = 11)
Glucose metabolism				
Fasting blood glucose	↓6%	↓14%	↓20%	↓20%
HbA1c	–	↓8%	ND	↓6%
Indices of beta cell function	–	–	–	–
Glucose fluxes				
Basal state: HGP	–	–	–	↓20%
Insulin-clamp: HGP	–	↓75%	↓38%	–
Glucose disposal	↑39%[c]	↑32%[c]	–	↑20%
Lipid metabolism				
Plasma total cholesterol	↓24%	–	ND	↓10%
Plasma triglycerides	ND	–	ND	–
Plasma FFA	ND	–	–	–
Serum or plasma V levels (ng/ml)	142	73	~83	104
Side-effects	Gastrointestinal disturbance requiring a reduction in V dosage in one patient	Transient and mild gastrointestinal disturbance	Transient gastrointestinal disturbance (one week)	Slight gastrointestinal disturbance requiring a reduction in V dosage in one patient

Notes: –, no effect; ↓, reduction; ↑, increase. ND, not done; HGP, hepatic glucose production. V treatment-induced changes were expressed as percentages of values obtained during the placebo period or in placebo-administered patients.
[a]This study also included another five (Type 1) diabetic patients whose results are not presented.
[b]Five of these patients served as a comparison group in another study.[64]
[c]Mainly explained by enhanced muscular glycogen synthesis.

Table 30.2
Effects of vanadium (V) treatment in Type 2 diabetic patients

novel insulin-like compounds with higher potency and low toxicity.

In this regard, the effects of several vanadium compounds complexed with organic ligands merit attention (for reviews see refs 4, 68). Bis(maltolato)oxovanadium (VM) has been the first of these complexes to be characterized in diabetic animals. Others have subsequently been described. Recently, a study has compared the efficacy of three organic vanadium complexes in STZ-diabetic rats (VM (cf. supra), vanadyl acetylacetonate (VAc) and vanadyl ethylacetonate (VEt)); a simple inorganic salt, vanadyl sulphate (VS) was also studied. Oral administration of the three organic forms of V for up to three months induced a faster and larger fall in glycaemia (VAc being the most potent) than VS. This greater efficacy of the organic forms, especially that of VAc, was not simply due improved intestinal absorption. Indeed, VAc retained its potency when the gastrointestinal tract was by-passed. When given as a single i.p. injection, VAc significantly decreased the hyperglycaemia of diabetic rats for up to five days, while the other forms were ineffective (Figure 30.5).[69] These data suggest that differences in potency between the compounds may, at least in part, be explained by differences in their insulin-like properties. Diarrhoea which occurred in 50% of rats chronically treated with VS, because inorganic vanadium is poorly absorbed by the intestinal tract, was not observed in animals receiving the organic forms.[69] Thus, organic V compounds, in particular VAc, may correct the hyperglycaemia of diabetic rats more safely and potently than VS. Other organic ligands for V (i.e. L-glutamic acid monohydroxamate;[23] reviewed in refs 4, 68) or agents co-administered with low doses of V (benzylamine)[70] were also found to potentiate the antidiabetic activity of the element. The chemical rules determining which ligands will generate the most suitable (most potent, less toxic) vanadium complexes are not completely

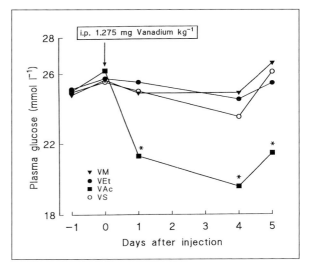

Figure 30.5
*Influence of a single intraperitoneal (i.p.) injection of vanadium compounds on plasma glucose levels in streptozotocin-diabetic rats. On day 0 (0930 h), either bis(maltolato)oxovanadium (VM), vanadyl ethylacetonate (VEt), vanadyl acetylacetonate (VAc), or vanadyl sulphate (VS) were injected into diabetic rats at a dose of 1.275 mg vanadium element per kg body weight. Values are the means for eight rats in each group (SEM which were always <10% of the mean were omitted for sake of clarity). *p <0.05 or less versus respective glycaemia on day 0. Source: data from Reul et al.[69]*

elucidated, but are relevant in view of their potential therapeutic value. Ideally, the use of one ligand should even direct the vanadium complex into one insulin-target tissue in preference to another.[71] Recently, clinical trials with KP-102, the ethyl derivative of VM, have begun.[68]

The peroxovanadium compounds are also a new class of powerful insulinomimetic derivatives that were discovered when two insulin-like agents, vanadate and H_2O_2 (hydrogen peroxide), were combined and found to be synergistic in their activities to produce insulin-like effects and activate the insulin receptor tyrosine kinase.[2,72] Although these compounds are highly potent inhibitors of PTP, their *in vivo* use is limited because of their degradation by the gastric environment, and their long-term toxicity has not been assessed. Testing of several organic ligands complexed with these compounds in order to improve their potential antidiabetic use is also under way.

Conclusions

Unravelling the insulin-like properties of vanadium and related metals has helped to elucidate the molecular mechanisms of insulin action and certain causes of its perturbations. These insulin-like agents have also opened new perspectives for the treatment of insulin-resistant subjects with Type 2 diabetes. Further work is now required to assess the long-term safety of these compounds before their use in clinical practice can be considered. Intensive search for optimized derivatives is also warranted.

Acknowledgements

Studies quoted from our laboratory were made possible by support from the FNRS, FRSM, FSR and the Belgian Association for Diabetes.

References

1. Brichard SM, Henquin JC. The role of vanadium in the management of diabetes. Trends Pharmacol Sci 1995; 16: 265–70.
2. Tsiani E, Fantus IG. Vanadium compounds. Biological actions and potential as pharmacological agents. Trends Endocrinol Metab 1997; 8: 51–8.
3. Cam MC, Brownsey RW, McNeill JH. Mechanisms of vanadium action: insulin-mimetic or insulin-enhancing agent? Can J Physiol Pharmacol 2000; 78: 829–47.
4. Goldwaser I, Gefel D, Gershonov E et al. Insulin-like effects of vanadium: basic and clinical implications. J Inorg Biochem 2000; 80: 21–5.
5. Nechay BR, Nanninga LB, Nechay PSE et al. Role of vanadium in biology. Fed Proc 1986; 45: 123–32.
6. Rehder D. The bioinorganic chemistry of vanadium. Angew Chem Int Ed 1991; 30: 148–67.
7. Lu B, Ennis D, Lai R et al. Enhanced sensitivity of insulin-resistant adipocytes to vanadate is associated with oxidative stress and decreased reduction of vanadate (+5) to vanadyl (+4). J Biol Chem 2001; 276: 35589–98.
8. Cantley LC, Jr, Josephson L, Warner R et al. Vanadate is a potent (Na,K)-ATPase inhibitor found in ATP derived from muscle. J Biol Chem 1977; 252: 7421–3.
9. Tolman EL, Barris E, Burns M et al. Effects of vanadium on glucose metabolism *in vitro*. Life Sci 1979; 25: 1159–64.
10. Dubyak GR, Kleinzeller A. The insulin-mimetic effects of vanadate in isolated rat adipocytes. Dissociation from effects of vanadate as a (Na+-K+)ATPase inhibitor. J Biol Chem 1980; 255: 5306–12.
11. Shechter Y, Karlish SJ. Insulin-like stimulation of glucose oxidation in rat adipocytes by vanadyl (IV) ions. Nature 1980; 284: 556–8.
12. Paquet MR, Romanek RJ, Sargeant RJ. Vanadate induces the recruitment of GLUT-4 glucose transporter to the plasma membrane of rat adipocytes. Mol Cell Biochem 1992; 109: 149–55.
13. Ueki H, Sera M, Tanaka K. Stimulatory release of lipoprotein lipase activity from rat fat pads by vanadate. Arch Biochem Biophys 1989; 272: 18–24.
14. Bosch F, Hatzoglou M, Park EA, Hanson RW. Vanadate inhibits expression of the gene for phosphoenolpyruvate carboxykinase (GTP) in rat hepatoma cells. J Biol Chem 1990; 265: 13677–82.
15. Bruck R, Prigozin H, Krepel Z et al. Vanadate inhibits glucose output from isolated perfused rat liver. Hepatology 1991; 14: 540–4.

16. Clark AS, Fagan JM, Mitch WE. Selectivity of the insulin-like actions of vanadate on glucose and protein metabolism in skeletal muscle. Biochem J 1985; 232: 273–6.

17. Munoz P, Guma A, Camps M et al. Vanadate stimulates system A amino acid transport activity in skeletal muscle. Evidence for the involvement of intracellular pH as a mediator of vanadate action. J Biol Chem 1992; 267: 10381–8.

18. Tsiani E, Abdullah N, Fantus IG. Insulin-mimetic agents vanadate and pervanadate stimulate glucose but inhibit amino acid uptake. Am J Physiol 1997; 272: C156–C162.

19. Fillat C, Rodriguez-Gil JE, Guinovart JJ. Molybdate and tungstate act like vanadate on glucose metabolism in isolated hepatocytes. Biochem J 1992; 282 (Pt 3): 659–63.

20. Goto Y, Kida K, Ikeuchi M et al. Synergism in insulin-like effects of molybdate plus H2O2 or tungstate plus H2O2 on glucose transport by isolated rat adipocytes. Biochem Pharmacol 1992; 44: 174–7.

21. Ezaki O. The insulin-like effects of selenate in rat adipocytes. J Biol Chem 1990; 265: 1124–8.

22. Swarup G, Speeg KV, Jr, Cohen S, Garbers DL. Phosphotyrosyl-protein phosphatase of TCRC-2 cells. J Biol Chem 1982; 257: 7298–301.

23. Goldwaser I, Li J, Gershonov E, Armoni M et al. L-Glutamic acid gamma-monohydroxamate. A potentiator of vanadium-evoked glucose metabolism *in vitro* and *in vivo*. J Biol Chem 1999; 274: 26617–24.

24. Tamura S, Brown TA, Whipple JH et al. A novel mechanism for the insulin-like effect of vanadate on glycogen synthase in rat adipocytes. J Biol Chem 1984; 259: 6650–8.

25. D'Onofrio F, Le MQ, Chiasson JL, Srivastava AK. Activation of mitogen activated protein (MAP) kinases by vanadate is independent of insulin receptor autophosphorylation. FEBS Lett 1994; 340: 269–75.

26. Shisheva A, Shechter Y. Role of cytosolic tyrosine kinase in mediating insulin-like actions of vanadate in rat adipocytes. J Biol Chem 1993; 268: 6463–9.

27. Elberg G, He Z, Li J et al. Vanadate activates membranous nonreceptor protein tyrosine kinase in rat adipocytes. Diabetes 1997; 46: 1684–90.

28. Ida M, Imai K, Hashimoto S, Kawashima H. Pervanadate stimulation of wortmannin-sensitive and -resistant 2-deoxyglucose transport in adipocytes. Biochem Pharmacol 1996; 51: 1061–7.

29. Tsiani E, Bogdanovic E, Sorisky A et al. Tyrosine phosphatase inhibitors, vanadate and pervanadate, stimulate glucose transport and GLUT translocation in muscle cells by a mechanism independent of phosphatidylinositol 3-kinase and protein kinase C. Diabetes 1998; 47: 1676–86.

30. Li J, Elberg G, Sekar N et al. Antilipolytic actions of vanadate and insulin in rat adipocytes mediated by distinctly different mechanisms. Endocrinology 1997; 138: 2274–9.

31. Fantus IG, Ahmad F, Deragon G. Vanadate augments insulin binding and prolongs insulin action in rat adipocytes. Endocrinology 1990; 127: 2716–25.

32. Heyliger CE, Tahiliani AG, McNeill JH. Effect of vanadate on elevated blood glucose and depressed cardiac performance of diabetic rats. Science 1985; 227: 1474–7.

33. Brichard SM, Okitolonda W, Henquin JC. Long term improvement of glucose homeostasis by vanadate treatment in diabetic rats. Endocrinology 1988; 123: 2048–53.

34. Ozcelikay AT, Becker DJ, Ongemba LN et al. Improvement of glucose and lipid metabolism in diabetic rats treated with molybdate. Am J Physiol 1996; 270: E344–E352.

35. Barbera A, Rodriguez-Gil JE, Guinovart JJ. Insulin-like actions of tungstate in diabetic rats. Normalization of hepatic glucose metabolism. J Biol Chem 1994; 269: 20047–53.

36. Becker DJ, Reul B, Ozcelikay AT et al. Oral selenate improves glucose homeostasis and partly reverses abnormal expression of liver glycolytic and gluconeogenic enzymes in diabetic rats. Diabetologia 1996; 39: 3–11.

37. McNeill JH, Delgatty HL, Battell ML. Insulinlike effects of sodium selenate in streptozocin-induced diabetic rats. Diabetes 1991; 40: 1675–8.

38. Dai S, Thompson KH, Vera E, McNeill JH. Toxicity studies on one-year treatment of non-diabetic and streptozotocin-diabetic rats with vanadyl sulphate. Pharmacol Toxicol 1994; 75: 265–73.

39. Barbera A, Gomis RR, Prats N et al. Tungstate is an effective antidiabetic agent in streptozotocin-induced diabetic rats: a long-term study. Diabetologia 2001; 44: 507–13.

40. Brichard SM, Desbuquois B, Girard J. Vanadate treatment of diabetic rats reverses the impaired expression of genes involved in hepatic glucose metabolism: effects on glycolytic and gluconeogenic enzymes, and on glucose transporter GLUT2. Mol Cell Endocrinol 1993; 91: 91–7.

41. Valera A, Rodriguez-Gil JE, Bosch F. Vanadate treatment restores the expression of genes for key enzymes in the glucose and ketone bodies metabolism in the liver of diabetic rats. J Clin Invest 1993; 92: 4–11.

42. Gil J, Miralpeix M, Carreras J, Bartrons R. Insulin-like effects of vanadate on glucokinase activity and fructose 2,6-bisphosphate levels in the liver of diabetic rats. J Biol Chem 1988; 263: 1868–71.

43. Pugazhenthi S, Khandelwal RL. Insulinlike effects of vanadate on hepatic glycogen metabolism in nondiabetic and streptozocin-induced diabetic rats. Diabetes 1990; 39: 821–7.

44. Bollen M, Miralpeix M, Ventura F et al. Oral administration of vanadate to streptozotocin-diabetic rats restores the glucose-induced activation of liver glycogen synthase. Biochem J 1990; 267: 269–71.

45. Blondel O, Simon J, Chevalier B, Portha B. Impaired insulin action but normal insulin receptor activity in diabetic rat liver: effect of vanadate. Am J Physiol 1990; 258: E459–E467.

46. Venkatesan N, Avidan A, Davidson MB. Antidiabetic action of vanadyl in rats independent of in vivo insulin-receptor kinase activity. Diabetes 1991; 40: 492–8.

47. Rossetti L, Lauglin MR. Correction of chronic hyperglycemia with vanadate, but not with phlorizin, normalizes in vivo glycogen repletion and in vitro glycogen synthase activity in diabetic skeletal muscle. J Clin Invest 1989; 84: 892–9.

48. Cam MC, Pederson RA, Brownsey RW, McNeill JH. Long-term effectiveness of oral vanadyl sulphate in streptozotocin-diabetic rats. Diabetologia 1993; 36: 218–24.

49. Brichard SM, Ongemba LN, Girard J, Henquin JC. Tissue-specific correction of lipogenic enzyme gene expression in diabetic rats given vanadate. Diabetologia 1994; 37: 1065–72.

50. Cordera R, Andraghetti G, DeFronzo RA, Rossetti L. Effect of in vivo vanadate treatment on insulin receptor tyrosine kinase activity in partially pancreatectomized diabetic rats. Endocrinology 1990; 126: 2177–83.

51. Shafrir E, Spielman S, Nachliel I et al. Treatment of diabetes with vanadium salts: general overview and amelioration of nutritionally induced diabetes in the Psammomys obesus gerbil. Diabetes Metab Res Rev 2001; 17: 55–66.

52. Brichard SM, Pottier AM, Henquin JC. Long term improvement of glucose homeostasis by vanadate in obese hyperinsulinemic fa/fa rats. Endocrinology 1989; 125: 2510–16.

53. Reul BA, Becker DJ, Ongemba LN et al. Improvement of glucose homeostasis and hepatic insulin resistance in ob/ob mice given oral molybdate. J Endocrinol 1997; 155: 55–64.

54. Munoz MC, Barbera A, Dominguez J et al. Effects of tungstate, a new potential oral antidiabetic agent, in Zucker diabetic fatty rats. Diabetes 2001; 50: 131–8.

55. Brichard SM, Bailey CJ, Henquin JC. Marked improvement of glucose homeostasis in diabetic ob/ob mice given oral vanadate. Diabetes 1990; 39: 1326–32.

56. Meyerovitch J, Rothenberg P, Shechter Y et al. Vanadate normalizes hyperglycemia in two mouse models of non-insulin-dependent diabetes mellitus. J Clin Invest 1991; 87: 1286–94.

57. Brichard SM, Ongemba LN, Henquin JC. Oral vanadate decreases muscle insulin resistance in obese fa/fa rats. Diabetologia 1992; 35: 522–7.

58. Brichard SM, Assimacopoulos-Jeannet F, Jeanrenaud B. Vanadate treatment markedly increases glucose utilization in muscle of insulin-resistant fa/fa rats without modifying glucose transporter expression. Endocrinology 1992; 131: 311–17.

59. Hallakou S, Doare L, Foufelle F et al. Pioglitazone induces in vivo adipocyte differentiation in the obese Zucker fa/fa rat. Diabetes 1997; 46: 1393–9.

60. Lyonnet B, Martz, Martin E. La Presse Médicale 1899; 1: 191–2.

61. Goldfine AB, Simonson DC, Folli F et al.

Metabolic effects of sodium metavanadate in humans with insulin-dependent and noninsulin-dependent diabetes mellitus *in vivo* and *in vitro* studies. J Clin Endocrinol Metab 1995; 80: 3311–20.

62. Cohen N, Halberstam M, Shlimovich P et al. Oral vanadyl sulfate improves hepatic and peripheral insulin sensitivity in patients with non-insulin-dependent diabetes mellitus. J Clin Invest 1995; 95: 2501–9.

63. Boden G, Chen X, Ruiz J et al. Effects of vanadyl sulfate on carbohydrate and lipid metabolism in patients with non-insulin-dependent diabetes mellitus. Metabolism 1996; 45: 1130–5.

64. Halberstam M, Cohen N, Shlimovich P et al. Oral vanadyl sulfate improves insulin sensitivity in NIDDM but not in obese nondiabetic subjects. Diabetes 1996; 45: 659–66.

65. Goldfine AB, Patti ME, Zuberi L et al. Metabolic effects of vanadyl sulfate in humans with non-insulin-dependent diabetes mellitus: *in vivo* and *in vitro* studies. Metabolism 2000; 49: 400–10.

66. Cusi K, Cukier S, DeFronzo RA et al. Vanadyl sulfate improves hepatic and muscle insulin sensitivity in Type 2 diabetes. J Clin Endocrinol Metab 2001; 86: 1410–17.

67. Curran GL, Azarnoff DL, Bolinger RE. Effect of cholesterol synthesis inhibition in normocholesterolemic young men. J Clin Invest 1959; 38: 1251–61.

68. Crans DC. Chemistry and insulin-like properties of vanadium(IV) and vanadium(V) compounds. J Inorg Biochem 2000; 80: 123–31.

69. Reul BA, Amin SS, Buchet JP et al. Effects of vanadium complexes with organic ligands on glucose metabolism: a comparison study in diabetic rats. Br J Pharmacol 1999; 126: 467–77.

70. Marti L, Abella A, Carpene C et al. Combined treatment with benzylamine and low dosages of vanadate enhances glucose tolerance and reduces hyperglycemia in streptozotocin-induced diabetic rats. Diabetes 2001; 50: 2061–8.

71. Bevan AP, Burgess JW, Yale JF et al. In vivo insulin mimetic effects of pV compounds: role for tissue targeting in determining potency. Am J Physiol 1995; 268: E60–E66.

72. Bevan AP, Drake PG, Yale JF et al. Peroxovanadium compounds: biological actions and mechanism of insulin-mimesis. Mol Cell Biochem 1995; 153: 49–58.

31

Contribution of pathophysiology of animal diabetes to the understanding of human diabetes

Eleazar Shafrir

Diabetes is one of the most common diseases in humans and animals alike. Apart from many species of rodents it has been found in non-human primates, dogs, cats, ruminants and fish. Animals with diabetes described in this chapter present an opportunity for research of the endocrine, metabolic, and morphologic changes in diverse phenotypic forms of Types 1 and 2 diabetes. None of the species exhibits the full spectrum of functional or structural lesions of human diabetes, but each offers an opportunity for investigating certain clusters of derangements that are common in diabetic animals and humans, particularly in their formative stages. Among the limitations in the use of diabetic animals as models of human diabetes is the nature of complications they develop probably because of their short life span. In addition, most species with diabetes due to mutations or environmental-nutritional influences do not develop atherosclerotic complications or CVD, most probably because of differences in the composition and metabolism of lipoproteins and the lipoprotein receptor pattern. A general overview of complications in diabetic animals and their relation to human disease is available.[1]

This chapter will deal with actively investigated models of spontaneous or nutritionally induced Type 1 and Type 2 diabetes, but not with cytotoxic diabetes induced by alloxan or streptozotocin. The diabetic animals may be divided into two general groups:

1. Insulin-dependent diabetes due to spontaneous autoimmune aggression of β-cells, most prominent in BB rats and NOD mice. The discovery of these two species contributed to the general acceptance of the etiologic role of autoimmunity in Type 1 diabetes.
2. Species developing Type 2-like syndromes with insulin resistance and obesity as a result of genetic mutation or an innate predisposition to affluent diets.

Animals with autoimmune etiology and insulin dependence

BB rats

Features of the diabetic syndrome in BB rats, with details on history and pathogenesis can be found in review publications.[2–4] The classic symptoms of polyuria, polydipsia, glucosuria, weight loss and marked hyperglycemia, hypoinsulinemia, insulitis, and β-cell loss occur at 60 to 100 days of age. Of the diabetes-prone (DP) rats 50 to 80% become diabetic and may show IGT (impaired glucose tolerance) a few days before the onset of overt symptoms; males and females are equally affected. Most diabetic BB rats require external insulin for protection from ketosis and for survival. Several sublines varying in incidence, severity, immunologic characteristics are known, including diabetes-resistant (DR) lines.[4] Because of variations in the incidence and severity of diabetes, which may be related to viral or microbial pathogens,[5] the BB derivation is denoted by a slash (e.g. BB/Wor for the Worcester, MA colony).

Diabetes in BB/Wor rats is probably inherited by autosomal recessive transmission, related to two genes at least. One non-MHC (major histocompatibility complex) linked gene expresses the T-cell lymphopenia which characterizes BB rats; the second is linked with RT+, the MHC of the rat.[4] This resembles human Type 1 diabetes without association with specific histocompatibility locus antigen (HLA) types. However, the permissive MHC haplotype and the recessive lymphopenic gene[6] are considered to be insufficient to account for the complete diabetes susceptibility.[7] A 'universal autoimmunity locus' on rat chromosome 4 has recently been postulated.[8]

Pancreas histology displays insulitis with striking lymphocytic islet infiltration, which precedes the onset of overt diabetes by several days. It disappears after β-cell loss, but it may reappear after β-cell transplantation. A varying extent of insulitis is also observed in 50–75% of non-hyperglycemic BB/Wor rats. Nitric oxide (NO) is involved in the lymphocyte-induced lesion. NO synthase activity is present in the pancreas of BB rats with insulitis,[9] derived from macrophages, and limited to areas of islet infiltration, in genetic association with T-lymphopenia.[10]

The autoimmune syndrome of BB rats is of polyendocrine nature as evident by the occurrence of lymphocytic thyroiditis and autoantibodies against smooth and skeletal muscle, gastric parietal cells, thyroglobulin, and thyroid cells. Islet cell cytoplasmic antibodies (ICA), thought to arise from cellular constituents after degradation, and islet cell-surface antibodies (ICSA), formed against specific membranal cell components, are often present in the circulation. Although not all rats with antibodies develop diabetes and not all rats with diabetes carry antibodies, a correlation of circulating antibodies with insulitis and diabetes in BB/Wor rats reveals that they are more frequent in DP than DR rats and are often already present at weaning.

One of the features of BB rats resembling human Type 1 diabetes is the pre-pubertal onset with a silent pre-diabetes period, which presents a treatment window based on the presence of early markers of the disorder. Plasma lymphocyte antibodies,[11] released by macrophages upon cytokine activation, have been proposed as predictors. Avoidance of wheat- and milk-derived dietary proteins[12] was suggested as beneficial for preventing the expression of diabetes in BB rats and humans. Bovine insulin ingested by infants in milk has been suggested to prime the humoral and T-cell immunity in individuals with genetic risk for Type 1 diabetes.[13]

The detection of ICSA, one to two months before the onset of diabetes in BB rats parallels their early presence in pre-diabetic children and their association with islet destruction. However, decisive proof of direct pathogenic role of ICSA *in vivo* is still lacking, despite correlations between the start of mononuclear islet infiltration and diabetes onset, and between the appearance of complement-fixing ICSA and β-cell destruction. ICA have not been conclusively found in BB rats. Moreover, GAD antibodies considered important for the prediction of human Type 1 diabetes, are absent in most lines of BB rats.[14] IA-2 antibodies have been detected only in some lines.

T-cell lymphopenia is the notable difference between the BB rat and human diabetes. The severe lymphopenia involves both primary and secondary lymphoid tissues, affects all subsets of T-cells and is permissive rather than obligatory for diabetes to occur. It is prevalent in all DP BB/Wor rats, originating either from a hematopoietic stem cell defect, or from a defective thymic maturation process.[4] Although the progression of the lymphocytic infiltration represents an intermediate stage of β-cell destruction, the initial events remain obscure. Altered β-cell antigenicity, resulting in activation of T- and NK-cells, and cytotoxic antibodies is possible. The nature and interaction of humoral antibodies and cell antigens remains to be elucidated. In this respect, it is intriguing that a membrane bound islet-specific 38-kd autoantigen[15] becomes expressed in DP BB rats at 30 days of age, when the immune effectors start to recognize β-cells. The delayed expression may be important for the breakdown of self-tolerance and for initiating autoimmunity.

Immunomodulation is another aspect of this immunologic approach.[4] In BB rats, not only the various β-cell-destroying effectors are present at the onset of diabetes, but the regulatory T-cells controling the system are defective or missing. These may be RT6+, post-thymic lymphocytes (carrying the RT6 rat alloantigen), detectable in peripheral lymphocytes of DR BB rats, but missing in the DP line. Removal of the RT6+ cells in DR rats with a monoclonal antibody frequently induces insulitis, and renders them diabetic. Immunomodulatory interventions may entail changing the balance between subsets of T-lymphocytes by cyclophosphamide, stimulation of lymphopoiesis by blood removal, dietary changes, and immunogenic stimulation. The novel corrective approaches to immunoregulatory defects (deletion of β-cell autoreactive Th1 lymphocytes and certain cytokines) and increasing the

regulatory Th2 lymphocytes and their cytokine products have been recently reviewed in depth.[16]

The NOD (non-obese diabetic) mice

The development, immunopathogenesis, and genetics of NOD mice has been well described.[17–20] They manifest insulitis starting at the age of four to five weeks, leading to overt diabetes at 13 to 30 weeks, with severe hyperglycemia and β-cell insulin deficiency. Unlike BB rats, the maintenance of NOD mice on insulin is not always obligatory. Despite prevalent insulitis both in males and females, overt diabetes occurs in 80% of females and in only 20% of males. The lines established outside the original colony at Shionogi Laboratories in Japan may differ in diabetes incidence, time of onset, and gender ratio.

The lymphocytes infiltrating the islets include CD4+ and CD8+ T-cells and B-cells. The initial invasion is localized in the periductular capillary spaces with a clear basement membrane boundary without overt contact with β-cells. Later, the lymphocytes penetrate the islet and destroy β-cells. NOD mice are not lymphopenic. Antibodies directed toward a variety of islet antigens are detectable soon after weaning and ICSA at six weeks with 50% prevalence between 12 and 18 weeks.

The contribution of multiple genes on different chromosomes to diabetes susceptibility has been demonstrated,[19–24] but like in humans, the environmental, hormonal and nutritional impact on the incidence of diabetes, in spite of the identical genetic background, affects the penetrance of genetic factors. Castration of males increases the incidence of diabetes, whereas implantation of testosterone to young females prevents diabetes, probably by inhibiting the production or action of autoimmune

	Humans	NOD mice	BB rats
β-cell loss, hyperglycemia, and insulin deficiency	+	+	+
Ketoacidosis	+	–	+
Insulitis	+	+	+
Polyendocrine involvement	Probably	Very strong	Very strong
Gender difference	No	Males/females 3:1	No
Genetic predisposition	+	+	+
Polygenicity	+	+	+
Disease transmission	+	+	+
via bone marrow	Not tested (ethics)	–	+
via T-lymphocytes	Not tested (ethics)	+	+
Lymphocytopenia	–	–	+
Defective immunoregulation	–	–	+
Insulin cell surface antibodies (ICSA)	+	+	–
Insulin cell antibodies (ICA)	+	+	+
IAA	+	+	–
Persistent aggression against implanted β-cells	+	+	+
Prevention by immunomodulation or free-radical scavengers	Possible	+	+
Effective immunotherapy	Possible	+	+
Virus induction	In certain cases	–	–
β-cells required for immune activation	Probably	+	+

Table 31.1
Features of autoimmune diabetes in human subjects, BB rats and NOD mice

effectors. This suggests that the expression of the genetically imprinted gender dimorphism can be manipulated.

The exposure of NOD mice to murine viral pathogens protects against diabetes, probably through general immunostimulation, because several exogenous immunomodulators, like complete Freund's adjuvant, various cytokines, polyinosinic-cytidylic RNA, or gangliosides, attenuate the diabetes development, as reviewed by Kolb.[25] These effects, more marked in NOD mice than in BB rats, are responsible for the genetic drift in various colonies and should be considered when comparing the experimental results.

The β-cell loss in NOD mice is attenuated by BCG inoculation stimulating the general immune reaction capacity, scavengers of free-radicals and inhibitors of the β-cell NAD consuming DNA repairing enzyme, poly (ADP-ribose) synthase.[26] Thus, the destructive processes in NOD mice exhibit similarities to the action of chemical cytotoxins. It is also of interest for the promising treatment of human subjects with insulin that, like in the BB rat, pre-treatment with insulin prevents the adoptive transfer of diabetes in NOD mice.[27] The mechanism of insulin treatment may be immunomodulatory rather than inducing a β-cell rest. Comparison of human Type 1 diabetes with that of BB rats and NOD mice is presented in Table 31.1.

LETL rats

The Long Evans Tokushima Lean (LETL) spontaneously diabetic strain of rats was isolated in Japan.[28] The onset of diabetes in inbred animals occurs at 8–20 weeks of age with an average incidence of 21% in males and 15% in females, influenced by whether one or two parents were diabetic. The clinical features are typical of Type 1 diabetes, LETL rats requiring insulin for survival. A control LETO strain, which exhibits Type 2-like diabetes, was inbred from non-diabetic animals of the same stock. The LETL rats are not lymphopenic and the distribution of thymocyte subsets is similar to control rats. Extensive insulitis is evident a few days before the onset of clinical diabetes, but is not seen in non-diabetic siblings and in the LETO control line. Other endocrine glands are also affected, similarly to BB rats and NOD mice. With regard to genetics, the LETL rats carry the RT1[u] haplotype, as does the DP BB rat. At least two recessive genes, one closely linked with RT1[u], seem to be involved in the pathogenesis of insulitis.

Insulin-resistant rodents with diabesity (diabetes and obesity)

Labile versus resilient β-cells: genetically endowed secretion capacity determines the ability of β-cells to compensate the insulin resistance

There exists a wide spectrum of β-cell response capacity to hyperphagia or to HE diets which result in syndromes of diabesity (diabetes + obesity). In some of them β-cells withstand and in some they succumb to the pressure of compensatory insulin hypersecretion. Several animal species are endowed with sturdy, robust β-cells like *ob/ob* mice, *fa/fa* rats, whereas other species are characterized by brittle, labile β-cells unable to sustain the protracted stimulation of insulin secretion (Table 31.2). Among the latter, the foremost are the mutant *db/db* mice, ZDF rats and the nutritionally diabetic gerbil *Psammomys obesus*, as well as rhesus monkeys. Animals with labile β-cells may transiently control their plasma glucose levels by insulin oversecretion until their insulin secretion apparatus collapses. Hyperinsulinemia in animals endowed with robust β-cells, often associated with hyperphagia, promotes lipogenesis. Shunting of glucose to fat, may protect β-cells from glucotoxicity by moderating the glycemia at the expense of obesity.

Type 2 diabetes has often been considered to result from combined β-cell malfunction and peripheral insulin resistance, involving a genetic failure of β-cells to accommodate for insulin insensitivity.[29] However, this statement does not mean that Type 2 diabetes, in humans or animals, is caused by primarily inferior β-cells. Hypoinsulinemia does not precede hyperglycemia in most cases of Type 2 diabetes, except if there is a specific genetic defect in β-cell function (e.g. glucokinase aberration). The reduced tissue (primarily muscle) sensitivity to insulin is generally considered to be the fundamental trigger of IGT and Type 2 diabetes.[30] To correct the insulin insensitivity, β-cells increase their output, responding even to marginal rises in the circulating glucose level. Most insulin-resistant subjects and many animal species are able to maintain normal glucose tolerance by durable, adaptive hypersecretion of insulin. However, when insulin resistance is unremitting, only a small decrease in the insulin secretion is sufficient to evoke overt diabetes. In

Species	Main phenotypic and metabolic features	Specific complications	Research opportunities
C57BL/KS db/db, leprdb mice	Transient hyperinsulinemia and obesity, hyperphagia, marked insulin resistance, genomic background modifiers, promoting β-cell destruction, sensitivity to carbohydrate diets, mutated leptin receptor	Vasculopathy, nephropathy, neuropathy	Insulin resistance amelioration, β-cell protection, glucotoxicity prevention
C57BL/6J ob/ob, lepob mice	Extreme obesity and hyperphagia, insulin resistance, long-lasting insulin oversecretion, neuroendocrine dysregulation, leptin deficiency, defective thermogenesis		Testing of antiobesity modalities
KK mice	Latent diabesity state, moderate hyperinsulinemia, and insulin resistance evoked on HE diets	Renal lesions similar to human nephropathy, including amyloidosis	Evaluation of antidiabetic and antiobesity drugs, e.g. PPARγ agonists
NZO mice	Diabesity syndrome with marked obesity heavily intra-abdominal, leptin resistance, multiple metabolic abnormalities	Nephropathy, IGG deposition	Investigation of polygenic nature of diabesity
fa/fa Zucker rats, leprfa	Extreme obesity and hyperphagia, long-standing β-cell oversecretion, high β-cell mass, hyperlipidemia, mutated leptin receptor, gender dimorphism	Nephropathy	Testing of anti-obesity and anti-lipidemic drugs
ZDF rats, substrain of leprfa	Diabesity superimposed on hyperlipidemia proceeding to β-cell depletion in males. In females diabesity HE diet induced, susceptibility to fat-rich diets	Vascular and retinal changes and β-cell loss	Testing of antidiabetic modalities, e.g. PPARγ agonists, protection of β-cell gluco- and lipo-toxicity
SHHF/Mcc-cpfa rats	Corpulent rat species group. Cardiomyocyte degeneration, vascular lesions, diabesity, hyperlipidemia, gender dimorphism	Unique in developing cardiomyopathy progressing to congestive heart failure; nephropathy	Anti-CHF modalities

Table 31.2
Comparative characteristics of models of Type 2 diabetes

Species	Main phenotypic and metabolic features	Specific complications	Research opportunities
JCR: LA-cp^{fa} rats	Insulin resistance, obesity, hypertriglyceridemia, atherosclerosis, cardiac ischemia, end-stage CVD, sensitivity to dietary cholesterol, leptin receptor deficiency	Severe vascular lesions, CVD	Antilipidemic, anti obesity modalities, prevention of atherosclerosis and vasculopathy, modulation of CVD
OLETF rats	Mild obesity, late onset but permanent diabesity, hyperlipidemia, bi-phasic changes similar to *db/db* mice	Nephropathy similar to human pathology	Control of nephropathy
Koletsky, SHROB fa^κ rats	Hypertension, hyperlipidemia, hyperphagia, marked obesity, lipogenesis, multiple metabolic abnormalities of insulin resistance syndrome	Nephropathy, vascular disease, cardiac hypertrophy	Angiotension II effects interaction of components of insulin resistance syndrome, antilipidemic drugs
WKY rats	Diabesity, hypertension, insulin resistance related to raised TNFα levels; reset sodium excretion threshold, hyperlipidemia, gender dimorphism	Early nephropathy, microangiopathy, neuropathy	Antidiabesity and antihypertension drugs
Torii rats	Diabesity	Retinopathy remarkably similar to human	Preventive measures against retinopathy
Psammomys obesus (sand rat)	Diet-induced diabesity based on genetic propensity, progressing to β-cell loss and PKCε overexpression detrimental to insulin signaling transduction	Cataracts	Study of insulin signaling pathway under/overnutrition and of innate insulin resistance
C57BL/6J mice	Diet-induced diabesity without hyperphagia, abnormalities in autonomic nervous system, β-cell and adipocyte function, hyperleptinemia	Uncoupling protein (UCP) abnormalities	Genetics of dietary obesity, role of UCP
Goto-Kakizaki (GK) rats	Non-obese Wistar substrain, abnormal islet morphology including reduced β-cell mass, mild hyperglycemia, impaired insulin release, mild insulin resistance	Glomerulopathy	Pathogenesis of islet changes and insulin release
Macaca mulatta rhesus monkeys	Spontaneous diabesity and β-cell loss with amyloid deposition in captivity on *ad libitum* diet during 10–12 years remarkable similarity to human pathophysiology of Type 2 diabetes in compressed time frame	Neuropathy, nephropathy, retinopathy, hypertension	Protection against insulin resistance syndrome during longitudinal progression to diabesity

these diabetic subjects the failure of β-cells is the main reason for hyperglycemia as reported in the UKPDS study.[30] It is apparent that, in these cases, β-cells are genetically not constructed to withstand the stress of oversecretion and may be affected by other genomic factors accentuating the β-cell exhaustion. However, there is no instance when β-cell dysfunction precedes the onset of insulin resistance. The lesson from animal diabetes, which applies also to humans, is that with controlled compensatory insulin oversecretion even labile β-cells may last for life.

db/db *mice now labeled* lepr[db]

The biphasic behavior of the mutant *db/db* mice to the imposed hyperglycemic stress is a good example of the initial diabesity induced by insulin oversecretion, followed by weight loss and ketosis due to β-cell demise. Diabetes in the *db/db* mice is a recessive, autosomal single gene mutation on chromosome 4, which occurred spontaneously in the inbred C57BL/KS mice in Bar Harbor, ME.[31] It is now considered to be a homologue of the rat *fa* gene on chromosome 5. Apart from genetic hyperphagia, the KS background potentiates insulin resistance and glucose overproduction, and damage to the insulin secretion apparatus. The genomic KS background factors of *db/db* mice are harmful by limiting β-cell replication and adversely sensitizing them to hyperglycemia. This is demonstrated by the abundant growth of spleen-implanted islets in non-diabetic BL/6J mice, which exceeds by far that of islets implanted in non-diabetic BL/Ks mice.[32] This is a cogent demonstration of the impact of deleterious genomic background modifiers on the course, severity, and final outcome of the diabesity syndrome, caused by a single abnormal gene.

The earliest abnormality of the *db/db* syndrome is hyperphagia at weaning. The mice gain weight, and become hyperglycemic, between 8 and 12 weeks, up to 400 mg/dl (33 mmol/l), in spite of six- to ten-fold increase in insulin levels. At three to six months, the insulinemia wanes to subnormal levels, β-cells necrotize and the mice do not survive longer than 10 months. The time course of diabetes development may differ in *db/db* mice raised in other colonies, and investigators should establish their local reference values.

The β-cell insulin oversecretion may last up to four months, irrespective of the islet content. The defective β-cell response to glucose, but sustained response to arginine, occurs concurrently with the loss of GLUT2 transporter. This is a reversible phenomenon, because *db* islets transplanted to non-diabetic *db/+* controls regain GLUT2 expression.[33] The reduced insulin secretion is concurrent with ultrastructural changes comprising dilatation of Golgi apparatus and of rough endoplasmic reticulum.[34] Although hyperinsulinemia initially compensates for insulin resistance, β-cells are unable to sustain the high secretion rate lapsing into drastic necrosis.

Tissue insulin resistance is already present in very young *db/db* mice. It is ameliorated by insulin treatment or by implantation of islets from isogeneic donors.[31] In older, hyperglycemic mice, glycolytic enzymes wane, while the gluconeogenic pathway escapes regulation, despite the high circulating insulin. Phosphoenolpyruvate carboxykinase (PEPCK) synthesis assessed by hepatic PEPCK mRNA levels, which is normally regulated by physiologic changes in insulin, is not suppressed in *db/db* mice. Reducing PEPCK transcription is achieved only by enormous amounts of exogenous insulin.[35] Regulatory failure of other liver systems is also evident: glycogen breakdown is not inhibited by glucose or insulin, while lipogenesis is enhanced in both the liver and intestine, accounting for the prevalent hyper-lipidemia.

Insulin binding to insulin receptors (IR) is reduced, tyrosine kinase (TK) activity in muscle, liver, and isolated fibroblasts is down-regulated.[36,37] A detailed review of the metabolic abnormalities in *db/db* mice and *ob/ob* mice has been provided by Herberg and Leiter.[38]

Db/db mice are highly sensitive to dietary carbohydrate. Dietary restriction does not induce normoinsulinemia in *db/db* mice, but total substitution of protein for carbohydrate has a beneficial effect.[39] The regimen of 83% casein substantially reduces the hyperglycemia by making it dependent on endogenously regulated hepatic gluconeogenesis rather than on external glucose. It also extends the life span, retards the decrease in islet insulin content[35] and delays β-cell glucotoxicity and necrosis. Inclusion of even 8% of carbohydrate in the diet, particularly sucrose, substantially aggravates the diabetes and shortens the life span. Such effective control of glycemia by high protein diet should be considered in human blood glucose control, and is advocated by the high protein diets of Atkins and Eades for prevention of diabesity.[40]

An improvement in glucose homeostasis by reducing blood glucose levels was obtained by transgenic overexpression of the insulin regulatable muscle GLUT4 transporter.[41] Inhibition of renal Na+ glucose co-transporter by a non-toxic derivative of phlorizin[42] also decreased the blood glucose level by enhancing glucose excretion, improved glucose tolerance and delayed the pancreatic insulin depletion. Inhibition of glycoalbumin formation reduced urinary collagen IV excretion and prevented renal insufficiency in *db/db* mice.[43]

Coleman[44] impressively demonstrated the hypothalamic defect in *db/db* mice eliciting hyperphagia by the failure to respond to satiety signals, when parabiosed with non-diabetic mice. The latter stopped eating and starved to death due to a massive inflow of the elevated satiety factor from *db/db* mice, now identified as leptin. The *db/db* mice gained weight and did not respond to the satiety factor of non-diabetic mice because of their truncated hypothalamic leptin receptor. Striking results were obtained when *db/db* mice were parabiosed with congenic *ob/ob* partners. The latter stopped eating, became lean and died from starvation because of the strong response to the satiety factor which they lacked. When *ob/ob* mice were parabiosed with normal mice, they lost weight themselves, showing that their own satiety systems reacted appropriately to leptin.

The molecular basis for the prescient hypothesis of Coleman on the nature of *db* and *ob* mutations was provided by Friedman and colleagues by the isolation of the *ob* gene product, leptin and of the hypothalamic leptin receptor.[45,46] This discovery revolutionized our approach to adipose tissue as not only a hormonally regulated fat depot, but also a lipostatic endocrine organ, the source of leptin. After the finding that *db* is the mutation of leptin receptor gene and *ob* is the mutation of leptin synthesis gene, the nomenclature of these two mice species has been changed to lepr[db] and lep[ob], respectively. Unfortunately, the early hope that treatment with leptin will prevent obesity in humans has not materialized. However, leptin administration was highly effective in the rare morbid obesity patients with mutations of the leptin gene producing an ineffective leptin protein. These data suggest an important, hitherto not well understood, role for leptin and its interaction with insulin, in human body weight regulation. However, it should be taken into consideration that the mode of action of leptin in mice may be quite different from that in humans as discussed by Himms-Hagen.[47]

Insulin-resistant mutant rodents with sustained insulin secretion

Ob/ob *mice now labeled lep[ob]*

In contradistinction to *db/db* mice, which lose their β-cells in the course of insulin-resistant diabetes, the C57BL/6J *ob/ob* mice, also originating from the Bar Harbor Jackson Laboratory,[34] are characterized by resilient, long lasting β-cells leading to remarkable obesity, up to 90 g body weight. The autosomal recessive, *ob* mutation is located on chromosome 6.

Ob/ob mice are hyperphagic, insulin-resistant, and only mildly hyperglycemic. The sustained β-cell hyperfunction results in 10- to 50-fold higher than normal insulin levels, which persist during their life and compensate, in large part, for the resistance, constrain the overactive gluconeogenesis and promote glucose incorporation into TG, despite an increased free fatty acids (FFA) turnover. Pancreatic insulin content is very high, the highest of any other mice mutants with diabesity. In contrast to *db/db*, β-cells exhibit a pronounced hypertrophy-hyperplasia. Insulin resistance in *ob/ob* mice, as in other diabese animals, appears to be due to impaired IR phosphorylation in the face of hyperinsulinemia, and consequently reduced insulin signal transduction.

The genetic defect in the *ob/ob* mice is the lack of satiety-controlling factors, as elegantly demonstrated by the parabiosis experiments (see *db/db* mice) and confirmed by the lack of leptin in *ob/ob* mice due to a mutation in the *ob* gene. The role of the associated hypothalamic peptides in neuroendocrine glucoregulation has been recently reviewed.[48,49] Levels of neuropeptide Y – a potent, insulin-suppressible appetite stimulant – are high in diabese animals, possibly as a result of leptin deficiency.

KK *mice*

The metabolic-endocrine features, and the pharmacologic utility of KK mice have been reviewed by Taketomi and Ikeda.[50] The KK strains and hybrids differ in the degree of obesity and glucose homeostasis, but obesity seems to be the primary factor precipitating the insulin resistance. The KK hybrids and the yellow KK mice develop overt diabetes along with weight gain on a regular diet, whereas the Japanese KK require HE diet for the expression of diabetes. The KK inheritance appears to be dominant with 25% penetrance, due to the association with a recessive modifier, but evidence for polygenic inheritance was also provided, as concluded from quantitative trait loci analysis.[51] Non-fasting hyperglycemia is <300 mg/dl (17 mmol/l), and weight reaches a peak of 50 g at five months, and is more marked in males than females. Non-fasting hyperinsulinemia may reach levels up to 1200 µU/ml. IGT is more marked in males than in females. KK mice have high plasma glucagon levels and deficient suppression of glucagon release by glucose.

The hyperglycemia in all KK strains is associated with high activities of glycolytic and lipogenic enzymes, concordant with the hyperinsulinemia, but the activity of gluconeogenesis enzymes also rises, similarly to the metabolic derangement in *db/db* mice. Insulin resistance in KK mice is due to downregulation of signal transduction components, among them IRS-1 and PI-3K.[52]

A prominent feature of the KK mice is β-cell hyperplasia and elevated insulin content, as well as an expanded endoplasmic reticulum, Golgi apparatus, and apparent neogenesis of β-cells from duct cells. Like other diabese rodents, KK mice exhibit high corticosterone levels and adrenal hyperplasia. However, obesity, glycemia, and insulinemia precede the adrenal changes, indicating that they are secondary. Hyperphagia is a common finding in all KK strains, but its onset is not as early as in other diabese mutants. Hyperglycemia, hyperinsulinemia, obesity, and sensitivity to exogenous insulin all tend to revert to normal with age, nevertheless, the life span of diabetic KK mice is significantly shorter.

New Zealand obese (NZO) mice

The polygenic New Zealand obese (NZO) strain was developed from a mixed colony of mice by selective breeding for heavy weight, until obesity with mild hyperglycemia and hyperinsulinemia became established. Body weight rises rapidly during the first two months of life conforming to the hyperphagia, reaching up to 90 g at ~14 months. Peak glycemia of ~250 mg/dl (14 mmol/l) occurs at ~5 months and is more pronounced in males than females. Hepatic gluconeogenesis is increased despite hyperinsulinemia. The features of the NZO diabesity have been reviewed in detail.[53,54] Hyperfunction of β-cells results in a wide spectrum of plasma insulin values, though less marked than in *ob/ob* or KK mice.

Insulin secretion pattern in NZO mice is abnormal. Plasma insulin level in fasted mice is similar to that of fed mice and two to three times higher than in controls. Islet responses to tolbutamide, cyclic AMP, or glucose are low, and effects of glucagon or aminophylline are delayed. The calcium ionophore IBMX promotes insulin release from islets of fasted mice but does not augment the effect of glucose. Arginine elicits a good response. The refractoriness to glucose may be related to limited islet glucose metabolism in relation to insulin

output with an impediment prior to the triose phosphate step, as glyceraldehyde provokes a potent insulin release. A single injection of a cyclic AMP elevating an 'islet activating protein' lowered the blood glucose level for as long as five days and improved the secretion of insulin *in vivo* and in isolated islets.

Insulin resistance is remarkable: large doses of exogenous insulin hardly affect the blood glucose level but intraperitoneally implanted islets of albino mice reverse the hyperglycemia. Basal- and insulin-stimulated muscle 2-deoxyglucose transport is reduced as is the glycogen content.[55] Adipose tissue was also found to be insulin resistant, evident from a defect in insulin stimulation of pyruvate dehydrogenase activity.[56] Hepatic glycolytic enzymes, glucokinase, and pyruvate kinase are elevated and the gluconeogenic PEPCK and glucose-6-phosphatase are reduced, as would be expected in a hyperinsulinemic state, which is in contrast to other diabese animals. However, the activity of fructose-1,6-bisphosphatase is not reduced by hyperinsulinemia, and the abnormal regulation of this enzyme was suggested to contribute to the increased hepatic glucose production.[57] Lipogenesis is increased both in the liver and adipose tissue, which responds to a fat-rich diet with hypercellularity. The ratio of total versus peritoneal adipose tissue is 2.5 in NZO and 3.5 in *ob/ob* mice[58] suggesting that the relative abundance of peritoneal fat may accentuate the metabolic disturbances, similarly to humans.

fa/fa (Zucker) rats now labeled lepr[fa]

The *fa* gene is a spontaneous autosomal recessive mutation on rat chromosome 5. On the basis of the flanking genetic markers the *fa* gene is now considered to be the rat homologue of the mouse *db* gene,[59] located on chromosome 4 which has been shown to produce a mutated leptin receptor. The pathophysiology of the *fa* mutation has been extensively reviewed.[60,61] *Fa/fa* rats develop hyperphagia and extreme obesity due to the prominent growth of all fat depots. This is accompanied by mild hyperglycemia, IGT, marked insulin resistance, hyperinsulinemia and pronounced hyperlipidemia. Phenotypically, the *fa/fa* rats appear similar to *ob/ob* mice. They exhibit early and persistent hyperphagia and obesity, but differ from *db/db* mice by long-lasting capacity of insulin hypersecretion.

Islets of *fa/fa* rats exhibit both hypertrophy and hyperplasia with pronounced microtubule formation, which is sustained through most of their life, despite lasting overstimulation. In these respects, *fa/fa* rats resemble *ob/ob* mice. The *fa/fa* rats oversecrete insulin even when fed a diet identical in carbohydrate content to their lean controls. Support for an intrinsic defect causing oversecretion comes from the observation that insulin release from isolated islets is not normalized after culturing for as long as 21 days, and that islets cultured at low glucose concentrations exhibit an exaggerated glucose-stimulated response, not inhibited by mannoheptulose.[62] The dissociation between hyperphagia and hyperinsulinemia is apparent in long-term experiments: food restriction does not preclude the development of hyperinsulinemia, obesity, hepatic lipogenesis and adipose tissue TG uptake.

The role of glucocorticoids was discussed in depth by York,[63] stressing that these hormones are required for the development of diabesity in *fa/fa* rats and other mutants by acting both at peripheral and central sites. The diabesity is characterized by increased availability of glucocorticoids from the enlarged adrenal glands. The hyperinsulinemia appears to be caused by CNS signals transmitted to the pancreas via the vagus.[64] Further evidence for the anomalous performance of the hypothalamo-pituitary axis is the dysregulation of NPY mRNA and CRF.

Abnormal cerebral glucose utilization has been found by Jeanrenaud and colleagues.[65] Tissue unresponsiveness to insulin is ameliorated by adrenalectomy, which also lowers food intake, decreases the efficiency of energy use, and depresses lipogenesis.

Insulin resistance is prominent in *fa/fa* rats. It is evident in perfused hind limb muscle both with respect to glucose transport and lactate oxidation. However, insulin sensitivity in the heart appears normal, although actual glucose transport and metabolism may be decreased. In an euglycemic-hyperinsulinemic clamp, the total glucose use, similar to lean rats, was achieved only at a 3.5-fold higher insulin level.[66] There is a substantial decrease in IRS-1 protein, insulin stimulated IRS-1 phosphorylation, and the expression of PI-3K,[67] consistent with deficient GLUT4 translocation.[68,69] These observations provide the molecular basis for muscle insulin resistance in the face of hyperinsulinemia, characteristic of *fa/fa* diabesity. Oxidative stress has also been implicated in the attenuated glucose transport in the skeletal muscle.[70] The hepatic VLDL secretion is not inhibited by insulin giving rise to marked VLDL hyperlipidemia,[71] and the activity of lipogenic enzymes and of lipoprotein lipase is increased in adipose tissue.[72,73]

The secretion of amylase by the exocrine pancreas is low. Amylase synthesis is insulin-dependent and its activity is reduced in insulinopenic conditions. Interestingly, amylase synthesis was found to be reduced in the hyperinsulinemic, but insulin-resistant *fa/fa* rats and *ob/ob* mice,[74] pointing out that insulin resistance is also manifested in proximal acinar cells, reducing the expression of the amylase gene.

Diabetic fa/fa *rat: ZDF*

A substrain of *fa/fa* rats, selectively inbred for hyperglycemia,[75] is popular in the the investigation of Type 2 diabetes. Non-fasting plasma glucose levels exceed 400 mg/dl (22 mmol/l) at 10 weeks of age in males. Females become diabetic on high energy diets. The hyperlipoproteinemia is similar to that seen in *fa/fa* rats, but the weight gain and insulin levels are lower. ZDF rats have a reduced expression of muscle GLUT4 transporter.[76] In contrast to *fa/fa* rats, the capacity to oversecrete insulin is limited, they manifest labile, glucose-sensitive β-cells proceeding to apoptosis.[77] They also demonstrate downregulation of β-cell GLUT2 transporters,[78] which impair glucose uptake and insulin synthesis, thus inducing severe Type-2-like diabetes. Food restriction in the pre-diabetic stage of ZDF rats may prevent β-cell deterioration and loss of GLUT2.[79] A lipotoxic effect of high plasma FFA and triglyceride (TG) levels on β-cell function has been described by Unger and collaborators,[80,81] which may have implications for humans with dyslipidemia or consuming fat-rich diets. PPARγ agonists had a diabetes attenuating effect, especially in the pre-diabetic stage.

Obese-hyperglycemic Wistar Kyoto fatty rat group

This group of rats with polygenic diabetes-obesity-hypertension was derived from reciprocal crosses between the *fa/fa* and Wistar Kyoto (WKY) rats in Japan.[82,83] The aim was to obtain an obese and hyperlipidemic animal with hypertension and hyperglycemia. After several crosses and inbreeding, insulin resistance and hyperinsulinemia became evident. Males are hyperglycemic and females become hyperglycemic on a sucrose-rich regimen. Several variants were developed and referred to as WDF/Ta-*fa* rats,[84] or Wistar diabetic rats, and WKY/N Drt-*fa*.[85]

The outbred males of the WDF/Ta-*fa* substrain are hyperglycemic on a sucrose-rich diet; females are not hyperglycemic, but both genders are hyperinsulinemic. Castration did not abolish the sexual dimorphism, but it did improve insulin sensitivity. Neonatal ovariectomy did not aggravate the diabesity, indicating no estrogen protection. Males are more hyperphagic than females, which could account, in part, for the sex difference. High hepatic glucose production with elevated PEPCK activity was abolished by adrenalectomy. Hypertrophic islets were prominent with pronounced insulin secretion, which did not diminish, however, the hyperglycemia. Insulin resistance was associated with downregulation of muscle IR, leading to decreased insulin binding and signaling. TK activity per receptor was also reduced demonstrating the detrimental effect of hyperinsulinemia on IR function.[86] The association of hypertension with insulin resistance was suggested to result from impaired vascular tone and growth of smooth muscle cells, as well as to the resetting of the natriuresis threshold by increased sodium reabsorption, with hypertension as a compensatory element for the sodium retention.[83]

The WKY fatty rats in Japan were reported to be spontaneously hypertensive and nephropathic.[85] Insulin resistance was attributed to enhanced muscle TNFα production, impairing insulin signaling. The WKY diabetic strain was also raised in the USA by crossing with the WKY/N stock.[84] The colony suffered from infections and had to be maintained in SPF condition. The animals delivered by cesarean section were more diabetic than those born naturally. It is interesting that infections reduced the incidence of Type-2-like diabetes, analogously to the effect of pathogens on diabetes in BB rats and NOD mice, even though the WKY fatty rats are without autoimmune background.

Diabetic corpulent cp rat group

Rats with Type-2-like diabesity and hypertension, were developed from two congenic strains, SHR/N and LA/N, at the NIH in Bethesda, MD (substrain code N). The SHR/N-*cp* and the LA/N-*cp* rats were obtained by introducing into these backgrounds the *cp* gene of the Koletzky SHR strain, which carries one *fa* allele. The investigators preferred the name 'corpulent' and symbol *cp*fa or *fa*cp over the proposed new designation *lepr*facp. Details on the backcrosses, which led to the different substrains[87] indicate the important feature of the *cp* gene: a small difference in the genomic background leads to substrains that markedly vary in the degree of hyperglycemia, hyperlipidemia, insulin resistance, hypertension nephropathy, propensity to myocardial lesions and atherosclerosis.

SHHF/Mcc-cp^fa rats

SHHF/Mcc-*cp*fa rats, maintained by McCune et al.[88] evolved on a genomic background conducive to the expression of cardiomyopathy, dramatically presenting as congestive heart failure (CHF) expressed in 100% of animals in association with hypertension and diabesity. Renal changes, similar to those in the SHR/N-*cp* strain, also occur, particularly in females. The mode of inheritance is polygenic, but the presence of the *cp*fa gene is essential. Sexual dimorphism is seen in the onset of CHF and diabesity. which includes also heterozygote littermates. Early death occurs in the following order: males, females, lean males, and lean females. Clinical symptoms resemble human CHF: pronounced cardiomegaly, edema, hydrothorax, ascites, dyspnea, and visceral hyperemia, changes in atrial natriuretic factor, norepinephrine, aldosterone, and renin. Morphologic observations indicate degeneration of myocytes

which begins long before hypertension or CHF.[89] Estrone treatment delays but does not prevent CHF. The calcium channel blocker nifedipine, reduces body weight, cardiac hypertrophy, and blood pressure, and improves glucose homeostasis mainly in females.[90]

JCR: LA-cp^fa corpulent rats

Backcrosses of LA/N-*cp* males with a hooded rat species produced an outbred substrain JCR: LA-*cp* with ~3% contribution of the SHR gene but the presence of the *fa* allele. Russell and Kelly[91] reported that these rats are not hypertensive but insulin-resistant, acquired at weaning, with pronounced hyperlipidemia, diabesity, and hepatic lipogenesis. Their prominent feature is early CVD with atherosclerotic lesions of major blood vessels, which do not appear in *fa/fa* or other *cp* strains. The lesions were morphologically classified into stages, assumed to represent the progression and repair of the ischemic damage, ranging from inflammatory cell infiltration, myocytolysis, to advanced focal infiltration with scavenging and collagen bands and scars at various stages of maturity.

JCR: LA-*cp* males show a greater CVD incidence than females, approaching 100% at nine months of age. The appearance of occlusive thrombi in coronary arteries indicates that the lesion is ischemic-atherosclerotic, although not related to plasma cholesterol concentration. Food restriction, strenuous exercise, alcohol intake, or suppression of lipogenesis delayed the progression of CVD and insulin resistance. Castration reduced the TG levels, but was without effect on vascular lesions, indicating that estrogens were not protective. Conversely, nifedipine prevented the formation of advanced lesions without improving insulin resistance. It was proposed that the frequency and severity of CVD is due to hyperinsulinemic stress-initiated primary endothelial injury, which in the face of hypertriglyceridemia, hyperphagia and genetic factors progresses to intimal atheroma and reduces the life span of JCR: LA-*cp* rats.[92]

OLETF rats

Male OLETF rats manifest a spontaneous IGT, hyperglycemia, and moderate hyperinsulinemia at about 18 weeks of age and are overweight. This mutation was discovered in the Otsuka Long Evans Tokushima colony, from which the LETL rats with Type 1-like disorder also originated, and was reviewed by Kawano et al.[93] β-cell infiltration with fibrotic tissue and mononuclear cells is seen around the time of onset, followed by β-cell enlargement due to the deposition of intra-islet fibrotic tissue and hemosiderin. Numerous fat droplets as a consequence of hyper-triglyceridemia were also observed.

The OLETF rats develop pronounced renal lesions, with clinical and pathological features resembling human diabetic nephropathy, characterized by thickening and rupture of the glomerular basement membrane, focal mesangial lesion, fibrin cap and aneurysmal dilatations of intraglomerular vessels.

Koletzky (SHROB) rats, now labeled fa^K

SHROB rats exhibit obesity, hyperinsulinemia, severe insulin resistance, with downregulated insulin signaling pathway, hypertriglyceridemia, nephropathy and hypertension.[94] The obesity is related to a mutation in the leptin receptor.[95] The designation *fa^K* implies that the genetic defect resides on the *fa/fa* allele. SHROB rats exhibit IGT and elevated corticosterone, but are normoglycemic in the fasting condition. Thus, they may represent a model for investigation of

human insulin-resistance syndrome and of gene modifiers, which dissociate obesity from hyperglycemia. Increased activity of the sympathetic nervous system was proposed to be responsible, by separate pathways, for both hypertension and insulin resistance.

Torii rats

A new spontaneously diabetic strain of Sprague Dawley rat has been established by Shinowara and colleagues.[96] Glucosuria appeared at ~20 weeks of age in males and ~45 weeks in females, followed by hyperglycemia, hyperinsulinemia and hypertriglyceridemia. Incidence of diabetes was 100% in males at 40 weeks and 33% in females at 65 weeks with survival of ~95% at 65 weeks in both genders. Fibrosis in the pancreatic islets was evident at 25 weeks, cataracts by 40 weeks, retinal detachment with fibrous proliferation by 70 weeks and hemorrhage in the anterior chamber at 77 weeks. It is remarkable that the ocular histopathological characteristics in the Torii rat closely resemble the retinopathy in human Type 2 diabetes at the stage of β-cell insufficiency.

Nutritionally induced diabetes: Psammomys obesus

Of particular relevance to the development of human Type 2 diabetes is the nutritionally induced IGT and β-cell collapse in the desert gerbil *Psammomys obesus* (often nicknamed sand rat). *Psammomys* is herbivorous and non-diabetic in its habitat, but develops fatal diabetes when transferred from the desert to the laboratory rodent diet, which is high energy (HE) for this animal. Maintaining the animals on a low energy (LE) diet was successful for establishing a reproducible colony.[97] The animals are not hyperphagic but on *ad libitum*

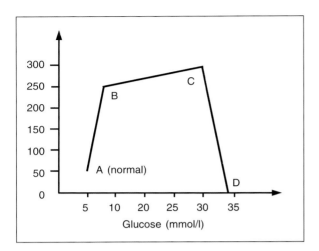

Figure 31.1
'Inverted U' pattern illustrating the progression of Psammomys *from normalcy (Stage A) to hyperinsulinemia (Stage B), hyperglycemia (Stage C) and hypoinsulinemia with marked hyperglycemia (stage D). Animals were selected at random from a large colony and kept on a regular rodent chow for two to four weeks. With time most of the animals progress to stages C and D.*

diet gradually lapse from normalcy (stage A) into hyperinsulinemia (stage B), hyperglycemia (stage C), and insulin deficiency with β-cell apoptosis (stage D).[98] The course of diabetes progress in Israeli *Psammomys* is shown in Figure 31.1 and is described in detail.[99–102] Similar observations were made on a branch of Israeli *Psammomys* colony bred in Australia.[102,103] Although insulin resistance and hyperinsulinemia appear before weight gain in *Psammomys*, they may contribute to adipose tissue accretion and diabesity. Tissue TG deposition is driven by the ample hepatic lipogenesis, which continues unabated despite insulin resistance. With regard to the genetic background of diabesity it is of special interest that the product of a hypothalamic gene,

termed beacon, discovered by Collier and colleagues[104,105] was found to increase the food intake and body weight after intracerebroventricular injection. It also induced a two-fold increase in hypothalamic NPY expression. The progress of *Psammomys* to diabesity may be reversed by reducing the nutrition in stage C, before apoptosis and β-cell degranulation set in, as described both in the Jerusalem and Australian colonies.[106,107]

Psammomys maintained on HE diet, undergoes massive β-cell degranulation, loss of insulin immunostaining, apoptosis and necrosis. Jörns and colleagues[108] have followed the β-cell changes during the progression of *Psammomys* to diabetes. A gradual loss of β-cell insulin, glucokinase and GLUT2 transporter immunoreactivities was visualized, subsequent to hyperglycemia. After one week on HE diet, the β-cell volume became reduced by ~one-third and immunostaining of glucokinase, and GLUT2 by >50%. After three weeks on HE diet this reduction became 70–95% in correlation with the rising blood glucose level. Ultrastructurally, different signs of necrotic destruction of pancreatic β-cells such as the pyknosis of nuclei and a massive vacuolization in the cytoplasm were evident, accompanied by swollen mitochondria and dilated cisternae of the Golgi complex and of the rough endoplasmic reticulum. When the pancreas was removed from hyperglycemic animals, after several weeks on a HE diet (stage D), β-cells exhibited apoptosis and DNA fragmentation (Figure 31.2).[109–111]

There is no direct evidence for the involvement of gluco- or lipotoxicity in the necrosis of β-cells in *Psammomys* unlike the findings in ZDF rats. An attempt to prevent the possible effect of advanced glycation end products or of nitrous oxide by including the glycation inhibitor, aminoguanidine, in the hyperglycemic incubation medium was not effective

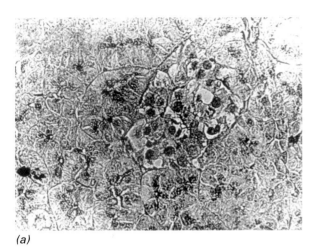

(a)

Figure 31.2
(a) β-cell apoptosis in the terminal stage D of hypoinsulinemic Psammomys *revealed by Tdt-mediated dUTP nick end labeling (TUNEL) and staining of the biotin labeled DNA cleavage nick ends with 3-aminoethyl carbazole. Note the nuclear fragmentation and spreading of nuclear fragments in the cytoplasm, indicated by the brownish flecks. Magnification 500×. (b) Two pancreas sections showing an islet with single β-cell apoptosis in the hyperglycemic-hyperinsulinemic stage C of* Psammomys *maintained on HE diet, preceding the pancreas degranulation in stage D. Magnification 500×. Source: adapted from ref. 113.*

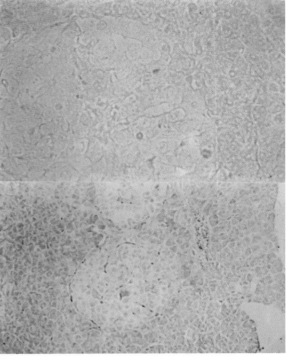

(b)

in protecting β-cells in *Psammomys*.[110] However, Kaneto et al.[112] reported that working with reducing sugars may trigger apoptosis in β-cells of streptozotocin-diabetic rats by provoking the oxidative stress of glycation products. In their hands, the antioxidant N-acetyl-L-cysteine and aminoguanidine inhibited the apoptosis. We presume that there may be species-difference in reaction to hyperglycemia. In *Psammomys* the prompt damage to β-cell architecture with loss of the insulin biosynthetic and secretory capacity is probably the result of exhaustion due to the hypersecre-

tion pressure prior to eventual glucotoxic effect. These findings may be compared with those in human subjects participating in the UKPDS study, in whom the rising blood glucose was mirrored by the decline in β-cell function without an appreciable decrease in insulin sensitivity, suggesting an ongoing glycation damage to β-cell proteins.[30]

Psammomys in stage C shows increased plasma proinsulin levels, up to one-half of the circulating immunoassayable total insulin.[113] The inordinate secretion pressure may cause a swift exocytosis of immature insulin granules escaping the C peptide cleavage before the release into the circulation. Similar disproportionate elevation of proinsulin in human subjects and in experimental Type 2 diabetes with insulin resistance has been observed.[114] This indicates that the compensation of the delayed glucose removal or suppression of gluconeogenesis are not effective because proinsulin has only a minute fraction of insulin activity. On the other hand, the high level of circulating proinsulin does not mean that its secretion is similar to that of insulin since the half-life of proinsulin is much longer than that of insulin.[115]

Insulin resistance and tyrosine kinase attenuation in Psammomys obesus

To investigate the development of insulin resistance, the activity of TK, the initiator of insulin signaling pathway, was studied in the liver and muscle of *Psammomys*. Kanety et al.[116] have found a low IR content in muscle and liver, about one-fifth of the laboratory albino rat. However, insulin binding and TK activity per receptor was normal, both *in vitro* and *in vivo*. The TK activity was measured in stages B and C of progression to diabetes, as compared to the normoglycemic stage A. Basal phosphorylation of the isolated IR was comparable in these stages to that in the normoglycemic stage A, but the extent of TK activation by insulin was pronouncedly lower in stages B and C in liver and muscle.[116] The reduced insulin activation was accompanied by a marked decrease in muscle GLUT4 protein and mRNA.[101] Both could be reversed by nutrition restriction to one-half of their daily food intake for a few days. The recovery of TK activity was not complete when hyperglycemia was corrected, and insulin levels were still elevated but full after the return to normoinsulinemia. These findings indicate that hyperinsulinemia is the basic event responsible for deficient IR function causing insulin resistance as a result of multisite phosphorylation of the receptor.

Deleterious effect of hyperinsulinemia on IR function

The deleterious effect of hyperinsulinemia, even in non-nutritionally induced conditions, can be demonstrated in several animal species and humans. A few cogent examples can be quoted. Transgenic mice enriched with 8 or 32 insulin gene copies, resulting in circulating hyperinsulinemia exhibited both IGT and high TG levels in correlation with the amount of insulin gene copies in their β-cells.[117] In other transgenic mice insulin oversecretion induced an overexpression of glutamine:fructose 6 phosphate amidotransferase associated with β-cell malfunction.[118] Hyperinsulinemia and insulin resistance was also achieved by targeted disruption of genes encoding the proteins participating in insulin signaling, glucose and lipid transport and metabolism in mice, recently reviewed by Sone et al.[119]

Miles et al.[120] have shown that protecting the insulin from hepatic degradation by diversion of pancreatic blood flow through anastomosis with vena cava in healthy dogs induced a sustained hyperinsulinemia. A marked insulin resistance resulted as evident from the 30% reduction in peripheral glucose disposal rate. The resistance was localized to IR/TK, the maximal activation of which (by insulin) decreased by ~40% compared to control dogs.

It was also found that hyperinsulinemia inhibits myocardial protein degradation in patients with CVD, which is a potential mechanism contributing to cardiomegaly.[121]

Hyperinsulinemia of endogenous or exogenous origin should be considered, also in humans, not only as a compensatory response to insulin resistance, but as an inhibitor of insulin action. In non-diabetic human volunteers, the infusion of insulin for several days followed by the euglycemic-hyperinsulinemic clamp, resulted in the reduction of non-oxidative whole-body glucose metabolism by up to 40%.[122] Also, patients with insulinoma exhibited insulin resistance that was related to the extent of their hyperinsulinemia.[123] Furthermore, fasting hyperinsulinemia in diabetes-prone Pima Indians has been found to be an antecedent of Type 2 diabetes, reflected by the decline in response to i.v. glucose load.[124]

Overexpression of PKCε – a negative feedback in insulin signal transduction

Protein kinase C (PKC) in the gastrocnemius muscle of hyperinsulinemic *Psammomys* was found to be pronouncedly overexpressed.[125,126] This enzyme group is now widely studied because of its preferential phosphorylation of serine and threonine residues on signaling pathway proteins, producing a negative feedback of this pathway.[127] The PKC group includes at least 11 isoenzymes, of which PKCε was most pronouncedly overexpressed in *Psammomys* muscle. These isoenzymes, including PKCε, have been termed 'lipid second messengers' because of their diacylglycerol (DAG) dependence.[128] PKCε was also translocated from the cytosol to muscle membrane to a larger extent than other PKC isoenzymes, which in addition to overexpression indicates an increased activity.[125] Other PKC isoenzymes tended also to be overexpressed, particularly PKCα and PKCζ.

The expression of PKCε was compared in DR and DP *Psammomys* lines. The DR line was isolated in the *Psammomys* colony by assortative mating of gerbils, which did not exhibit hyperglycemia and hyperinsulinemia on HE diet.[129] PKCε showed the highest over-

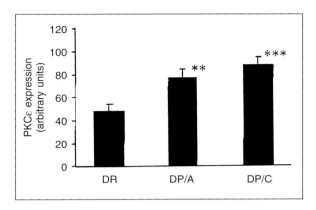

Figure 31.3
Overexpression of PKCε in stages A and C of the DP Psammomys *muscle compared with the DR line. Note a significant overexpression of PKCε in the hyperglycemic–hyperinsulinemic stage C (p <0.001), as well as already in the normoglycemic–normoinsulinemic stage A of Psammomys (p <0.01), indicating the innate insulin resistance preceding the onset of diabetes. Courtesy of Dr Luitgard Mosthaf-Seedorf.*

expression in the skeletal muscle of *Psammomys*, in the hyperglycemic-hyperinsulinemic stage C compared with the DR line.

Figure 31.3 points out a significant overexpression of PKCε in the normoglycemic stage A of DP *Psammomys* compared with the DR line, which indicates that PKCε overexpression precedes the onset of overt hyperglycemia. Thus, PKCε overexpression in stage A may be considered as a marker of 'pre-diabetic' or 'pre-insulinemic' stage and of propensity of a given individual to progress to overt diabetes on affluent nutrition. It is, however, without untoward consequences as long as the diet is LE.

Additional evidence of the innate insulin resistance in stage A *Psammomys* was demonstrated by the failure of external insulin to produce hypoglycemia.[130] Insulin also failed to suppress in stage A *Psammomys* the activity of

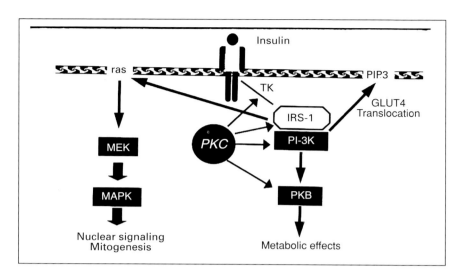

Figure 31.4
Insulin signaling scheme pointing to the PKCε effects on tyrosine kinase, PI-3K and PKB activities. The latter is responsible for activation of multiple metabolic systems.

hepatic PEPCK, the rate limiting enzyme of gluconeogenesis,[54] as well as the hepatic glucose output. This appears to be a typical characteristic of a desert animal in which muscle insulin resistance saves glucose for the support of other glucose obligatory tissues.

Because PKCε overexpression resulted in impaired TK activation by insulin and reduced GLUT4 mRNA and protein, which indicates an impaired PI-3K activation, it was of interest to investigate whether PKC overexpression induces a further negative downstream effect on insulin signaling. The activity of PKB/Akt, an enzyme regarded as responsible for the activation of pleiotropic metabolic systems, was determined. The transfection of HEK 293 cells with IR and/or PKCε plasmids, followed by stimulation with insulin or TPA respectively, showed that the activation of PKCε by TPA caused a reduction of PKB expression and inhibition of PKB activation.[125] These results indicate that the inhibition of PKB activity by PKCε may have a far-reaching negative effect on insulin signaling as presented in Figure 31.4.

The increased activity of PKC isoenzymes in muscle membrane, in IR proximity, suggested the involvement of PKCε in the attenuation of IR/TK activation, as described before,[116] as several PKC isoenzymes were known to reduce the TK catalyzed phosphorylation of the IR and IRS-1.[131–134] It was found that PKCε overexpression was associated with reduced binding of insulin by muscle IR due to the reduction in the number of IR per cell. The downregulation of IR was demonstrated in HEK 293 cells, which were transfected with human IR and PKCε plasmids. Activation of the PKCε by phorbolester (TPA) reduced the amount of IR to ~40% of the original number.[125] This finding is in accord with observations of degradation of IR, by PKCε and possibly other DAG-sensitive PKC enzymes.[134–136] It is therefore likely that serine/threonine phosphorylation of IR and/or IRS-1, inhibits the TK activity via a feedback loop, and is responsible for the deficient TK activation by insulin and IR degradation, leading to insulin resistance accentuation at stages B and C in *Psammomys* on HE diet.[116]

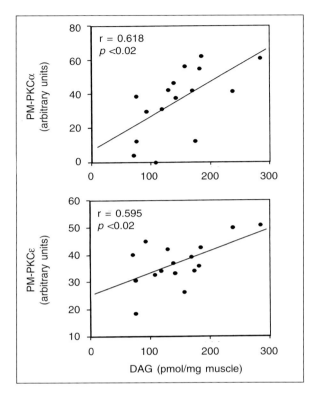

Figure 31.5
PKCε activity correlated to intracellular content of diacylglycerol (DAG) in the gastrocnemius muscle of Psammomys. *Note a high correlation coefficient of membrane associated PKCε and PCKα with muscle DAG content. There was no significant correlation with other PKC isoenzymes. Reproduced with permission from Ziv et al. In: Animal Models of Diabetes (Sima and Shafrir, eds). Harwood Academic Publishers, 2000: 327–42.*[129]

PKCε overexpression and muscle lipid content

The enhanced PKCε activity and/or expression in *Psammomys* was found to be correlated with the increased muscle content of DAG[125] (Figure 31.5). DAG is an intermediate of both fatty acid esterification to TG and TG breakdown to fatty

acids and glycerol. The raised muscle concentration of DAG results from increased TG turnover in muscle, which occurs in the situation of hyper-insulinemia and hyper- glycemia, characteristic of stages B and C of *Psammomys*. Also, the general rise in plasma FFA in diabetic subjects contributes to muscle TG deposition. Indeed, *in vitro* uptake of saturated FFA was recently reported by Yu et al.[137] to raise rat muscle DAG levels and lead to PKC activation. Exogenous lipid infusion in rats resulted in the deposition of a significant fraction of fatty acids in muscle, particularly in the fasted state, and FFA infusion to human subjects was found to elicit insulin resistance and activation of PKCθ.[138]

TG deposition in muscles was studied extensively in rats maintained on a fat-rich diet, and reviewed by Kraegen and colleagues.[139–141] Insulin resistance developed in these rats both in muscles and liver. The hepatic insulin resistance was associated with increased gluconeogenesis, whereas the muscle insulin resistance markedly reduced the insulin stimulated glucose uptake. The accumulation of muscle fat was also inversely correlated with insulin resistance and delayed glucose disposal in human subjects.[142] Intramyocellular lipid excess, particularly in red muscle may reduce glucose uptake by enzyme changes active in the classic Randle glucose-fatty acid cycle. Zierath et al. have shown that high fat feeding impairs the recruitment of GLUT4 and produces a defect in PI-3K function in muscle of mice.[143] However, Schmitz-Pfeiffer et al.[140] demonstrated that in high fat-fed rats, TG and DAG accumulated in muscle and activated PKC isoenzymes interfering with IR function. The total expression of PKCα, -ε and -ζ isoenzymes was not increased in muscles of these rats but their activity and distribution was shifted from cytosolic to membrane compartment. This was particularly prominent in the case of PKCε, showing a six-fold increase in the membrane/ cytosol ratio in correlation with muscle TG content. There was no accumulation of TG and DAG in rats fed a starch diet. Also in *Psammomys*, the muscle and liver TG and DAG content increased on HE diet,[144] but the increase was moderate versus fat-fed rats and evidence is forthcoming that it is generally occurring in diabese animals and humans.

C57BL/6J mice

The non-obese, non-diabetic BL/6J mice, the genomic host of the *ob/ob* mutation, are susceptible to diabesity when placed on an affluent fat- and sucrose-rich diet. They become hypertensive and exhibit an insulin-resistant syndrome: increased outflow from the sympathetic nervous system, deranged β-cell function and adipocyte metabolism hyperleptinemia but without hyperphagia or elevation in corticosterone secretion.[145] Genetic mapping has identified differences in the expression of uncoupling protein UCP2 in adipocytes which may have a role in the development of diabesity.[146] Thus, inbred laboratory mice, without overt metabolic disturbance, were demonstrated to be vulnerable to metabolic abnormalities on HE diet. The hyperinsulinemia most probably interferes with the action of catecholamines on β_1 and β_3 adrenergic receptors, thereby affecting the uptake of glucose by adipocytes and increasing the sympathetic outflow. Thus, the C57BL/6J mice present an attractive model for the study of multiple endocrine abnormalities induced by dietary hyperinsulinemia.

Diabetes obtained by selective inbreeding of normal rodents: Goto-Kakizaki (GK) rats

Apart from animals with spontaneous alterations leading to inappropriate hyperglycemia

and β-cell loss, it was possible to isolate a diabetic line by selective, repetitive breeding of animals from a normal pool, with minimal deviation from the mean response to a glucose load. This underscores the requirement for environmental influences to make the genetic predisposition clinically overt and emphasizes the polygenic basis of diabetes within the 'normal' genetic mosaic.

GK diabetic rat line was obtained by breeding of Wistar rats for >35 generations in Japan, using relative intolerance to a 2 g/kg glucose load as a selection index.[147] The 10% of rats within the 'hyperglycemic zone' were mated in each generation until the offspring had an IGT at F_{10} and fasting hyperglycemia at F_{35}. The GK rats are non-obese, and their diabetes is inheritable and stable with age. Moderate insulin resistance and decreased hepatic IR numbers were noted with normal TK activity per receptor.[148] The reason for insulin resistance remains to be clarified, but it is of interest that PKCε overexpression was seen in GK liver and muscles.[149]

Neuropathy, glomerulopathy and retinopathy were observed despite only moderate hyperglycemia. GK islets are oval or round until two months of age, and then become 'starfish-shaped' due to the accumulation of fibrous material. Insulin secretion in response to glucose is impaired, but progression to diabetes may be also related to low β-cell mass.[150] The response of ATP-sensitive K+ channels to glucose is impaired as is the action of various secretagogues,[151] pointing to a dysfunction in β-cell glycolysis preceding the triose phosphate step. GLUT2 is also underexpressed in GK rat islets,[152] but not enough to explain the deficient insulin secretion, as is seen in *db/db* mice or ZDF rats. It is of interest that treatment of GK rats with GLP-1 or exendin-4 resulted in expansion of the low β-cell mass, improved insulin secretion and restored plasma glucose to normal.[153] The diabetes pathogenesis in the GK rat has been extensively reviewed.[154]

Diabetic non-rodents

A preference has been voiced for animal models other than rodents in diabetes research. The advantages of using large animals is the possibility to perform catheterizations and clamp studies with multiple sampling across organs, as well as long-term longitudinal follow-up of changes and complications that may not be expressed during the short life of rodents. Rodents have a higher rate of metabolic fuel turnover than humans and differ in patterns of growth, but they have the advantage of performing statistically reliable observations in large cohorts. Large mammals have metabolic, nutritional and digestive characteristics not necessarily similar to humans and require lengthy observations with considerable expenses for facilities and maintenance. It may take years to record the complications of diabetes in dogs or monkeys, which live much longer than rodents but are sometimes close to the productive life span of the investigator. There is also difficulty with terminal experiments. Thus, both non-rodents and rodents offer a wide range of research opportunities and the choice of a model depends on the specific aims of the investigator. In this chapter, only the non-human primates will be described, the reader is referred to ref. 155 for information on diabetes in dogs and cats.

Primates with diabetes

Howard[156] found among Celebes black ape (*Macaca nigra*) and other simian species, hyperglycemia without hyperinsulinemia with varying degrees of IGT, weight loss, morpho-logic and functional β-cell defects, total β-cell loss and amyloidosis. Amyloidosis was also seen in other monkey species with overt diabetes including *Macaca fascicularis*, *Macaca radiata* and a baboon *Papo anubis*.[157] Although amyloid was restricted to islet tissue, there is no certainty whether this is a result of primary reaction or a secondary deposit related to antigen–antibody interaction. The islet amyloid content correlates with the intensity of diabetes and the cessation of insulin secretion and is usually not seen in rodent species, in which insulin and amyloid polypeptide oversecretion occur in parallel.[158] Type 1 diabetes in monkeys is severe, associated with hyperlipidemia, xanthomatosis and ketosis.

Circulating antibodies to islet cells ICSA and ICA are found in the majority of macaques with islet dysfunction. Although a correlation between the antibody titers and islet pathology exists, their role in the initiation of insulitis awaits confirmation. The presence of antibodies may reflect a response to antigens released from β-cells. The overt diabetes requires insulin treatment.[156]

Type 2 diabetes occurs in several monkey species in captivity, but was also found in free ranging monkeys. In Mauritius, 4 of 30 investigated *Macaca fascicularis* exhibited IGT without correlation to age or overweight.[159]

Primates with obesity and pronounced insulin resistance leading to β-cell loss

Studies spanning over many years were performed by Hansen and colleagues with rhesus monkeys (*Macaca mulatta*), in a colony maintained on an *ad libitum* ration, which develop a Type 2 diabetes-like syndrome.[160,161] Several phases were identified, in the progression to diabesity, by metabolic and endocrine indices. In the first phase no appreciable elevations of fasting blood glucose and insulin were noted, except IGT after a glucose load. In phase 4, plasma insulin amounted to ~160 versus 2 µU/ml in phase 1. In phases 5–6 body weight peaked at ~19 kg and plasma insulin at ~400 µU/ml and the monkeys were found to be leptin resistant.[162] β-Cells became exhausted with further progression to overt diabetes and plasma insulin dropped to very low levels. At this time, blood glucose levels were two- to three-fold higher than in phase 1. Overt diabetes was prevalent in monkeys 10 to 20 years old, with pronounced weight loss and β-cell malfunction associated with the deposition of amyloid[163] (Figure 31.6). The deposition of amyloid in monkeys, but not in rodents[158] is of interest, since amyloidosis is known to occur in human Type 2 diabetes and is implicated to accentuate β-cell malfunction.[164]

Hyperinsulinemia in the diabetic obese monkeys was associated with altered muscle insulin receptor mRNA splicing,[165] assumed to be related to the nutritionally induced insulin resistance. Long-term dietary restriction was beneficial in extending the life span and preventing diabetes[166] and offset the effect of sedentary life in captivity.

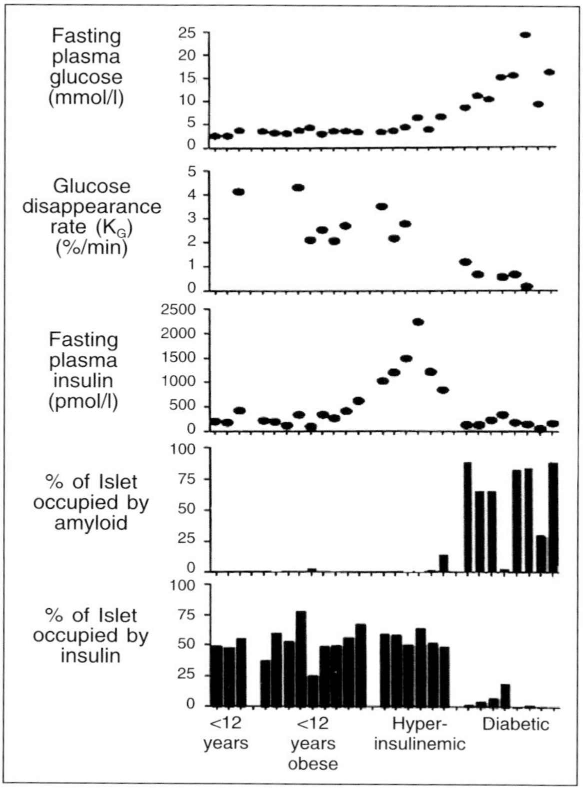

Figure 31.6
Progression of rhesus monkeys Macaca mulatta *to diabetes on* ad libitum *laboratory diet during 12 years of observation. Courtesy of Dr Barbara Hansen.*

Conclusions and overview

Research into animal diabetes has importantly contributed to the understanding of the etiology of the two types of diabetes and continues to offer new opportunities for the elucidation of yet latent mechanisms. A unified theory emerges now on the autoimmune aggression of β-cells and destruction of the insulin secretion apparatus. Animal models of Type 1 diabetes have revealed several mechanisms of lethal insulitis and means for its possible prevention. Modulation of improper β-cell antigen presen-

tation and/or faulty function of T-lymphocyte subsets is under active investigation.

Animal species with Type 2-like syndromes present an opportunity for investigation of the endocrine, metabolic and morphologic changes in the diverse phenotypic forms. A distinction should be made between those endowed with long-lasting secretion of β-cells, sustaining the huge insulin requirements to accommodate the resistance during the whole life span, and those with labile β-cells failing in the protracted compensation. The animals of the second group initially oversecrete and present the full picture of typical diabesity. Later their β-cells succumb to overtaxation, nuclear DNA fragmentation and necrosis. They are vulnerable to hyperglycemia, either because of the diabetogenic genomic background or due to gluco- and lipotoxicity.

Loss of β-cells is preventable if the secretion pressure can be reduced either by preventive treatment or restriction of nutrient intake. This is particularly evident in the gerbil *Psammomys* and *Macaca mulatta* monkeys. It is worth emphasizing that in the progression to diabetes, the finding of a few apoptotic β-cells in an islet may serve as a marker of an imminent irreversible loss of insulin secretion. Pancreas screening at this stage might be a useful procedure for detecting the onset of apoptosis and launching of preventive measures. Although human pancreatic biopsy is seldom clinically recommended, except in suspected pancreatic malignancy,[167] the development of procedures for accurately targeted biopsy is justified in light of the rise in incidence of nutritional diabetes and the need for institution of measures for correction of insulin sensitivity. The detection of autoimmune lesions in human Type 1 diabetes in its pre-clinical stage by pancreatic biopsy has now been reported.[168]

A feature common to most animal models of Type 2 diabetes is hyperinsulinemia, which develops early in life, often prior to obesity, as a result of a hypothalamic aberration causing hyperphagia, transmitting direct signals to the pancreas through the vagus or to the availability of affluent nutrition. The hyperinsulinemia and the later developing hyperglycemia are the hallmark of diabesity. When this appears, it signifies an already advanced stage of β-cell malfunction. Hyperinsulinemia per se is also detrimental. Insulin excess impairs hepatic and muscle IR function by modifying the intracel-

lular phosphorylations along the cascade of signaling sequences. The inability to restrain the expression of PEPCK, the rate-limiting enzyme of gluconeogenesis, contributes importantly to the hyperglycemia. It is intriguing that, in almost all animals with hyperinsulinemia, lipogenesis continues along with gluconeogenesis, resulting in hyperlipidemia and exacerbating obesity. By shunting the glucose excess to lipids, many of the diabese species are able to maintain moderate hyperglycemia.

Psammomys is a model of human nutritionally induced diabetes, which now reaches epidemic proportions in certain populations. The underlying cause is increased food availability and consumption, promoting the transition of indigenous populations from traditional to supermarket lifestyle. However, the latent propensity to diabetes among these populations is related to their inborn metabolic capacity which is preponderably not adjustable to the dietary surplus. Some authors refer to such a socioeconomic perspective as leading to nutritional genocide of global proportions (see Chapter 1). The elements of insulin resistance in *Psammomys* represent the antecedents of the development of worldwide diabetes epidemic in human populations emerging from food scarcity to food abundance.

Insulin resistance and β-cell dysfunction are considered two interrelated factors in the pathogenesis of IGT and Type 2 diabetes. Although a debate is still continuing on the relative impact of each factor, the evidence from *Psammomys* and other animals clearly demonstrates that insulin resistance with hyperinsulinemia precede the β-cell lesion. In contrast to many rodents with genetically determined diabetes, in which the diet constitutes only an ancillary factor, in *Psammomys* and other animals subsisting on scarce nutrition, the β-cell dysfunction occurs only on HE diet. There is no β-cell lesion in animals consuming their native nutrients or laboratory LE diets. The onset of insulin resistance and hyperinsulinemia in *Psammomys* precedes an appreciable weight gain, precluding any contribution of obesity to IGT. If β-cells oversecrete long enough, the expansion of adipose tissue may secondarily occur. A return to normalcy is possible even after a period on HE diet, either by a short-term fasting, or by restricting the food intake. It is most probable that similar triggering of IGT and diabetes applies to the affected human populations.

The aberrant activity of PKC isoenzymes, especially of PKCε, is the potential causative mechanism in the generation of insulin resistance by phosphorylation of serine/threonine residues on IR and proteins of the signaling pathway. This may lead to TK, PI-3K and PKB attenuation with negative feedback, as well as to IR degradation. Thus, the compensatory hyperinsulinemia precludes the adequate function of insulin signaling. The common aspect of this overexpression with *Psammomys* and fat-fed rats is tissue accumulation of DAG. DAG is directly related to tissue TG content and this may be an especially important inducer of insulin resistance in non-adipose tissues. Insulin resistance and its corollaries may then result from enhanced muscle TG deposition, not necessarily from hyperlipidemia. The initial fat deposition may also be promoted by hyperinsulinemia with hyperglycemia and the following diabesity.

The therapeutic effort should be therefore based on the prevention of muscle insulin resistance. Preventive strategies should be directed to avoiding muscle TG deposition and DAG elevation, which are the most probable causes of attenuated insulin signaling and the ensuing insulin resistance. DAG breakdown may be achieved by the use of modalities activating DAG kinase, which converts DAG into phosphatidic acid, or by specific inhibition of DAG-sensitive PKC isoenzymes. Among poten-

tial modalities is H7 – a piperazine derivative, polymyxin B, bisindoxylmaleimide and staurosporine which are inhibitory to PKC isoenzymes *in vitro*.[169] Herbimycin was also shown to have PKC inhibitory properties.[170] Inhibition of PKCβ, appealing for the treatment of the glycation-mediated chronic complications and developing in insulin independent renal and neural tissues,[171] has been achieved by LY33353 and high dose vitamin E treatment.[172,173] It is also remarkable that the recently reported PKCθ knockout in mice improved insulin action and signaling defects induced by lipid infusion.[174] Potentiating insulin sensitivity at its prevalent concentrations would also lead to lowering of insulin resistance as shown by the application of IR activators.[175] Increased insulin sensitivity can be likewise accomplished by the treatment with vanadyl sulfate and other vanadium compounds[176–179] which were effective in *Psammomys* maintained on HE diet. Vanadyl sulfate restoration of normoglycemia and normoinsulinemia and increase in muscle metabolic activity appears to be distal to IR/TK signaling.[176]

The overexpression of PKC isoenzymes may be the result of genetic susceptibility exemplified by *Psammomys* or by 'thrifty gene' characteristics of desert animals or individuals in the affected populations, activated by the changing environmental influences. This course of events is illustrated by Figure 31.7. The inherent muscle insulin resistance aimed to spare glucose for obligatory tissues (such as the brain) fails when confronted with excess of nutrients. It turns the beneficial innate insulin resistance to misuse of the surplus energy by promoting lipogenesis and diabesity, hyperlipidemia and other complications. Such a situation is most probably an integral component of the insulin-resistance syndrome in animals and humans alike and may be therefore considered as 'PKC overexpression syndrome'.

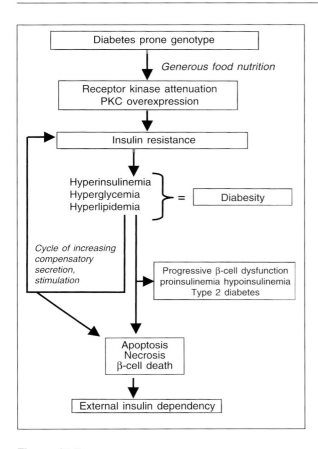

Figure 31.7
Schematic presentation of the development of nutritional diabetes in Psammomys obesus *valid for other subjects with a 'thrifty gene' background consuming an abundant energy diet. Initially marginal hyperglycemia promotes β-cell insulin secretion resulting in compensatory hyperinsulinemia and propels a vicious cycle, which in time may lead to exhaustion of labile β-cells as insulin resistance and PKCε overexpression develop. Hyperinsulinemia and PKCε overexpression attenuate the function of insulin receptor and IRS as well as the glucose transport and PKB activity. Tissue TG deposition ensues with raised levels of intracellular DAG, which in turn exacerbates the expression of PKCε and possibly other PKC isoenzymes. The permanent secretion pressure on β-cells causes apoptosis and β-cell death, requiring support with external insulin for survival.*

Acknowledgements

My sincere thanks are due to my colleagues, Drs Ehud Ziv, Luitgard Mosthaf-Seedorf and Yukio Ikeda for their extensive contribution to the research of diabetes in animals.

References

1. Shafrir E, Sima AAF. Diabetic animals for research into the complications: a general review. In: Sima AAF, ed. Chronic Complications in Diabetes, Frontiers in Animal Diabetes, Harwood Academic Press, 2000: 1–42.
2. Boitard C, Carnaud C. Lessons from animal models regarding pathogenesis of insulin-dependent diabetes mellitus. In: Leslie RDG, ed. Molecular Pathogenesis of Diabetes Mellitus (Series: Frontiers of Hormone Research) Basel: Karger, 1997; 22: 109–30.
3. Crisa L, Mordes JP, Rossini AA. Autoimmune diabetes in the BB rat. Diabetes Metab Rev 1992; 8: 9–37.
4. Mordes JP, Bortell R, Groen H et al. Autoimmune diabetes mellitus in the BB rat. In: Sima AAF, Shafrir E, eds. Primer on Animal Models of Diabetes, Harwood Academic Press, 2000: 1–41.
5. Ellerman KE, Richards CA, Guberski DL et al. Kilham rat virus triggers T-cell dependent autoimmune diabetes in multiple strains of rat. Diabetes 1996; 45: 557–62.
6. Jacob HJ, Patterson A, Wilson D et al. Genetic dissection of autoimmune type I diabetes in the BB rat. Nat Genet 1992; 2: 56–60.
7. Colle E, Fuks A, Poussier P et al. Polygenic nature of spontaneous diabetes in the rat. Diabetes 1992; 41: 1617–23.
8. Martin A-M, Maxson MN, Leif J et al. Diabetes-prone and diabetes-resistant BB rats share a common major diabetes susceptibility locus, iddm4. Additional evidence for a 'univeral autoimmunity locus' on rat chromosome 4. Diabetes 1999; 48: 2138–44.
9. Kolb H, Worz-Pagenstert U, Kleeman R et al. Cytokine gene expression in the BB rat pancreas: natural course and impact of bacterial vaccines. Diabetologia 1996; 39: 1448–54.

10. Lau A, Ramanthan, Poussier P. Excessive productuion of nitric oxide by macrophages from DP-BB rats is secondary to the T-lymphopenic state of these animals. Diabetes 1998; 47: 197–205.

11. Bertrand S, Vigeant C, Yale JF. Predictive value of lymphocyte antibodies for the appearance of diabetes in BB rats. Diabetes 1994; 43: 137–42.

12. Scott FW, Cloutier HE, Kleeman R et al. Potential mechanisms by which certain foods promote or inhibit the development of spontaneous diabetes in BB rats – dose, timing early effect on islet area and switch in infiltrate from TH1 to TH2 cells. Diabetes 1997; 46: 589–98.

13. Paronen J, Knip M, Savilahti E et al. Effect of cow's milk exposure and maternal Type 1 diabetes on cellular and humoral immunization to dietary insulin in infants at genetic risk for Type 1 diabetes. Diabetes 2000; 49: 1657–65.

14. Mackay IR, Bone A, Tuomi T et al. Lack of autoimmune serological reactions in rodent models of insulin dependent diabetes mellitus. J Autoimmun 1996; 9: 705–11.

15. Ko IY, Jun HS, Kim GS, Yoon JW. Studies on autoimmunity for initiation of beta-cell destruction, 10. Delayed expression of a membrane bound islet cell specific 38 kDa autoantigen that precedes insulitis and diabetes in the diabetes-prone BB rat. Diabetologia 1994; 37: 460–5.

16. Suarez-Pinzon WL, Rabinovitch A. Approaching to Type 1 diabetes prevention by intervention in cytokine immunoregulatory circuits. Int J Exp Diabetes Res 2001; 2: 3–17.

17. Leiter EH. The nonobese diabetic (NOD) mouse: A model for analyzing the interplay between hereditary and environment in development of autoimmune disease. ILAR News 1993; 35: 4–14.

18. Ikegami H, Makino S. The NOD Mouse and its related strains. In: Sima AAF, Shafrir E, eds. Primer on Animal Models of Diabetes, Harwood Academic Press, 2000: 43–62.

19. Baxter AG, Cooke A. The genetics of the NOD mouse. Diabetes Metab Rev 1995; 11: 315–35.

20. Tisch R, McDevitt H. Insulin-dependent diabetes mellitus. Cell 1996; 85: 291–7.

21. Benoist C, Mathis D. Cell death mediators in autoimmune diabetes – no shortage of suspects. Cell 1997; 89: 1–3.

22. Todd JA. A protective role of the environment in the development of Type 1 diabetes? Diab Med 1991; 8: 906–10.

23. Wicker L, Todd J, Peterson L. Genetic control of autoimmune diabetes in the NOD mouse. Annu Rev Immunol 1995; 13: 179–200.

24. Ikegami H, Makino S, Ogihara T. Molecular genetics of insulin-dependent diabetes mellitus: analysis of congenic strains. In: Shafrir E, ed. Lessons from Animal Diabetes, Boston: Birkhauser,1996; 6: 33–46.

25. Kolb H. Mouse models of insulin dependent diabetes: low-dose streptozotocin-induced diabetes and nonobese diabetic (NOD) mice. Diabetes Metab Rev 1987; 3: 751–78.

26. Okamoto H. The molecular basis of experimental diabetes. In: Okamoto H, ed. Molecular Biology of the Islets of Langerhans. Cambridge: Cambridge University Press, 1990.

27. Thivolet CH, Goillot E, Bedosa P et al. Insulin prevents adaptive cell transfer of diabetes in the autoimmune non-obese diabetic mouse. Diabetologia 1991; 34: 314–19.

28. Natori T, Kawano K. The LETL rat: a model for IDDM without lymphopenia. ILAR News 1993; 35: 15–18.

29. Polonsky K, Sturis J, Bell GJ. Non-insulin-dependent diabetes mellitus – a genetically programmed failure of the beta cell to compensate for insulin resistance. N Engl J Med 1996; 334: 777–83.

30. Matthews DR. Insulin resistance and β-cell function – a clinical perspective. Diabetes Obes Metab, 2001; Suppl 1: S28–33.

31. Coleman DL. Lessons from studies with genetic forms of diabetes in the mouse. Metabolism 1983; 32: 162–4.

32. Shafrir E, Ben-Sasson R, Ziv E, Bar-On H. Insulin resistance, β-cell survival and apoptosis in Type 2 diabetes; animal models and human implications. Diabetes Rev 1999; 7: 114–23.

33. Thorens B, Wu YJ, Leahy JL, Weir GC. The loss of GLUT2 expression by glucose-unresponsive beta-cells of db/db mice is reversible and is induced by the diabetic environment. J Clin Invest 1992; 90: 77–85.

34. Like AA, Chick WL. Studies on the diabetic mutant mouse, 2. Electron microscopy of pancreatic islets. Diabetologia 1970; 6: 216–42.

35. Shafrir E. Nonrecognition of insulin as gluconeogenesis suppressant. A manifestation of

selective hepatic insulin resistance in several animal species with type II diabetes: sand rats, spiny mice and db/db mice. In: Shafrir E, Renold AE, eds. Lessons from Animal Diabetes. London: Libbey, 1988; 2: 304–15.

36. Shargill NS, Tatoyan A, El-Refai MF et al. Impaired insulin receptor phosphorylation in skeletal muscle membranes of db/db mice: the use of a novel skeletal muscle plasma membrane preparation to compare insulin binding and stimulation of receptor phosphorylation. Biochem Biophys Res Commun 1986; 137: 286–94.

37. Le Marchand-Brustel Y, Tanti JF, Rochet N et al. Insulin receptor alterations in noninsulin-dependent diabetes. In: Shafrir E, Renold AE, eds. Lessons from Animal Diabetes. London: Libbey, 1988; 2: 362–6.

38. Herberg L, Leiter EH. Obesity/diabetes in mice with mutations in the leptin or leptin receptor genes. In: Sima AAF, Shafrir E, eds. Animal Models of Diabetes. A Primer. Harwood Academic Publishers, 2001: 63–108.

39. Leiter EH, Coleman DL, Ingram DK, Reynold MA. Influence of dietary carbohydrate on the induction of diabetes in C57BL/KsJ-*db/db* diabetes mice. J Nutr 1983; 113: 184–95.

40. Eades MR, Eades MP. Protein Power. Bantam Books, 1996.

41. Gibbs, EM, Stock JL, McCoid SC et al. Glycemic improvement in diabetic db/db mice by overexpression of the human insulin-regulatable glucose transporter (GLUT4). J Clin Invest 1995; 95: 1512–18.

42. Arakawa K, Ishihara T, Oku A et al. Improved diabetic syndrome in C57BL/KsJ-db/db mice by oral administration of the Na(+)-glucose cotransporter inhibitor T-1095. Br J Pharmacol 2001; 132: 578–86.

43. Cohen MP, Hud E, Shea E, Shearman CW. Normalizing glycated albumin reduces increased urinary collagen IV and prevents renal insufficiency in diabetic *db/db* mice. Metabolism 2002; 51: 901–5.

44. Coleman DL. Effects of parabiosis of obese with diabetic and normal mice. Diabetologia 1973; 9: 294–8.

45. Friedman JM, Halaas JL. Leptin and the regulation of body weight in mammals. Nature 1998; 395: 763–70.

46. Maffei M, Fei H, Lee GH et al. Increased expression in adipocytes of Ob RNA in mice with lesions of the hypothalamus and with mutations of the db locus. Proc Natl Acad Sci USA 1995; 92: 6957–60.

47. Himms-Hagen J. Physiological roles of the leptin endocrine system: differences between mice and humans. Crit Rev Clin Lab Sci 1999; 36: 575–655.

48. Caro JF, Sinha MK, Kolaczynski JW et al. Leptin: the tale of an obesity gene. Diabetes 1996; 45: 1455–62.

49. Wang Q, Bing C, Al-Barazanji K, et al. Interactions between leptin and hypothalamic neuropeptide Y neurons in the control of food intake and energy homeostasis in the rat. Diabetes 1997; 46: 335–41.

50. Taketomi S, Ikeda H. KK and KKAy mice. In: Sima AAF, Shafrir E, ed. Primer on Animal Models of Diabetes, Harwood Academic Press, 2000: 129–42.

51. Suto JS, Matsuura S, Imamura K et al. Genetic analysis of non-insulin-dependent diabetes mellitus in KK and yellow KK mice with various diabetic states. Eur J Endocrinol 1998; 139: 654–61.

52. Bonini JA, Colca JR, Dailey C et al. Compensatory alterations for insulin signal transduction and glucose transport in insulin resistant diabetes. Am J Physiol 1995; 269: E759–E765.

53. Proietto J, Larkins RG. A perspective on the New Zealand obese mouse. In: Shafrir E, ed. Lessons From Animal Diabetes. London: Smith-Gordon, 1992; 4: 65–74.

54. Andrikopoulos S, Thorburn AWE, Proietto J. The New Zealand obese mouse: a polygenic model of Type 2 diabetes. In: Sima AAF, Shafrir E, ed. Primer on Animal Models of Diabetes, Harwood Academic Press, 2000: 171–84.

55. Veroni MC, Proietto J, Larkins RG. Evolution of insulin resistance in New Zealand obese mice. Diabetes 1991; 40: 1480–7.

56. Macaulay SL, Larkins RG. Impaired insulin action in adipocytes of New Zealand obese mice: A role for postbinding defects in pyruvate dehydrogenase and insulin mediator activity. Metabolism 1988; 37: 958–65.

57. Andrikopoulos S, Proietto J. The biochemical basis of increased hepatic glucose production in a mouse model of Type 2 (non-insulin-dependent) diabetes mellitus. Diabetologia 1995; 38: 1389–96.

58. Herberg L. Insulin resistance in abdominal and subcutaneous obesity: comparison of C57BL/6J ob/ob with New Zealand obese mice. In: Shafrir E, Renold AE, eds. Lessons from Animal Diabetes, London: Libbey, 1988; 2: 367–73.

59. Truett G, Bahary N, Friedman JM, Leibel RL. The Zucker rat obesity gene fatty (fa) maps to chromosome 5 and is a homolog of the mouse diabetes (db) gene. Proc Natl Acad Sci USA 1991; 88: 7806–9.

60. Kava R, Greenwood MRC, Johnson PR. Zucker (fa/fa) rat. ILAR News 1990; 32: 4–8.

61. Bray GA, York DA, Fisler JS. Experimental obesity: A homeostatic failure due to defective nutrient stimulation of the sympathetic nervous system. Vitam Horm 1989; 45: 1–126.

62. Chan CB, MacPhail RM, Mitton K. Evidence for defective glucose sensing by islets of fa/fa obese Zucker rats. Can J Physiol Pharmacol 1993 71: 34–9.

63. York DA. Role of glucocorticoids in the development of obesity and diabetes in experimental animal models. In: Shafrir E, ed. Lessons from Animal Diabetes, London: Smith-Gordon, 1992; 4: 229–39.

64. Lee HC, Curry DL, Stern JS. Direct effect of CNS on insulin hypersecretion in obese Zucker rats: involvement of vagus nerve. Am J Physiol 1989; 256: E439–E444.

65. Bchini-Hooft van Huijsduijnen O, Rohner-Jeanrenaud F, Jeanrenaud B. Hypothalamic neuropeptide Y messenger ribonucleic acid levels in preobese and genetically obese (fa/fa) rats; potential regulation thereof by corticotropin-releasing factor. J Neuroendocrinol 1993; 5: 381–6.

66. Terretaz J, Assimacopoulos-Jeannet F, Jeanrenaud B. Severe hepatic and peripheral insulin resistance as evidenced by euglycemic clamps in genetically obese fa/fa rats. Endocrinology 1986; 118: 674–8.

67. Anai M, Funaki M, Ogihara T et al. Altered expression levels and impaired steps in pathways of phosphatidylinositol-3-kinase activation via insulin receptor substrates. Diabetes 1998; 47: 13–23.

68. King PA, Horton EO, Hirshman MP, Hortion ES. Insulin resistance in obese Zucker rat (fa/fa) skeletal muscle is associated with a failure of glucose transporter translocation. J Clin Invest 1992; 90: 1568–75.

69. Uphues I, Kolter T, Goud B, Eckel J. Failure of insulin regulated recruitment of the glucose transporter GLUT4 in cardiac muscle of obese Zucker rats is associated with alterations of small molecular-mass GTP-binding proteins. Biochem J 1995; 311: 161–6.

70. Henriksen EJ. Oxidative stress and antioxidant treatment: effects on muscle glucose transport in animal models of Type 1 and Type 2 diabetes. In: Packer L, Rosen P, Tritscher HJ et al. eds. Antioxidants in Diabetes Management. New York: Marcel Decker, 2000: 303–17.

71. Bourgeois C, Wiggins D, Hioms R, Gibbions GF. VLDL output by hepatocytes from obese Zucker rats is resistant to the inhibitory effect of insulin. Am J Physiol 1995; 269: E206–E215.

72. Penicaud L, Ferre P, Assimacopoulos-Jeannet F et al. Increased gene expression of lipogenic enzymes and glucose transporter in white adipose tissue of suckling and weaned obese Zucker rats. Biochem J 1991; 279: 303–8.

73. Terrettaz J, Cusin I, Etienne J, Jeanrenaud B. In vivo regulation of adipose tissue lipoprotein lipase in normal rats made hyperinsulinemic and in hyperinsulinemic genetically-obese (fa/fa) rats. Int J Obesity 1994; 18: 9–15.

74. Trimble ER, Bruzzone R, Belin D. Insulin resistance is accompanied by impairment of amylase gene expression in the exocrine pancreas of the obese Zucker rat. Biochem J 1986; 237: 807–12.

75. Peterson RG. The Zucker diabetic fatty (ZDF) rat. In: Sima AAF, Shafrir E, ed. Animal Diabetes of Diabetes. A Primer, Harwood Academic Press, 2000: 109–28.

76. Friedman JE, Devente JE, Peterson RG, Dohm GL. Altered expression of muscle glucose transporter GLUT-4 in diabetic fatty Zucker rats (ZDF/Drt-fa). Am J Physiol 1991; 261: E782–788.

77. Pick A, Clark J, Kubstrup C et al. Role of apoptosis in failure of β-cell mass compensation for insulin resistance and β-cell defects in the male Zucker diabetic rat. Diabetes 1998; 47: 358–64.

78. Orci L, Ravazzola M, Baetens D et al. Evidence that down-regulation of B-cell glucose transporters in non-insulin-dependent diabetes may be the cause of diabetic hyperglycemia. Proc Natl Acad Sci USA 1990; 87: 9953–7.

79. Ohneda M, Inman LR, Unger RH. Caloric restriction in obese prediabetic rats prevents beta-cell depletion, loss of beta-cell GLUT2 and glucose incompetence. Diabetologia 1995; 38: 173–9.

80. Unger RH. Lipotoxicity in the pathogenesis of obesity-dependent NIDDM. Genetic and clinical implications. Diabetes 1995; 44: 863–70.

81. Unger RH. How obesity causes diabetes in Zucker Diabetic Fatty rats. Trends Endocrinol Metab 1998; 7: 276–82.

82. Odaka H, Sugiyama Y, Ikeda H. Characteristics of Wistar fatty rat. In: Sima AAF, Shafrir E, ed. Animal Diabetes of Diabetes. A Primer, Harwood Academic Press, 2000: 159–70.

83. Suzuki M, Odaka H, Sugiyama Y. Hypertension and insulin resistance in the Wistar fatty rat. In: Hansen B, Shafrir E, eds. Insulin Resistance Syndrome, Taylor & Francis, UK, 2002.

84. Albright AL, Gregoire F, Green S et al. Studies in the Wistar diabetic fatty rat (WDF fa/fa). A model of non-insulin-dependent diabetes mellitus. In: Shafrir E, ed. Lessons from Animal Diabetes. London: Smith-Gordon, 1994; 5: 75–82.

85. Yamakawa T, Tanaka S, Tamura K et al. Wistar fatty rat is obese and spontaneously hypertensive. Hypertension 1995; 25: 146–50.

86. Karasik A, Shafrir E. Function and regulation of insulin receptor in animal models of diabetes and insulin resistance. In: Shafrir E, ed. Lessons from Animal Diabetes. London: Smith-Gordon, 1995; 5: 161–8.

87. Greenhouse DD, Hansen CT, Michaelis OE. Development of fatty and corpulent rat strains. ILAR News 1990; 32: 2–4.

88. McCune SA, Radin MJ, Jenkins JE et al. SHHF/Mcc-facp rat model: effects of gender and genotype on age of expression of metabolic complications and congestive heart failure and on response to drug therapy. In: Shafrir E, ed. Lessons from Animal Diabetes. London: Smith-Gordon, 1994; 5: 255–70.

89. Ondera T, Tamura T, Said S et al. Maladaptive remodeling of cardiac myocyte shape begins long before failure in hypertension. Hypertension 1998; 32: 753–7.

90. Radin MJ, Chu YY, Hoepf MM, McCune SA. Treatment of obese female and male SHHF/Mcc-fa^{cp} rats with antihypertensive drugs, nifedipine and enalapril: effects on body weight, fat distribution, insulin resistance and

91. systolic pressure. Obes Res 1993; 1: 433–42.

91. Russell JC, Kelly SE. Cardiovascular disease in the insulin-resistant, atherosclerosis-prone JCR: LA-cp rat. In: Hansen B, Shafrir E, eds. Insulin Resistance and Insulin Resistance Syndrome. Taylor & Francis, UK, 2002.

92. Russel JC, Graham SE. The JCR: LA-cp rat: an animal; model of obesity and insulin resistance with spontaneous cardiovascular disease. In: Sima AAF, Shafrir E, eds. Models of Animal Diabetes. A Primer, Harwood Academic Press, 2000: 227–46.

93. Kawano S, Hirashima T, Mori S et al. The OLETF rat. In: Sima AAF, Shafrir E, eds. Models of Animal Diabetes. A Primer, Harwood Academic Press, 2000: 213–26.

94. Koletzky RJ, Friedman JE, Ernsberger P. The obese spontaneously hypertensive rat (SHROB, Koletzky rat): a model of metabolic syndrome X. In: Sima AAF, Shafrir E, eds. Models of Animal Diabetes. A Primer, Harwood Academic Press, 2000: 143–58.

95. Ishizuka T, Ernsberger S, Liu D et al. Phenotypic consequences of a nonsense mutation in the leptin receptor gene (fa^k) in obese spontaneously hypertensive Koletzky rat (SHROB). J Nutr 1998; 128: 2299–306

96. Shinohara M, Masuyama T, Shoda T et al. A new spontaneously diabetic non-obese Torii rat strain with severe ocular complications. Intl J Exp Diabetes Res 2000; 1: 89–100.

97. Adler JH, Kalman R, Lazarovici G et al. Achieving predictable model of Type 2 diabetes in sand rats. In: Shafrir E, ed. Lessons from Animal Diabetes, London: Smith-Gordon, 1991; 3: 212–14.

98. Kalderon B, Gutman A, Shafrir E, Adler JH. Characterization of stages in the development of obesity-diabetes syndrome in sand rat. (*Psammomys obesus*). Diabetes 1986; 35, 717–24.

99. Shafrir E, Gutman A. *Psammomys obesus* of the Jerusalem colony: a model for nutritionally induced, non-insulin-dependent diabetes. J Basic Clin Physiol Pharmacol 1993; 4, 83–99.

100. Ziv E, Shafrir E. *Psammomys obesus*: nutritionally induced NIDDM-like syndrome on a 'thrifty gene' background. In: Shafrir E, ed. Lessons from Animal Diabetes, London: Smith-Gordon, 1995; 5: 285–300.

101. Shafrir E, Ziv E. Cellular mechanism of nutritionally induced insulin resistance: the desert rodent *Psammomys obesus* and other animals in which insulin resistance leads to detrimental outcome. J Basic Clin Physiol Pharmacol 1998; 9: 347–85.

102. Barnett M, Collier GR, Collier FMcL et al. A cross-sectional and short-term longitudinal characterization of NIDDM in Psammomys obesus. Diabetologia 1994; 37: 671–6.

103. Barnett M, Collier GR, Zimmet P, O'Dea K. Energy intake with respect to the development of diabetes mellitus in Psammomys obesus. Diabetes Nutr Metab 1995; 8: 1–6.

104. Collier GR, McMillan JS, Windmill K et al. Beacon: a novel gene involved in regulation of energy balance. Diabetes 2000; 49: 1766–71.

105. Walder K, Ziv E, Kalman R et al. Elevated hypothalamic gene expression in *Psammomys obesus* prone to develop obesity and type 2 diabetes. Int J Obes 2002; 26: 605–9.

106. Bar-On H, Ben-Sasson R, Ziv E et al. Irreversibility of nutritionally induced NIDDM in *Psammomys obesus* is related to β-cell apoptosis. Pancreas 1999; 18: 259–65.

107. Barnett M, Collier GR, Zimmet P, O'Dea K. The effect of restricting energy intake on diabetes in Psammomys obesus. Int J Obes 1994; 18: 789–94.

108. Jörns A, Tiedge M, Ziv E, Shafrir E, Lenzen S. Gradual loss of pancreatic beta-cell insulin, glucokinase and GLUT2 glucose transporter immunoreactivities during the time course of nutritionally-induced Type 2 diabetes in Psammomys obesus (sand rat). Virchows Arch 2002; 440: 63–9.

109. Shafrir E, Ben-Sasson R, Ziv E, Bar-On H. Insulin resistance, β-cell survival, and apoptosis in Type 2 diabetes: animal models and human implications. Diabetes Rev 1991; 7: 114–23.

110. Donath MY, Gross D, Cerasi E, Kaiser, N. Hyperglycemia-induced β-cell apoptosis in pancreatic islets of *Psammomys obesus* during development of diabetes. Diabetes 1999; 48: 738–44.

111. Nesher R, Gross D, Donath MY et al. Interaction between genetic and dietary factors determines β-cell function in *Psammomys obesus*, an animal model of Type 2 diabetes. Diabetes 1999; 48: 731–7.

112. Kaneto H, Fujii J, Myint TM et al. Reducing sugars trigger oxidative modification and apoptosis in pancreatic beta-cells by provoking oxidative stress through the glycation reaction. Biochem J 1996; 320: 855–63.

113. Gadot MG, Leibowitz G, Shafrir E et al. Hyperproinsulinemia and insulin deficiency in the diabetic *Psammomys obesus*. Endocrinology 1994; 135: 610–16.

114. Ward WK, Lacava EC, Paquette TL et al. Disproportionate elevation of immunoreactive proinsuin in Type 2 (non-insulin) diabetes mellitus and in experimental insulin resistance. Diabetologia 1987; 30: 698–702.

115. Glauber HS, Revers RR, Henry R et al. In vivo deactivation of proinsulin action on glucose disposal and hepatic glucose production in normal man. Diabetes 1986; 35: 311–17.

116. Kanety H, Moshe S, Shafrir E et al. Hyperinsulinemia induces a reversible impairment in insulin receptor function leading to diabetes in the sand rat model of non-insulin-dependent diabetes mellitus. Proc Natl Acad Sci USA 1994; 91: 1853–57.

117. Marban SL, De Loia JA, Gearhart JD. Hyperinsulinemia in transgenic mice carrying multiple copies of the human insulin gene. Dev Genet 1989; 19: 356–64.

118. Tang J, Neldigh JL, Cooksey RC, McClain DA. Transgenic mice with increased hexosamine flux specifically targeted to β-cells exhibit hyperinsulinemia and peripheral insulin resistance. Diabetes, 2000; 49, 1492–9.

119. Sone H, Suzuki H, Takahashi A, Yamada N. Disease model: hyperinsulinemia and insulin resistance. Part A. Targeted disruption of insulin signaling or glucose transport. Part B. Polygenic and other animal models. Trends Mol Med 2001; 7: 320–2; 373–6.

120. Miles PDG, Li S, Hart M et al. Mechanisms of insulin resistance in experimental hyperinsulinemic dogs. J Clin Invest 1998; 101: 202–11.

121. McNulty PH, Louard R, Deckelbaum RJ et al. Hyperinsulinemia inhibits myocardial protein degradation in patients with cardiovascular disease and insulin resistance. Circulation, 1995; 92: 2151–6.

122. Del Prato S, Leonetti F, Simonson DC et al.

Effect of sustained physiologic hyperinsuli-naemia and hyperglycaemia on insulin secretion and insulin sensitivity in man. Diabetologia 1994; 27: 1025–35.

123. Pontiroli AE, Alberetto M, Pozza G. Patients with insulinoma show insulin resistance in the absence of arterial hypertension. Diabetologia 1992; 35: 294–5.

124. Weyer C, Hanson RL, Tataranni PA et al. A high fasting plasma insulin concentration predicts Type 2 diabetes independent of insulin resistance. Diabetes 2000; 49: 2094–101.

125. Ikeda Y, Olsen GS, Ziv E et al. Cellular mechanism of nutritionally induced insulin resistance in *Psammomys obesus*. Over-expression of protein kinase Cε in skeletal muscle precedes the onset of hyperinsulinemia and hyperglycemia. Diabetes, 2001; 50: 584–92.

126. Shafrir E, Ziv E, Mosthaf L. Nutritionally induced insulin resistance and receptor defect leading to β-cell failure in animal models. Ann NY Acad Sci 1999; 892: 223–46.

127. Haring HU, Kellerer M, Mosthaf L. Modulation of insulin signaling in non-insulin-dependent diabetes mellitus: significance of altered receptor isoform patterns and mechanisms of glucose-induced receptor modulation. Horm Res 1994; 41 Suppl. 2: 87–92.

128. Nishizuka Y. Protein kinase C and lipid signaling for sustained cellular responses. FASEB J 1995; 9: 484–96.

129. Ziv E, Kalman R. Primary insulin resistance leading to nutritionally induced Type 2 diabetes. In: Sima AEF, Shafrir E, eds. Animal Models of Diabetes: A Primer. Harwood Academic Publishers, 2000: 327–42.

130. Ziv E, Kalman R, Hershkop K et al. Insulin resistance in the NIDDM model Psammomys obesus in the normoglycemic, normoinsulinemic state. Diabetologia, 1996; 39: 1269–75.

131. Berti L, Mosthaf L, Kroder G et al. Glucose-induced translocation of protein kinse C isoforms in rat-1 fibroblasts is paralleled by inhibition of the insulin receptor tyrosine kinase. J Biol Chem 1994; 369: 3381–6.

132. Danielsen AG, Liu F, Hosomi Y et al. Activation of protein kinase Cα inhibits

signaling by members of the insulin receptor family. J Biol Chem 1995; 270: 21600–5.

133. Bossenmaier B, Mosthaf L, Mischak H et al. Protein kinase C isoforms β1 and β2 inhibit the tyrosine kinase activity of the insulin receptor. Diabetologia 1997; 40: 863–6.

134. Seedorf K, Shearman M, Ullrich A. Rapid and long term effects of protein kinase C on receptor tyrosine kinase phosphorylation and degradation. J Biol Chem 1995; 270: 18953–60.

135. Chin JE, Liu F, Roth RA. Activation of protein kinase Cα inhibits insulin-stimulated tyrosine phosphorylation of insulin receptor substrate-1. Molec Endocr 1994; 8: 51–8.

136. deVente JE, Carey JO, Bryant WO et al. Transcriptional regulation of insulin receptor substrate 1 by protein kinase C. J Biol Chem 1996; 271: 32276–80.

137. Yu HY, Inoguchi T, Kakimoto M et al. Saturated non-esterified fatty acids stimulate de novo diacylglycerol synthesis and protein kinase C activity in cultured aortic smooth muscle cells. Diabetologia 2001; 44: 614–20.

138. Griffin ME, Marcucci Mj, Cline GW et al. Free fatty-induced insulin resistance is associated with activation of protein kinase Cθ and alterations in the insulin signaling cascade. Diabetes 1999; 48: 1270–4.

139. Kraegen EW, Clark PW, Jenkins AB et al. Muscle insulin resistance develops after liver insulin resistance in the high fat fed rat. Diabetes, 1991; 40: 1397–403.

140. Schmitz-Pfeiffer C, Browne CL, Oakes ND et al. Alterations in the expression and cellular localization of protein kinase C isozymes ε and θ are associated with insulin resistance in skeletal muscle of the high-fat-fed rat. Diabetes, 1997; 46: 169–78.

141. Kraegen EW, Cooney G, Ye J, Furler SM. Fat feeding and muscle fat deposition eliciting insulin resistance. In: Hansen B, Shafrir E, eds. Insulin Resistance and Insulin Resistance Syndrome. London: Taylor & Francis, 2002.

142. Pan DA, Lillioja S, Kriketos AD et al. Skeletal muscle triglyceride levels are inversely related to insulin action. Diabetes 1997; 46: 983–8.

143. Zierath JR, Krook A, Wallberg-Henriksson H. Insulin action and insulin resistance in human

skeletal muscle. Diabetologia 2000; 43: 821–35.

144. Shafrir E, Ziv E, Saha AK, Ruderman NB. Regulation of muscle malonyl-CoA levels in the nutritionally insulin-resistant gerbil, *Psammomys obesus*. Diabetes Metab Res Rev 2002; 18: 217–23.

145. Martin-Dixon T, Collins S, Surwit RS. The C57BL/6J mouse as a model of insulin resistance and hypertension. In: Hansen B, Shafrir E, eds. Insulin Resistance and Insulin Resistance Syndrome, Taylor & Francis, UK, 2002: 73–86.

146. Petro AE, Surwit RS. The C57BL/6J mouse as a model of diet induced Type 2 diabetes and obesity. In: Sima AAF, Shafrir E, eds. Models of Animal Diabetes. A Primer, Harwood Academic Press, 2000: 337–50.

147. Suzuki KI, Goto Y, Toyota T. Spontaneously diabetic GK (Goto-Kakizaki) rats. In: Shafrir E, ed. Lessons from Animal Diabetes. London: Smith-Gordon, 1992; 4: 107–16.

148. Bisbis S, Bailbe D, Tormo MA et al. Insulin resistance in the GK rat: decreased receptor number but normal kinase activity in liver. Am J Physiol 1993; 265: E807–E813.

149. Avignon A, Yamada K, Zhou X et al. Chronic activation of protein kinase C in soleus muscle and other tissues of insulin resitant type II diabetuic Goto Kakizaki (GK) obese/aged and obese Zucker rats: a mechanism for inhibiting glycogen synthesis. Diabetes 1996; 45: 1396–404.

150. Movassat J, Saulnier C, Serradas P, Portha B. Impaired development of pancreatic beta-cell mass is a primary event during the progression of to diabetes in the GK rat. Diabetologia 1997; 40: 916–25.

151. Tsuura Y, Ishida H, Okamoto Y et al. Glucose sensitivity of ATP-sensitive K+ channels is impaired in B-cells of the GK rat. A new genetic model of IDDM. Diabetes 1993; 41: 1446–53.

152. Sener A, Malaisse-Lagae F, Ostenson CG, Malaisse WJ. Metabolism of endogenous nutrients in islets of Goto-Kakizaki (GK) rats. Biochem J 1993; 296: 329–34.

153. Tourrel C, Baitbe D, Lacorne M et al. Persistent improvement of Type 2 diabetes in the Goto Kakisoki rat model by expansion of β-cell mass during the prediabetic period with glucagon-like peptide-1 or exendin-4. Diabetes 2002; 31: 1443–52.

154. Ostenson CG. The Goto-Kakizaki rat. In: Sima AAF, Shafrir E, eds. Models of Animal Diabetes. A Primer, Harwood Academic Press, 2000: 197–212.

155. Shafrir E. Diabetes in Animals. In: Porte D, Sherwin R, Baron AD, eds. Diabetes Mellitus, McGraw-Hill Publishers, 2002.

156. Howard CF Jr. Use of nonhuman primates to gain insight into diabetes mellitus, related hormonal and metabolic controls, and secondary complications. In: Shafrir E, Renold AE, eds. Lessons from Animal Diabetes. London: Libbey, 1988; 2: 272–8.

157. Howard CF Jr. Longitudinal studies on the development of diabetes in individual Macaca nigra. Diabetologia 1986; 29: 301–6.

158. Leckstrom A, Ziv E, Shafrir E, Westermark P. Islet amyloid polypeptide in Psammomys obesus (sand rat). Effects of nutritionally induced diabetes and recovery on low energy diet or vanadyl sulfate treatment. Pancreas 1922; 15: 358–66.

159. Dunaif A, Tattersall I. Prevalence of glucose intolerance in free-ranging Macaca fascicularis of Mauritius. Am J Perinatol 1987; 13: 435–42.

160. Hansen BC, Ortmeyer HK, Bodkin NL. Obesity, insulin resistance, and noninsulin-dependent diabetes mellitus in aging monkeys: Implications for NIDDM in humans. In: Shafrir E, ed. Lessons from Animal Diabetes. London: Smith-Gordon, 1994; 5: 93–105.

161. Bodkin NL. The rhesus monkey (Macaca mulatta): a unique and valuable model for the study of spontaneous diabetes mellitus and associated conditions. In: Sima AAF, Shafrir E, eds. Primer on Animal Diabetes, Harwood Academic Press, 2000: 303–20.

162. Bodkin NL, Nicolson M, Ortmeyer HK, Hansen BC. Hyperleptinemia: relationship to adiposity and insulin resistance in the spontaneously obese rhesus monkeys. Horm Metab Res 1996; 28: 674–8.

163. De Koning EJP, Bodkin NL, Hansen BC, Clark A. Diabetes mellitus in Macaca mulatta monkeys is characterized by islet amyloidosis and reduction in beta-cell population. Diabetologia 1993; 36: 374–8.

164. Kahn SE, Andrikopoulos S, Verchere CB. Islet amyloid: a long-recognized but underappreciated pathological feature of Type 2 diabetes. Diabetes 1999; 48: 241–53.

165. Huang Z, Bodkin NL, Ortmeyer HK et al. Hyperinsulinemia is associated with altered insulin receptotr mRNA splicing in muscle of the spontaneously obese diabetic rhesus monkey. J Clin Invest 1994; 94: 1289–96.

166. Hansen BC, Bodkin NL. Primary prevention of diabetes mellitus by prevention of obesity in monkeys. Diabetes 1993; 42: 1809–14.

167. Kerr J, Winterford C, Harmon B. Apoptosis, its significance in cancer and cancer therapy. Cancer 1994; 33: 596–603.

168. Imagawa A, Hanafusa T, Tamura S. et al. Pancreatic biopsy as a procedure for detecting in situ autoimmune phenomena in Type 1 diabetes. Close correlation between serological markers and histological evidence of cellular autoimmunity. Diabetes 2001; 50: 1269–73.

169. Muller HK, Kellerer M, Ermel B et al. Prevention by protein kinase C inhibitors of glucose-induced insulin-receptor tyrosine kinase resistance in rat fat cells. Diabetes 1991; 40: 1440–8.

170. Taher, M.M. Herbimycin A inhibits protein kinase C in vascular smooth muscle cells. Biochem Molec Biol Int 1996; 39: 267–77.

171. Ways DK, King GL. Glucotoxicity: a role for protein kinase activation? In: Diabetes Current Perspectives, Betteridge DJ, ed. London: Martin Dunitz, 2000.

172. Koya D, King GL. Protein kinase C activation and the development of diabetic complications. Diabetes, 1998; 47: 859–66.

173. Bursell S-E, King GL. Protein kinase C activation, development of diabetic vascular complications, and role of vitamin E in preventing these abnormalities. In: Packer L, et al., eds, Antioxidants in Diabetes Management, New York: Marcel Dekker, Inc, 2000: 241–64.

174. Kim JK, Fillmore J, Sunshine MJ et al. Transgenic mice with inactivation of PKC-θ are protected from lipid-induced defects in insulin action and signaling in skeletal muscle. Diabetes 2001; 50 Suppl. 1: A58.

175. Qureshi SA, Ding V, Li ZH et al. Activation of insulin signal transduction pathway and anti-diabetic activity of small molecule insulin receptor activators. J Biol Chem 2000; 275: 3543–9.

176. Shafrir E, Spielman S, Nachliel I et al. Treatment of diabetes with vanadium salts: general overview and amelioration of nutritionally induced diabetes in the Psammomys obesus gerbil. Diabetes Metab Res Rev 2001; 17: 55–66.

177. Cam MD, Brownsey RW, McNeill JH. Mechanisms of vanadium action: insulin-mimetic or insulin-enhancing agent? Can J Physiol Pharmacol 2000; 78: 829–47.

178. Goldwaser I, Li J, Gershonov E et al. L-Glutamic acid γ-monohydroxamate. A potentiator of vanadium evoked glucose metabolism in vitro and in vivo. J Biol Chem 1999; 27: 26617–24.

179. Brichard SM, Henquin JC. The role of vanadium in the management of diabetes. Trends Pharmacol Sci 1995; 16: 265–79.

32

A view of the future

Jay S Skyler

The management of patients with diabetes – both diagnosis and treatment – has radically changed over the past three decades.

In the early 1970s, the vast majority of patients with Type 1 diabetes took only one daily injection of insulin. That insulin was mixed beef/pork insulin, usually just NPH or Lente. The preparations were not highly purified, containing as many as 80,000 parts per million of impurities. Meal plans and diabetic diets were difficult. Patients resented being confined to three strict meals a day, never being able to skip meals, never being able to alter meal times, never being able to sleep late on weekends. Moreover, they needed to take snacks whether convenient or not. This was because the insulin program dictated the lifestyle of the patient, with need to adhere to a strict schedule in order to avert hypoglycemia. Monitoring of diabetes was carried out by messy urine testing and the debate was whether this should be a 'first void' or a 'double void'. Physicians caring for these patients had no easy way to assess overall chronic glycemic control. Meanwhile, the management of Type 2 diabetes was clouded in controversy. The report of the University Group Diabetes Program (UGDP) had suggested that neither sulfonylureas nor the then-available biguanide phenformin were safe pharmaceutical agents in the management of Type 2 diabetes. Physicians were in a quandary wondering how to manage these patients. Physicians struggled with the management of diabetic patients, providing their diets by tear sheets obtained from pharmaceutical companies, feebly instructing the patients to take their injections, and contending with their frequent episodes of either hypoglycemia or ketoacidosis. The concept of the diabetes educator was non-existent and dietitians were deemed as individuals from another planet.

Also in the early 1970s, diabetic complications were difficult, and available treatments were virtually non-existent. The only treatment for diabetic retinopathy was the desperate procedure of pituitary ablation. Laser photocoagulation was in its infancy and the Diabetic Retinopathy Study was just getting underway. Treatment of end-stage renal disease in individuals with diabetes was problematic while hemodialysis was considered verboten and renal transplantation too dangerous. Peritoneal dialysis had not yet emerged as chronic therapy. Few, if any, pharmaceutical agents could control the symptoms of diabetic neuropathy. The management of hyperlipidemia in diabetes was difficult at best, with patients not being able to tolerate nicotinic acid and with compliance problems associated with bile acid sequestrants. The management of hypertension in diabetes was complicated by the use of thiazide diuretics and beta-blockers as mainstays of therapy, since both of these classes of drugs may aggravate hyperglycemia.

During the early 1970s, there were also vigorous debates as to whether or not glycemic control was important in reducing the chronic complications of diabetes. Many chose to ignore the vast and accumulating evidence on this subject – evidence from animal studies, from epidemiological studies, from retrospective clinical studies, and from studies defining biochemical mechanisms. All of these lines of evidence clearly suggested that the degree of glucose elevation is the crucial factor influencing the appearance of complications.

Over the past three decades, we have advanced dramatically from the situation described in the early 1970s.

Current insulin preparations are highly purified recombinant (genetically engineered) human insulin and specially designed insulin analogues. 'Medical Nutrition Therapy' has replaced 'meal plans' and 'diabetic diets' – emphasizing the importance of a comprehensive individualized nutritional plan as the cornerstone of effective diabetes management. Contemporary insulin programs permit total flexibility in timing and composition of meals and the ability to skip meals. Monitoring of diabetes is carried out by patients at home on a daily basis using readily available test strips and glucose meters. Glycated hemoglobin (HBA_{IC}) provides chronic assessment of integrated glycemic control. Targeted glucose control – with the goal of near normal glycemia – has become a reality in Type 2 diabetes due to the emergence of classes of pharmaceuticals with complementary mechanisms of action – insulin secretagogues (sulfonylureas and glinides), insulin sensitizers (metformin and thiazolidinediones), and alpha-glucosidase inhibitors – that can be used safely in combination as effective orally administered glucose-lowering agents.

Laser photocoagulation is the mainstay of the management of diabetic retinopathy, and there are specific criteria for its use. Renal transplantation is the norm in the management of diabetic end-stage renal disease, often accompanied by simultaneous or subsequent pancreas transplantation. Dialysis – both hemodialysis and peritoneal dialysis – are accepted practice when transplantation is not feasible. Progression of renal disease – both incipient nephropathy and overt nephropathy – can be slowed by use of angiotensin converting enzyme inhibitors or angiotensin receptor blockers. For diabetic neuropathy, symptoms are better treated, disability can be decreased, and amputations have become preventable. Sildenafil has revolutionized treatment of erectile dysfunction in diabetes. Fibric acid derivatives and HMG-CoA reductase inhibitors permit effective management of dyslipidemia.

The beneficial effects and impact of effective glycemic control on chronic complications of diabetes has been firmly established by results from the Diabetes Control and Complications Trial (DCCT) and the Stockholm Diabetes Intervention Study (SDIS) in Type 1 diabetes, and by the United Kingdom Prospective Diabetes Study (UKPDS) and the Kumamoto Intervention Study in Type 2 diabetes. These studies have ended the long-standing debate on whether or not glycemia is important and refocused the debate on the best means of attaining effective glycemic control.

Yet, we must bear in mind that in some parts of the world, crucial diabetes supplies – including insulin – may be either in short supply or priced beyond the fiscal means of many patients with diabetes.

Research progress over the past three decades has been unparalleled. Nonetheless, our treatments are imperfect and diabetes still exacts a massive burden on patients, families and the health care system. In the USA, diabetic retinopathy remains the leading cause of new blindness in adults of 20 to 65 years of age; diabetes is the leading cause of end-stage renal disease, accounting for 42% of new cases; diabetes is the leading cause (accounting for 45% to 70%) of non-traumatic lower extremity amputations; and diabetes is the largest single health care expense, consuming 12–15% of the overall health care budget.

Diabetes: From Research to Diagnosis and Treatment is designed to provide the reader with a contemporary view of advances in diabetes research that have had an impact or have the potential to impact on management of patients. An array of highly respected international contributors have provided detailed analyses of the subjects they were charged to address. Yet, not all exciting research progresses to clinical application. In this chapter, I will summarize where we are and speculate on where research advances will take us in the future management of diabetes. The operative word is 'speculate' as this represents personal opinion. At times, it differs with that presented in earlier chapters or with 'conventional wisdom'.

Insulin therapy

The present

Physiologic insulin secretion is of two types: continuous basal insulin secretion and incremental meal-related prandial insulin secretion, controlling meal-related glucose excursions. Designing insulin treatment programs that mimic the physiological insulin secretion profile has been a vexing problem for clinicians and researchers. This has led to a number of advances designed to approximate more closely an ideal insulin absorption pattern. One approach to improving the timing of prandial insulin is the development of rapid-acting genetically engineered insulin analogues,

designed to have both a rapid onset of action and a short duration of action when injected subcutaneously (e.g. an onset of action in 15–30 min, a peak effect that occurs 30–90 min after administration, and an effective duration of action of no more than 3–4 h). The medical rationale for such analogues is that they more closely mimic physiological insulin profiles, they may be administered at meal-time rather than 20–40 min prior to meals, and they result in improved postprandial glycemic control with a lower risk of late hypoglycemia. Three such analogues have been developed, all of which either exist as monomers in solution or rapidly dissociate into monomers, thus speeding absorption from subcutaneous tissue. The first rapid-acting insulin analogue to become available is (Lys(B28), Pro(B29))-human insulin (insulin lispro), in which the amino acid sequence of the B-chain at positions 28 and 29 is inverted. The second rapid-acting insulin analogue introduced is (Asp(B28))-human insulin (insulin aspart), in which aspartic acid is substituted for proline at position 28 of the B-chain. The third such analogue, still in clinical development, is (Lys(B3), Glu(B29))-human insulin (insulin glulisine), an analogue in which there are two substitutions in the B-chain: lysine for asparagine at position 3 and glutamic acid for lysine at position 29.

A second approach to improving the timing of prandial insulin is the development of pulmonary insulin delivery systems, or inhaled insulin. Since the alveolar mucosa is but one cell thick, insulin administered via the pulmonary route is rapidly absorbed and thus has rapid biological availability similar to the rapid-acting insulin analogues. Several studies have demonstrated that aerosolized insulin appears to be well tolerated, with about 10–40% of an inhaled dose of insulin absorbed into the circulation, depending on the system used. As of the Summer of 2002, there are several alliances developing pulmonary insulin delivery systems. Farthest ahead is Exubera (in development by a collaboration of Pfizer, Aventis, and Inhale Therapeutics) which consists of a dry powder aerosol delivery system packaged as a unit dose in blister packs, and a simple mechanical delivery device from which the patient inhales the dispersed insulin. In Phase 2 and Phase 3 human trials, it has been demonstrated that Exubera may be used for prandial insulin delivery for the achievement of good glycemic control. It must be accompanied by subcutaneous basal insulin in insulin-deficient patients, but has been used either alone or together with oral hypoglycemic agents in patients with Type 2 diabetes who are not severely insulin deficient. The AERx insulin diabetes management system (in development by a collaboration of Novo Nordisk and Aradigm) uses an electronic inhalation device to deliver liquid insulin aerosol droplets to the lung. Its electronic features guide the patient to breathe at an optimal speed for delivery, and also maintains a record of insulin delivery. Another approach (in development by MannKind's PDC Division) uses a small organic molecule, 3,6-bis-N-fumaryl-N(n-Butyl)amino-2,5-di-ketopiperazine, which self-assembles into microspheres in an acid environment, microencapsulating any peptide present, in this case insulin. This is then lyophilized, with delivery of a dry powder formulation by a simple device, the microspheres dissolving upon absorption and the ketopiperazine being rapidly excreted in the urine. With this approach, there is more rapid insulin availability and higher bioavailability of insulin. Yet another approach is the AIR insulin delivery system (in development by a collaboration of Eli Lilly and Alkermes), in which a dispersion chamber delivers a powder of porous microparticles with large surface but low cohesion forces into the deep lung.

Another pulmonary insulin system (in development by a collaboration of Aerogen and Disetronic) uses small liquid droplets of insulin. A program (in development by the Aeropharm Division of Kos) uses a novel but simple delivery device to facilitate deep lung absorption. A program involving insulin with a bile acid to enhance absorption appears to have been abandoned by its developer (AstraZeneca).

Confounders of pulmonary insulin delivery include cigarette smoking, upper respiratory tract infections, and airway hyper-reactivity. Long-term safety studies are in progress and their outcome will determine the viability of the pulmonary route for insulin delivery although efficacy has been demonstrated. Administration of insulin via the pulmonary route should improve patient compliance and facilitate earlier insulin initiation without compromising the benefits achieved with multiple injection programs.

Another goal is to improve reproducibility and duration of action of basal insulin by the development of long-acting soluble insulins. These more closely mimic physiological insulin profiles, provide more reducible insulin delivery, and have a lower risk of unexpected hypoglycemia. One long-acting insulin analogue is (Gly(A21), Arg(B31), Arg(B32))-human insulin (insulin glargine), in which glycine is substituted for asparginine at position 21 of the A-chain, and two arginines are appended to the carboxy terminal of the B-chain. These changes alter the isoelectric point of the molecule, causing precipitation at neutral tissue pH, resulting in retardation of the absorption rate and a corresponding longer duration of action. Unfortunately, because it is an acid formulation, insulin glargine cannot be mixed with either regular insulin or any of the rapid-acting insulin analogues, all of which are formulated at neutral pH. Another approach to extend the duration of action of insulin is to cause it to bind to a serum carrier protein (e.g. albumin), thus prolonging its time in the circulation. This is accomplished by constructing acylated insulin analog, e.g. (Lys(B29)-N-ε-tetradecanoyl, Des(B30))-human insulin (insulin detemir), which currently is in clinical trials. Another approach to basal insulin availability, also in development, is the use of a transdermal delivery system, in which micropores are created to allow insulin to be delivered through a transdermal patch. Finally, one system for basal insulin delivery involves a disposable pump system that provides continuous basal insulin infusion for several days.

View of the future

My predictions are:

- Insulin analogues – both rapid-acting and basal – will replace conventional human insulin preparations as the primary insulins used in injection therapy.
- Meal-related prandial insulin will be provided by analogue injections or by pulmonary delivery. The latter will principally be used by patients with Type 2 diabetes who are reluctant to take injections, and thus facilitate glycemic control in these individuals, since they otherwise might not take insulin when needed.
- Basal insulin will be provided by insulin analogues or the transdermal patch/microporation system. The disposable pump will be a novelty.
- Oral insulin, nasal insulin, and buccal insulin delivery approaches will all fail.
- Insulin mixtures will remain on the market because of stubbornness on the part of the pharmaceutical industry, even though they fail to provide optimal insulin replacement.

Insulin delivery systems

The present

Currently, insulin may be administered via conventional needle and syringe, via insulin pens (both prefilled disposable pens and durable reusable pens using insulin cartridges), and via infusion pump (continuous subcutaneous insulin infusion or CSII). (As noted, pulmonary and transdermal systems are in development.)

In most parts of the world (the USA uniquely excepted), insulin pens have overtaken syringes as the preferred method of insulin delivery. Although the USA lags far behind, there is a growing array of pens available and pen usage is increasing. Moreover, particularly amongst patients with Type 1 diabetes, growing numbers are using insulin infusion pumps for CSII, with usage in the USA now estimated at approximately 200,000 individuals. Many new features have made CSII easier for patients to use: multiple basal rates; profiling of meal-related prandial insulin to allow a square-wave or extended delivery to correspond better with food; a mode for suspending insulin delivery for exercise, if appropriate; automatic inserters; quick release valves to separate the electronics from indwelling catheters, thus facilitating such activities as showering, swimming, shopping, and sexual intercourse; and remote control activators to initiate meal-related prandial insulin delivery. Implantable insulin pumps (IIP), which provide peritoneal insulin delivery, are available in France, and are expected to become available elsewhere in 2003–2004, pending regulatory approval.

The current generation of insulin pumps (for both CSII and IIP) utilize open looped insulin delivery, with the patient taking action to alter the insulin delivery profile. Closed loop insulin delivery systems have been tested on a short-term basis both in experimental animals and in human beings, using both IIP and to a lesser extent CSII. The obstacle to closed loop insulin delivery has been the lack of reliable continuous glucose sensing systems (glucose sensing is discussed in the next section).

View of the future

My predictions are:

- Conventional needle and syringe delivery of insulin will become progressively obsolete. Pen delivery will become the dominant mode of subcutaneous insulin injection delivery.
- CSII use will continue to grow, facilitated in part by the use of rapid-acting insulin analogues in pumps.
- IIP will become readily available and its usage will grow rapidly amongst patients with Type 1 diabetes in spite of high costs.
- Closed loop CSII and IIP systems will make their appearance when continuous glucose sensing systems are perfected (vide infra). This will radically change the face of diabetes management.

Glucose monitoring systems

The present

There are many systems available for patient self-monitoring of blood glucose – using tiny drops of blood obtained either from fingers or alternative sites with automated lancets. Instrument response time to provide a reading is as short as a few seconds. Most instruments store readings, calculate averages, and have download capability to allow a variety of displays of accumulating data. Yet, all of these are designed for sporadic testing. Although

highly motivated pregnant women (and some engineers or accountants) may perform readings 8 or 10 or 12 times daily, most patients measure blood glucose anywhere from 1 to 4 times daily. Thus, the readings provide but a snapshot of the day.

Recently, a continuous glucose monitoring system (CGMS) has become available. The CGMS is comprised of a disposable subcutaneous glucose sensing device connected by a cable to a pager-sized glucose monitor. The system takes a glucose measurement every 10 seconds and stores an average value every five minutes, for a total of 288 measurements each day. A communication device enables the data stored in the monitor to be downloaded and reviewed on a personal computer. The current version is used for a three-day period for diagnostic purposes, and has provided better understanding of glycemic fluctuations, and detection of unsuspected problems. With the available information, physicians may suggest specific changes in the timing and dosage of insulin infusion or injections, dietary changes and changes in the timing and frequency of blood glucose measurements. Future versions will provide patients with continuous glucose measurements over three days, and, provide feedback to control insulin infusions automatically and, thus provide a basis for closed loop delivery of insulin.

Other glucose monitoring systems include the Glucowatch Biographer, which samples interstitial fluid glucose intermittently during the day and provides readings over a 12–14 hour period; it may also help identify hypoglycemia in some patients.

There are a number of continuous glucose monitoring systems in various stages of development. Some are implantable in subcutaneous tissue, others in an intravascular location, e.g. inferior vena cava. These have provided readings for weeks, months, or years in preclinical testing. These are substantially longer intervals than the 12–14 hours for the Glucowatch or three days for the CGMS and its variants. One intravascular long-term glucose sensor has been linked to an implantable insulin pump, providing closed loop insulin delivery. This has been tested in dogs and is being used in clinical trials in human beings.

View of the future

My predictions are:

- Self-monitoring blood glucose systems will become more sophisticated: storing information about insulin doses, food intake, exercise, and stress; interpreting glucose patterns; and providing automated recommendations to patients.
- Continuous glucose monitoring systems will become widely available.
- Closed loop systems – both subcutaneous and implantable – will become a reality and will forever change diabetes management.
- Non-invasive glucose monitoring systems will continue to be elusive, but will nonetheless attract investors with a 'dream beam' mentality. Hope and hype differ by but one letter.

Controlling glycemia

The present

In addition to insulin, a number of classes of oral antidiabetic agents are currently available. These include drugs that enhance insulin secretion (insulin secretagogues), drugs that enhance insulin action (biguanides and thiazolidinediones), and drugs that retard glucose absorption from the gastrointestinal tract (alpha-glucosidase inhibitors).

There are two classes of insulin secretagogues currently available: sulfonylureas and 'glinides' (repaglinide and nateglinide). These act to close the ATP-dependent potassium channel on beta-cells, resulting in increased insulin secretion. The problem is that to a greater or lesser degree they stimulate insulin secretion independent of the prevailing plasma glucose level, potentially creating hypoglycemia. They are also associated with weight gain, to a greater or lesser degree. It is interesting that the newer secretagogues include two extremes – those designed to be rapid-acting, in order to stimulate meal-related insulin secretion (the glinides) and those designed to last 24 hours, i.e. the 'third generation' sulfonylureas (glipizide-GITS and glimiperide). Both strategies appear to play a role, but they are very different approaches; insulin secretagogues that facilitate glucose-mediated insulin secretion without spontaneous insulin secretion, thus avoiding the risk of hypoglycemia are very much needed. GLP-1 is a gastrointestinal peptide that achieves this (vide infra).

There are two classes of insulin sensitizers currently available: biguanides (e.g. metformin) and thiazolidinediones (TZDs or glitazones). Both classes enhance insulin sensitivity and action. Metformin has been thought to work principally in the liver to suppress hepatic glucose production, with less effect in the periphery on stimulating glucose disposal. Yet, recent studies suggest that the molecular action of metformin may be through stimulation of AMP-activated protein kinase (AMPK), an enzyme implicated in stimulation of glucose uptake into skeletal muscle and inhibition of liver gluconeogenesis. Thus, AMPK has become a major target for future drug development.

In contrast to metformin, the TZDs have been thought to lower glucose principally by enhancing insulin sensitivity with regards to glucose uptake into skeletal muscle, with less effect in the liver to suppress hepatic glucose production. Their molecular action is by activating PPARγ, a nuclear transcription factor, resulting in adipogenesis, alteration in circulating free fatty acids (FFAs), and consequent stimulation of glucose uptake into skeletal muscle and inhibition of liver gluconeogenesis. Unfortunately, PPARγ activation results in weight gain and fluid retention, neither of which is desirable in patients with diabetes. PPARγ activators with other chemical structures (non-TZD) have been tested, but unfortunately also result in weight gain and fluid retention, which appear to be directly related to the mechanism of action. Thus, major efforts are underway to find other molecular targets that will result in improved insulin sensitivity. These include vanadium derivatives and other agents that interact with the insulin action cascade, such as PTP1B phosphatase inhibitors and PKC θ inhibitors.

Alpha-glucosidase inhibitors (acarbose, miglitol, voglibose) work by slowing digestion of starches and oligosaccharides, thus retarding gastrointestinal glucose absorption and minimizing post-prandial glycemic excursions. In doing so, there is significant gas formation in the intestine, resulting in socially unacceptable flatulence and meteorism. This has resulted in their use being minimal in many fastidious societies, although they are otherwise devoid of appreciable side effects.

Retarding gastrointestinal glucose availability (by modulating gastric emptying) is one of the mechanisms of action of pramlintide, a soluble synthetic version of amylin, the partner hormone of insulin also produced in the pancreatic islet beta-cell. Pramlintide also decreases appetite and glucagon secretion. In clinical trials, it has been shown to facilitate glucose lowering, particularly when used with insulin. It should become available in 2003.

The most exciting prospect on the horizon is that of drugs that work by enhancing glucagon-like peptide-1 (GLP-1)-like actions. GLP-1 stimulates insulin secretion and decreases glucagon secretion in a glucose-dependent manner, improves insulin sensitivity, delays gastric emptying, decreases appetite, and has the potential to increase pancreatic beta-cell mass by stimulating neogenesis and proliferation of beta-cells and inhibiting apoptosis of these cells. In theory, one could stimulate GLP-1 secretion from the gut, replace GLP-1 directly or with an analog, or prolong GLP-1 activity in the circulation by inhibiting dipeptidase-IV (DPP-IV, the enzyme that rapidly inactivates circulating GLP-1), or by creating GLP-1 receptor agonists. All of these approaches are being attempted. One of the most exciting molecules is synthetic exendin-4, which is both highly potent and has a prolonged half-life to make it a viable pharmaceutical agent. Exendin-4 is a peptide contained in the salivary venom of the gila monster (*Heloderma suspectum*) which although not a GLP-1 analog does activate the GLP-1 receptor as well as having other biological effects. In clinical studies, synthetic exendin-4 has been shown to lower fasting and postprandial glycemia through stimulation of insulin secretion in a glucose-dependent manner, suppression of postprandial glucagon secretion, and coordination of insulin secretion to the rate of nutrient delivery to the small intestine.

View of the future

My predictions are:

- New AMPK activators will be developed and these will play an important role in diabetes management, particularly because they may achieve the same effect as exercise.

- Other approaches to increasing insulin sensitivity will be exploited, while PPARγ activators while have decreasing use due to their promotion of weight gain.
- Pramlintide will become available first for use as a partner hormone with insulin, and because of its effect on suppressing appetite, will also be used for treatment of obesity.
- Synthetic exendin-4 will emerge as a mainstay in Type 2 diabetes management, by addressing all of the fundamental defects, including progressive loss of beta-cell mass.
- DPP-IV inhibitors will prove to be too promiscuous to be pharmacologically viable to enhance GLP-1 availability.

Interdicting the diabetes disease process

The present

The Type 1 diabetes disease process is a selective immunologically-mediated destruction of the insulin-producing beta-cells in the pancreatic islets of Langerhans with consequent insulin deficiency. This occurs in genetically susceptible individuals and is a cell-mediated (T-lymphocyte) process, generally thought to be influenced by environmental factors, which may trigger the process or modify the rate or intensity of autoimmunity. The disease process is insidious, evolving over a period of years, during which there is progressive decline of beta-cell function and mass, offering an opportunity to intervene. A variety of potential interventions are available to interdict the immune processes that eventuate in Type 1 diabetes, based on work in animal models of spontaneous diabetes. These include antigen-based therapies, immunosuppression, immuno-

modulation, and interventions designed to afford some beta-cell protection. Recently formed is 'Type 1 Diabetes TrialNet', an NIH-funded network of clinical sites conducting an ongoing series of clinical trials aimed at preserving pancreatic beta-cell function and preventing Type 1 diabetes as well as better understanding the natural history and immunopathogenesis of Type 1 diabetes.

The Type 2 diabetes disease process involves defect(s) in insulin secretion, almost always with a major contribution from insulin resistance, probably with separate genetic defects responsible for altered insulin secretion and for insulin resistance. In addition, environmental factors – particularly adiposity and a sedentary lifestyle – create further insulin resistance. Type 2 diabetes is a progressive disease with a relentless decline in insulin secretion irrespective of conventional oral therapy. Adequate beta-cell function with preservation of insulin secretory capacity sufficient to compensate for the insulin resistance determines whether or not a patient progresses with Type 2 diabetes. Over time, insulin secretion further declines, presumably accelerated by glucotoxicity and lipotoxicity. Any therapeutic strategy that corrects hyperglycemia and reduces free fatty acid levels can potentially improve insulin action and increase insulin secretion. GLP-1 therapy may correct all of the defects and permit expansion of islet cells. INGAP has similar therapeutic potential.

View of the future

My predictions are:

- Type 1 diabetes will be able to be prevented or substantially delayed. This may require a combination of several agents rather than relying on one. Ultimately, a vaccine may be possible.

- Type 2 diabetes management will be dramatically altered by the availability of both exendin-4 (and/or GLP-1 analogs) and islet neogenesis associated protein (INGAP).

Thwarting diabetic complications

The present

Although a number of pathways are involved in the evolution of the chronic complications of diabetes, all of these are driven by glucose excess resulting from chronic hyperglycemia, particularly in cells where insulin-mediated glucose transport is not rate limiting and glucose is freely permeable (nervous system, retina, kidneys). Thus, perfect control of glycemia should thwart these complications. That, however, is not yet achievable. Attention is therefore being paid to develop agents that interrupt the putative pathways involved in the progression of complications. These certainly have been demonstrated to do so in animal models of diabetes. Yet, to date there are no ringing successes available for use in human beings.

The pathways most under examination include the polyol pathway, the protein kinase C (PKC) pathway, non-enzymatic glycation of proteins, the dicarbonyl pathway, and oxidative stress.

The polyol pathway is that in which glucose is converted to its sugar alcohol sorbitol by the enzyme aldose reductase, with further conversion to fructose catalyzed by sorbitol dehydrogenase – resulting in intracellular accumulation of sorbitol and fructose in direct proportion to degree of hyperglycemia. The reaction consumes NADPH, altering intracellular redox potential. In animal models, these abnormalities are reversible with aldose reductase inhibitors

(ARIs). They are currently being tested in clinical trials.

Hyperglycemia results in increased levels of diacylglycerol (DAG) and activation of PKC-β in retinal endothelial, renal mesangial, aortic endothelial and smooth muscle cells. A number of subsequent pathways are activated, eventuating in complications. For example, PKC-β activation regulates vascular permeability and neovascularization via expression of growth factors. Clinical trials are being conducted to test the effects of an orally effective inhibitor of PKC-β.

Non-enzymatic glycation of proteins occurs in virtually all tissues, and leads to many functional changes. Glycated proteins then may undergo cross-linking to form 'advanced glycation end products' (AGEs), an essentially irreversible transformation which disrupts protein function and structure. Glycation reaction inhibitors (GRIs), which block cross-linking or actually break cross-links, have been developed. Reactive α-dicarbonyl compounds may contribute to diabetic complications either as direct toxins or as precursors for AGE formation. Their formation may be blocked. Antioxidants, including simple vitamins, have been used to decrease oxidative stress.

There has been a logjam in regulatory approval of drugs that thwart the complications of diabetes both due to difficulty in establishing appropriate end-points, particularly for neuropathy, and to reluctance on the part of corporate sponsors to commit the resources needed to conduct the necessary long-term clinical trials with true clinical end-points. Nonetheless, that there are several agents in clinical trials which may yet emerge as effective therapies.

View of the future

My predictions are:

- The logjam will be broken and several classes of agents will win approval to attempt to thwart the complications of diabetes. These may well need to be used in combination, if success is to be attained.

Islet replacement therapy

The present

Pancreas transplantation, especially when performed together with kidney transplantation, leads to sustained reversal of hyperglycemia and normalization of metabolic control in approximately 80–90% of individuals who receive such grafts. This has led to the routine use of combined kidney–pancreas transplantation in diabetic patients with end-stage renal disease, when both organs are available. Yet, the adverse effects of conventional immunosuppressive drugs has limited the use of pancreas transplantation in the absence of end-stage renal disease and the compelling need for immunosuppression to sustain renal allograft function. Moreover, the approach is limited by the supply of organs available for transplantation.

Islet isolation and implantation offers the hope of a simple implantation procedure with minimal risk. Clinically, until recently, islet cell transplantation rarely resulted in reversal of hyperglycemia and normalization of metabolic control without the occurrence of hypoglycemia. Currently, at the University of Alberta in Edmonton, amongst 33 consecutive islet transplants, 85% have been free of insulin therapy at one year, and 70% at two years. Other centers are experiencing similar rates of success.

The problem of organ and tissue availability limits potential wide-scale application of islet cell transplantation. Protecting islets from rejection by encapsulation might permit use of animal islets for human implantation. Another alternative is to induce stem cells – either embryonic or adult – to become beta-cells. This has been successful to some degree in animals and is the subject of intense investigation. Another alternative is genetically engineered pseudo-'beta' cells, which have glucose-mediated insulin secretion. By gene transfer approaches, it is possible to program cells to synthesize and secrete insulin. The challenge is to develop cell lines that both respond to glucose and secrete insulin in a physiologic manner. Ideally, such cells would also be designed to be non-immunogenic and thus not rejected. It is too early to tell which, if any, of these approaches will progress to success in human beings.

In experimental models, both *in vitro* and in animals, a number of molecules – including INGAP, exendin-4, and GLP-1 – have been shown to stimulate both beta-cell replication and neogenesis. In animals, this results in increased beta-cell mass and improved glucose tolerance. When used prior to the onset of diabetes, the frequency of diabetes can be reduced. Thus, the use of these substances may help stimulate beta-cell growth of transplanted cells, stem cells, or genetically engineered cells.

View of the future

My predictions are:

- There will be continued success in islet transplantation.
- It will be possible to induce immune tolerance so that islets will survive without the need for lifelong immunosuppressive therapy.
- An inexhaustible source of islets will be developed – either through stem cell differentiation or through genetic engineering.
- Diabetes will be conquered.

This chapter has provided a brief odyssey through contemporary diabetes issues, and a perspective of where research in these areas might take us.

Index